MEMMLER'S

Structure and Function of the Human Body

10TH EDITION

MEMMLER'S

Structure and Function of the Human Body

10TH EDITION

Jason James Taylor
Instructor
Department of Nursing
Red River College
Winnipeg, Manatoba, Canada

Barbara Janson Cohen

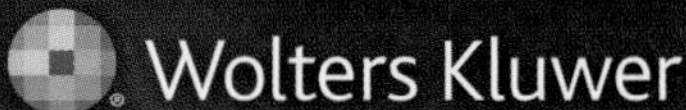
Wolters Kluwer | Lippincott Williams & Wilkins
Health

Philadelphia • Baltimore • New York • London
Buenos Aires • Hong Kong • Sydney • Tokyo

Executive Editor: David Troy
Senior Product Manager: Eve Malakoff-Klein
Designer: Terry Mallon
Artist: Christine Vernon/Hearthside and Dragonfly Media Group
Cover Art: Imagineering
Compositor: SPi Global
Printer: C&C Offset Printing

10th Edition

351 West Camden Street
Baltimore, MD 21201

Two Commerce Square
2001 Market Street
Philadelphia, PA 19103

Printed in China

Library of Congress Cataloging-in-Publication Data
Taylor, Jason J.
Memmler's structure and function of the human body. — 10th ed. / Jason James Taylor, Barbara Janson Cohen.
p. ; cm.
Structure and function of the human body
Rev. ed. of: Memmler's structure and function of the human body / Barbara Cohen. 9th ed. c2009.
Includes bibliographical references and index.
ISBN 978-1-60913-900-1
I. Memmler, Ruth Lundeen. II. Cohen, Barbara J. Memmler's structure and function of the human body. III. Title. IV. Title: Structure and function of the human body.
[DNLM: 1. Anatomy. 2. Physiology. QS 4]
612—dc23

2011053417

To purchase additional copies of this book, call our customer service department at (800) 638-3030 or fax orders to (301) 223-2320. International customers should call (301) 223-2300.

Visit Lippincott Williams & Wilkins on the Internet: http://www.lww.com. Lippincott Williams & Wilkins customer service representatives are available from 8:30 am to 6:00 pm, EST.

9 8 7 6 5 4 3 2 1

CCS0212

Preface

Memmler's Structure and Function of the Human Body is a textbook for introductory-level health professions and nursing students who need a basic understanding of anatomy and physiology, and the interrelationships between structure and function.

Like preceding editions, the 10th edition remains true to Ruth Memmler's original vision. The features and content specifically meet the needs of those who may be starting their health career preparation with little or no science background. This book's primary goals are:

- To provide the essential knowledge of human anatomy, and physiology at an ideal level of detail and in language that is clear and understandable.
- To illustrate the concepts discussed with anatomic art that depicts the appropriate level of detail with accuracy, simplicity, and elegance, and that is integrated seamlessly with the narrative.
- To incorporate the most recent scientific findings into the fundamental material on which Ruth Memmler's classic text is based.
- To include pedagogy designed to enhance interest in and understanding of the concepts presented.
- To teach the basic anatomic and medical terminology used in healthcare settings, preparing students to function efficiently in their chosen health career.
- To present an integrated teaching–learning package that includes all of the elements necessary for a successful learning experience.

This revision is the direct result of in-depth market feedback solicited to tell us what instructors and students at this level most need. We listened carefully to the feedback, and the results we obtained are integrated into many features of this book and into the ancillary package accompanying it. The text itself has been revised and updated where needed to improve organization of the material and to reflect current scientific thought.

Because visual learning devices are so important to students at this level, this edition includes a new section, "The Body Visible," a series of illustrations and transparent overlays of the major body major systems that are presented in the text. In addition to being a learning tool, these illustrations provide enrichment and are a valuable general reference.

The 10th edition retains its extensive art program with updated versions of figures from previous editions. These features appear in a modified design that makes the content more user-friendly and accessible than ever. Our innovative PASSport to Success® ancillary package helps students match their learning styles to a wealth of resources, while the comprehensive package of instructor resources provides instructors with maximum flexibility and efficiency.

Organization and Structure

Like previous editions, the 10th edition uses a body systems approach to the study of the normal human body. The book is divided into six units, grouping related information and body systems together as follows:

- Unit I, The Body as a Whole (Chapters 1–5), focuses on the body's organization; basic chemistry needed to understand body functions; cells and their functions; tissues, glands, and membranes; and the skin.
- Unit II, Movement and Support (Chapters 6 and 7), includes the skeletal and muscular systems.
- Unit III, Coordination and Control (Chapters 8–11), focuses on the nervous system, the sensory system, and the endocrine system.
- Unit IV, Circulation and Body Defense (Chapters 12–15), includes the blood, the heart, blood vessels and circulation, and the lymphatic system and immunity.
- Unit V, Energy: Supply and Use (Chapters 16–19), includes the respiratory system; the digestive system; metabolism, nutrition, and temperature control; and the urinary system and body fluids.
- Unit VI, Perpetuation of Life (Chapters 20 and 21), covers the male and female reproductive systems, as well as development, birth, and heredity.

The main Glossary defines the chapters' boldfaced terms. An additional Glossary of Word Parts is a reference tool that not only teaches basic anatomic and physiologic terminology but also helps students learn to recognize unfamiliar terms. Appendices include a variety of supplementary information that students will find useful as they work with the text, including a photographic dissection atlas (Appendix 3) and answers to the Chapter Checkpoint questions and Zooming In illustration questions (Appendix 2) that are found in every chapter.

Pedagogic Features

Every chapter contains pedagogy that has been designed with the health professions and nursing student in mind.

- **Learning Outcomes:** Chapter objectives at the start of every chapter help the student organize and prioritize learning.
- **Ancillaries At-A-Glance:** Learning Tools, Learning Resources, and Learning Activites are highlighted in a one-stop overview of the supplemental materials available for the chapter.

- **A&P in Action:** Familiar scenarios transport chapter content into a real-life setting, bringing the information to life for students and, through a discussion of the disease process, helping them to better understand normal anatomy and physiology.
- **A Look Back:** With the exception of Chapter 1, each chapter starts with a brief review of how its content relates to prior chapters.
- **Chapter Checkpoints:** Brief questions at the end of main sections test and reinforce the student's recall of key information in that section. Answers are in Appendix 2.
- **Key Points (NEW to this edition):** Critical information highlighted in figure legends spotlights essential aspects of the illustrations.
- **"Zooming In" questions:** Questions in the figure legends test and reinforce student understanding of concepts depicted in the illustration. Answers are in Appendix 2.
- **Phonetic pronunciations:** Easy-to-learn phonetic pronunciations are spelled out in the narrative, appearing in parentheses directly following many terms—no need for students to understand dictionary-style diacritical marks. (See the "Guide to Pronunciation" below.)
- **Special interest boxes:** Each chapter contains three special interest boxes focusing on topics that augment chapter content. The book includes five kinds of boxes altogether:
  - > **A&P in Action Revisited:** Traces the outcome of the real-life scenario that opens each chapter and shows how the cases relate to material in the chapter and to others in the book.
  - > **A Closer Look:** Provides additional in-depth scientific detail on topics in or related to the text.
  - > **Clinical Perspective:** Focuses on diseases and disorders relevant to the chapter, exploring what happens to the body when the normal structure–function relationship breaks down.
  - > **Hot Topic:** Focuses on current trends and research, reinforcing the link between anatomy and physiology and related news coverage that students may have seen.
  - > **Health Maintenance:** Offers supplementary information on health and wellness issues.
- **Figures:** The art program includes full-color anatomic line art, some new or revised, with a level of detail that matches that of the narrative. Photomicrographs, radiographs, and other scans give students a preview of what they might see in real-world healthcare settings. Supplementary figures are available on the companion Web site as well as on the Student DVD included with this text.
- **Tables:** The numerous tables in this edition summarize key concepts and information in an easy-to-review form. Additional summary tables are available on the companion Web site as well as on the Student DVD included with this text.
- **Color figure and table callouts:** Figure and table numbers appear in color in the narrative, helping students quickly find their place after stopping to look at an illustration or table.
- **Word Anatomy:** This chart defines and illustrates the various word parts that appear in terms within the chapter. The prefixes, roots, and suffixes presented are grouped according to chapter headings so that students can find the relevant text. This learning tool helps students build vocabulary and promotes understanding of even unfamiliar terms based on a knowledge of common word parts.
- **Chapter Wrap-Up (NEW to this edition):** A graphic outline at the end of each chapter provides a concise overview of chapter content, aiding in study and test preparation.
- **Key Terms:** Selected boldface terms throughout the text are listed at each chapter's end and defined in the book's glossary.
- **Questions for Study and Review:** Study questions are organized hierarchically into three levels. (Note that answers appear in the Instructor's Manual as well as on the instructor resource Web site):
  - > **Building Understanding:** Includes fill-in-the-blank, matching, and multiple choice questions that test factual recall.
  - > **Understanding Concepts:** Includes short-answer questions (define, describe, compare/contrast) that test and reinforce understanding of concepts.
  - > **Conceptual Thinking:** Includes short-essay questions that promote critical thinking skills. New in this edition are thought questions related to the A&P in Action case stories.

PASSport to Success® for Students

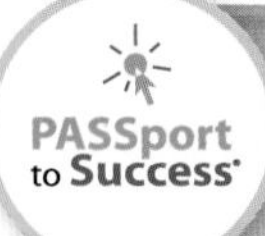

Look for this icon throughout the book for pertinent supplementary material on the companion Web site and student resource DVD

The PASSport to Success® is a practical system that lets students learn faster, remember more, and achieve success. Students discover their unique learning styles—visual, auditory, or kinesthetic—with a simple online assessment, then choose from a wealth of resources for each learning style, including animations, a pre-quiz, and 10 different types of online learning activities; an audio glossary; and other supplemental materials such as health professions career information, additional charts and images, answers to the "Questions for Study and Review" from the text, and study and test-taking tips and resources. Throughout the textbook, the graphic icon shown above alerts students to pertinent supplementary material.

The PASSport to Success® is available on the DVD bound into this textbook as well as on the book's companion Web site at http://thePoint.lww.com/MemmlerStructureFunction10e. On the companion Web site, students can also access the fully searchable online version of the text. See the inside front cover of this text for the passcode you will need to gain access to the Web site, and see pages ix–xvii for details about the PASSport to Success® and a complete listing of student resources.

Instructor Ancillary Package

All instructor resources are available to approved adopting instructors and can be accessed online at http://thePoint.lww.com/MemmlerStructureFunction10e:

- **Instructor's Manual** is available in print format as well as online as a PDF.
- **Using the PASSport to Success® in Your Course** provides practical tips for integrating this innovative approach.
- **Brownstone Test Generator** allows you to create customized exams from a bank of questions.
- **PowerPoint Presentations** include multiple choice and true/false questions for use with Student Response System technology.
- **Image Bank** includes labels-on and labels-off options.
- **Supplemental Image Bank** with additional images can be used to enhance class presentations.
- **Lesson Plans** are organized around the learning objectives and include lecture notes, in-class activities, and assignments, including student activities from the PASSport to Success®.
- **Answers to "Questions for Study and Review"** provide responses to the quiz material found at the end of each chapter in the textbook.
- **Strategies for Effective Teaching** provide sound, tried-and-true advice for successful instruction.
- **WebCT/Blackboard/Angel Cartridge** allows easy integration of the ancillary materials into learning management systems.

Instructors also have access to all student ancillary assets, including the PASSport to Success®, via *thePoint* Web site.

Guide to Pronunciation

The stressed syllable in each word is shown with capital letters. The vowel pronunciations are as follows:

Any vowel at the end of a syllable is given a long sound, as follows:

a as in say
e as in be
i as in nice
o as in go
u as in true

A vowel followed by a consonant and the letter e (as in rate) also is given a long pronunciation.

Any vowel followed by a consonant receives a short pronunciation, as follows:

a as in absent
e as in end
i as in bin
o as in not
u as in up

Summary

The 10th edition of *Memmler's Structure and Function of the Human Body* builds on the successes of the previous nine editions by offering clear, concise narrative into which accurate, aesthetically pleasing anatomic art has been woven. We have made every effort to respond thoughtfully and thoroughly to reviewers' and instructors' comments, offering the ideal level of detail for students preparing for a career in the health professions and nursing and the pedagogic features that best support them. With the PASSport to Success®, we have provided students with an integrated system for understanding and using their unique learning styles—and ultimately succeeding in the course. We hope you will agree that the 10th edition of *Memmler's* suits your educational needs.

User's Guide

For today's health careers, a thorough understanding of human anatomy and physiology is more important than ever. *Memmler's Structure and Function of the Human Body,* 10th edition, not only provides the conceptual knowledge you'll need but also teaches you how to apply it. This User's Guide introduces you to the features and tools that will help you succeed as you work through the materials.

Your journey begins with your textbook, ***Memmler's Structure and Function of the Human Body***. Newly updated and fully illustrated, this easy-to-use textbook is filled with resources and activities that will enhance your personal learning style.

- **A&P in Action** provides an interesting case story that uses a familiar, real-life scenario to illustrate key concepts in anatomy and physiology. Later in the chapter, the case story is revisited in more detail—improving your understanding and helping you remember the information.
- **Ancillaries At-A-Glance** highlight the Learning Tools, Learning Resources, and Learning Activities available for the chapter.
- **Learning Outcomes** help you identify learning goals and familiarize yourself with the materials covered in the chapter.

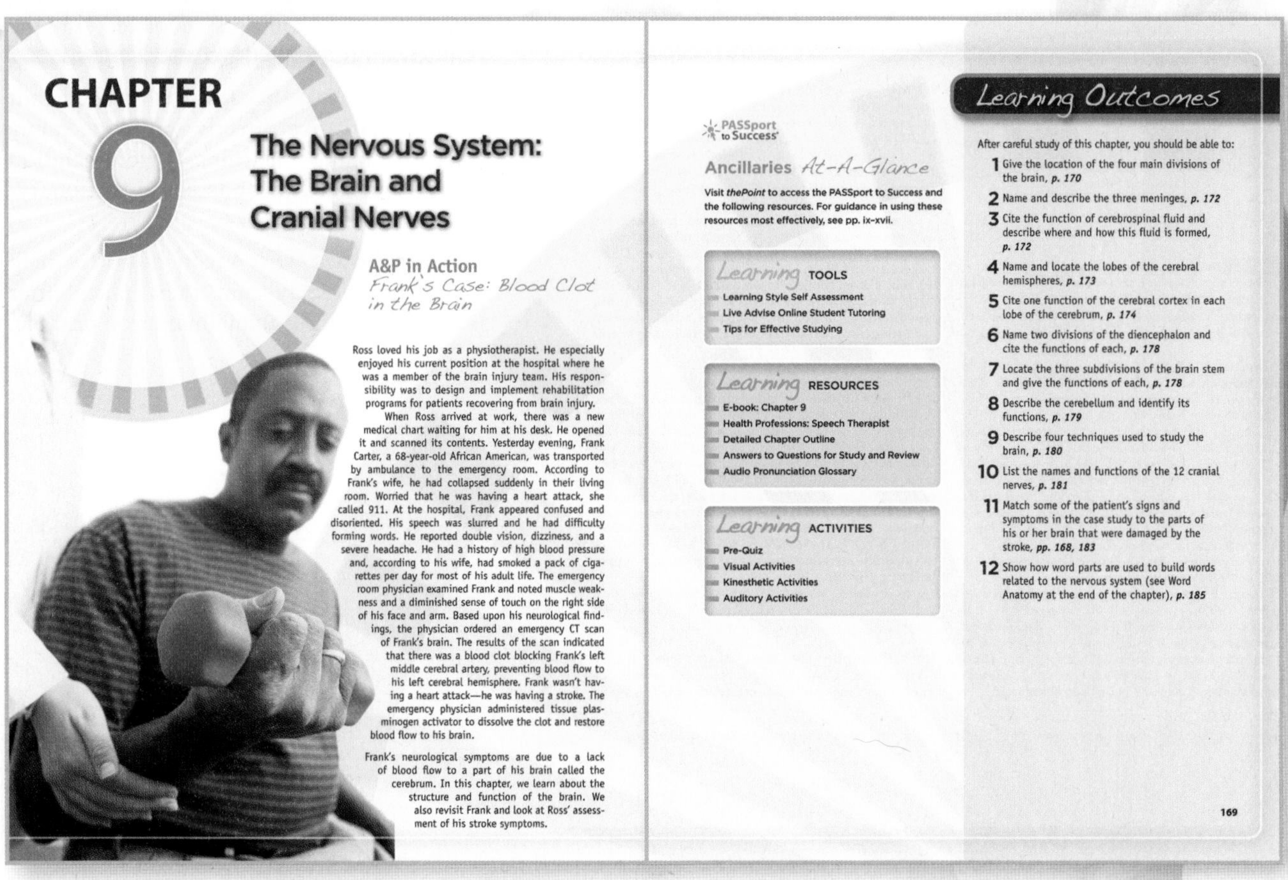

CHAPTER 9

The Nervous System: The Brain and Cranial Nerves

A&P in Action

Frank's Case: Blood Clot in the Brain

Ross loved his job as a physiotherapist. He especially enjoyed his current position at the hospital where he was a member of the brain injury team. His responsibility was to design and implement rehabilitation programs for patients recovering from brain injury.

When Ross arrived at work, there was a new medical chart waiting for him at his desk. He opened it and scanned its contents. Yesterday evening, Frank Carter, a 68-year-old African American, was transported by ambulance to the emergency room. According to Frank's wife, he had collapsed suddenly in their living room. Worried that he was having a heart attack, she called 911. At the hospital, Frank appeared confused and disoriented. His speech was slurred and he had difficulty forming words. He reported double vision, dizziness, and a severe headache. He had a history of high blood pressure and, according to his wife, had smoked a pack of cigarettes per day for most of his adult life. The emergency room physician examined Frank and noted muscle weakness and a diminished sense of touch on the right side of his face and arm. Based upon his neurological findings, the physician ordered an emergency CT scan of Frank's brain. The results of the scan indicated that there was a blood clot blocking Frank's left middle cerebral artery, preventing blood flow to his left cerebral hemisphere. Frank wasn't having a heart attack—he was having a stroke. The emergency physician administered tissue plasminogen activator to dissolve the clot and restore blood flow to his brain.

Frank's neurological symptoms are due to a lack of blood flow to a part of his brain called the cerebrum. In this chapter, we learn about the structure and function of the brain. We also revisit Frank and look at Ross' assessment of his stroke symptoms.

PASSport to Success

Ancillaries *At-A-Glance*

Visit *thePoint* to access the PASSport to Success and the following resources. For guidance in using these resources most effectively, see pp. ix–xvii.

Learning TOOLS
- Learning Style Self Assessment
- Live Advise Online Student Tutoring
- Tips for Effective Studying

Learning RESOURCES
- E-book: Chapter 9
- Health Professions: Speech Therapist
- Detailed Chapter Outline
- Answers to Questions for Study and Review
- Audio Pronunciation Glossary

Learning ACTIVITIES
- Pre-Quiz
- Visual Activities
- Kinesthetic Activities
- Auditory Activities

Learning Outcomes

After careful study of this chapter, you should be able to:

1 Give the location of the four main divisions of the brain, ***p. 170***

2 Name and describe the three meninges, ***p. 172***

3 Cite the function of cerebrospinal fluid and describe where and how this fluid is formed, ***p. 172***

4 Name and locate the lobes of the cerebral hemispheres, ***p. 173***

5 Cite one function of the cerebral cortex in each lobe of the cerebrum, ***p. 174***

6 Name two divisions of the diencephalon and cite the functions of each, ***p. 178***

7 Locate the three subdivisions of the brain stem and give the functions of each, ***p. 178***

8 Describe the cerebellum and identify its functions, ***p. 179***

9 Describe four techniques used to study the brain, ***p. 180***

10 List the names and functions of the 12 cranial nerves, ***p. 181***

11 Match some of the patient's signs and symptoms in the case study to the parts of his or her brain that were damaged by the stroke, ***pp. 168, 183***

12 Show how word parts are used to build words related to the nervous system (see Word Anatomy at the end of the chapter), ***p. 185***

169

148 **Unit III** Coordination and Control

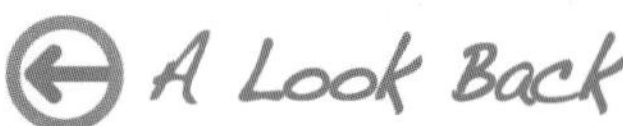

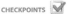

In Chapter 3, we learned about the electric charge, potential, on the plasma membrane. In Chapter 7, discussed synapses between cells, the importance of n rotransmitters, and generation of an action poten to activate muscle cells. Now, we put this informat together in describing the nervous system's activities it transmits information and coordinates responses changes in the environment.

- **A Look Back** relates each chapter's content to concepts in the preceeding chapters.

Chapter 6 The Skeleton: Bones and Joints 95

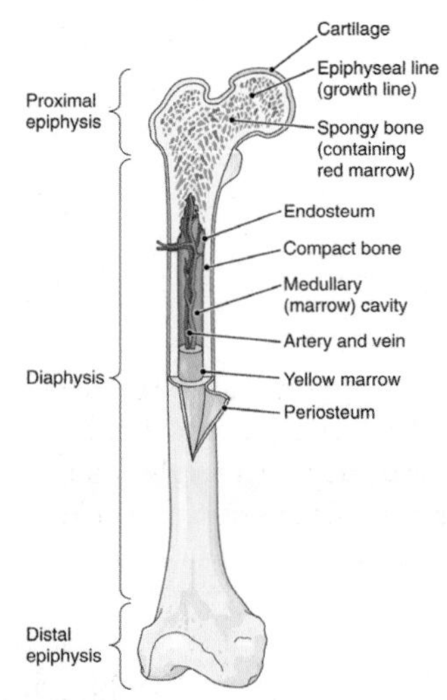

Figure 6-2 **The structure of a long bone.** KEY POINT A long bone has a long, narrow shaft, the diaphysis, and two irregular ends, the epiphyses. The medullary cavity has yellow marrow. Red marrow is located in spongy bone. ZOOMING IN What are the membranes on the outside and the inside of a long bone called?

There are two types of osseous tissue: compact and spongy. **Compact bone** is hard and dense (Fig. 6-3). This tissue makes up the main shaft of a long bone and the outer layer of other bones. The cells in this type of bone are located in rings of bone tissue around a **central canal**, also called a *haversian* (ha-VER-shan) *canal* containing nerves and blood vessels. The bone cells live in spaces (lacunae) between the rings and extend out into many small radiating channels so that they can be in contact with nearby cells. Each ringlike unit with its central canal makes up an **osteon** (OS-te-on) or haversian system (see Fig. 6-3B). Forming channels across the bone, from one side of the shaft to the other, are many **perforating** (Volkmann) **canals**, which also house blood vessels and nerves.

The second type of bone tissue, called **spongy bone**, or cancellous bone, has more spaces than compact bone. It is made of a meshwork of small, bony plates filled with red marrow. Spongy bone is found at the epiphyses (ends) of the long bones and at the center of other bones. It also lines the medullary cavity of long bones. Figure 6-3C shows a photograph of both compact and spongy bone tissue.

CHECKPOINTS 

6-1 What are the scientific names for the shaft and the ends of a long bone?

6-2 What are the two types of osseous (bone) tissue and where is each type found?

BONE GROWTH, MAINTENANCE, AND REPAIR

The process of bone formation begins in the earliest weeks of embryonic life and continues until young adulthood. Even after skeletal growth is complete, bone cells actively maintain and repair bone tissue.

Fetal Ossification During early development, the embryonic skeleton is at first composed almost entirely of cartilage. (Portions of the skull and a few other bones develop from fibrous connective tissue.) The conversion of cartilage to bone, a process known as **ossification,** begins during the second and third months of embryonic life. At this time, bone-building cells, called **osteoblasts** (OS-te-o-blasts), become active. First, they begin to manufacture the **matrix,** which is the material located between the cells. This intercellular substance contains large quantities of **collagen** (KOL-ah-jen), a fibrous protein that gives the tissue strength and resilience. Then, with the help of enzymes, calcium compounds are deposited within the matrix.

Once this intercellular material has hardened, the cells remain enclosed within the lacunae (small spaces) in the matrix. These cells, now known as **osteocytes** (OS-te-o-sites), are still living and continue to maintain the existing bone matrix, but they do not produce new bone tissue. When bone has to be remodeled or repaired later in life, new osteoblasts develop from stem cells in the endosteum and periosteum. You will see the importance of these cells in Reggie's case study.

Formation of a Long Bone In a long bone, the transformation of cartilage into bone begins at the center of the shaft during fetal development. Around the time of birth, secondary bone-forming centers, or **epiphyseal** (ep-ih-FIZ-e-al) **plates**, develop across the ends of the bones. The long bones continue to grow in length at these centers by calcification of new cartilage through childhood and into the late teens. Finally, by the late teens or early 20s, the bones stop growing in length. Each epiphyseal plate hardens and can be seen in x-ray films as a thin line, the epiphyseal line, across the end of the bone (see Figs. 6-2 and 6-3C). Physicians can judge a bone's future growth by the appearance of these lines on x-ray films.

As a bone grows in length, the shaft is remodeled as well, becoming wider as the central marrow cavity increases in size.

Bone Resorption One other cell type found in bone develops from a type of white blood cell (monocyte). These large, multinucleated **osteoclasts** (OS-te-o-klasts)

- **Chapter Checkpoints** pose brief questions at the end of main sections that test and reinforce student recall.
- **Key Points** spotlight essential aspects of the illustrations.
- **"Zooming In" questions** in the figure legends test and reinforce student understanding of concepts depicted in the illustration.
- **Phonetic pronunciations** spelled out in the narrative directly following many terms make learning pronunciation easy—no need to understand dictionary-style diacritical marks.
- **Color figure and table callouts** help students quickly find their place after stopping to look at an illustration or table.

- **Special interest boxes** focus on topics that augment chapter content.

A&P in Action Revisited

Adam's Colonoscopy

At his scheduled time, Adam reported to the hospital as an outpatient for his colonoscopy. He had stayed on a clear liquid diet for a day and done the required laxative prep to clear his colon. He met with Dr. Clarkson, a gastroenterologist (a physician who specializes in disorders of the gastrointestinal tract). Dr. Clarkson described the procedure. "We'll give you light sedation, and then use a flexible lighted endoscope with a camera to examine the entire colon. The procedure should take only about half an hour and has a very low risk. You have made arrangements for someone to go home with you, haven't you?" Adam said his brother was coming.

After the test, Dr. Clarkson reported that everything looked fine and that he would send the results to Dr. Michaels. "The good news, Adam, is that you have 10 years before you have to do this again. Maybe next time we'll be able to get our pictures with a small camera in a pill that you can swallow. That's already being tested. Scientists are also working on developing a screening test done by genetic study of cells sloughed off in the stool—and that won't require a prep."

Adam's case shows the importance of anatomic studies in the diagnosis and treatment of disease. Box 1-2 has general information on medical imaging, and various methods are mentioned in chapters and cases throughout t... We will visit Adam again in Chapter 19 when he ... that his prostate gland is affecting his urinary sys...

- **A&P in Action Revisited** provides the outcome of the real-life scenario that opens each chapter.

Box 4-2 *A Closer Look*

Collagen: The Body's Scaffolding

The most abundant protein in the body, making up about 25% of total protein, is collagen. Its name, derived from a Greek word meaning "glue," reveals its role as the main structural protein in connective tissue.

Fibroblasts secrete collagen molecules into the surrounding matrix, where the molecules are then assembled into fibers. These fibers give the matrix its strength and its flexibility. Collagen fibers' high tensile strength makes them stronger than steel fibers of the same size, and their flexibility confers resilience on the tissues that contain them. For example, collagen in skin, bone, tendons, and ligaments resists pulling forces, whereas collagen found in joint cartilage and between vertebrae resists compression. Based on amino acid structure, there are at least 19 types of collagen, each of which imparts a different property to the connective tissue containing it.

The arrangement of collagen fibers in the... much about the tissue's function. In the skin a... covering muscles and organs, collagen fibers irregularly, with fibers running in all directions... tissue that can resist stretching forces in many... tions. In tendons and ligaments, collagen fibers arrangement, forming strong ropelike cords... longitudinal pulling forces. In bone tissue, c... meshlike arrangement promotes deposition o... into the tissue, which gives bone strength whi... ing flexibility.

Collagen's varied properties are also evide... ration of a gelatin dessert. Gelatin is a collage... by boiling animal bones and other connective t... cous liquid in hot water but forms a semisolid g...

- **A Closer Look** gives in-depth scientific detail on topics in or related to the text.

Box 11-2 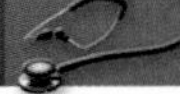 *Clinical Perspectives*

Seasonal Affective Disorder: Seeing the Light

Most of us find that long, dark days make us blue and sap our motivation. Are these learned responses or is there a physical basis for them? Studies have shown that the amount of light in the environment does have a physical effect on behavior. Evidence that light alters mood comes from people who are intensely affected by the dark days of winter—people who suffer from **seasonal affective disorder**, aptly abbreviated SAD. When days shorten, these people feel sleepy, depressed, and anxious. They tend to overeat, especially carbohydrates. Research suggests that SAD has a genetic basis and may be associated with decreased levels of the neurotransmitter serotonin.

As light strikes the retina of the eye, it sends impulses that decrease the amount of melatonin produced by the pineal gland in the brain. Because melatonin depresses mood, the final effect of light is to elevate mood. Daily exposure to bright lights has been found to improve the mood of most people with SAD. Exposure for 15 minutes after rising in the morning may be enough, but some people require longer sessions both morning and evening. Other aids include aerobic exercise, stress management techniques, and antidepressant medications.

- **Clinical Perspectives** focuses on diseases and disorders relevant to the chapter, exploring what happens to the body when the normal structure-function relationship breaks down.

Box 10-1 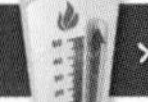 *Hot Topics*

Eye Surgery: A Glimpse of the Cutting Edge

Cataracts, glaucoma, and refractive errors are the most common eye disorders affecting Americans. In the past, cataract and glaucoma treatments concentrated on managing the diseases. Refractive errors were corrected using eyeglasses and, more recently, contact lenses. Today, laser and microsurgical techniques can remove cataracts, reduce glaucoma, and allow people with refractive errors to put their eyeglasses and contacts away. These cutting-edge procedures include

- *Laser in situ keratomileusis (LASIK)* to correct refractive errors. During this procedure, a surgeon uses a laser to reshape the cornea so that it refracts light directly onto the retina, rather than in front of or behind it. A microkeratome (surgical knife) is used to cut a flap in the cornea's outer layer. A computer-controlled laser sculpts the middle layer ...ea and then the flap is replaced. The procedure ... few minutes and patients recover their vision ... usually with little postoperative pain.
- *Laser trabeculoplasty* to treat glaucoma. This procedure uses a laser to help drain fluid from the eye and lower intraocular pressure. The laser is aimed at drainage canals located between the cornea and iris and makes several burns that are believed to open the canals and allow fluid to drain better. The procedure is typically painless and takes only a few minutes.
- *Phacoemulsification* to remove cataracts. During this surgical procedure, a very small incision (approximately 3 mm long) is made through the sclera near the cornea's outer edge. An ultrasonic probe is inserted through this opening and into the center of the lens. The probe uses sound waves to emulsify the lens' central core, which is then suctioned out. Then, an artificial lens is permanently implanted in the lens capsule. The procedure is typically painless, although the patient may feel some discomfort for 1 to 2 days afterward.

- **Hot Topics** examines current trends and research.

Box 6-2 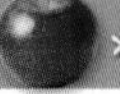 *Health Maintenance*

Three Steps toward a Strong and Healthy Skeleton

The skeleton is the body's framework. It supports and protects internal organs, helps to produce movement, and manufactures blood cells. Bone also stores nearly all of the body's calcium, releasing it into the blood when needed for processes such as nerve transmission, muscle contraction, and blood clotting. Proper nutrition, exercise, and a healthy lifestyle can help the skeleton perform all these essential roles.

A well-balanced diet supplies the nutrients and energy needed for strong, healthy bones. Calcium, phosphorus, and magnesium make up the mineral crystals of bone and confer strength and rigidity. Foods rich in both calcium and phosphorus include dairy products, fish, beans, and leafy green vegetables. When body fluids become too acidic, bone releases calcium and phosphate and is weakened. Both magnesium and potassium help regulate the pH of body fluids, with magnesium also helping bone absorb calcium. Foods rich in magne-...

Protein supplies the amino acids needed to make collagen, which gives bone tissue flexibility. Meat, poultry, fish, eggs, dairy, soy, and nuts are excellent sources of protein.

Vitamin C helps stimulate collagen synthesis, and vitamin D helps the digestive system absorb calcium into the bloodstream, making it available for bone. Most fruits and vegetables are rich in vitamin C. Few foods supply vitamin D. Reliable sources include fatty fish and fortified milk. Liver, butter, and eggs also contain very small amounts.

Like muscle, bone becomes weakened with disuse. Consistent exercise promotes a stronger, denser skeleton by stimulating bone to absorb more calcium and phosphate from the blood, reducing the risk of osteoporosis. A healthy lifestyle also includes avoiding smoking and excessive alcohol consumption, both of which decrease bone calcium and ...

- **Health Maintenance** offers supplementary information on health and wellness issues.

- **Figures:** The art program includes full-color anatomic line art, some new or revised, with a level of detail that matches that of the narrative. Photomicrographs, radiographs, and other scans give students a preview of what they might see in real-world healthcare settings. Supplementary figures are available on the companion Web site as well as on the Student DVD included with this text.

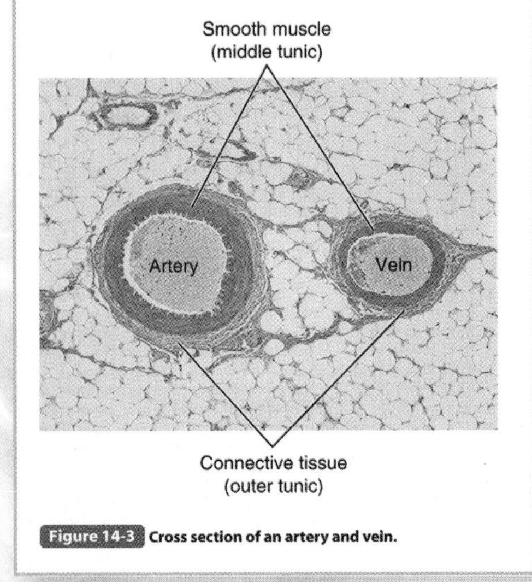

Figure 14-3 Cross section of an artery and vein.

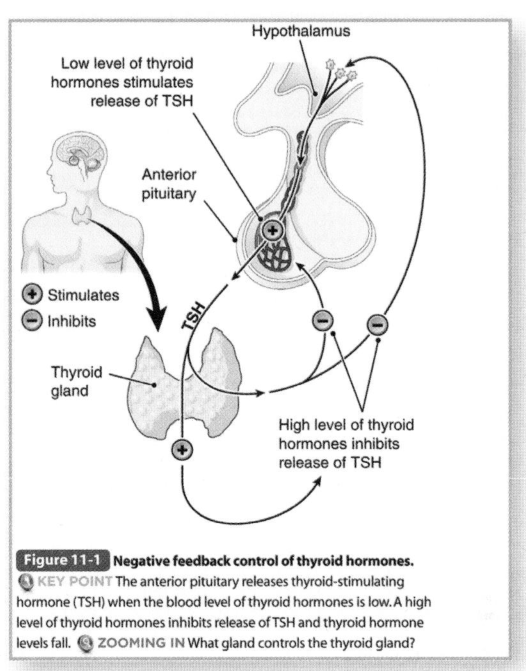

Figure 11-1 Negative feedback control of thyroid hormones. KEY POINT The anterior pituitary releases thyroid-stimulating hormone (TSH) when the blood level of thyroid hormones is low. A high level of thyroid hormones inhibits release of TSH and thyroid hormone levels fall. ZOOMING IN What gland controls the thyroid gland?

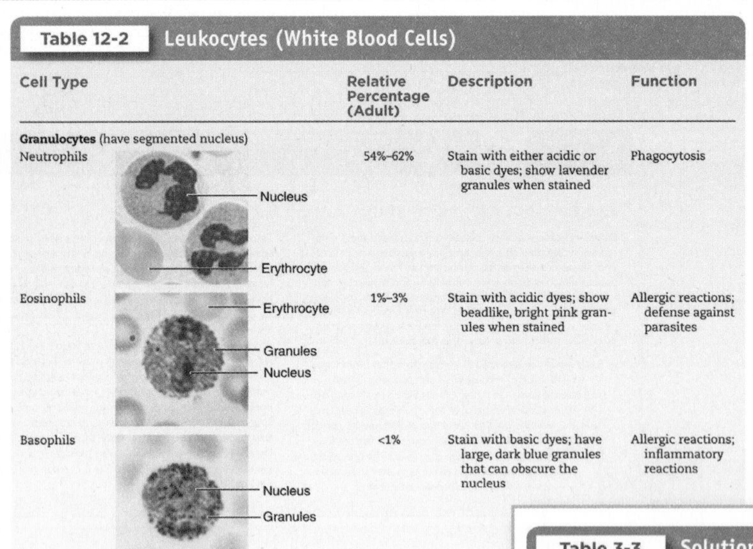

Table 12-2 Leukocytes (White Blood Cells)

Cell Type	Relative Percentage (Adult)	Description	Function
Granulocytes (have segmented nucleus)			
Neutrophils Nucleus Erythrocyte	54%–62%	Stain with either acidic or basic dyes; show lavender granules when stained	Phagocytosis
Eosinophils Erythrocyte Granules Nucleus	1%–3%	Stain with acidic dyes; show beadlike, bright pink granules when stained	Allergic reactions; defense against parasites
Basophils Nucleus Granules	<1%	Stain with basic dyes; have large, dark blue granules that can obscure the nucleus	Allergic reactions; inflammatory reactions
Agranulocytes (have unsegmented nucleus)			

- **Tables:** The numerous tables in this edition summarize key concepts and information in an easy-to-review form. Additional summary tables are available on the companion Web site as well as on the Student DVD included with this text.

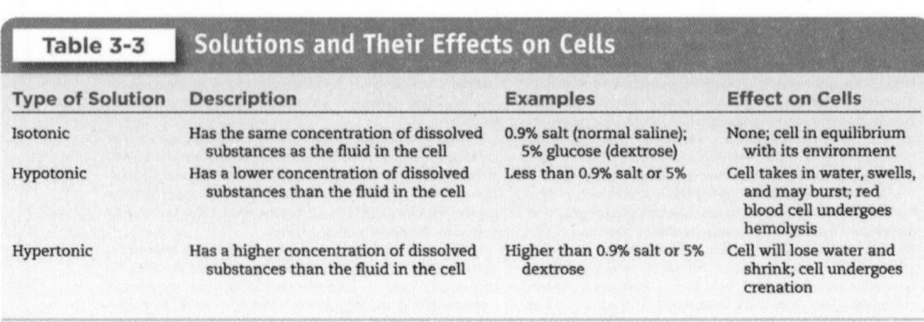

Table 3-3 Solutions and Their Effects on Cells

Type of Solution	Description	Examples	Effect on Cells
Isotonic	Has the same concentration of dissolved substances as the fluid in the cell	0.9% salt (normal saline); 5% glucose (dextrose)	None; cell in equilibrium with its environment
Hypotonic	Has a lower concentration of dissolved substances than the fluid in the cell	Less than 0.9% salt or 5%	Cell takes in water, swells, and may burst; red blood cell undergoes hemolysis
Hypertonic	Has a higher concentration of dissolved substances than the fluid in the cell	Higher than 0.9% salt or 5% dextrose	Cell will lose water and shrink; cell undergoes crenation

- **Chapter Wrap-Up** at the end of each chapter outlines the chapter content.

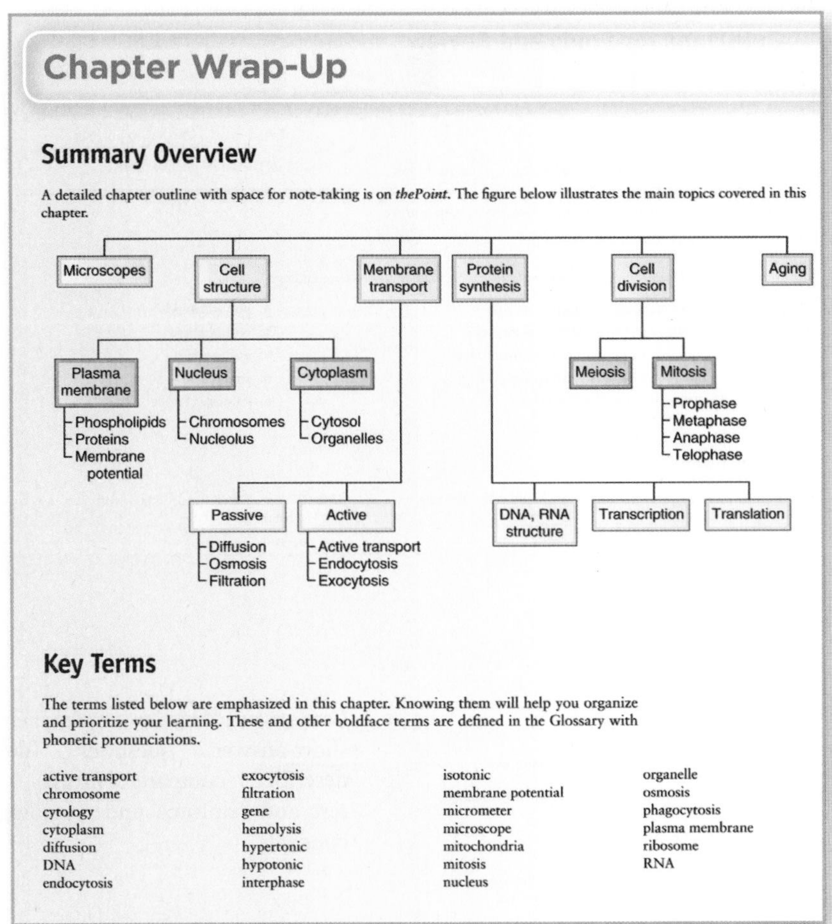

Chapter Wrap-Up

Summary Overview

A detailed chapter outline with space for note-taking is on *thePoint*. The figure below illustrates the main topics covered in this chapter.

Key Terms

The terms listed below are emphasized in this chapter. Knowing them will help you organize and prioritize your learning. These and other boldface terms are defined in the Glossary with phonetic pronunciations.

active transport	exocytosis	isotonic	organelle
chromosome	filtration	membrane potential	osmosis
cytology	gene	micrometer	phagocytosis
cytoplasm	hemolysis	microscope	plasma membrane
diffusion	hypertonic	mitochondria	ribosome
DNA	hypotonic	mitosis	RNA
endocytosis	interphase	nucleus	

- **Key Terms** provides a concise list at the end of each chapter of selected boldface terms used in the text and defined in the book's glossary.

- **Word Anatomy** defines and illustrates the various word parts that appear in terms within the chapter, helping to build vocabulary and promote understanding of unfamiliar terms.

Word Anatomy

Scientific terms are built from standardized word parts (prefixes, roots, and suffixes). Learning the meanings of these parts can help you remember words and interpret unfamiliar terms.

WORD PART	MEANING	EXAMPLE
Microscopes		
cyt/o	cell	*Cytology* is the study of cells.
micr/o	small	*Microscopes* are used to view structures too small to see with the naked eye.
Cell Structure		
bi-	two	The lipid *bilayer* is a double layer of lipid molecules.
-some	body	*Ribosomes* are small bodies in the cytoplasm that help make proteins.
chrom/o-	color	*Chromosomes* are small, threadlike bodies that stain darkly with basic dyes.
end/o-	in, within	The *endoplasmic* reticulum is a membranous network within the cytoplasm.
lys/o	loosening, dissolving, separating	*Lysosomes* are small bodies (organelles) with enzymes that dissolve materials (*see also hemolysis*).

- **Questions for Study and Review** organizes study questions hierarchically into three levels.

  - **Building Understanding:** Includes fill-in-the-blank, matching, and multiple choice questions that test factual recall.

Questions for Study and Review

BUILDING UNDERSTANDING

Fill in the blanks

1. The subunits of elements are _____.
2. The atomic number is the number of_____ in an atom's nucleus.
3. A mixture of solute dissolved in solvent is called a(n) _____.
4. Blood has a pH of 7.35 to 7.45. Gastric juice has a pH of about 2.0. The more alkaline fluid is _____.
5. Proteins that catalyze metabolic reactions are called _____.

Matching > Match each numbered item with the most closely related lettered item.

___ 6. A simple carbohydrate such as glucose
___ 7. A complex carbohydrate such as glycogen
___ 8. An important component of cell membranes
___ 9. Examples include DNA, RNA, and ATP
___10. The basic building block of protein

a. polysaccharide
b. phospholipid
c. nucleotide
d. amino acid
e. monosaccharide

Multiple Choice

___11. What type of mixture is red blood cells "floating" in plasma?
a. compound

___14. Which chemical can donate hydrogen ions to other substances?
a. acid

UNDERSTANDING CONCEPTS

___16. Compare and contrast the following terms:
a. element and atom
b. molecule and compound
c. proton, neutron, and electron
d. anion and cation
e. ionic bond and covalent bond
f. acid and base

17. What are some of the properties of water that make it an ideal medium for living cells?

18. What is pH? Discuss the role of buffers in maintaining pH

19. What are the characteristics of organic compounds?

20. Compare and contrast carbohydrates, proteins, and nucleotides.

21. Describe three different types of lipids.

22. Define the term *enzyme* and discuss the relationship between enzyme structure and enzyme function.

  - **Understanding Concepts:** Includes short-answer questions (define, describe, compare/contrast) that test and reinforce understanding of concepts.

CONCEPTUAL THINKING

23. Based on your understanding of strong acids and bases, why does the body have to be kept at a close-to-neutral pH?

24. In Margaret's case, she was hypotensive when she arrived at the hospital. Explain the link between dehydration and low blood pressure.

25. In Margaret's case, an aqueous solution of 5% dextrose was used to rehydrate her. Name the solution's solute and solvent.

  - **Conceptual Thinking:** Includes short-essay questions that promote critical thinking skills. New in this edition are thought questions related to the A&P in Action case stories.

Getting Started with the Student Resources and the PASSport to Success® for Students

Your journey begins with your textbook, *Memmler's Structure and Function of the Human Body,* 10th edition. The textbook has icons that guide you to resources and activities designed for your personal learning style.

Look for this icon throughout the book for pertinent supplementary material on the companion Web site and student resource DVD

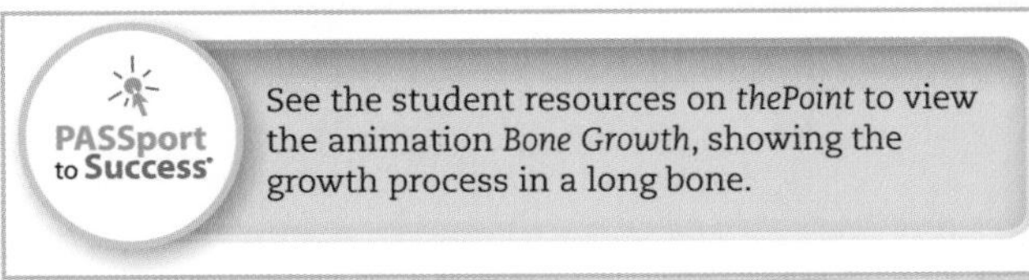
PASSport to Success
See the student resources on thePoint to view the animation Bone Growth, showing the growth process in a long bone.

Here's how to begin:

1. Scratch off the personal access code inside the front cover of your textbook.
2. Log on to *http://thePoint.lww.com/MemmlerStructureFunction10e*, the companion Web site for *Memmler's Structure and Function of the Human Body,* 10th Edition, on *thePoint.*
3. Click on "Student Resources" and then "PASSport to Success®."
4. Once you are on the PASSport to Success® site, click on "MyPowerLearning."
5. Take the online self-assessment. *(Don't worry - There are no wrong answers!).*
6. Read your own personal learning styles report to better understand how to study most effectively and efficiently.

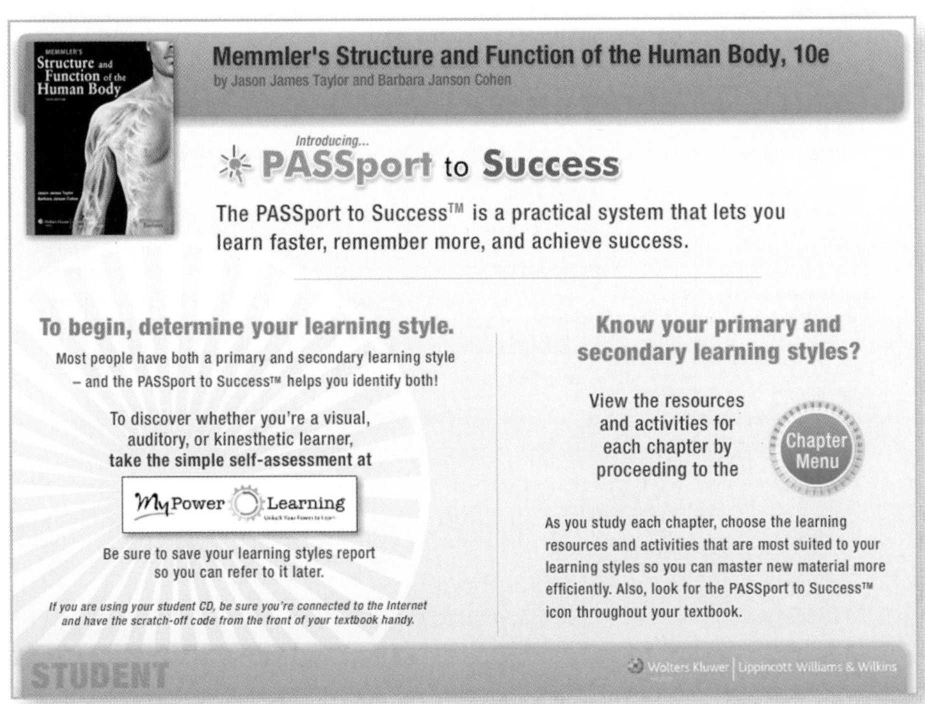
Memmler's Structure and Function of the Human Body, 10e
by Jason James Taylor and Barbara Janson Cohen
Introducing...
PASSport to Success
The PASSport to Success™ is a practical system that lets you learn faster, remember more, and achieve success.
To begin, determine your learning style.
Most people have both a primary and secondary learning style – and the PASSport to Success™ helps you identify both!
To discover whether you're a visual, auditory, or kinesthetic learner, take the simple self-assessment at
MyPower Learning
Be sure to save your learning styles report so you can refer to it later.
If you are using your student CD, be sure you're connected to the Internet and have the scratch-off code from the front of your textbook handy.
Know your primary and secondary learning styles?
View the resources and activities for each chapter by proceeding to the
Chapter Menu
As you study each chapter, choose the learning resources and activities that are most suited to your learning styles so you can master new material more efficiently. Also, look for the PASSport to Success™ icon throughout your textbook.
STUDENT
Wolters Kluwer | Lippincott Williams & Wilkins

Once you know your personal learning style, click on the "Chapter Menu" button on the PASSport to Success® home screen. Within each chapter, you can search and sort PASSport to Success® activities by learning style to choose the most effective way for you to learn the material.

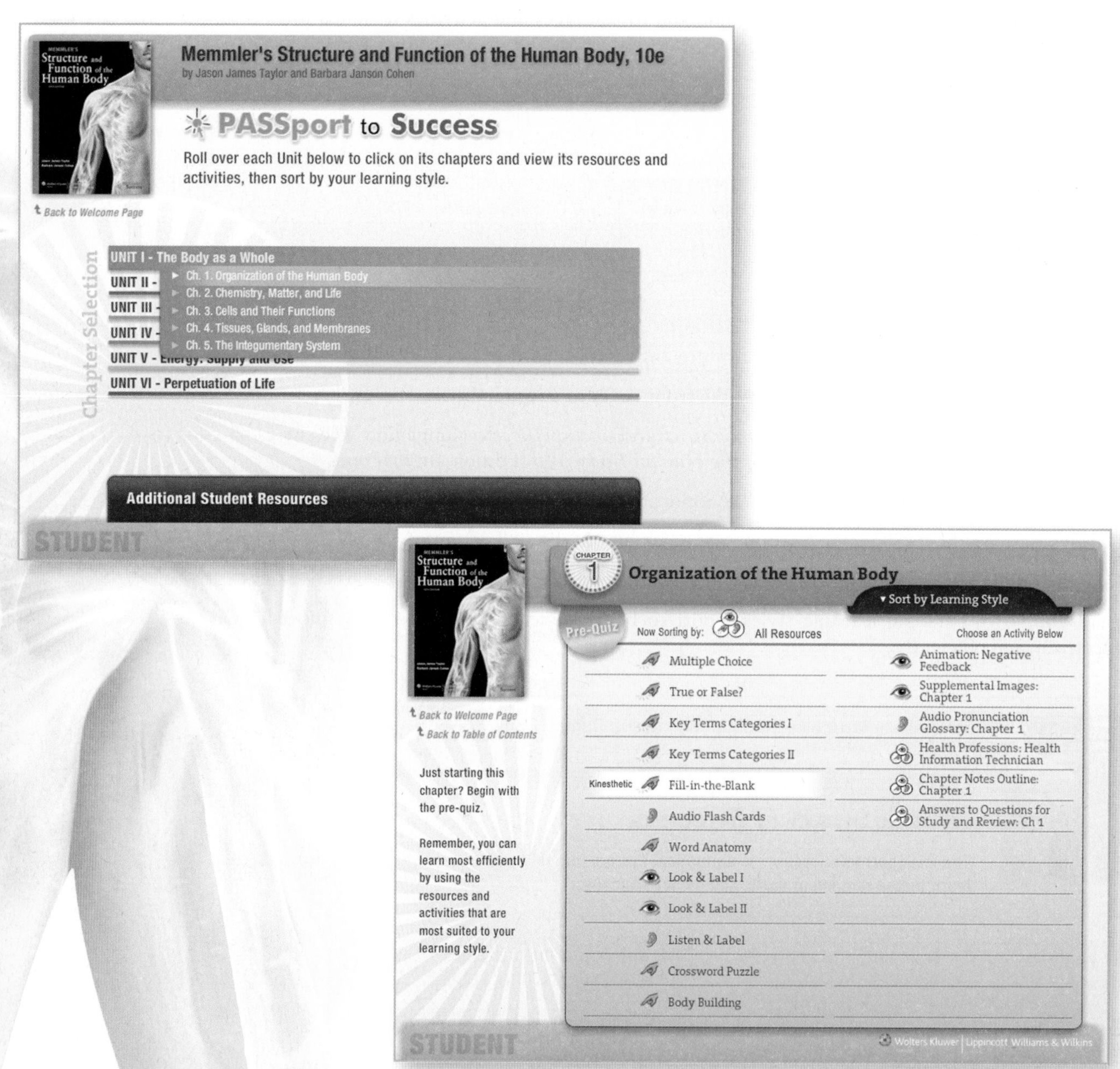

Resources and activities available to students include the following:

Pre-Quiz
True or False?
Key Terms Categories
Fill-in-the-Blank
Crossword Puzzle *NEW*!
Audio Flash Cards
Word Anatomy
Look & Label
Listen & Label
Zooming In
Body Building
Animations
Supplemental Images
Audio Pronunciation Glossary
Answers to "Questions for Study and Review"
Health Professions Career Information
Tips for Effective Studying
Student Note-Taking Guides

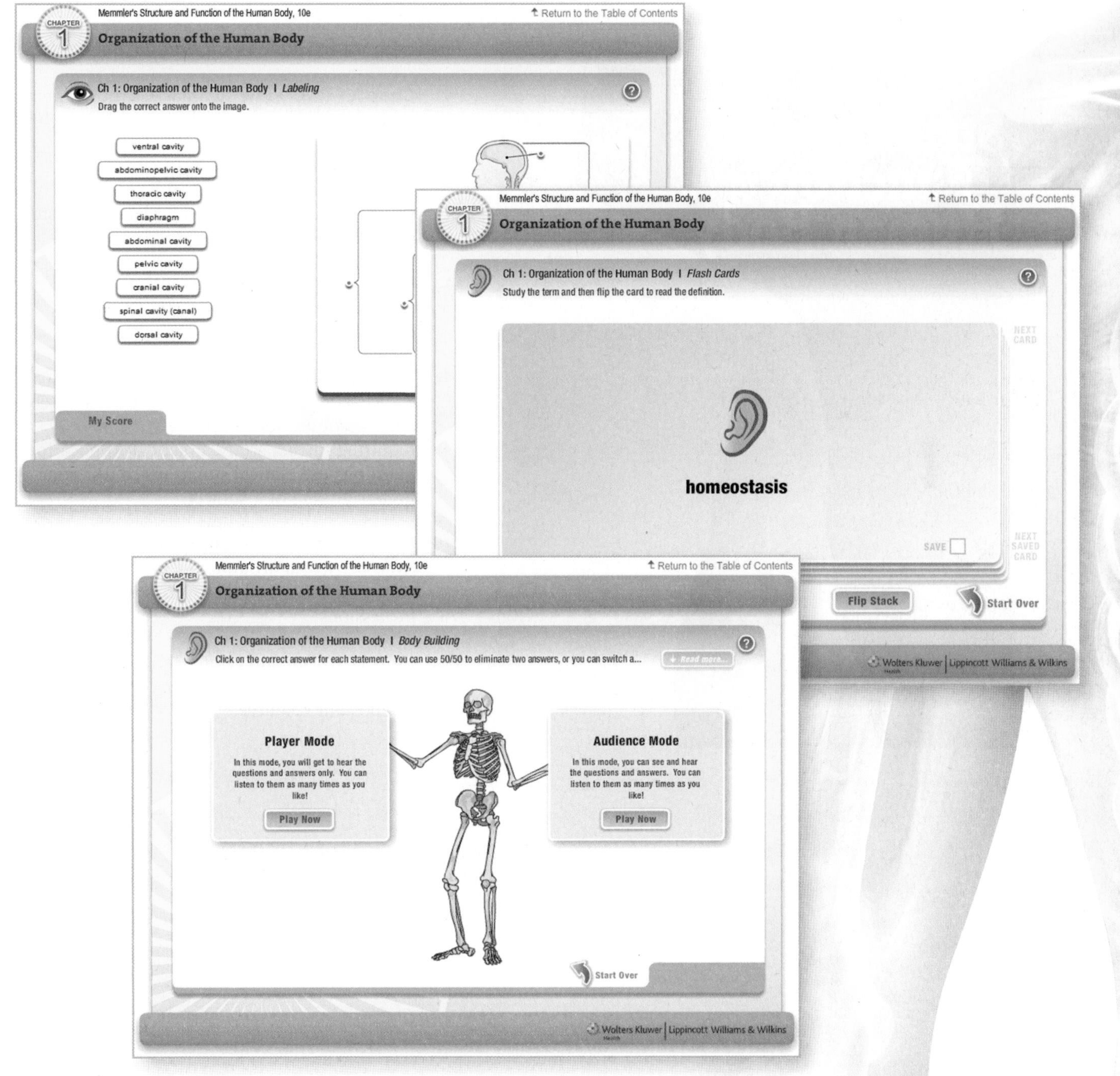

- ***Study Guide* for *Memmler's Structure and Function of the Human Body,*** 10th edition
  Kerry L. Hull, BSC, PhD
  Barbara Janson Cohen, BA, MSEd

  Along with the PASSport to Success®, this *Study Guide* is the ideal companion to the 10th edition of *Memmler's Structure and Function of the Human Body*. Following the text's organization chapter by chapter, the *Study Guide* provides a full range of self-study aids that actively engage you in learning and enable you to assess and build your knowledge as you advance through the text. Most importantly, the *Study Guide* allows you to get the most out of your study time, with a variety of exercises that meet the needs of all types of learners.

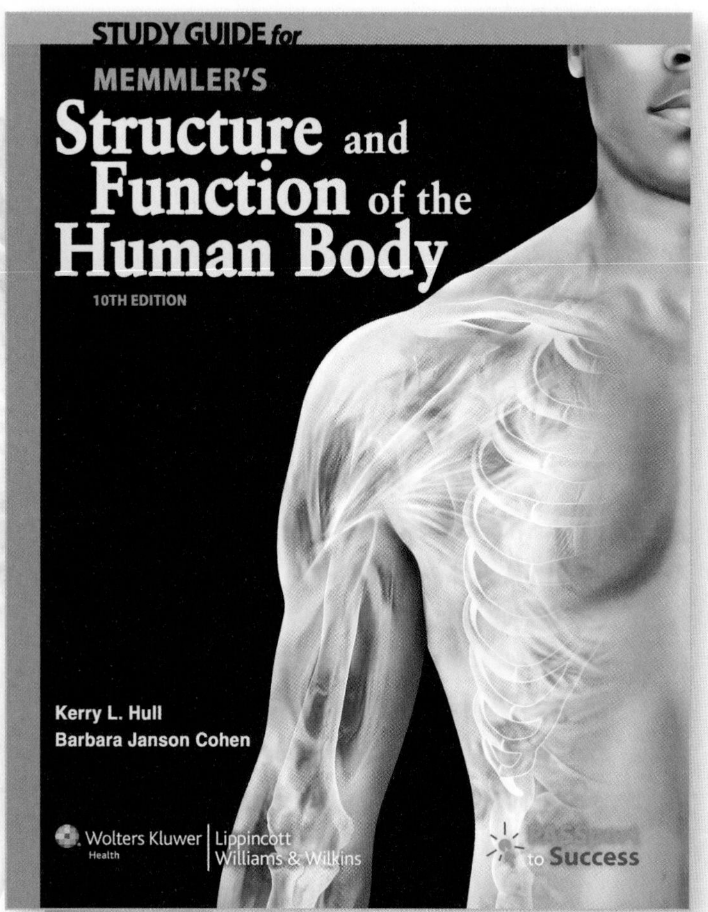

Inside the Study Guide you'll find the following:

- **Chapter Overview** summarizes the chapter's critical concepts.
- **Addressing the Learning Outcomes** includes labeling, coloring, matching, and short-answer questions, all designed to foster active learning.
- **Making the Connections** integrates information from each chapter's learning outcomes into concept mapping exercises.
- **Testing Your Knowledge** provides multiple choice, true/false, completion, short- answer, and essay questions to identify areas requiring further study. Practical Applications questions use clinical situations to test your understanding of a subject.
- **Expanding Your Horizons** helps you learn from the world around you, and highlights emerging issues and discoveries in the health professions.

Visit www.lww.com *and reference* ISBN 978-1-6091-3901-8 to order your copy of this important resource.

Reviewers

We gratefully acknowledge the generous contributions of the reviewers whose names appear in the list that follows.

Brian Blumhorst, BS, MA
Science Chairperson
Mendota High School
Mendota, IL

Michael Broughton, DC
Faculty Member
Department of General Education
Bohecker College
Cincinnati, OH

Joyce B. Ceresini, RN, BSN
Med-Surg Instructor
LPN Program
Lebanon County Career and Technical Center
Lebanon, PA

Lane Miller, MBA/HCM
LMS Administrator
Department of LMS and Continuing Education
Medical Careers Institute
Virginia Beach, VA

Julie K. Pepper, CMA (AAMA), BS
Instructor
Chippewa Valley Technical College
Medical Assistant Department
Eau Claire, WI

Terri Rutzen, Masters Adult Education
Faculty Member
Department of Health Science
Baker College—Muskegon
Muskegon, MI

Michael Vogel, MA, Education; MS, Biology
Instructor, Anatomy and Physiology, Microbiology, Nursing/Allied Health
Fortis College
Cincinnati, OH

Acknowledgments

Thanks to the many dedicated and talented professionals who worked tirelessly on this project. Above all, my thanks go to Barbara Cohen, whose skill and experience guided this revision from start to finish. After almost a decade of working together, Barbara has had a great impact on my teaching and writing career. Special thanks must also go to David Troy and Eve Malakoff-Klein for their endless support and guidance.

Many thanks to the students I have taught over the years at Red River College. Like Barbara, they have helped me hone my teaching and writing skills. There are many examples of their insight within this 10th edition of *Memmler's Structure and Function of the Human Body*

I am also deeply indebted to my wife, Nicole. Without her support, I could not have finished this project. Lastly, thanks to my kids, Alek, Emily, and Wren, who, in addition to insisting that they be included in the case stories, continue to remind me to look at the world around and within me with the eyes of a child.

—Jason James Taylor

Major credit for this 10th edition of *Memmler's Structure and Function of the Human Body* goes to the lead author, Jason James Taylor. Consulting editor Kerry Hull has contributed throughout to the preparation of this revision and has written the *Study Guide* and the *Instructor's Manual* that accompany the book.

The skilled staff at Lippincott Williams & Wilkins, as always, has been instrumental in the development of these texts. Consistently striving for improvements and high quality, they have helped achieve the great success of these books over their long history. Specifically, I'd like to acknowledge David Troy, Executive Editor; Laura Bonazzoli, Development Editor; and Matt Hauber, Senior Product Manager. Special recognition is reserved for Eve Malakoff-Klein, Senior Product Manager, who took on the guidance of this project with vigor and contributed enormously to the final product.

Thanks to the reviewers, listed separately, who made valuable comments on the text. Their suggestions and insights formed the basis for this revision.

As always, thanks to my husband, Matthew, an instructor in anatomy and physiology, who not only gives consistent support but also contributes advice and suggestions for the text.

—Barbara Janson Cohen

Brief Contents

Contents

The Body Visible

New to this 10th edition of *Memmler's Structure and Function of the Human Body* is *The Body Visible*, a unique study tool designed to enhance your learning of the body's systems in this course and in your future work.

The Body Visible illustrates the systems discussed in the text in the same sequence in which they appear in the text. Each full-color detailed illustration also contains numbers and lines for identifying the structures in the illustration. A transparent overlay with labels for all of the numbered structures in the art accompanies each image.

With the labels in place, *The Body Visible* allows you to study each illustration and helps you to learn the body's structures. When you view each system without the overlay in place, *The Body Visible* becomes a self-testing resource. As you test your knowledge and identify each numbered part, you can easily check your answers with the overlay.

Many of the images in *The Body Visible* have somewhat more detail than is covered in the text. We encourage you to keep *The Body Visible* available as a general reference and as a useful study tool as you progress to more advanced levels in your chosen healthcare career.

*The Body Visible** begins on the next page.

---

*The images in *The Body Visible* are adapted with permission from Anatomical Chart Company, *Rapid Review: A Guide for Self-Testing and Memorization*, 3rd ed. Philadelphia: Lippincott Williams & Wilkins, 2010.

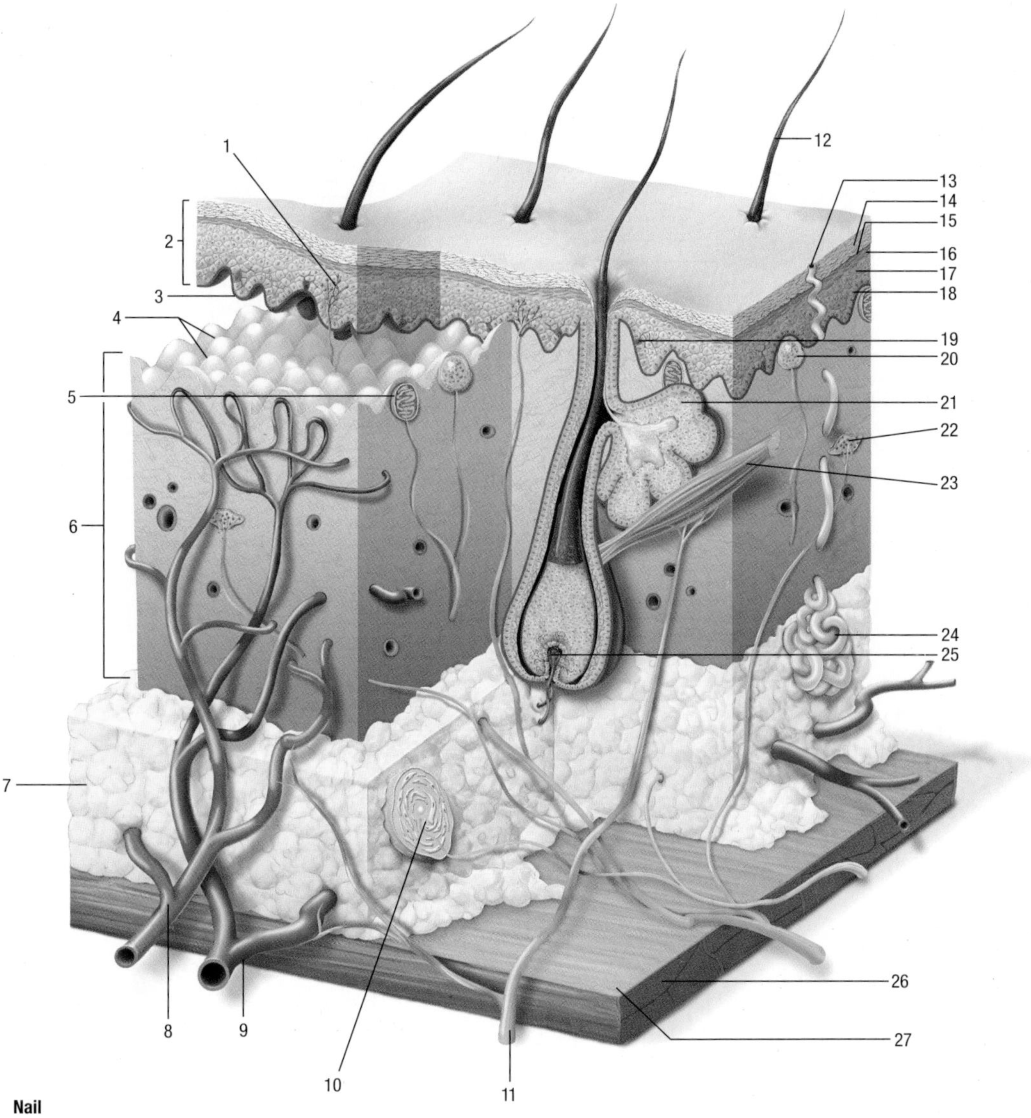

1 2 3 4 5 6 7 8 9 10 11 12 13 14 15 16 17 18 19 20 21 22 23 24 25 26 27

Nail

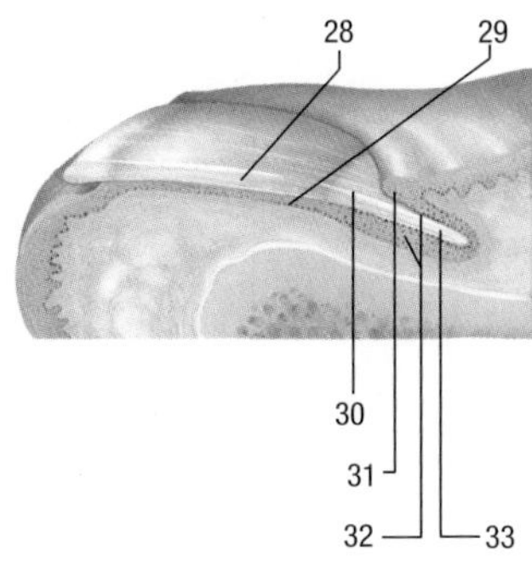

The Skeletal System

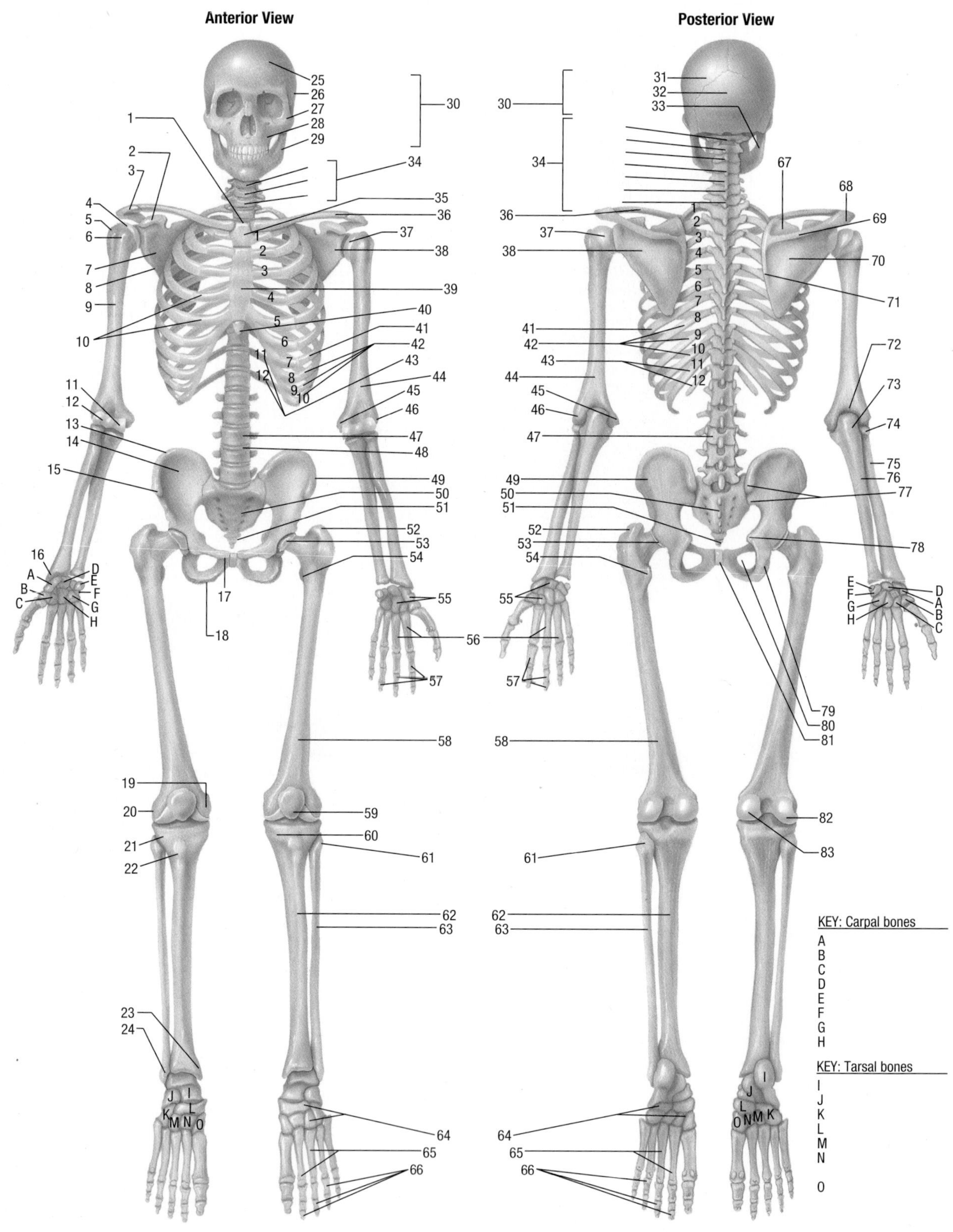

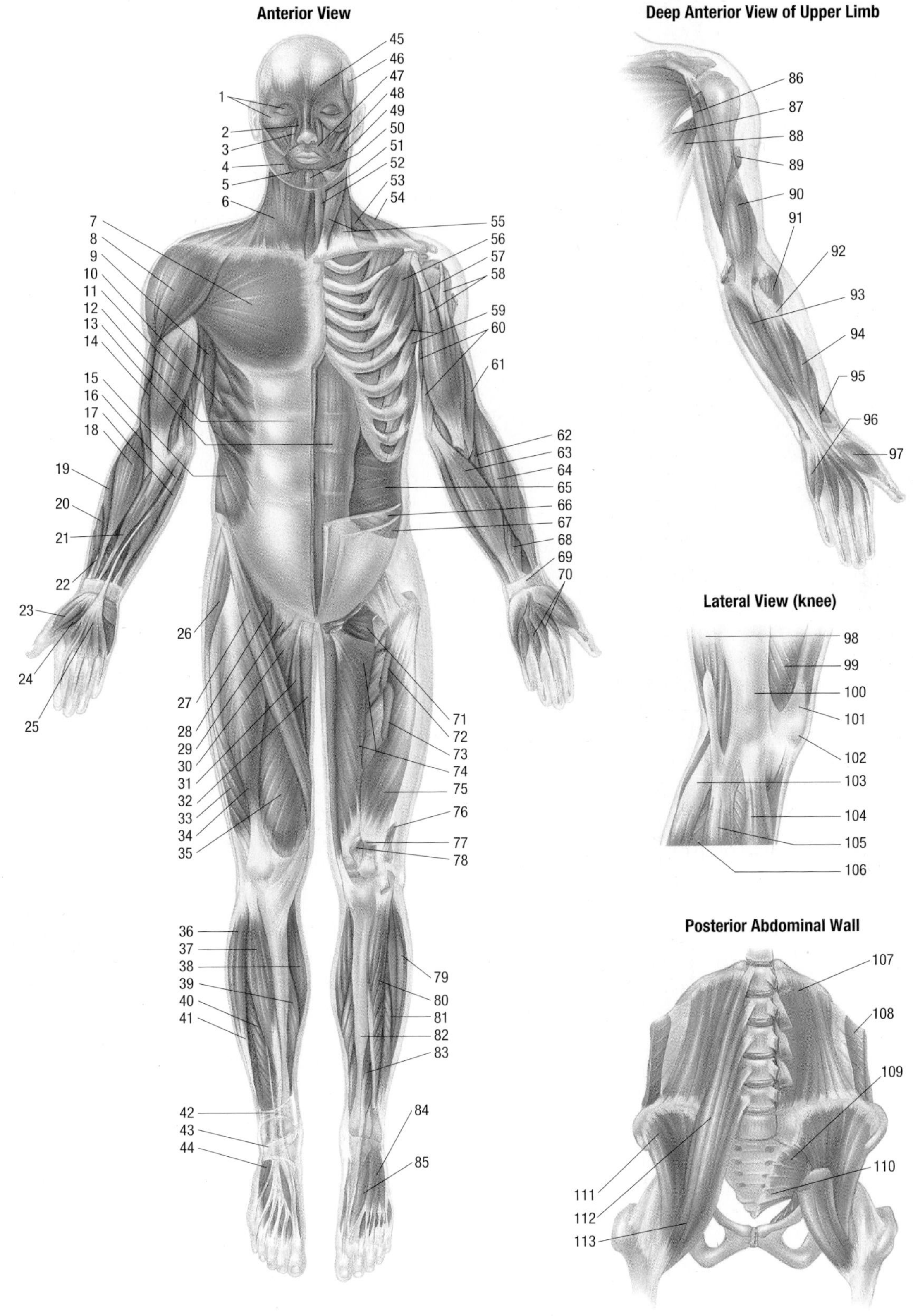
Anterior View
1
2
3
4
5
6
7
8
9
10
11
12
13
14
15
16
17
18
19
20
21
22
23
24
25
26
27
28
29
30
31
32
33
34
35
36
37
38
39
40
41
42
43
44
45
46
47
48
49
50
51
52
53
54
55
56
57
58
59
60
61
62
63
64
65
66
67
68
69
70
71
72
73
74
75
76
77
78
79
80
81
82
83
84
85
Deep Anterior View of Upper Limb
86
87
88
89
90
91
92
93
94
95
96
97
Lateral View (knee)
98
99
100
101
102
103
104
105
106
Posterior Abdominal Wall
107
108
109
110
111
112
113

The Muscular System—Posterior View

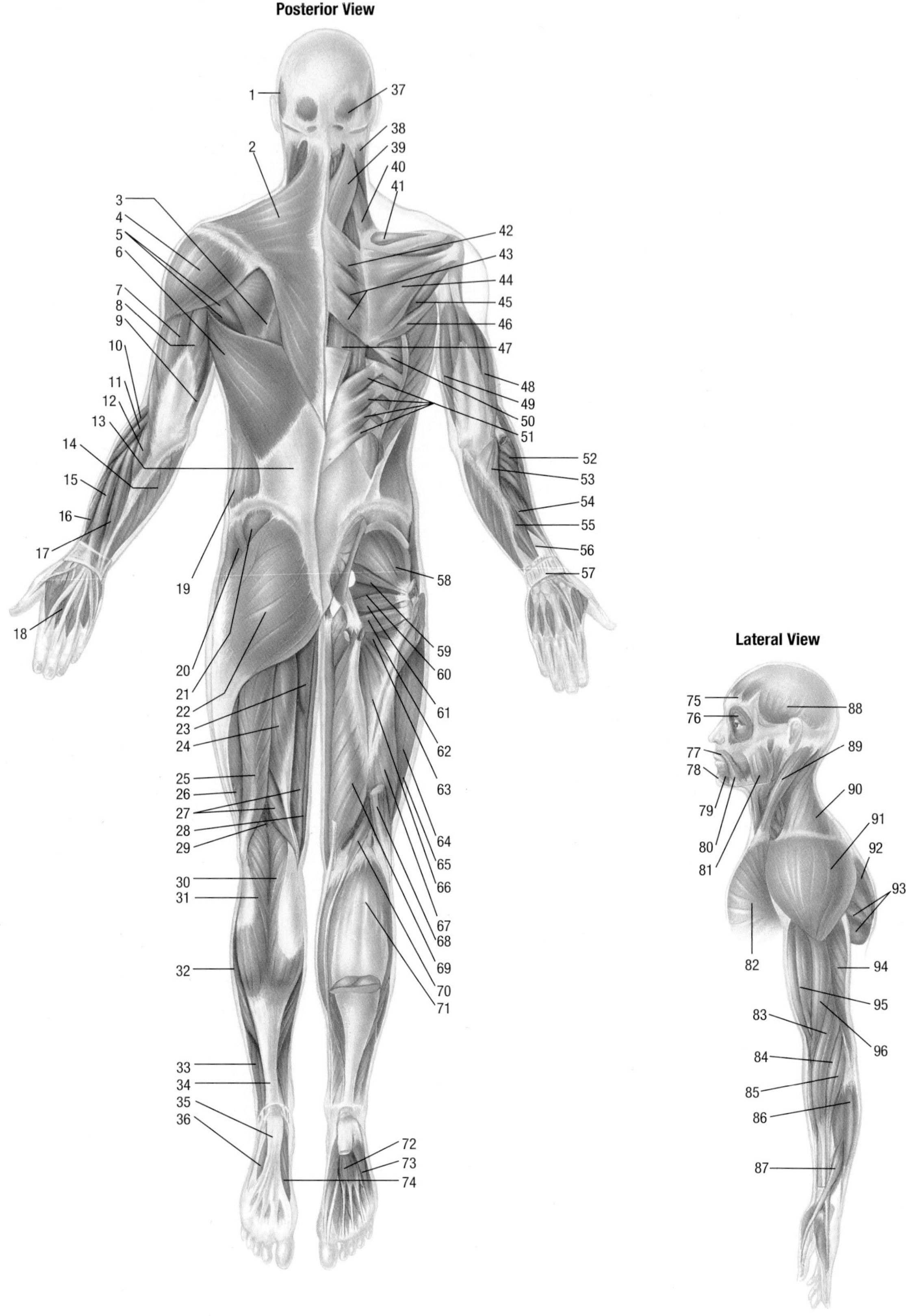

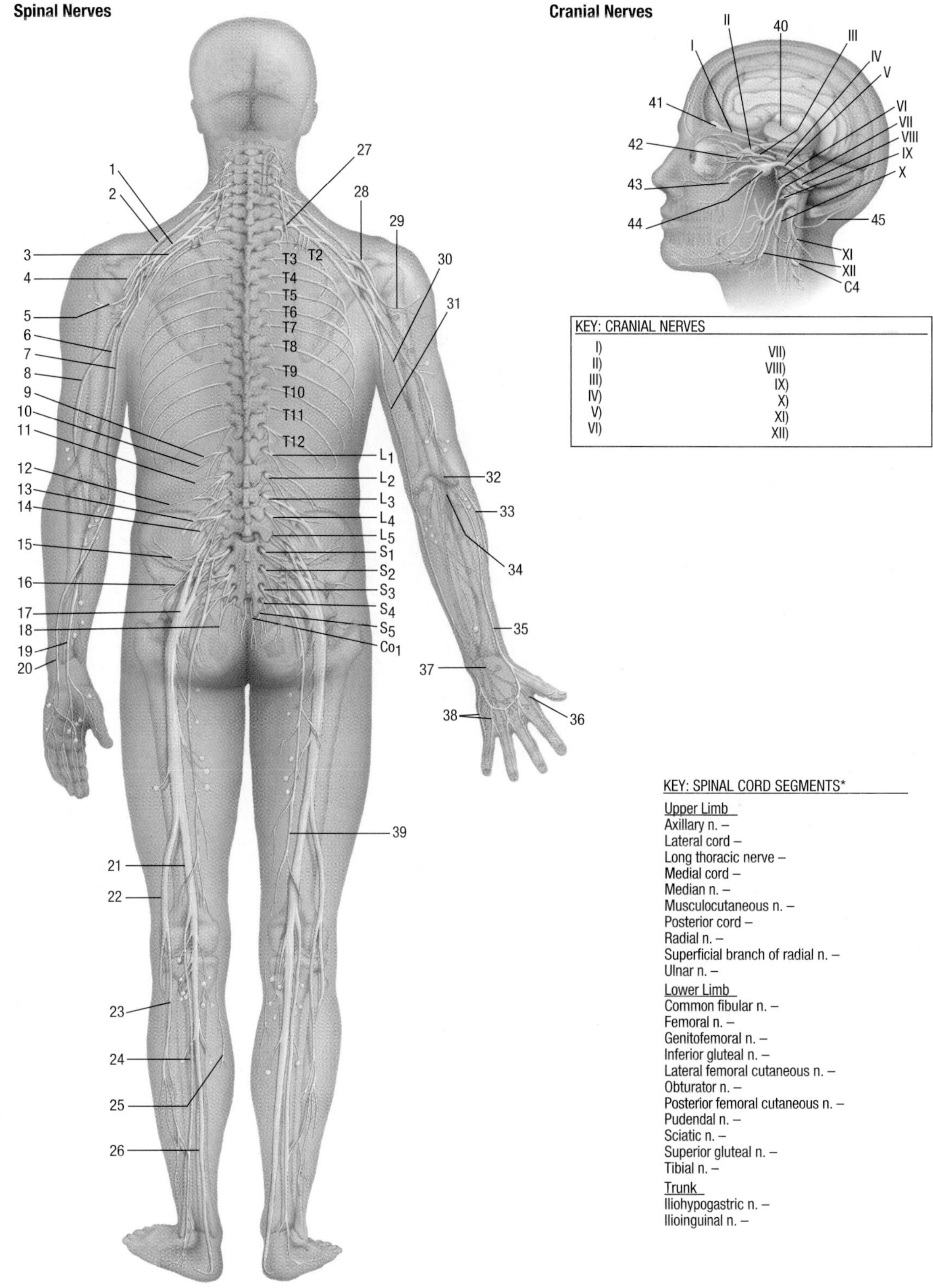
Spinal Nerves
Cranial Nerves
1
2
3
4
5
6
7
8
9
10
11
12
13
14
15
16
17
18
19
20
21
22
23
24
25
26
27
28
29
30
31
32
33
34
35
36
37
38
39
40
41
42
43
44
45
T2
T3
T4
T5
T6
T7
T8
T9
T10
T11
T12
L_1
L_2
L_3
L_4
L_5
S_1
S_2
S_3
S_4
S_5
Co_1
I
II
III
IV
V
VI
VII
VIII
IX
X
XI
XII
C4
KEY: CRANIAL NERVES
I)
II)
III)
IV)
V)
VI)
VII)
VIII)
IX)
X)
XI)
XII)
KEY: SPINAL CORD SEGMENTS*
Upper Limb
Axillary n. –
Lateral cord –
Long thoracic nerve –
Medial cord –
Median n. –
Musculocutaneous n. –
Posterior cord –
Radial n. –
Superficial branch of radial n. –
Ulnar n. –
Lower Limb
Common fibular n. –
Femoral n. –
Genitofemoral n. –
Inferior gluteal n. –
Lateral femoral cutaneous n. –
Obturator n. –
Posterior femoral cutaneous n. –
Pudendal n. –
Sciatic n. –
Superior gluteal n. –
Tibial n. –
Trunk
Iliohypogastric n. –
Ilioinguinal n. –

The Brain

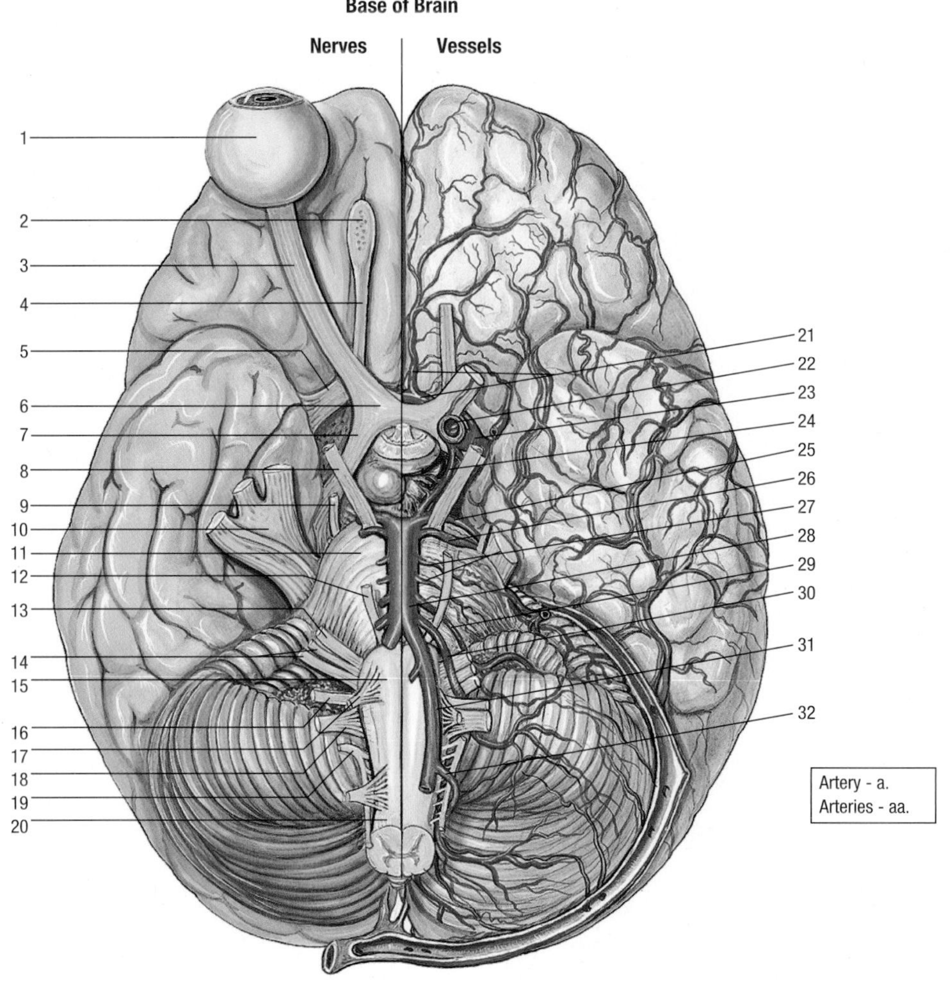
Base of Brain
Nerves
Vessels
1
2
3
4
5
6
7
8
9
10
11
12
13
14
15
16
17
18
19
20
21
22
23
24
25
26
27
28
29
30
31
32
Artery - a.
Arteries - aa.

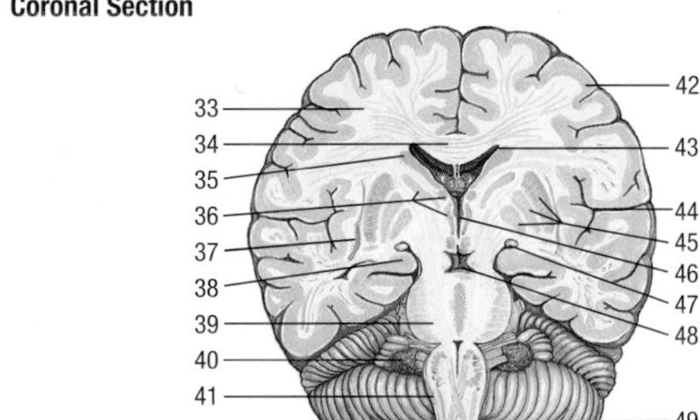
Coronal Section
33
34
35
36
37
38
39
40
41
42
43
44
45
46
47
48
49

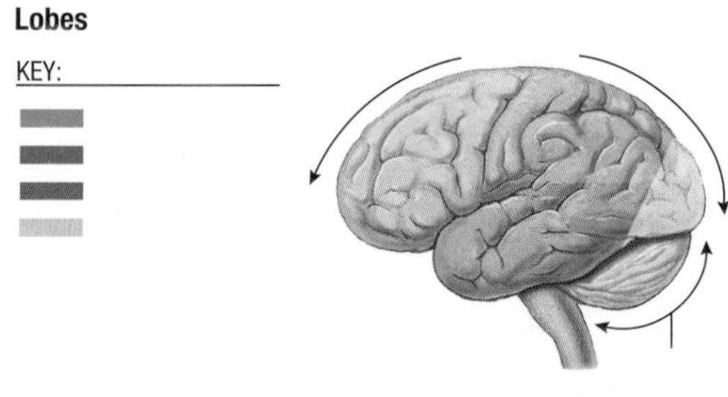
Lobes
KEY:

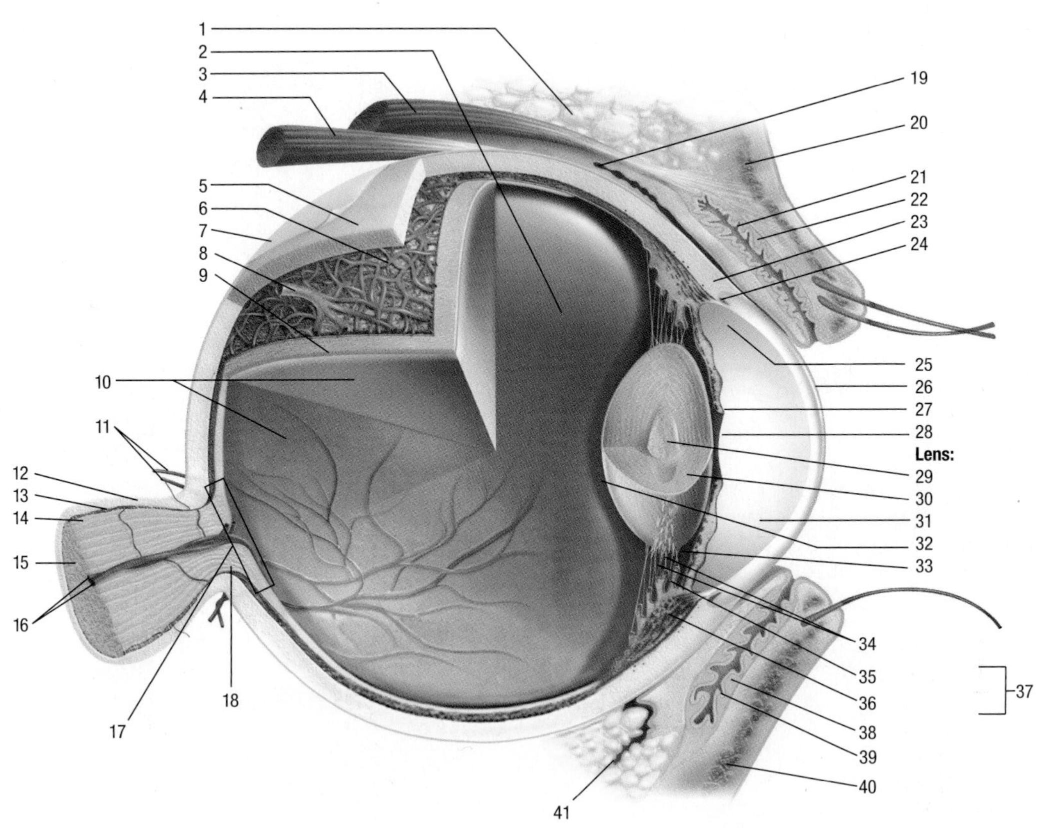

Lacrimal Gland:

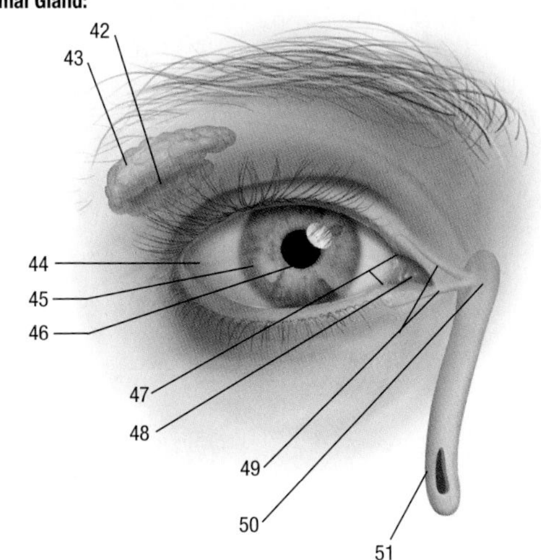

Eye Muscles Superior View

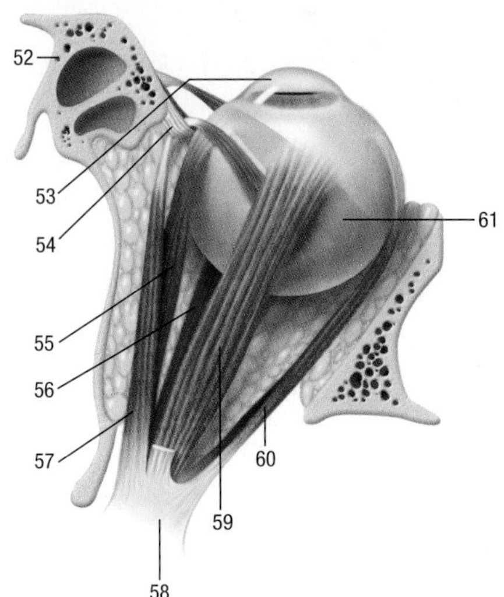

The Ear

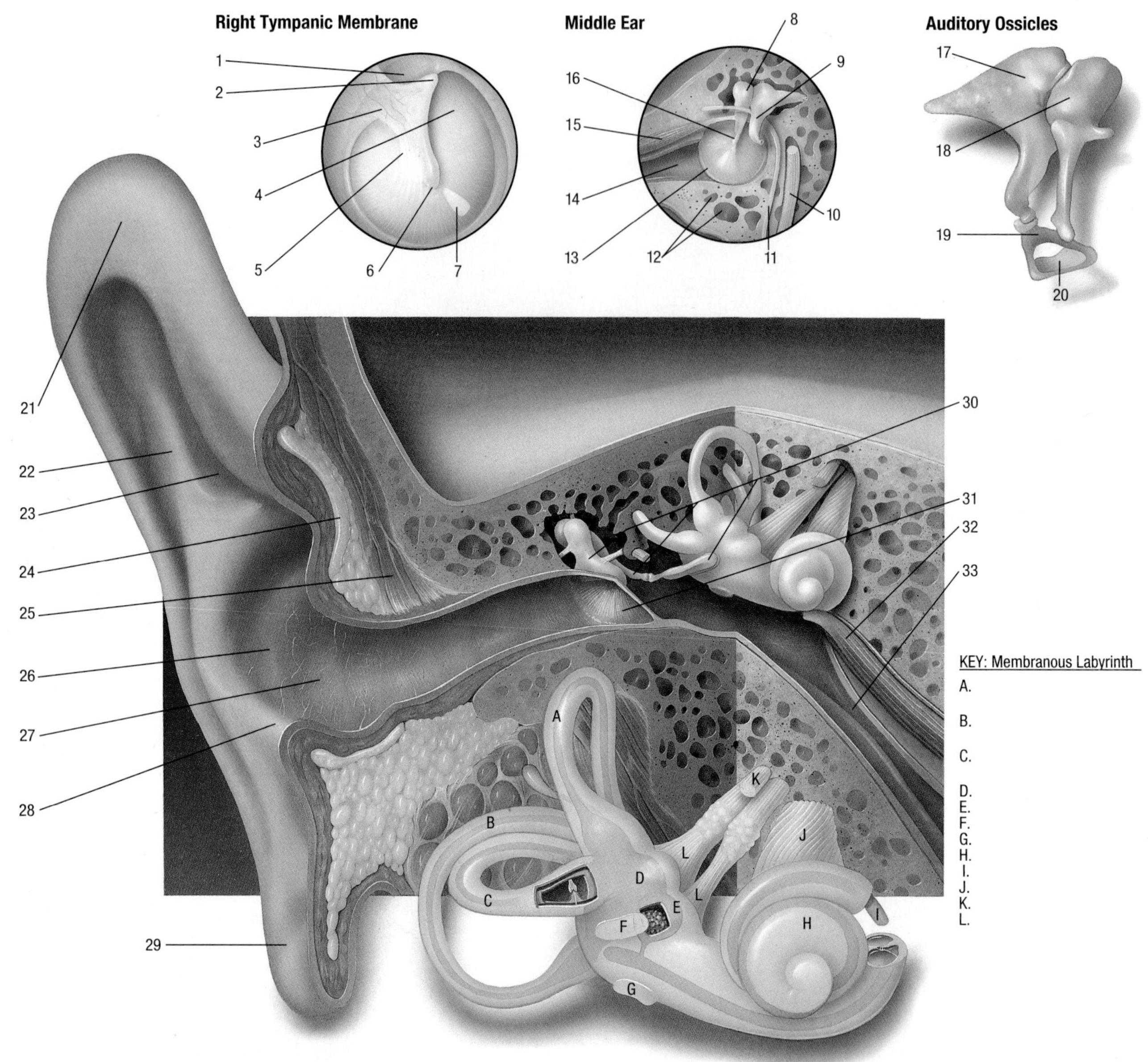

KEY: Membranous Labyrinth

A.

B.

C.

D.
E.
F.
G.
H.
I.
J.
K.
L.

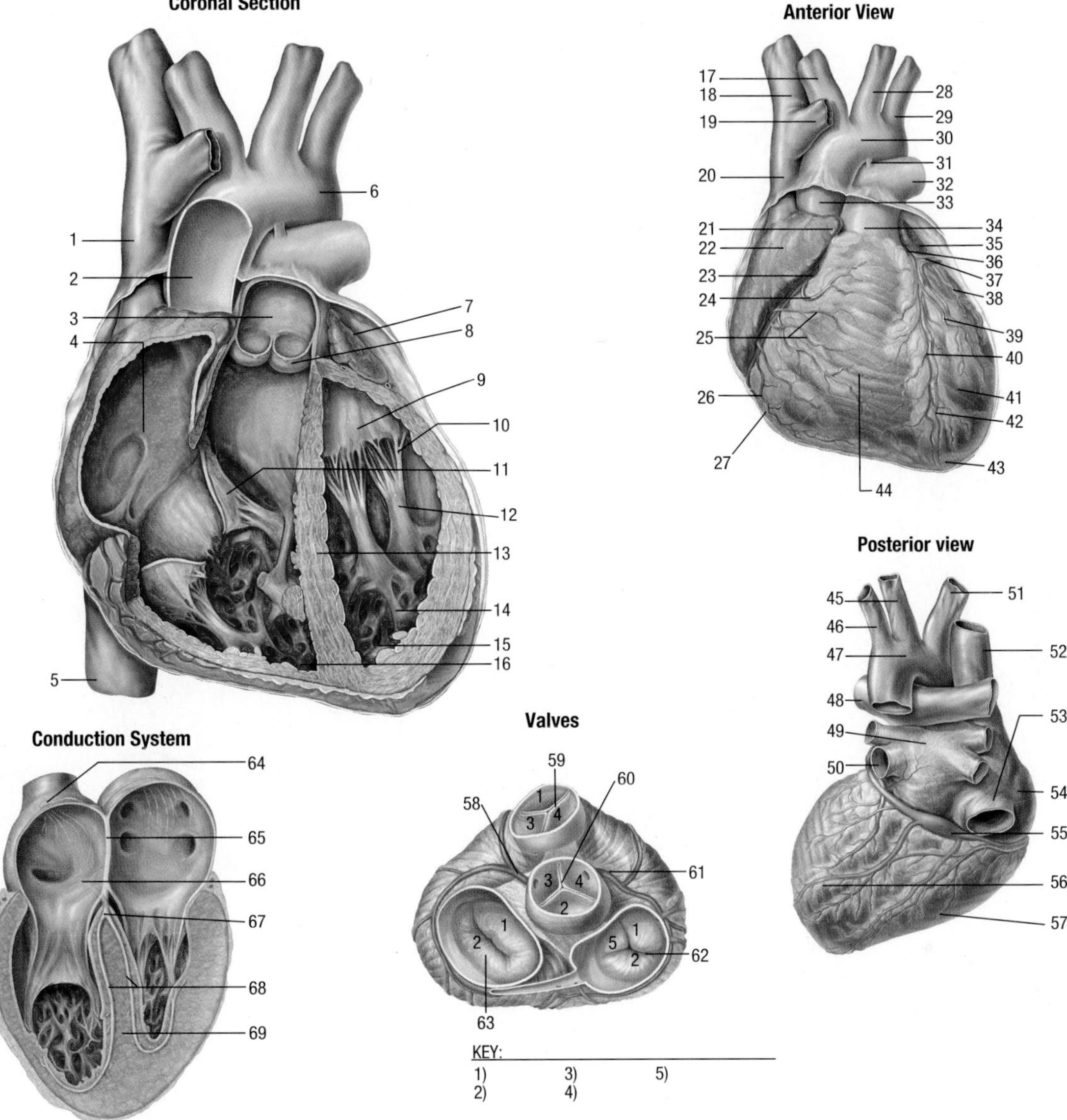
Coronal Section
1
2
3
4
5
6
7
8
9
10
11
12
13
14
15
16
Anterior View
17
18
19
20
21
22
23
24
25
26
27
28
29
30
31
32
33
34
35
36
37
38
39
40
41
42
43
44
Posterior view
45
46
47
48
49
50
51
52
53
54
55
56
57
Conduction System
64
65
66
67
68
69
Valves
58
59
60
61
62
63
KEY:
1)
2)
3)
4)
5)

The Arteries

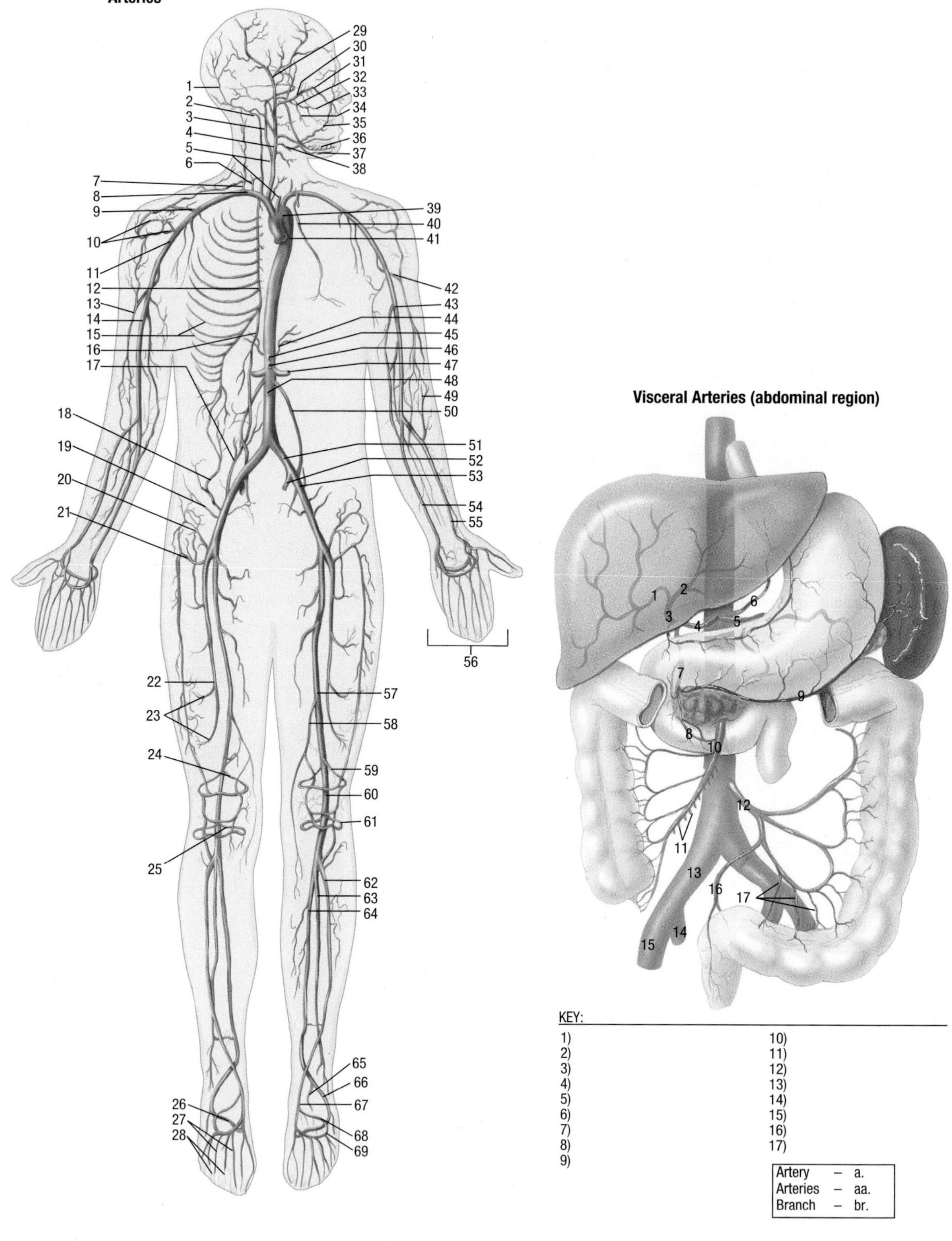

KEY:

1)
2)
3)
4)
5)
6)
7)
8)
9)
10)
11)
12)
13)
14)
15)
16)
17)

Artery	–	a.
Arteries	–	aa.
Branch	–	br.

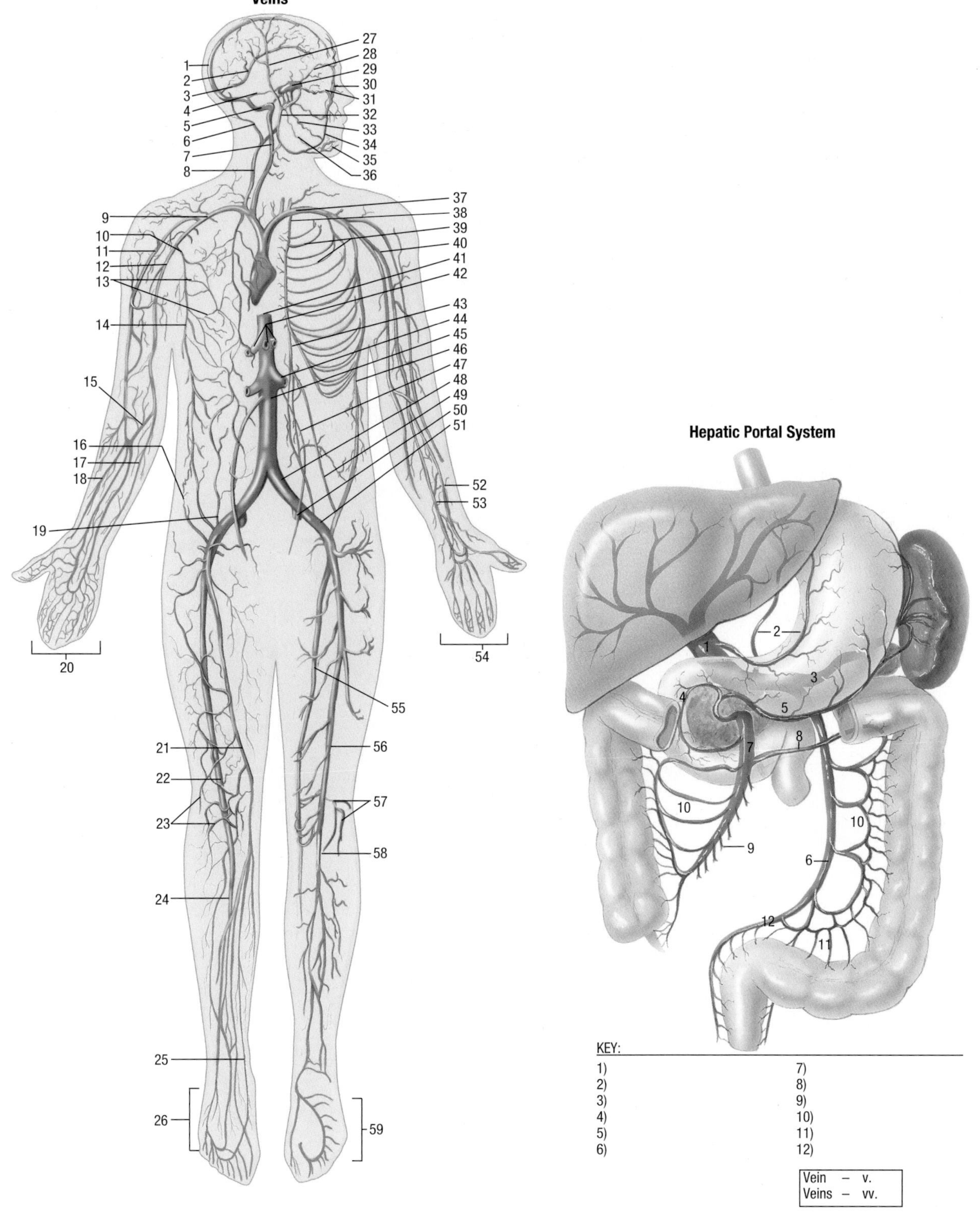

KEY:

1)
2)
3)
4)
5)
6)
7)
8)
9)
10)
11)
12)

Vein – v.
Veins – vv.

The Respiratory System

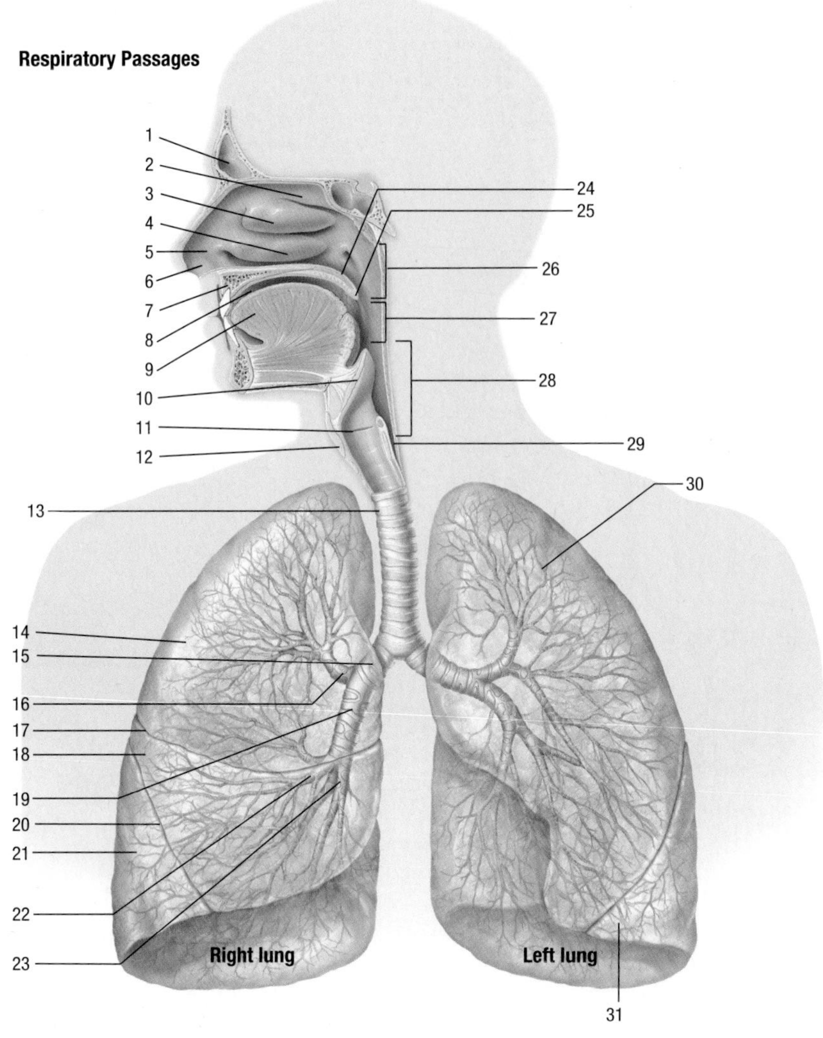

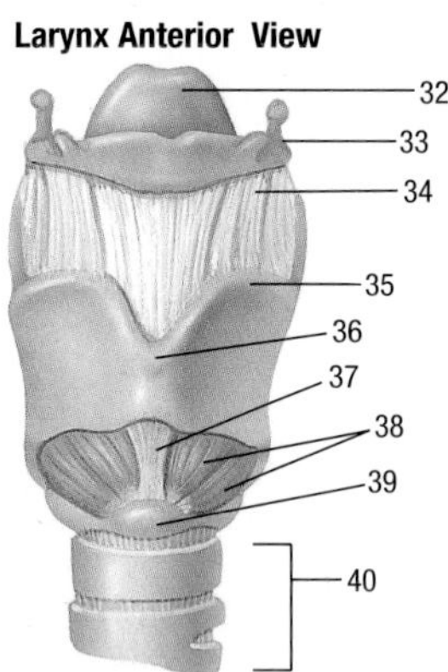

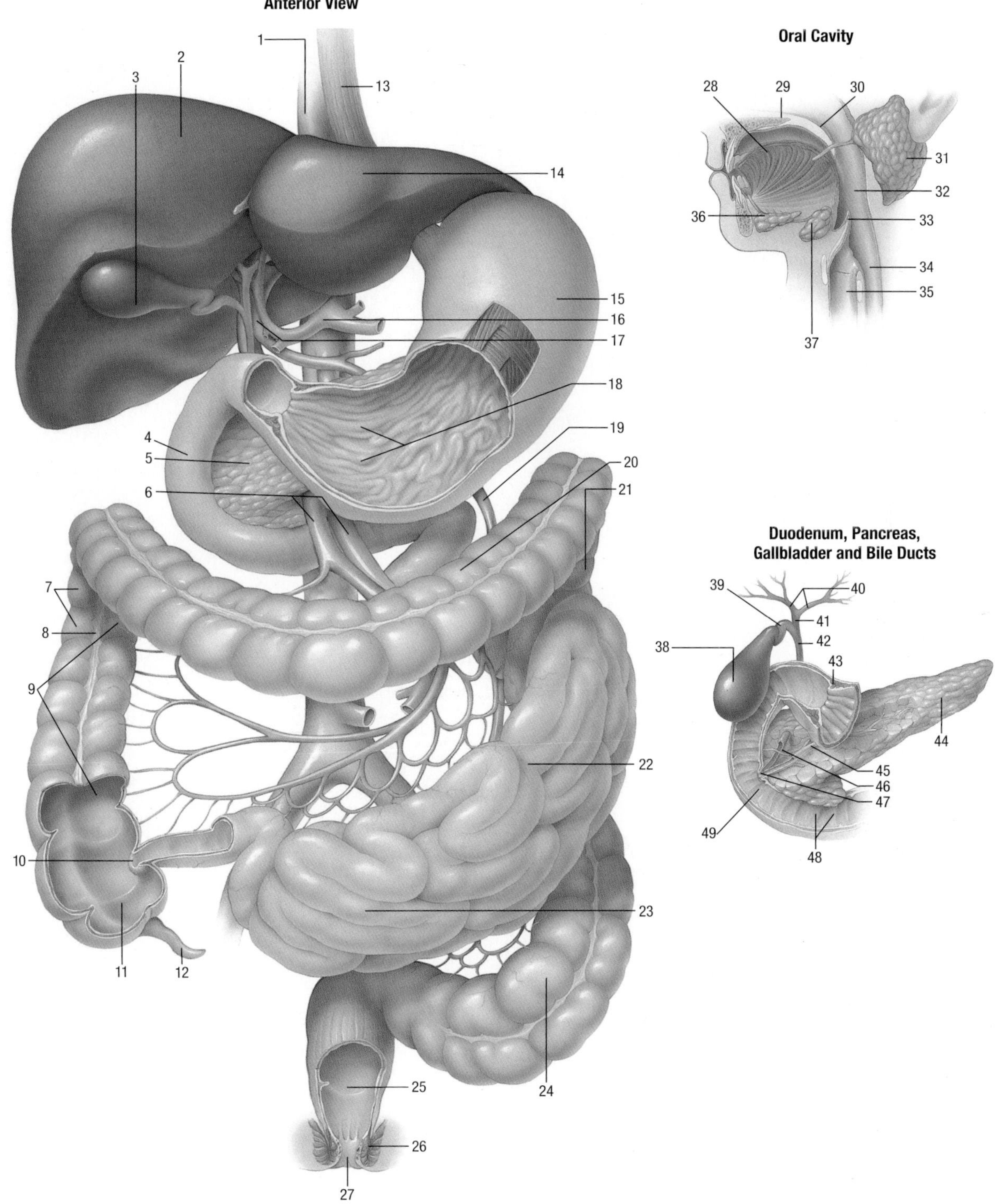
Anterior View
1
2
3
4
5
6
7
8
9
10
11
12
13
14
15
16
17
18
19
20
21
22
23
24
25
26
27
Oral Cavity
28
29
30
31
32
33
34
35
36
37
Duodenum, Pancreas,
Gallbladder and Bile Ducts
38
39
40
41
42
43
44
45
46
47
48
49

The Urinary System

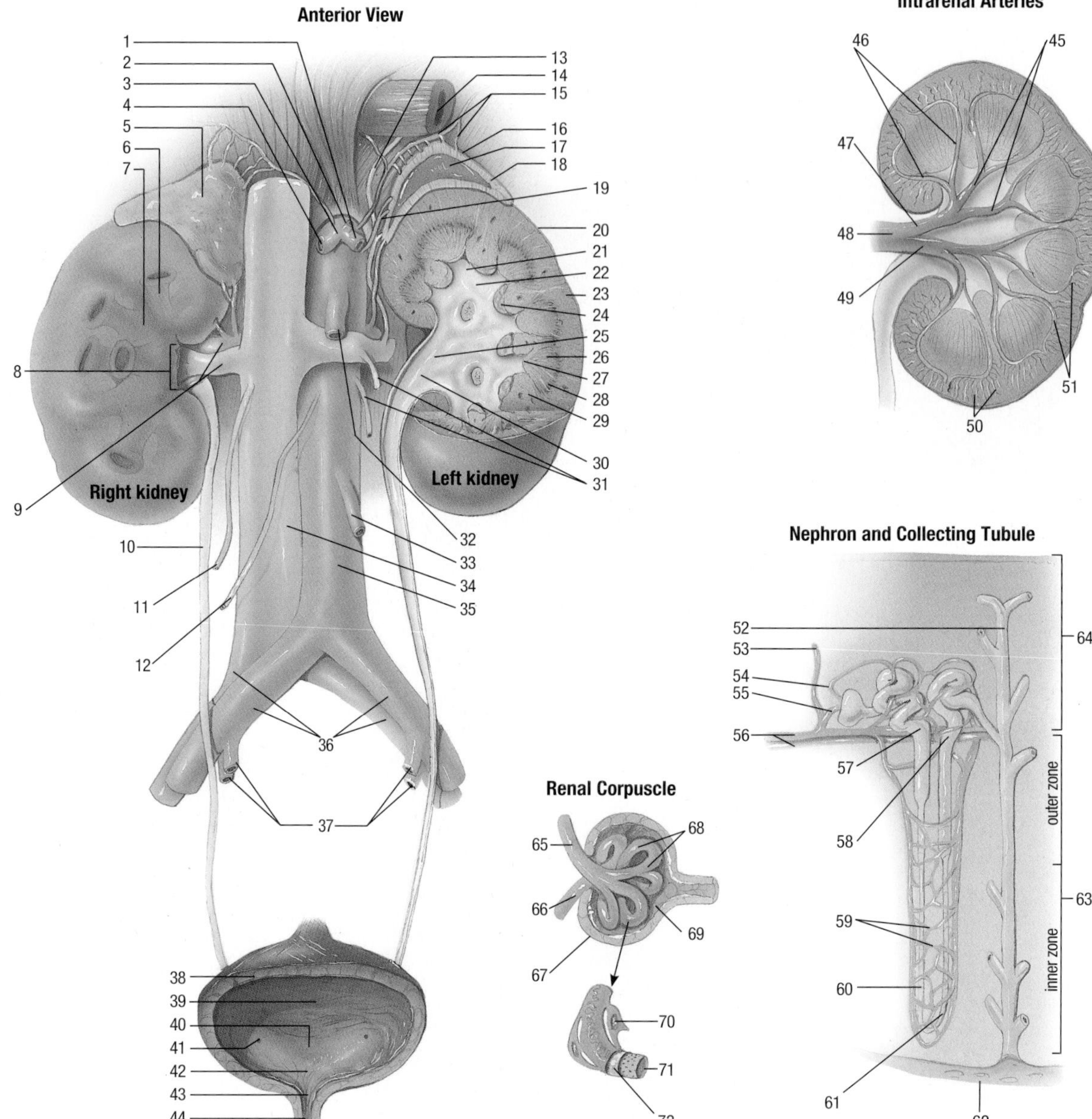

Pelvic Organs (median section)

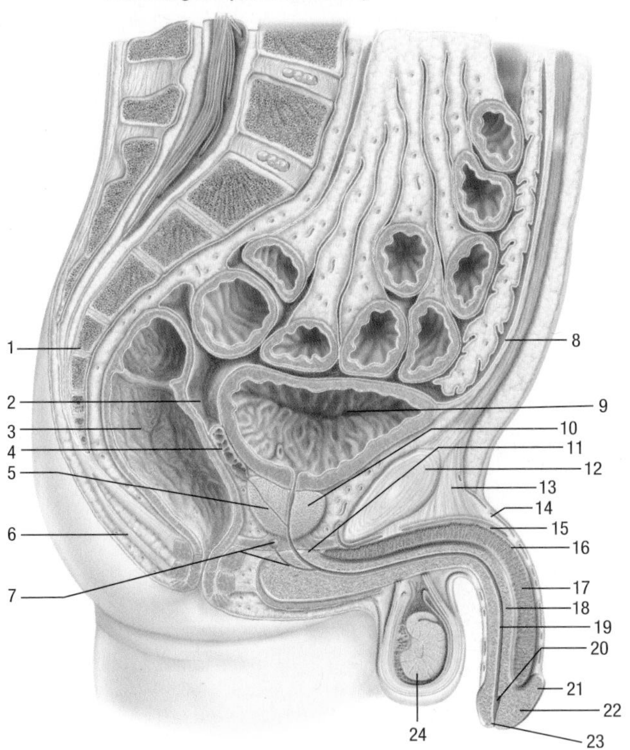

Anterior View (oblique section)

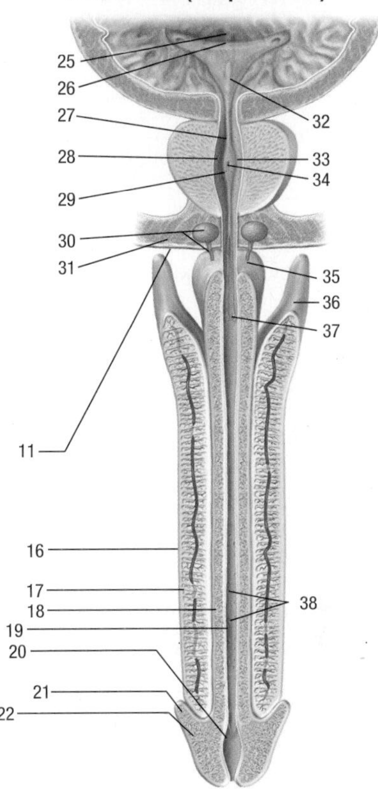

The Female Reproductive System

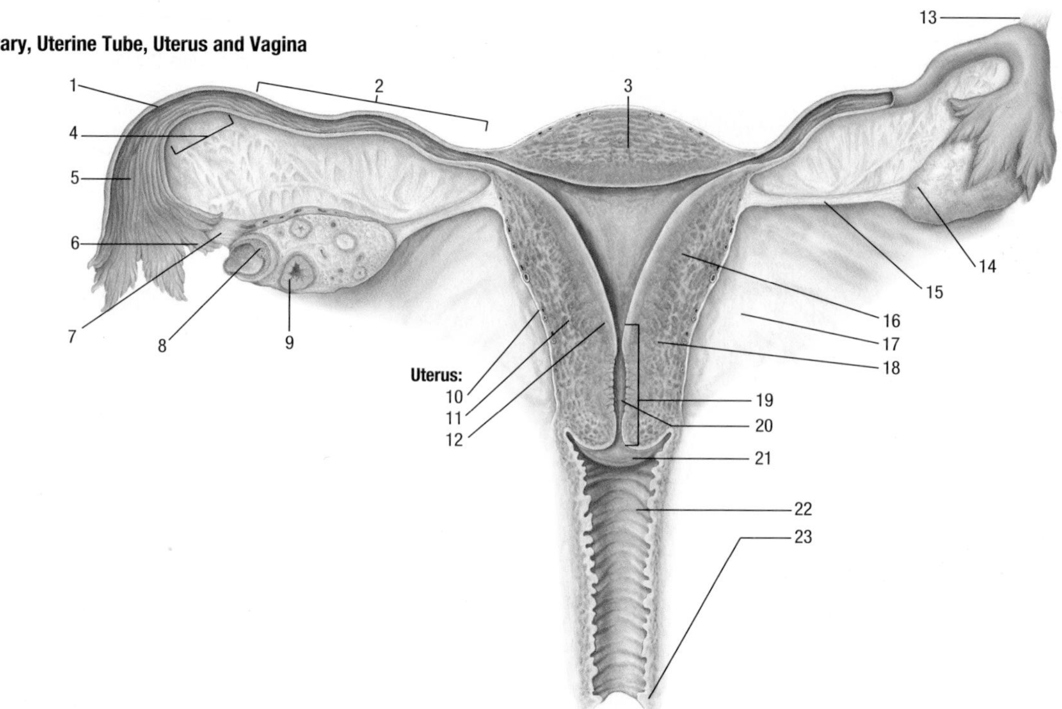

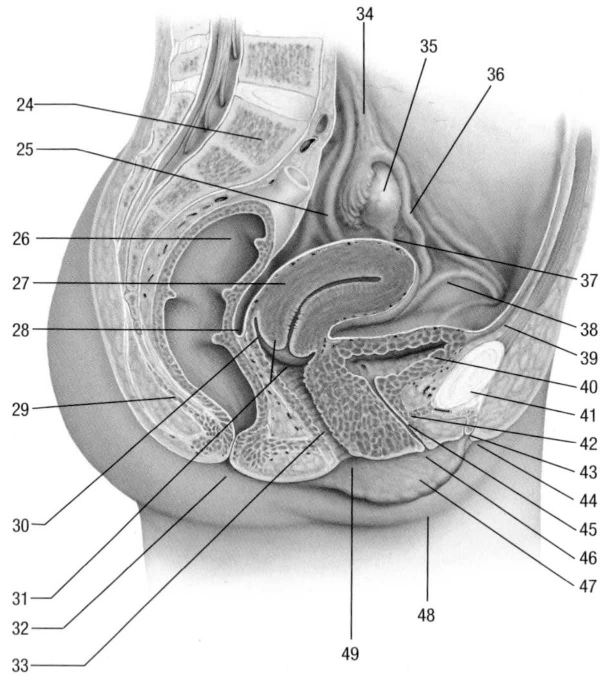

UNIT I

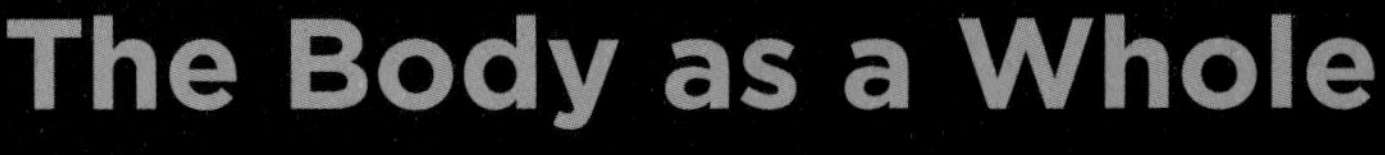

The Body as a Whole

This unit presents the basic levels of organization within the human body. Included is a description of the smallest units of life called cells. Similar cells are grouped together as tissues, which are combined to form organs. Organs, in turn, work together in the various body systems, which together satisfy the needs of the entire organism. A short survey of chemistry, which deals with the composition of all matter and is important for the understanding of human physiology, is incorporated into this unit. The final chapter in the unit illustrates some of these basic principles with a study of the skin and its associated structures.

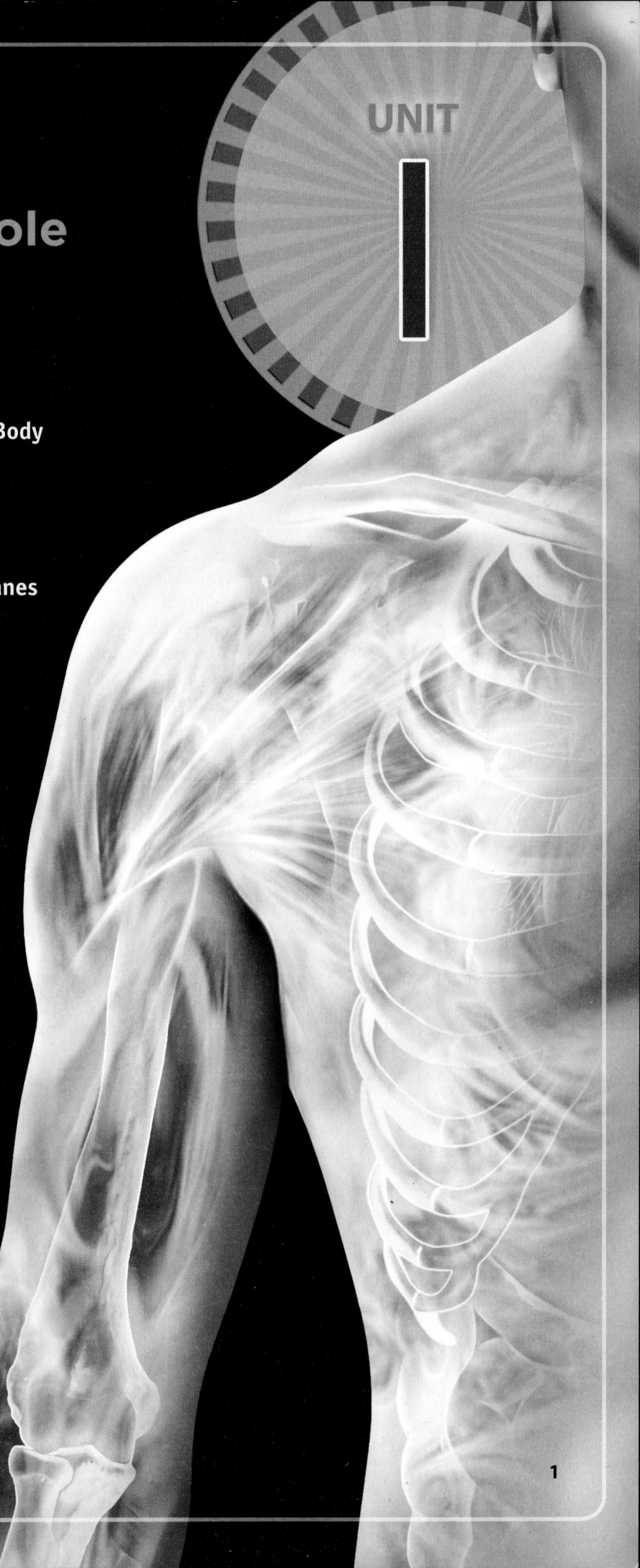

CHAPTER

Organization of the Human Body

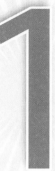

A&P in Action

Mike's Case: Emergency Care and Homeostatic Imbalance

"Location—Belle Grove Road. Single MVA. Male. Early 20s. Fire and police on scene," crackled the radio. "Medic 12. Respond channel 2."

"Medic 12 responding. En route to Belle Grove Road," Ed radioed back, while his partner, Samantha, flipped the switch for the lights and siren and hit the accelerator. When they arrived at the scene, police officers were directing traffic and a fire crew was at work on the vehicle. Samantha parked the ambulance just as the crew breached the door of the crumpled minivan. Samantha and Ed grabbed their trauma bags and approached the wreck.

Ed bent down toward the injured man. "I hear your name is Mike. Mine is Ed. I'm a paramedic. My partner and I are going to take a quick look at you and then get you out of here."

Samantha inspected the vehicle. "Looks like the impact sent him up and over the steering wheel. Guessing from the cracked windshield, he may have a head injury. The steering column is bent, so I wouldn't rule out thorax or abdomen either."

Ed agreed. "He's got forehead lacerations and he's disoriented. Chest seems fine, but his abdominal cavity could be a problem. There is significant bruising across the left lumbar and umbilical regions—probably from the steering wheel. When I palpated his left upper quadrant, it caused him considerable pain."

Samantha and Ed carefully immobilized Mike's cervical spine and, with the help of the fire crew, transferred him to a stretcher. Samantha started a saline IV while Ed performed a detailed physical examination beginning at the head and working inferiorly. Mike's blood pressure was very low and his heart rate was very high—both signs of a cardiovascular emergency. In addition, he had become unresponsive to questions.

Ed shared his findings with Samantha while she placed an oxygen mask on Mike's nose and mouth. "He's hypotensive and tachycardic. With the pain he reported earlier, signs are pointing to intraabdominal hemorrhage. We've got to get him to the trauma center right now."

Ed depends on his understanding of anatomy and physiology to help his patient and communicate with his partner. He suspects that Mike is bleeding internally and that his heart is working hard to compensate for the drastic decrease in blood pressure. As we will see later, Mike's state of internal balance, known as homeostasis, must be restored, or his body systems will fail.

PASSport to Success

Ancillaries *At-A-Glance*

Visit *thePoint* to access the PASSport to Success and the following resources. For guidance in using these resources most effectively, see pp. ix–xviii.

Learning TOOLS

- Learning Style Self-Assessment
- Live Advise Online Student Tutoring
- Tips for Effective Studying

Learning RESOURCES

- E-book: Chapter 1
- Web Figure: Abdominal Regions
- Web Figure: Abdominal Quadrants
- Web Chart: Body Systems and Their Functions
- Web Chart: Directional Terms
- Web Chart: The Metric System
- Animation: Negative Feedback
- Health Professions: Health Information Technician
- Detailed Chapter Outline
- Answers to Questions for Study and Review
- Audio Pronunciation Glossary

Learning ACTIVITIES

- Pre-Quiz
- Visual Activities
- Kinesthetic Activities
- Auditory Activities

Learning Outcomes

After careful study of this chapter, you should be able to:

1. Define the terms *anatomy* and *physiology*, ***p. 4***
2. Describe the organization of the body from chemicals to the whole organism, ***p. 4***
3. List 11 body systems and give the general function of each, ***p. 4***
4. Define *metabolism* and name the two types of metabolic reactions, ***p. 5***
5. Define and give examples of homeostasis, ***p. 6***
6. Explain how negative feedback maintains homeostasis, ***p. 6***
7. List and define the main directional terms for the body, ***p. 7***
8. List and define the three planes of division of the body, ***p. 8***
9. Name the subdivisions of the dorsal and ventral cavities, ***p. 10***
10. Name and locate the subdivisions of the abdomen, ***p. 10***
11. Cite some anterior and posterior body regions along with their common names, ***p. 13***
12. Find examples of anatomic and physiologic terms in a case study, ***pp. 2, 14***
13. Show how word parts are used to build words related to the body's organization (see Word Anatomy at the end of the chapter), ***p. 16***

Studies of the body's normal structure and functions are the basis for all medical sciences. It is only from understanding the normal that we can analyze what is going wrong in cases of disease. These studies give us an appreciation for the design and balance of the human body and for living organisms in general.

Studies of the Human Body

The scientific term for the study of body structure is **anatomy** (ah-NAT-o-me). The *-tomy* part of this word in Latin means "cutting," because a fundamental way to learn about the human body is to cut it apart, or **dissect** (dis-sekt) it. **Physiology** (fiz-e-OL-o-je) is the term for the study of how the body functions; *physio* is based on a Latin term meaning "nature" and *logy* means "study of." Anatomy and physiology are closely related—that is, structure and function are intertwined. The stomach, for example, has a pouch-like shape for storing food during digestion. The cells in the lining of the stomach are tightly packed to prevent strong digestive juices from harming underlying tissue.

LEVELS OF ORGANIZATION

All living things are organized from very simple levels to more complex levels (**Fig. 1-1**). Living matter is derived from simple chemicals. These chemicals are formed into the complex substances that make living **cells**—the basic units of all life. Specialized groups of cells form **tissues**, and tissues may function together as **organs**. Organs working together for the same general purpose make up the body **systems**. All of the systems work together to maintain the body as a whole organism.

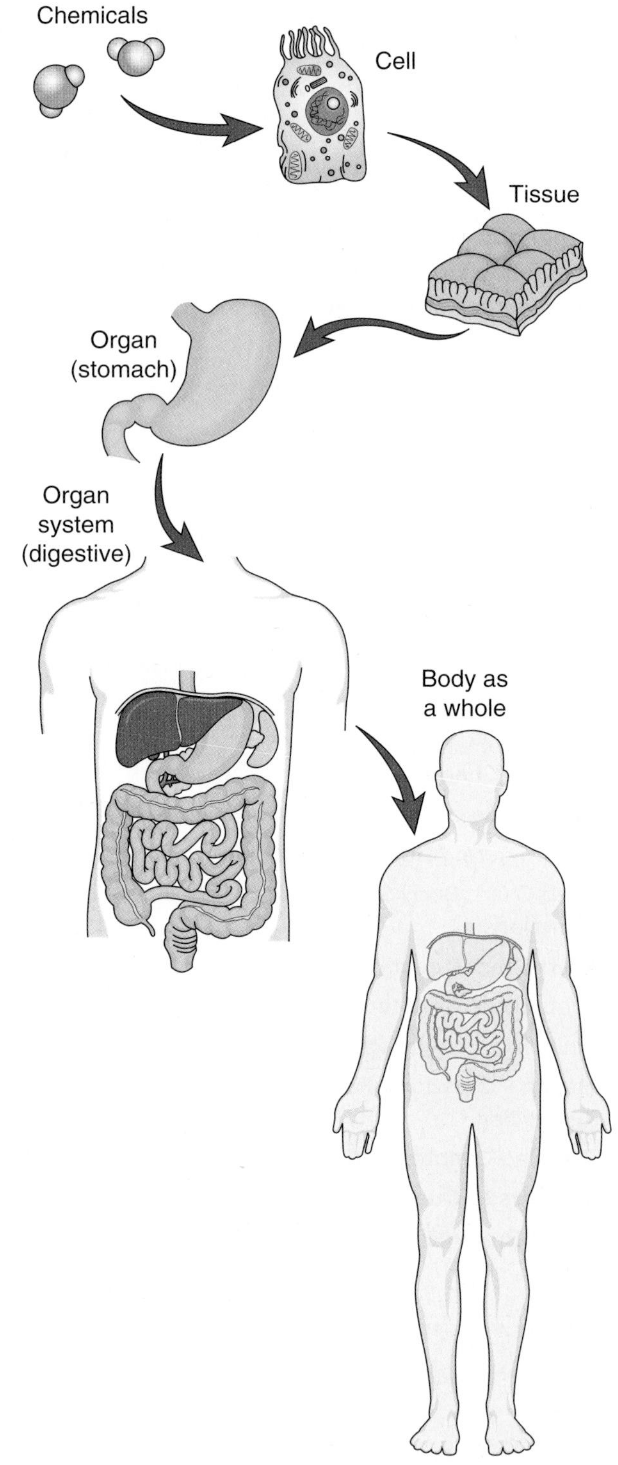

Figure 1-1 **Levels of organization.** KEY POINT The body is organized from the level of simple chemicals by increasing levels of complexity to the whole organism. The organ shown here is the stomach, which is part of the digestive system.

BODY SYSTEMS

We can think of the human body as organized according to the individual systems, as listed below, grouped according to their general functions.

- Protection, support, and movement
  - The **integumentary** (in-teg-u-MEN-tar-e) **system.** The word ***integument*** (in-TEG-u-ment) means "skin." The skin with its associated structures is considered a separate body system. The skin's associated structures include the hair, nails, sweat glands, and oil glands.
  - The **skeletal system.** The body's basic framework is a system of 206 bones and the joints between them, collectively known as the **skeleton.**
  - The **muscular system.** The muscles in this system are attached to the bones and produce movement of the skeleton. These skeletal muscles also give the body structure, protect organs, and maintain posture. The two other muscle types are smooth muscle, present in the walls of body organs, such as the stomach and intestine, and cardiac muscle, which makes up the wall of the heart.

- Coordination and control
  - > The **nervous system**. The brain, spinal cord, and nerves make up this complex system by which the body is controlled and coordinated. The nervous system also includes the special sense organs (the eyes, ears, taste buds, and organs of smell) and the receptors of the general senses, such as pain and touch. When sense organs or receptors detect changes in the external and internal environments, electrical signals are transmitted along nerves to the brain, which directs responses.
  - > The **endocrine** (EN-do-krin) **system**. The scattered organs known as endocrine glands are grouped together because they share a similar function. All produce special substances called hormones, which regulate such body activities as growth, nutrient utilization, and reproduction. Examples of endocrine glands are the thyroid, pituitary, and adrenal glands.
- Circulation and immunity
  - > The **cardiovascular system**. The heart and blood vessels make up the system that pumps blood to all body tissues, bringing with it nutrients, oxygen, and other needed substances. This system then carries waste materials away from the tissues to points where they can be eliminated.
  - > The **lymphatic system**. Lymphatic vessels assist in circulation by returning fluids from the tissues to the blood. Lymphatic organs, such as the tonsils, thymus gland, and spleen, play a role in immunity, protecting against disease. The lymphatic system also aids in the absorption of dietary fats. The fluid that circulates in the lymphatic system is called *lymph*.
- Energy supply and fluid balance
  - > The **respiratory system**. This system includes the lungs and the passages leading to and from the lungs. This system takes in air and conducts it to the areas in the lungs designed for gas exchange. Oxygen passes from the air into the blood and is carried to all tissues by the cardiovascular system. In like manner, carbon dioxide, a gaseous waste product, is taken by the circulation from the tissues back to the lungs to be expelled through the respiratory passages.
  - > The **digestive system**. This system is composed of all the organs that are involved with taking in nutrients (foods), converting them into a form that body cells can use, and absorbing them into the circulation. Organs of the digestive system include the mouth, esophagus, stomach, small and large intestine, liver, gallbladder, and pancreas.
  - > The **urinary system**. The chief purpose of the urinary system is to rid the body of waste products and excess water. This system's main components are the kidneys, the ureters, the bladder, and the urethra. (Note that some waste products are also eliminated by the digestive and respiratory systems and by the skin.)
- Production of offspring
  - > The **reproductive system**. This system includes the external sex organs and all related internal structures that are concerned with the production of offspring.

References may vary in the number of body systems cited. For example, some separate the sensory system from the nervous system. Others have a separate entry for the immune system, which protects the body from foreign matter and invading organisms. The immune system is identified by its function rather than its structure and includes elements of both the cardiovascular and lymphatic systems. Bear in mind that, even though you will study the systems as separate units, they are interrelated and must cooperate to maintain health.

CHECKPOINTS 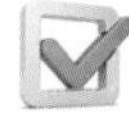

1-1 What are the studies of body structure and body function called?

1-2 What do organs working together combine to form?

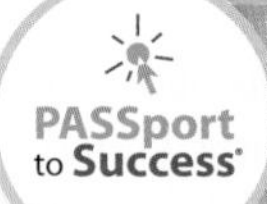

See the Student Resources on *thePoint* for a chart summarizing the body systems and their functions.

Metabolism and Its Regulation

All the life-sustaining reactions that occur within the body systems together make up **metabolism** (meh-TAB-o-lizm). Metabolism can be divided into two types of activities:

- In **catabolism** (kah-TAB-o-lizm), complex substances are broken down into simpler compounds **(Fig. 1-2)**. The breakdown of food, for example, yields simple chemical building blocks and energy to power cellular activities.
- In **anabolism** (ah-NAB-o-lizm), simple compounds are used to manufacture materials needed for growth, function, and tissue repair. Anabolism consists of building, or synthesis, reactions.
- The energy obtained from the breakdown of nutrients is used to form a compound often described as the cell's "energy currency." It has the long name of **adenosine triphosphate** (ah-DEN-o-sene tri-FOS-fate) but is commonly abbreviated ATP. Chapter 2 (see Figure 2-12)

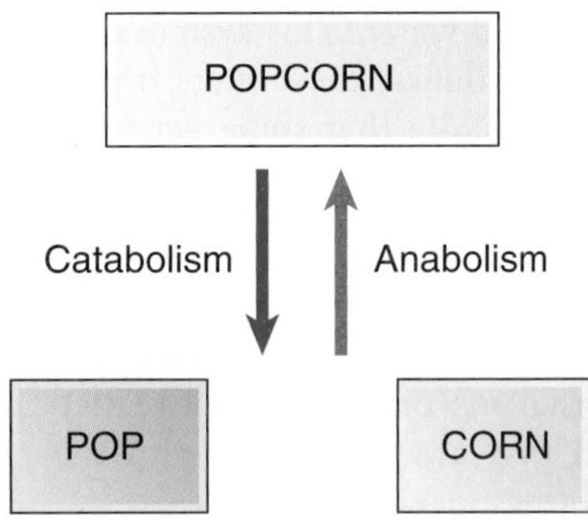

Figure 1-2 Metabolism. KEY POINT Metabolism includes two types of reactions. In catabolism, substances are broken down into their building blocks. In anabolism, simple components are built into more complex substances. We use the breakdown and building of a simple word here as an example of these reactions.

and Chapter 18 have more information on metabolism and ATP.

HOMEOSTASIS

Normal body function maintains a state of internal balance, an important characteristic of all living things. Such conditions as body temperature, the composition of body fluids, heart rate, respiration rate, and blood pressure must remain within a somewhat narrow range if we are to stay healthy. This steady state within the organism is called **homeostasis** (ho-me-o-STA-sis), which literally means "staying (stasis) the same (homeo)." Mike's case study illustrates the dangers of homeostatic imbalance.

Body Fluids Our bodies are composed of large amounts of fluids. The volume and composition of these fluids must be kept in homeostatic balance at all times. One type of fluid bathes the cells, carries nutrients to and from the cells, and transports nutrients into and out of the cells. This type is called **extracellular fluid** because it includes all body fluids outside the cells (the prefix *extra-* means "outside"). Examples of extracellular fluids are the blood plasma (the fluid portion of blood), lymph, and the fluid between the cells in tissues. A second type of fluid, **intracellular fluid**, is contained within the cells (the prefix *intra-* means "within"). Body fluids are discussed in more detail in Chapter 19.

Negative Feedback The main method for maintaining homeostasis is **negative feedback**, a control system based on information returning to a source. We are all accustomed to getting feedback about the results of our actions and using that information to regulate our behavior. Grades on tests and assignments, for example, may inspire us to work harder if they're not so great or "keep up the good work" if they are good.

Negative feedback systems keep body conditions within a set normal range by reversing any upward or downward shift. Note that negative feedback doesn't always mean less response; it just means an opposite response to a stimulus. A familiar example of negative feedback is the thermostat in a house (Fig. 1-3). When the house temperature falls, the thermostat triggers the furnace to turn on and increase the temperature; when the house temperature reaches an upper limit, the furnace is shut off. In the body, a brain center detects changes in temperature and starts mechanisms for cooling or warming if the temperature deviates too far above or below the average set point of 37°C (98.6°F) (Fig. 1-4).

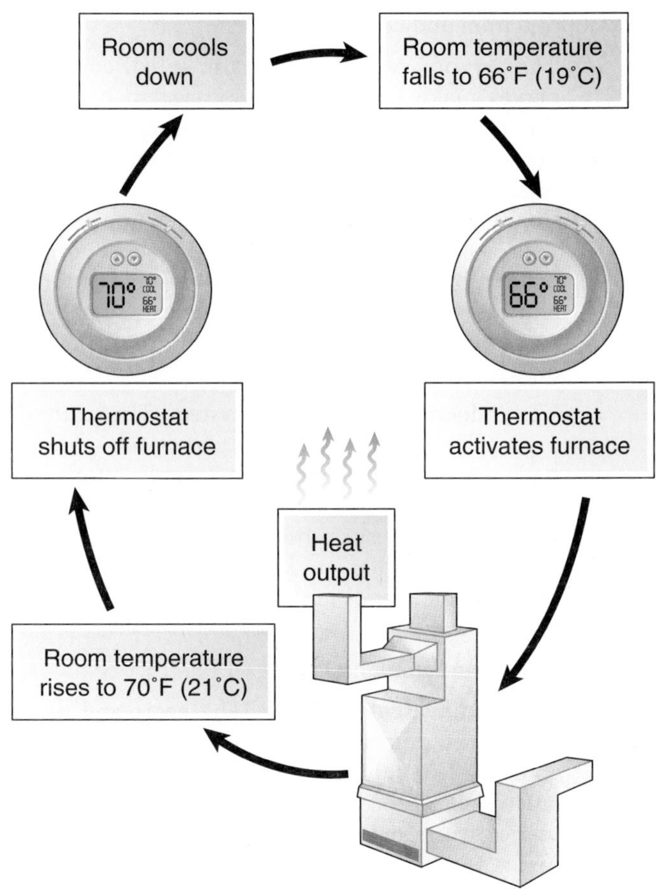

Figure 1-3 Negative feedback. KEY POINT A home thermostat illustrates how negative feedback keeps temperature within a set range. This thermostat is set to keep the average temperature at 68°F.

As another example, let's say you've just finished eating breakfast—a bowl of cereal and a glass of orange juice. As a result, the level of glucose (a simple sugar) increases in your bloodstream. This increase prompts endocrine cells in your pancreas to secrete insulin, a hormone that causes body cells to use more glucose. Increased glucose uptake and the subsequent drop in the blood glucose level signal the pancreas to reduce insulin secretion (Fig. 1-5). As a result of insulin's action, the secretion of insulin is inhibited. This type of self-regulating feedback loop is used in the endocrine system to maintain proper hormone levels,

1

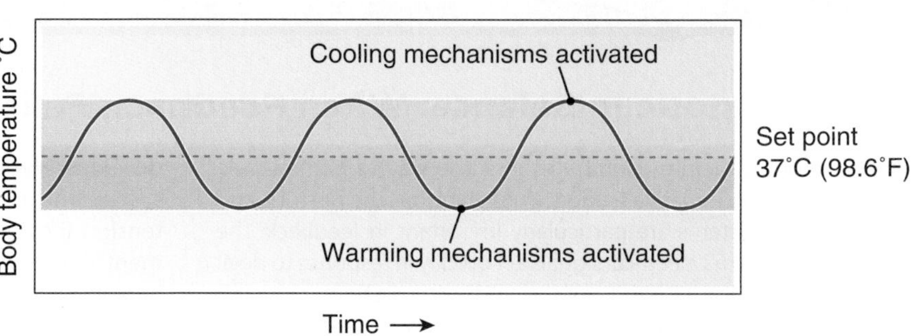

Figure 1-4 Negative feedback and body temperature. KEY POINT Body temperature is kept within a narrow range by negative feedback acting on a center in the brain. The set point is 37°C.

as described in Chapter 11. Many more examples of internal regulation by negative feedback will appear throughout this book. Clearly, negative feedback systems are critical for maintaining our health **(see Box 1-1)**.

PASSport to Success® See the Student Resources on *thePoint* to view an animation on negative feedback.

THE EFFECTS OF AGING

With age, changes occur gradually in all body systems. Some of these changes, such as wrinkles and gray hair, are obvious. Others, such as decreased kidney function, loss of bone mass, and formation of deposits within blood vessels, are not visible. However, they may make a person more subject to injury and disease. Changes due to aging are described in chapters on the body systems.

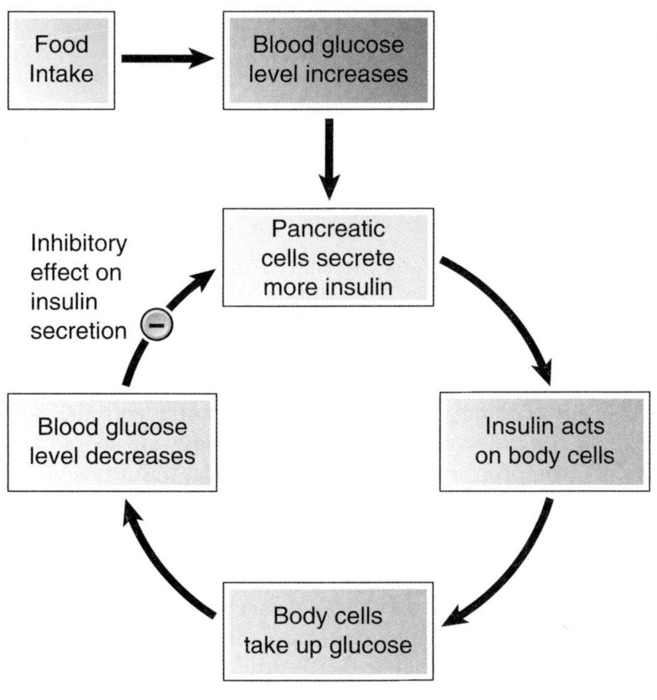

Figure 1-5 Negative feedback in the endocrine system. KEY POINT Glucose intake and use regulate insulin production by means of negative feedback.

CHECKPOINTS 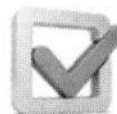

☐ **1-3** What are the two types of metabolic reactions and what happens during each?

☐ **1-4** Compare the locations of extracellular and intracellular fluids.

☐ **1-5** What is the main method used to maintain homeostasis?

Body Directions

Because it would be awkward and inaccurate to speak of bandaging the "southwest part" of the chest, for example, a number of terms are used universally to designate body positions and directions. For consistency, all descriptions assume that the body is in the **anatomic position**. In this posture, the subject is standing upright with face front, arms at the sides with palms forward, and feet parallel, as shown in **Figure 1-6**.

DIRECTIONAL TERMS

The main terms for describing directions in the body are as follows **(see Fig. 1-6)**:

- **Superior** is a term meaning above, or in a higher position. Its opposite, **inferior**, means below, or lower. The heart, for example, is superior to the intestine.
- **Anterior** and **ventral** have the same meaning in humans: located toward the belly surface or front of the body. Their corresponding opposites, **posterior** and **dorsal**, refer to locations nearer the back.
- **Medial** means nearer to an imaginary plane that passes through the midline of the body, dividing it into left and right portions. **Lateral**, its opposite, means farther away from the midline, toward the side. For example, your nose is medial to your ears.
- **Proximal** means nearer to the origin of a structure, such as a limb, or nearer to a given reference point, such as

Box 1-1 *Clinical Perspectives*

Homeostatic Imbalance: When Feedback Fails

Each body structure contributes in some way to homeostasis, often through negative feedback mechanisms. The nervous and endocrine systems are particularly important in feedback. The nervous system's electrical signals act quickly in response to deviations from normal, whereas the endocrine system's chemical signals (hormones) act more slowly but over a longer time. Often both systems work together to maintain homeostasis.

As long as feedback keeps conditions within normal limits, the body remains healthy, but if feedback cannot maintain these conditions, the body enters a state of homeostatic imbalance. Moderate imbalance causes illness and disease, while severe imbalance causes death. At some level, all illnesses and diseases can be linked to homeostatic imbalance.

For example, feedback mechanisms closely monitor and maintain normal blood pressure. When blood pressure rises, negative feedback mechanisms lower it to normal limits. If these mechanisms fail, hypertension (high blood pressure) develops. Hypertension further damages the cardiovascular system and, if untreated, may lead to death. With mild hypertension, lifestyle changes in diet, exercise, and stress management may lower blood pressure sufficiently, whereas severe hypertension often requires drug therapy. The various types of antihypertensive medication all help negative feedback mechanisms lower blood pressure.

Feedback mechanisms also regulate body temperature. When body temperature falls, negative feedback mechanisms raise it back to normal limits, but if these mechanisms fail and body temperature continues to drop, hypothermia develops. The main effects of hypothermia are uncontrolled shivering, lack of coordination, decreased heart and respiratory rates, and, if left untreated, death. Cardiac surgeons use hypothermia to their advantage during open heart surgery. Cooling the heart reduces its need for oxygen, which allows surgeons more time to operate without damaging it.

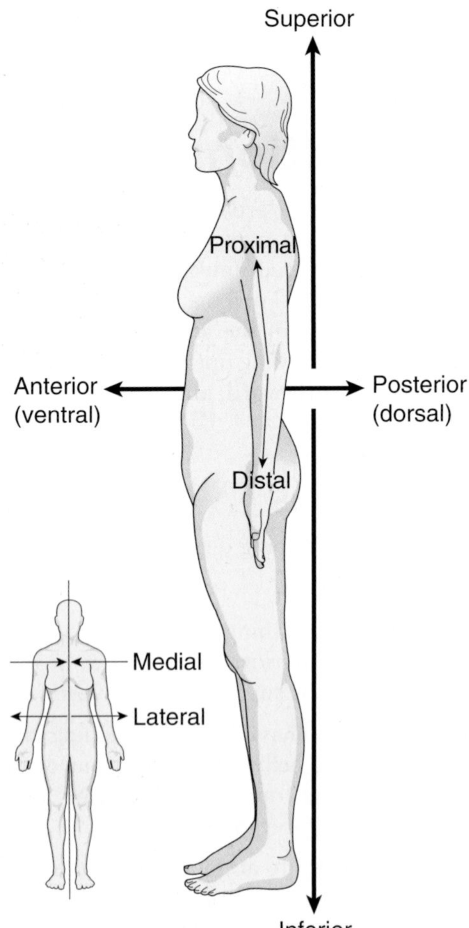

Figure 1-6 Directional terms. KEY POINT Standardized terms are used to describe body directions. ZOOMING IN What is the scientific name for the position in which the figures are standing?

the beginning of a system; **distal** means farther from that point. For example, the part of your thumb where it joins your hand is its proximal region; the tip of the thumb is its distal region. Considering the mouth as the start of the digestive system, the small intestine is distal to the stomach.

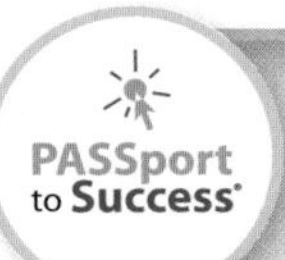

See the Student Resources on *thePoint* for a chart of directional terms with definitions and examples.

PLANES OF DIVISION

To visualize the various internal structures in relation to each other, anatomists can divide the body along three planes, each of which is a cut through the body in a different direction (Fig. 1-7), as follows:

- **Frontal plane.** If the cut were made in line with the ears and then down the middle of the body, you would see an anterior, or ventral (front), section and a posterior, or dorsal (back), section. Another name for this plane is *coronal plane*.
- **Sagittal** (SAJ-ih-tal) **plane.** If you were to cut the body in two from front to back, separating it into right and left portions, the sections you would see would be sagittal sections. A cut exactly down the midline of the body, separating it into equal right and left halves, is a **midsagittal plane.**
- **Transverse plane.** If the cut were made horizontally, across the other two planes, it would divide the body

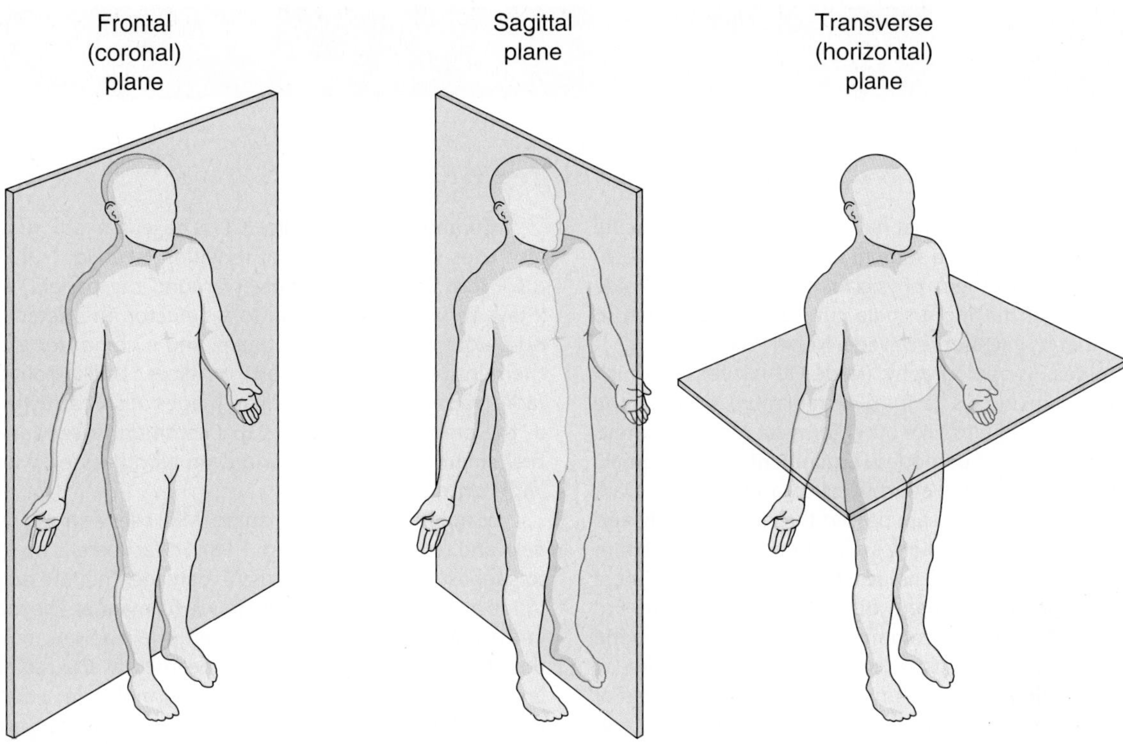

Figure 1-7 Planes of division. KEY POINT The body can be divided along three different planes. ZOOMING IN Which plane divides the body into superior and inferior parts? Which plane divides the body into anterior and posterior parts?

into a superior (upper) part and an inferior (lower) part. A transverse plane is also called a *horizontal plane*.

Some additional terms are used to describe sections (cuts) of tissues, as used to prepare them for study under the microscope. A cross section **(Fig. 1-8)** is a cut made perpendicular to the long axis of an organ, such as a cut made across a banana to give a small round slice. A longitudinal section is made parallel to the long axis, as in cutting a banana from tip to tip to make a slice for a banana split. An oblique section is made at an angle. The type of section used will determine what is seen under the microscope, as shown with a blood vessel in **Figure 1-8**.

These same terms are used for images taken by techniques such as computed tomography (CT) or magnetic resonance imaging (MRI) **(see Box 1-2)**. In imaging studies, the term *cross section* is used more generally to mean any two-dimensional view of an internal structure obtained by imaging, as shown in **Figure 1-9**.

CHECKPOINTS 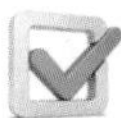

- 1-6 What term describes a location closer to an origin, such as the elbow in comparison to the wrist?
- 1-7 What are the three planes in which the body can be cut?

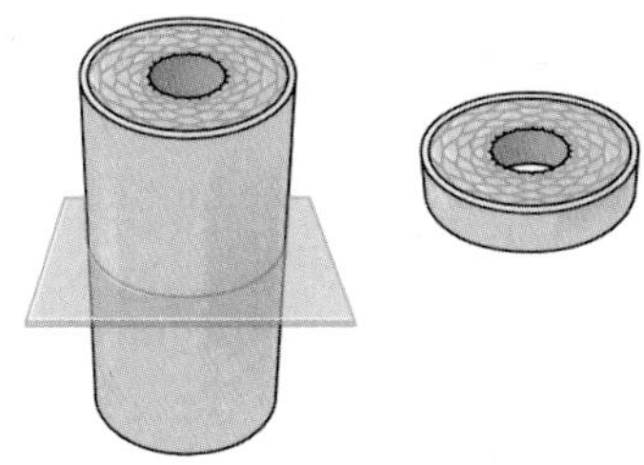

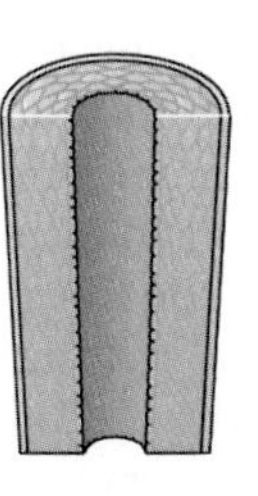

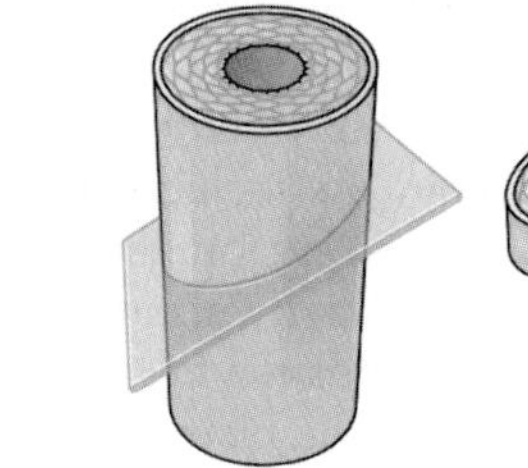

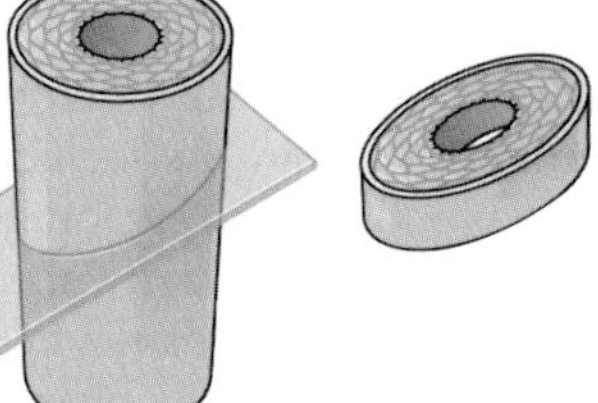

Figure 1-8 Tissue sections. 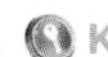 KEY POINT The direction in which tissue is cut affects what is seen under the microscope.

Box 1-2 *Hot Topics*

Medical Imaging: Seeing without Making a Cut

Three imaging techniques that have revolutionized medicine are radiography, computed tomography, and magnetic resonance imaging. With them, physicians today can "see" inside the body without making a single cut. Each technique is so important that its inventor received a Nobel Prize.

The oldest is radiography (ra-de-OG-rah-fe), in which a machine beams x-rays (a form of radiation) through the body onto a piece of film. Like other forms of radiation, x-rays damage body tissues, but modern equipment uses extremely low doses. The resulting picture is called a radiograph. Dark areas indicate where the beam passed through the body and exposed the film, whereas light areas show where the beam did not pass through. Dense tissues (bone, teeth) absorb most of the x-rays, preventing them from exposing the film. For this reason, radiography is commonly used to visualize bone fractures and tooth decay as well as abnormally dense tissues like tumors. Radiography does not provide clear pictures of soft tissues because most of the beam passes through and exposes the film, but contrast media can help make structures like blood vessels and hollow organs more visible. For example, radiologists use ingested barium sulfate (which absorbs x-rays) to coat the digestive tract for imaging.

Computed tomography (CT) is based on radiography and also uses very low doses of radiation (see Fig. 1-9A). During a CT scan, a machine revolves around the patient, beaming x-rays through the body onto a detector. The detector takes numerous pictures of the beam, and a computer assembles them into transverse sections, or "slices." Unlike conventional radiography, CT produces clear images of soft structures such as the brain, liver, and lungs. It is commonly used to visualize brain injuries and tumors, and even blood vessels when used with contrast media.

Magnetic resonance imaging (MRI) uses a strong magnetic field and radio wave (see Fig. 1-9B). So far, there is no evidence to suggest that MRI causes tissue damage. The MRI patient lies inside a chamber within a very powerful magnet. The molecules in the patient's soft tissues align with the magnetic field inside the chamber. When radio waves beamed at the region to be imaged hit the soft tissue, the aligned molecules emit energy that the MRI machine detects, and a computer converts these signals into a picture. MRI produces even clearer images of soft tissue than does computed tomography and can create detailed pictures of blood vessels without contrast media. MRI can visualize brain injuries and tumors that might be missed using CT.

Body Cavities

Internally, the body is divided into a few large spaces, or cavities, which contain the organs. The two main cavities are the **dorsal cavity** and **ventral cavity** (Fig. 1-10).

DORSAL CAVITY

The dorsal body cavity has two subdivisions: the **cranial cavity**, containing the brain, and the **spinal cavity (canal)**, enclosing the spinal cord. These two areas form one continuous space.

VENTRAL CAVITY

The ventral cavity is much larger than the dorsal cavity. It has two main subdivisions, which are separated by the **diaphragm** (DI-ah-fram), a muscle used in breathing. The **thoracic** (tho-RAS-ik) **cavity** is superior to (above) the diaphragm. Its contents include the heart, the lungs, and the large blood vessels that join the heart. The heart is contained in the pericardial cavity, formed by the pericardial sac, the tissue that surrounds the heart; the lungs are in the pleural cavity, formed by the pleurae, the membranes that enclose the lungs (Fig. 1-11). The **mediastinum** (me-de-as-TI-num) is the space between the lungs, including the organs and vessels contained in that space.

The **abdominopelvic** (ab-dom-ih-no-PEL-vik) **cavity** (see Fig. 1-10) is inferior to (below) the diaphragm. This space is further subdivided into two regions. The superior portion, the **abdominal cavity**, contains the stomach, most of the intestine, the liver, the gallbladder, the pancreas, and the spleen. The inferior portion, set off by an imaginary line across the top of the hip bones, is the **pelvic cavity**. This cavity contains the urinary bladder, the rectum, and the internal parts of the reproductive system. See Figures A3-5 and A3-7 in Appendix 3, Dissection Atlas, for dissection photographs showing organs of the ventral cavity.

DIVISIONS OF THE ABDOMEN

It is helpful to divide the abdomen for examination and reference into nine regions (Fig. 1-12).

The three central regions, from superior to inferior, are the following:

- **epigastric** (ep-ih-GAS-trik) **region**, located just inferior to the breastbone
- **umbilical** (um-BIL-ih-kal) **region**, around the umbilicus (um-BIL-ih-kus), commonly called the *navel*
- **hypogastric** (hi-po-GAS-trik) **region**, the most inferior of all the midline regions

The regions on the right and left, from superior to inferior, are the following:

- **hypochondriac** (hi-po-KON-dre-ak) **regions**, just inferior to the ribs

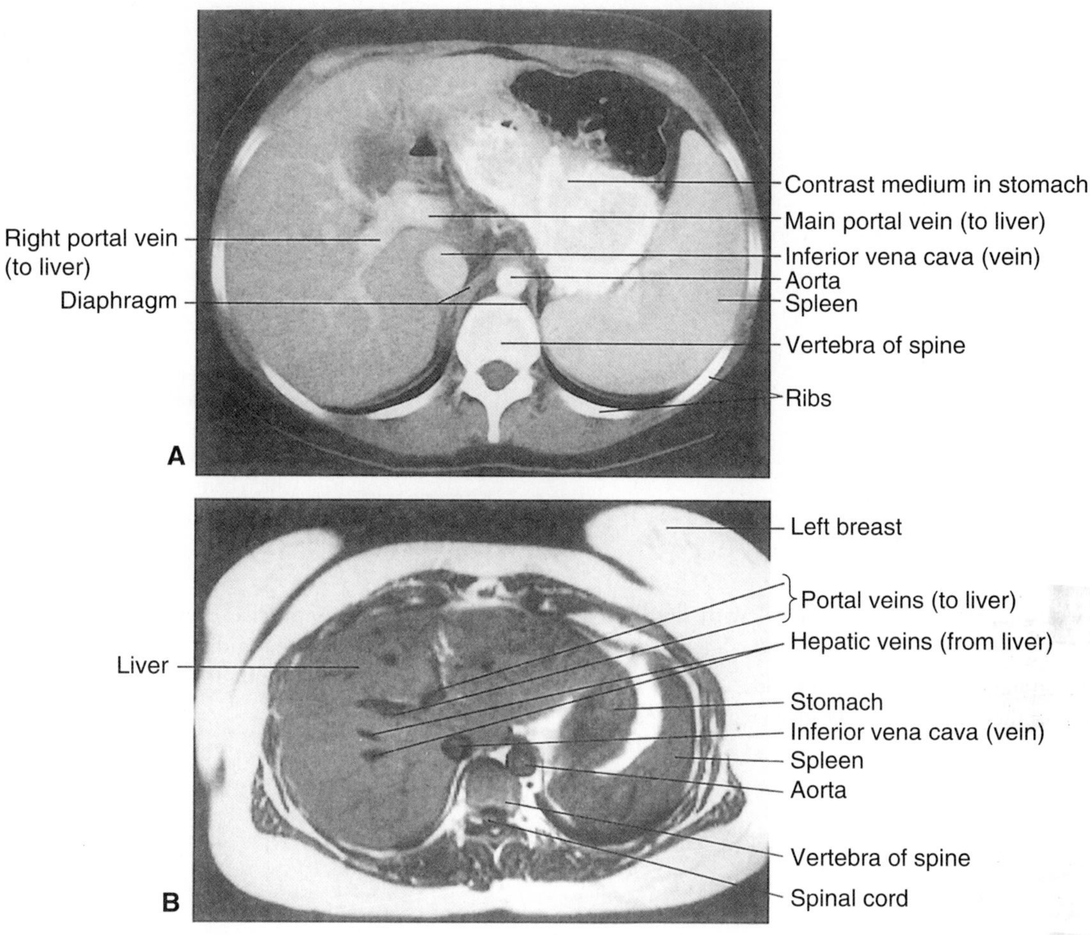

Figure 1-9 **Cross sections in imaging.** Images taken across the body through the liver and spleen by (A) computed tomography and (B) magnetic resonance imaging. (Reprinted with permission from Erkonen WE, Smith WL. *Radiology 101: Basics and Fundamentals of Imaging*. 3rd ed. Philadelphia, PA: Lippincott Williams & Wilkins, 2010.)

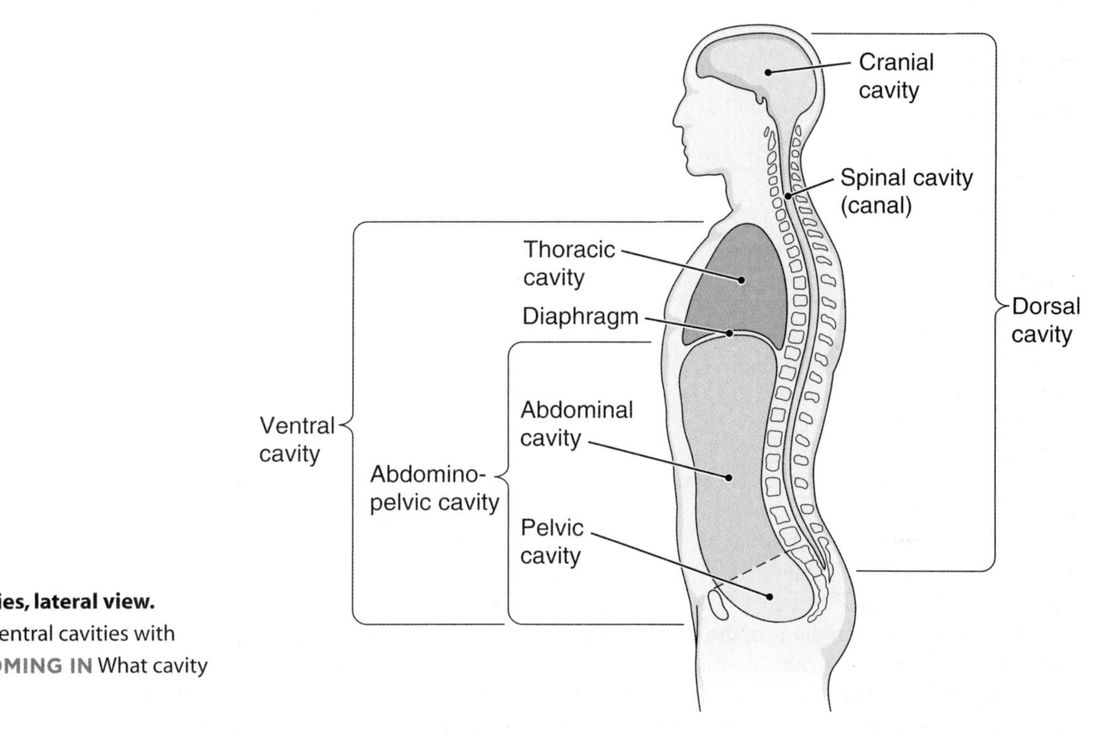

Figure 1-10 **Body cavities, lateral view.** Shown are the dorsal and ventral cavities with their subdivisions. ZOOMING IN What cavity contains the diaphragm?

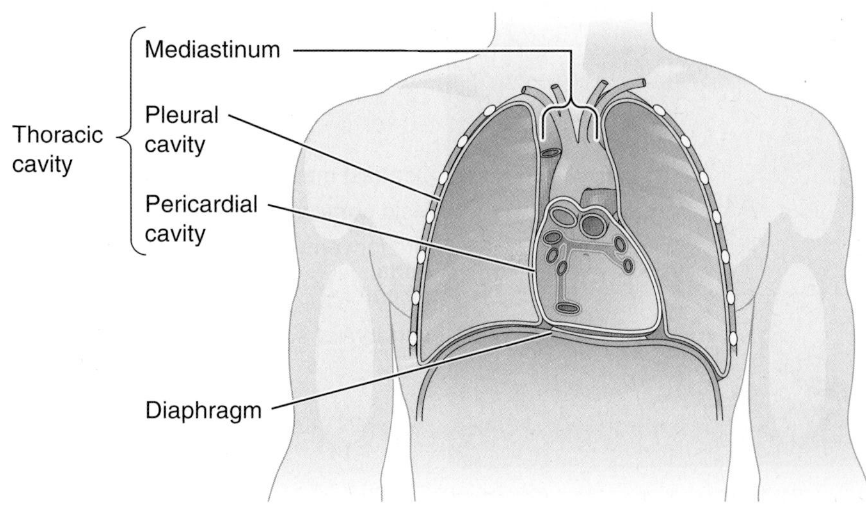

Figure 1-11 The thoracic cavity. KEY POINT Among other structures, the thoracic cavity encloses the pericardial cavity, which contains the heart, and the pleural cavity, which contains the lungs.

- **lumbar regions**, which are on a level with the lumbar regions of the spine
- **iliac**, or **inguinal** (IN-gwih-nal), **regions**, named for the upper crest of the hip bone and the groin region, respectively

A simpler but less precise division into four quadrants is sometimes used. These regions are the right upper quadrant, left upper quadrant, right lower quadrant, and left lower quadrant **(Fig. 1-13)**.

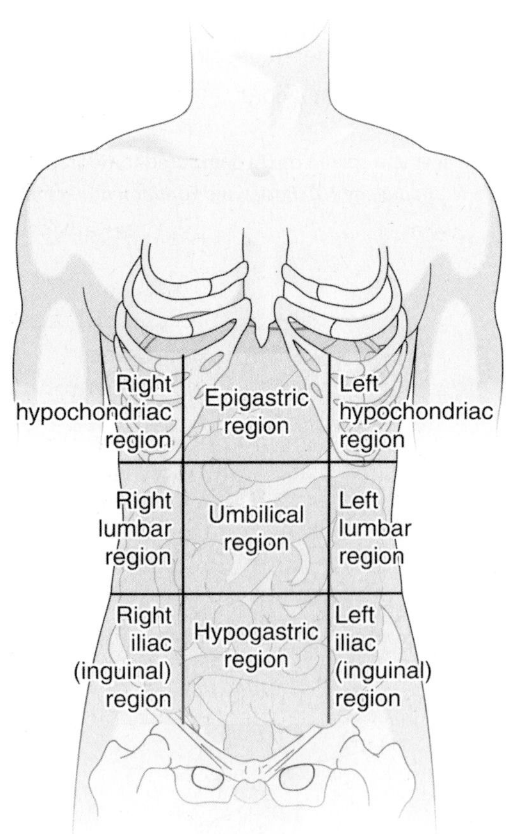

Figure 1-12 The nine regions of the abdomen. KEY POINT Internal structures can be localized within nine regions of the abdomen.

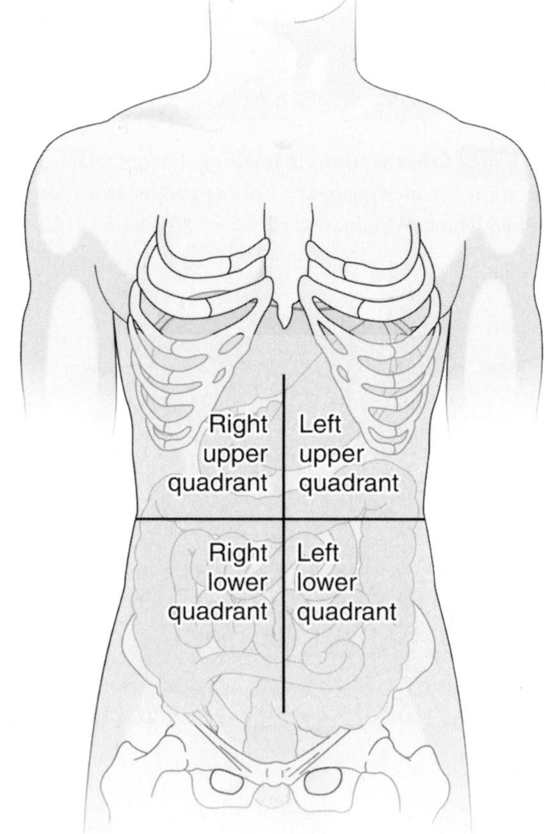

Figure 1-13 Quadrants of the abdomen. The organs within each quadrant are shown. ZOOMING IN Which four abdominal regions are represented in the left lower quadrant?

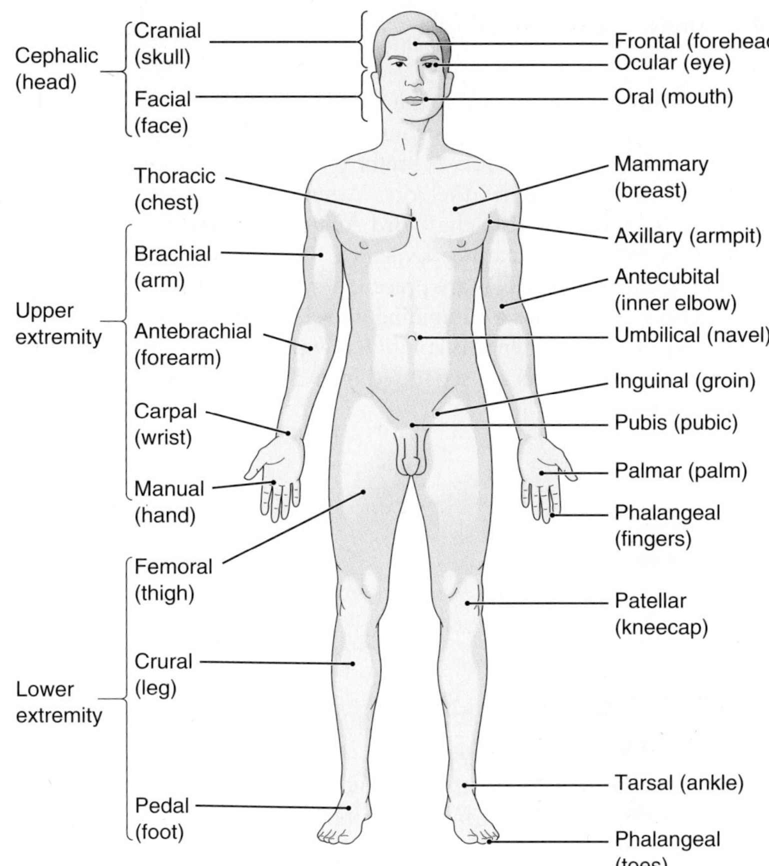

Figure 1-14 Adjectives for some anterior body regions. The names of the regions are in parentheses.

For your reference, **Figures 1-14** and **1-15** give anatomic adjectives for some other body regions along with their common names.

CHECKPOINTS 

1-8 Name the two main body cavities.

1-9 Name the three central regions and the three left and right lateral regions of the abdomen.

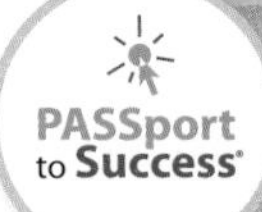

See the Student Resources on *thePoint* for photographic versions of Figures 1.12 and 1.13 and a list of the organs in each quadrant. You may also refer there to information on the metric system, which is used for all scientific measurements.

Medical Terminology

In Mike's case, we saw that health professionals speak the same language: medical terminology. This special scientific vocabulary is based on word parts with consistent meanings that are combined to form different words. Each chapter in this book has a section near the end entitled "Word Anatomy." Here, you will find definitions of word parts commonly used in scientific and medical terms with examples of their usage.

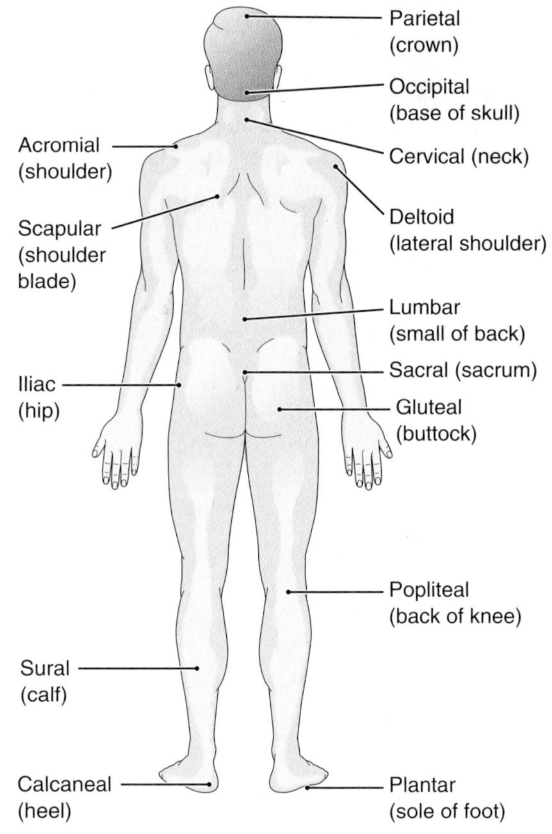

Figure 1-15 Adjectives for some posterior body regions. The names of the regions are in parentheses.

The main part of a word is the **root.** Some compound words, such as wheelchair, gastrointestinal, and lymphocyte, use more than one root. A **prefix** is a short part that starts a word and modifies the root. A **suffix** follows the root and also modifies it. In the Word Anatomy charts, the word parts follow the chapter sequence. Prefixes are followed by a dash and suffixes are preceded by a dash. A root has no dash but often has a combining vowel added to make pronunciation easier when it is combined with another root or a suffix. These vowels are separated from the root with a slash, as in physi/o.

By using the Word Anatomy charts, the Glossary, and the Glossary of Word Parts (the last two found at the back of this text), you too can learn to speak this language of science and medicine.

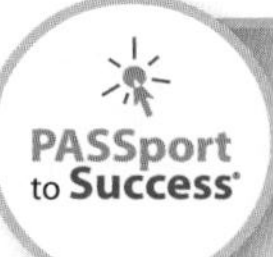

See the box Health Information Technicians in the Student Resources on *thePoint* for description of a profession that requires knowledge of medical terminology.

A&P in Action Revisited

Mike's Homeostatic Emergency

The dispatch radio crackled to life in the ER. "This is Medic 12. We have Mike. 21 years old. Involved in a head-on collision. Patient is on oxygen and an IV of normal saline running wide open. ETA is 15 minutes."

When they arrived at the ER, Samantha and Ed wheeled their unconscious patient into the trauma room. Immediately, the emergency team sprang into action. The trauma nurse measured Mike's vital signs while a technician drew blood from a vein in Mike's antecubital region for testing in the lab. The emergency physician inserted an endotracheal tube into Mike's pharynx to keep his airway open and then carefully examined his abdominopelvic cavity.

"Blood pressure is 80 over 40. Heart rate is 146. Respirations are shallow and rapid," said the nurse.

"We need to raise his blood pressure—let's start a second IV of plasma. His abdomen is as hard as a board. I think he may have a bleed in there—we need an ultrasound," replied the doctor. The sonographer wheeled the ultrasound machine into position and placed the transducer onto Mike's abdomen. Immediately, she located the cause of Mike's symptoms—blood in the left upper quadrant.

"OK. We have a ruptured spleen here," said the doctor. "Call surgery—they need to operate right now."

In Chapter 15, we'll visit Mike again as doctors save his life by removing his spleen, an important organ of the lymphatic system.

Chapter Wrap-Up

Summary Overview

A detailed chapter outline with space for note-taking is on *thePoint*. The figure below illustrates the main topics covered in this chapter.

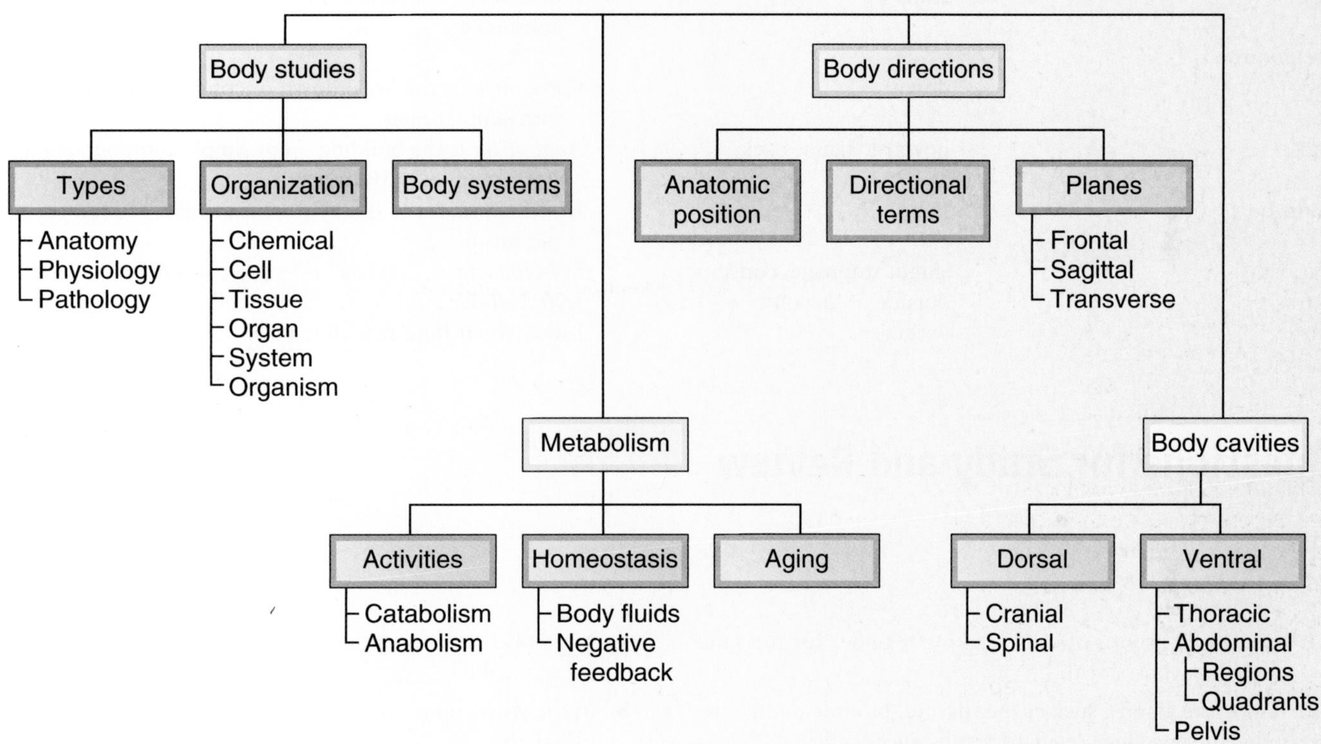

Key Terms

The terms listed below are emphasized in this chapter. Knowing them will help you organize and prioritize your learning. These and other boldface terms are defined in the Glossary with phonetic pronunciations.

anabolism
anatomic position
anatomy
catabolism
cell
extracellular fluid
homeostasis
intracellular fluid
metabolism
negative feedback
organ
physiology
system
tissue

Word Anatomy

Scientific terms are built from standardized word parts (prefixes, roots, and suffixes). Learning the meanings of these parts can help you remember words and interpret unfamiliar terms.

WORD PART	MEANING	EXAMPLE
Studies of the Human Body		
-tomy	cutting, incision of	*Anatomy* can be revealed by cutting the body.
dis-	apart, away from	To *dissect* is to cut apart.
physi/o	nature, physical	*Physiology* is the study of how the body functions.
-logy	study of	*Radiology* is the study and use of radioactive substances.
Metabolism		
cata-	down	*Catabolism* is the breakdown of complex substances into simpler ones.
ana-	upward, again, back	*Anabolism* is the building up of simple compounds into more complex substances.
home/o-	same	*Homeostasis* is the steady state (sameness) within an organism.
stat, -stasis	stand, stoppage, constancy	In *homeostasis,* "-stasis" refers to constancy.
extra-	outside of, beyond	*Extracellular* fluid is outside the cells.
intra-	within	*Intracellular* fluid is within a cell.

Questions for Study and Review

BUILDING UNDERSTANDING

Fill in the blanks

1. Specialized groups of cells working together for the same general purpose form _____.
2. Endocrine glands, such as the thyroid, pituitary, and adrenal glands produce regulatory substances called _____.
3. In location, the eyes are _____ to the nose.
4. Normal body function maintains a state of internal balance called _____.
5. In the word anatomy, *-tomy* is an example of a word part called a(n) _____.

Matching > Match each numbered item with the most closely related lettered item.

___ **6.** One of two systems that control and coordinate other systems
___ **7.** The system that brings needed substances to the body tissues
___ **8.** The system that converts foods into a form that body cells can use
___ **9.** The cavity that contains the liver
___ **10.** The cavity that contains the urinary bladder

a. nervous system
b. abdominal cavity
c. cardiovascular system
d. pelvic cavity
e. digestive system

Multiple Choice

____ **11.** Which science studies normal body structure?

a. homeostasis
b. anatomy
c. physiology
d. biology

____ **12.** Where is intracellular fluid located?

a. between body cells
b. in blood plasma
c. in lymph
d. within body cells

____ **13.** What is the main way of regulating homeostasis?

a. anabolism
b. biofeedback
c. catabolism
d. negative feedback

____ **14.** Which cavity contains the mediastinum?

a. abdominal
b. dorsal
c. pelvic
d. ventral

____ **15.** In location, the foot is _____ to the knee.

a. distal
b. inferior
c. proximal
d. superior

UNDERSTANDING CONCEPTS

16. What do you study in anatomy? In physiology? Would it be wise to study one without the other?

17. List in sequence the levels of organization in the body from simplest to most complex. Give an example for each level.

18. Compare and contrast the anatomy and physiology of the nervous system with that of the endocrine system.

19. What is the difference between catabolism and metabolism?

20. What is the difference between intracellular and extracellular fluids?

21. How does the body maintain a state of internal balance?

22. List the subdivisions of the dorsal and ventral cavities. Name some organs found in each subdivision.

CONCEPTUAL THINKING

23. The human body is organized from very simple levels to more complex levels. With this in mind, describe why a disease at the chemical level can have an effect on organ system function.

24. In Mike's case, the paramedics and emergency team injected several liters of saline and blood plasma into Mike's cardiovascular system. How might the addition of IV fluids stabilize Mike's blood pressure?

25. In Mike's case, the paramedics discovered bruising of the skin over Mike's left lumbar region and umbilical region. Mike also reported considerable pain in his upper left quadrant. Locate these regions on your own body. Why is it important for health professionals to use medical terminology when describing the human body?

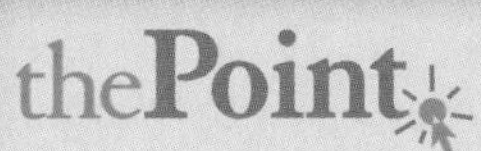

For more questions, see the learning activities on *thePoint*.

CHAPTER 2

Chemistry, Matter, and Life

A&P in Action

Margaret's Case: Chemistry's Role in Homeostasis

"Ugghh," sighed Angela as she pulled into her hospital parking spot. The heat wave was into its second week and she was getting tired of it. It was beginning to take its toll on the city too, especially on its infants and older residents. As Angela walked toward the hospital, she thought back to yesterday's ICU shift. One elderly patient stood out in her mind, probably because she reminded Angela of her own grandmother.

The patient, Margaret Ringland, a 78-year-old widow, lived alone in her apartment on New York's Upper East Side. Yesterday, her niece found Margaret collapsed on the floor, weak and confused. She called 911, and Margaret was rushed to the emergency room. According to her medical chart, Margaret presented with flushed dry skin, a sticky oral cavity, and a furrowed tongue. She was confused and disoriented. She also had hypotension (low blood pressure) and tachycardia (an elevated heart rate). All were classic signs of dehydration, a severe deficiency of water. Without adequate water, Margaret's body was unable to perform essential metabolic processes and her tissues and organs were not in homeostatic balance.

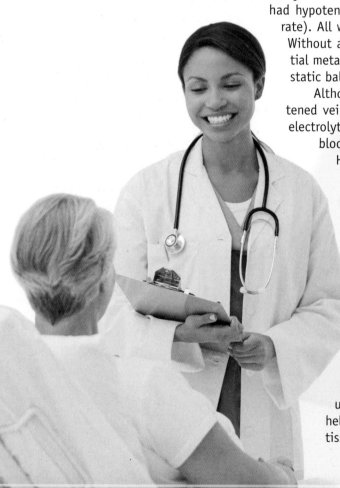

Although it was difficult to get a blood sample from Margaret's flattened veins, her blood work confirmed the initial diagnosis. Margaret's electrolyte levels were out of balance—specifically, she had a high blood sodium ion concentration, a condition called hypernatremia. Her hematocrit was also high, indicating low blood volume. This decrease was seriously affecting her cardiovascular system. Margaret's blood pressure had dropped, which forced her heart to beat faster to ensure proper delivery of blood to her tissues.

The emergency team started an IV line in Margaret's antebrachium. An aqueous solution of 5% dextrose (a sugar) was delivered through the IV at a rate of 500 mL/hour. A catheter was inserted into Margaret's urethra to allow for urinary drainage. Once stabilized, Margaret was moved to ICU for recovery.

Angela depends on her knowledge of chemistry to make sense of the signs and symptoms she observes in her patients. As you read Chapter 2, keep in mind that a firm understanding of the chemistry presented in this chapter will help you understand the anatomy and physiology of the cells, tissues, and organ systems discussed in subsequent chapters.

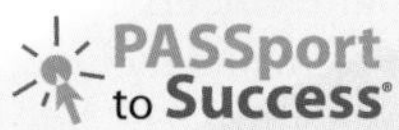

Ancillaries *At-A-Glance*

Visit *thePoint* to access the PASSport to Success and the following resources. For guidance in using these resources most effectively, see pp. ix–xviii.

Learning TOOLS

- Learning Style Self-Assessment
- Live Advise Online Student Tutoring
- Tips for Effective Studying

Learning RESOURCES

- E-book: Chapter 2
- Animation: Enzymes
- Health Professions: Pharmacist and Pharmacy Technician
- Detailed Chapter Outline
- Answers to Questions for Study and Review
- Audio Pronunciation Glossary

Learning ACTIVITIES

- Pre-Quiz
- Visual Activities
- Kinesthetic Activities
- Auditory Activities

Learning Outcomes

After careful study of this chapter, you should be able to:

1. Define a chemical element, ***p. 20***
2. Describe the structure of an atom, ***p. 20***
3. Differentiate between ionic and covalent bonds, ***p. 22***
4. Define an electrolyte, ***p. 22***
5. Differentiate between molecules and compounds, ***p. 23***
6. Define *mixture*; list the three types of mixtures and give two examples of each, ***p. 24***
7. Explain why water is so important in metabolism, ***p. 25***
8. Compare acids, bases, and salts, ***p. 25***
9. Explain how the numbers on the pH scale relate to acidity and alkalinity, ***p. 25***
10. Explain why buffers are important in the body, ***p. 26***
11. Define *radioactivity* and cite several examples of how radioactive substances are used in medicine, ***p. 26***
12. Name the three main types of organic compounds and the building blocks of each, ***p. 27***
13. Define *enzyme*; describe how enzymes work, ***p. 29***
14. List the components of nucleotides and give some examples of nucleotides, ***p. 30***
15. Use the case study to discuss the importance of body fluid quantity and composition, ***pp. 18, 31***
16. Show how word parts are used to build words related to chemistry, matter, and life, ***p. 33***

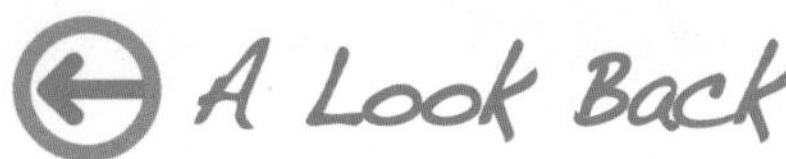

In Chapter 1, we learned that chemicals are the fundamental components of living organisms. In this chapter, we explore chemicals—some of their properties and how they react.

Greater understanding of living organisms has come to us through **chemistry**, the science that deals with the composition and properties of matter. Knowledge of chemistry and chemical changes helps us understand the body's normal and abnormal functioning. Food digestion in the intestinal tract, urine production by the kidneys, the regulation of breathing, and all other body activities involve the principles of chemistry. The many drugs used to treat diseases are also chemicals. Chemistry is used for their development and for understanding their actions in the body.

To provide some insights into the importance of chemistry in the life sciences, this chapter briefly describes elements, atoms, molecules, compounds, and mixtures, which are fundamental forms of matter. We also describe the chemicals that characterize organisms—organic chemicals.

Elements

Matter is anything that takes up space, that is, the materials from which the entire universe is made. **Elements** are the unique substances that make up all matter. The food we eat, the atmosphere, and water—everything around us and everything we can see and touch—are made from just 92 naturally occurring elements. (Twenty additional elements have been created in the laboratory.) Examples of elements include various gases, such as hydrogen, oxygen, and nitrogen; liquids, such as mercury used in barometers and other scientific instruments; and many solids, such as iron, aluminum, gold, silver, and zinc. Graphite (the so-called lead in a pencil), coal, charcoal, and diamonds are different forms of the element carbon.

Elements can be identified by their names or their chemical symbols, which are abbreviations of their modern or Latin names. Each element is also identified by its own number, which is based on its atomic structure, discussed shortly. The periodic table is a chart used by chemists to organize and describe the elements. Appendix 1 shows the periodic table and gives some information about how it is used. **Table 2-1** lists some elements found in the human body along with their functions.

ATOMIC STRUCTURE

The smallest units of elements are **atoms**. As such, atoms are the smallest complete units of matter. They cannot be broken down or changed into another form by ordinary chemical and physical means. Atoms are so small that millions of them could fit on the sharpened end of a pencil.

Despite the fact that the atom is so tiny, chemists have studied it extensively and have found that it has a definite structure composed of even smaller, or subatomic, particles. At the center of each atom is a nucleus composed of positively charged particles called **protons** (PRO-tonz) and noncharged particles called **neutrons** (NU-tronz) **(Fig. 2-1)**. Together, the protons and neutrons contribute nearly all of the atom's weight.

In orbit around the nucleus are **electrons** (e-LEK-tronz). These nearly weightless particles are negatively charged. It is

Table 2-1 Some Common Elements[a]

Name	Symbol	Function
Oxygen	O	Part of water; needed to metabolize nutrients for energy
Carbon	C	Basis of all organic compounds; component of carbon dioxide, the gaseous by-product of metabolism
Hydrogen	H	Part of water; participates in energy metabolism, acid–base balance
Nitrogen	N	Present in all proteins, ATP (the energy-storing compound), and nucleic acids (DNA and RNA)
Calcium	Ca	Builds bones and teeth; needed for muscle contraction, nerve impulse conduction, and blood clotting
Phosphorus	P	Active ingredient in ATP; builds bones and teeth; in cell membranes and nucleic acids
Potassium	K	Nerve impulse conduction; muscle contraction; water balance and acid–base balance
Sulfur	S	Part of many proteins
Sodium	Na	Active in water balance, nerve impulse conduction, and muscle contraction
Chlorine	Cl	Active in water balance and acid–base balance; found in stomach acid
Iron	Fe	Part of hemoglobin, the compound that carries oxygen in red blood cells

[a]*The elements are listed in decreasing order by weight in the body.*

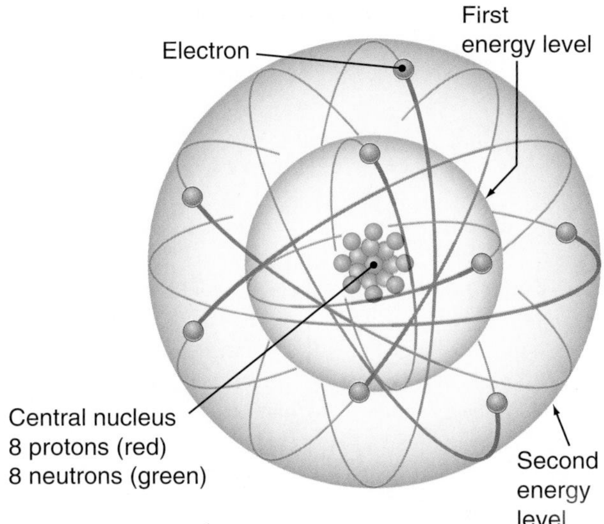

Figure 2-1 **Representation of the oxygen atom.** KEY POINT Eight protons and eight neutrons are tightly bound in the central nucleus. The eight electrons are in orbit around the nucleus, two in the first energy level and six in the second. ZOOMING IN How does the number of protons in this atom compare with the number of electrons?

the electrons that determine how (or if) the atom will react chemically. The protons and electrons of an atom always are equal in number, so that the atom as a whole is electrically neutral **(see Fig. 2-1)**.

The **atomic number** of an element is equal to the number of protons that are present in the nucleus of its atoms. Because the number of protons is equal to the number of electrons, the atomic number also represents the number of electrons orbiting the nucleus. As you can see in **Figure 2-1**, oxygen has an atomic number of 8. No two elements share the same atomic number. Oxygen is the only element with the atomic number of 8. As another example, a carbon atom has six protons in the nucleus and six electrons orbiting the nucleus, so the atomic number of carbon is six. In the Periodic Table of the Elements (see Appendix 1), the atomic number is located at the top of the box for each element. The atomic weight (mass), the sum of the protons and neutrons, is the number at the bottom of each box.

The positively charged protons keep the negatively charged electrons in orbit around the nucleus by means of the opposite charges on the particles. Positively (+) charged protons attract negatively (–) charged electrons.

Energy Levels An atom's electrons orbit at specific distances from the nucleus in regions called energy levels. The first energy level, the one closest to the nucleus, can hold only two electrons. The second energy level, the next in distance away from the nucleus, can hold eight electrons. More distant energy levels can hold more than eight electrons, but they are stable (nonreactive) when they have eight.

The electrons in the energy level farthest away from the nucleus determine how the atom will react chemically. Atoms can donate, accept, or share electrons with other atoms to make their outermost level complete. In so doing, they form chemical bonds, as described shortly.

If the outermost energy level has more than four electrons but less than its capacity of eight, the atom typically completes this level by sharing or gaining electrons from one or more other atoms. The oxygen atom in **Figure 2-2**, illustrated with only the protons in the nucleus and the electrons in fixed position in their energy levels, has six electrons in its second, or outermost, level. When oxygen enters into chemical reactions, it must gain or share two electrons to achieve a complete outermost level.

In contrast, if an atom's outermost energy level has fewer than four electrons, the atom typically loses those electrons to empty the level. Magnesium **(see Fig. 2-2B)** has two electrons in the outermost energy level. In chemical reactions, it gives up those electrons, leaving the second level, complete with eight electrons, as the outermost level. Hydrogen **(see Fig. 2-2C)**, having just one electron, can lose or share that one electron.

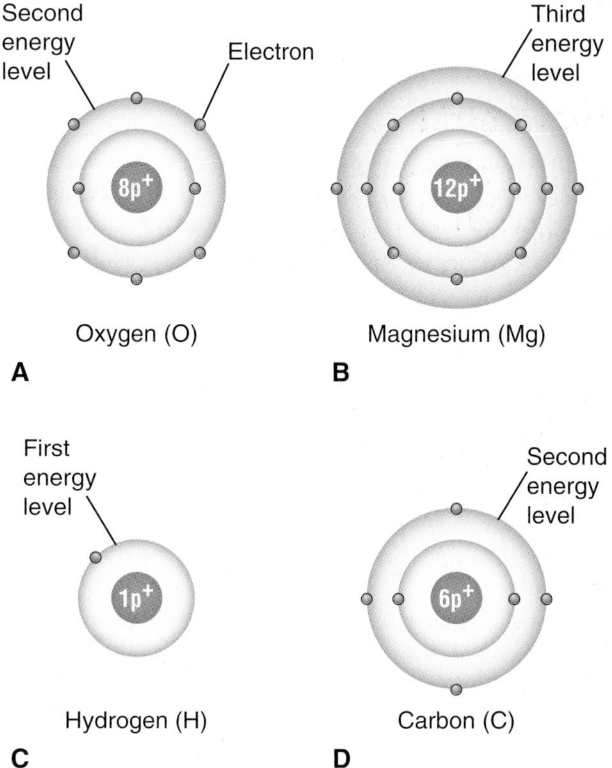

Figure 2-2 **Examples of atoms.** KEY POINT The first energy level can hold two electrons, the second and third can hold eight. The outermost energy level determines chemical reactivity. ZOOMING IN How many electrons does oxygen need to complete its outermost energy level? How does magnesium achieve a stable outermost energy level?

Carbon, which has four electrons in its outermost energy level, usually shares its electrons with multiple atoms in order to complete its outer energy level **(see Fig. 2-2D)**. Atoms with a stable number of electrons in the outermost energy level are not reactive. Examples are the inert or "noble" gases, including helium, neon, and argon.

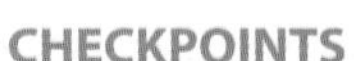 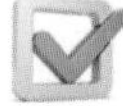

CHECKPOINTS

- 2-1 What are atoms?
- 2-2 What are three types of particles found in atoms?

Chemical Bonds

When atoms interact with other atoms to stabilize their outermost energy levels, a bond is formed between the atoms. In these chemical reactions, electrons may be transferred from one atom to another or may be shared between atoms. The number of bonds an atom needs to form in order to stabilize its outermost energy level is called its **valence** (from a Latin word that means "strength"). An atom needs to form one bond for every electron it donates, accepts, or shares, so valence can also be defined as the number of electrons lost, gained, or shared by atoms of an element in chemical reactions.

IONIC BONDS

When electrons are transferred from one atom to another, the type of bond formed is called an **ionic** (i-ON-ik) **bond**. The sodium atom, for example, tends to lose the single electron in its outermost shell leaving the now outermost shell with a stable number of electrons (8) **(Fig. 2-3)**. Removal of a single electron from the sodium atom leaves one more proton than electrons, and the sodium then has a single net positive charge. The sodium in this form is symbolized as Na+.

Alternately, atoms can gain electrons so that there are more electrons than protons. Chlorine, which has seven electrons in its outermost energy level, tends to gain one electron to fill the level to its capacity. The resultant chlorine is negatively charged (Cl^-) **(see Fig. 2-3)**. (Chemists refer to this charged form of chlorine as *chloride*.) An atom or group of atoms that has acquired a positive or negative charge is called an **ion** (I-on). Any ion that is positively charged is a **cation** (CAT-i-on). Any negatively charged ion is an **anion** (AN-i-on).

Let us imagine a sodium atom coming in contact with a chlorine atom. The sodium atom gives up its outermost electron to the chlorine and becomes positively charged; the chlorine atom gains the electron and becomes negatively charged. The two newly formed ions (Na^+ and Cl^-), because of their opposite charges, attract each other to produce sodium chloride, ordinary table salt **(see Fig. 2-3)**. The attraction between the oppositely charged ions forms an ionic bond. Sodium chloride and other ionically bonded substances tend to form crystals when solid and to dissolve easily in water.

Electrolytes When ionically bonded substances go into solution, the atoms separate as ions. Compounds formed by ionic bonds that release ions when they are in solution are called **electrolytes** (e-LEK-tro-lites). Note that in practice, the term *electrolytes* is also used to refer to the ions themselves in body fluids. Electrolytes include a variety of salts, such as sodium chloride and potassium chloride. They also include acids and bases, which are responsible for the acidity or alkalinity of body fluids, as described shortly. Electrolytes must be present in the proper quantities in the intracellular and extracellular fluids, or very damaging

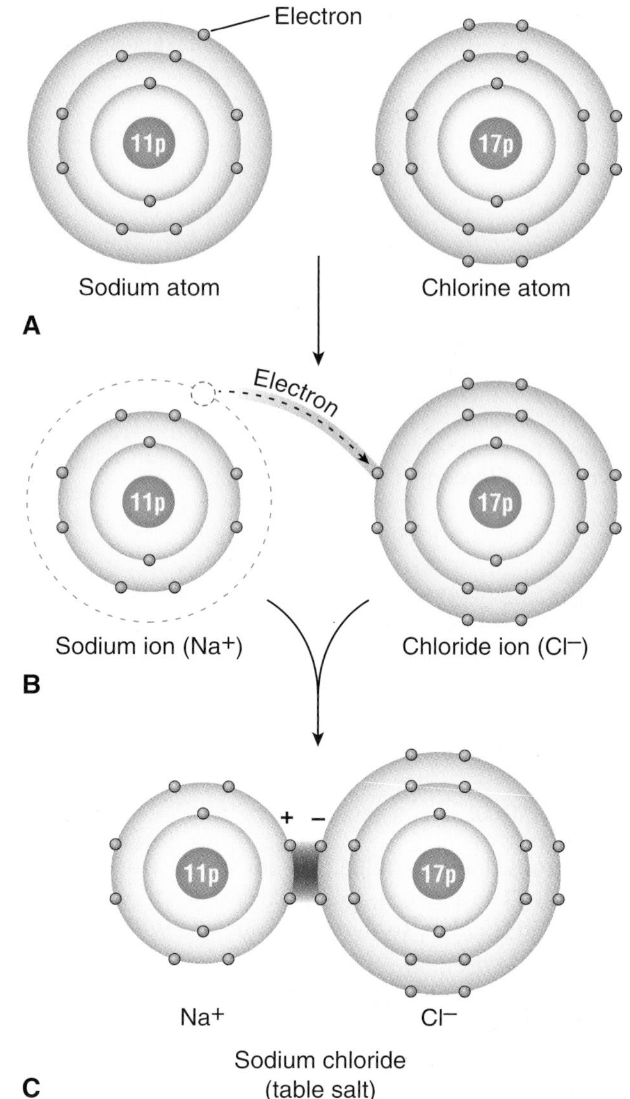

Figure 2-3 Ionic bonding. A. A sodium atom has 11 protons and 11 electrons. A chlorine atom has 17 protons and 17 electrons. **B.** A sodium atom gives up one electron to a chlorine atom in forming an ionic bond. The sodium atom now has 11 protons and 10 electrons, resulting in a positive charge of one. The chlorine becomes negatively charged by one, with 17 protons and 18 electrons. **C.** The ionic bond between the sodium ion (Na^+) and the chloride ion (Cl^-) forms the compound sodium chloride (table salt). **ZOOMING IN** How many electrons are in the outermost energy level of a sodium atom? Of a chlorine atom?

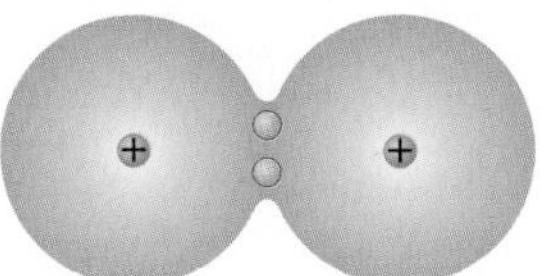

Figure 2-4 A nonpolar covalent bond. KEY POINT The electrons involved in the bonding of two hydrogen atoms are equally shared between the two atoms. The electrons orbit evenly around the two. ZOOMING IN How many electrons are needed to complete the energy level of each hydrogen atom?

effects will result, as seen in Margaret's case study, which opens this chapter.

Ions in the Body Many different ions are found in body fluids. Calcium ions (Ca^{2+}) are necessary for blood clotting, muscle contraction, and the health of bone tissue. Bicarbonate ions (HCO_3^-) are required for the regulation of acidity and alkalinity of body fluids. An organism's normally stable condition, homeostasis, involves the balance of ions.

Because ions are charged particles, electrolytic solutions can conduct an electric current. Records of electric currents in tissues are valuable indications of the functioning or malfunctioning of tissues and organs. The **electrocardiogram** (e-lek-tro-KAR-de-o-gram) and the **electroencephalogram** (e-lek-tro-en-SEF-ah-lo-gram) are graphic tracings of the electric currents generated by the brain and heart muscle, respectively (see Chapters 9 and 13).

COVALENT BONDS

Although ionic bonds form some chemicals, many more are formed by another type of chemical bond. This bond involves not the exchange of electrons but a sharing of electrons between the atoms and is called a **covalent bond.** This name comes from the prefix *co-*, meaning "together," and *valence*, referring to the electrons involved in chemical reactions between atoms. In a covalently bonded substance, the shared electrons orbit around both of the atoms, making both of them stable. Covalent bonds may involve the sharing of one, two, or three pairs of electrons between atoms.

In some covalent bonds, the electrons are equally shared, as in the case of hydrogen bonding to itself (Fig. 2-4) or when other identical atoms, such as those of oxygen or nitrogen, combine with each other. Electrons may also be shared equally in some bonds involving different atoms, methane (CH_4), for example. If electrons are equally shared in forming a bond, the electric charges are evenly distributed around the atoms and the bond is described as a *nonpolar covalent bond*. That is, no part of the combined particle is more negative or positive than any other part. More commonly, the electrons are held closer to one atom than the other, as in the case of water (H_2O), shown in Figure 2-5. In water, the shared electrons are actually closer to the oxygen atom than the hydrogen atoms at any one time, making that region more negative. Such bonds are called *polar covalent bonds*, because one region of the combination is more negative and one part is more positive at any one time.

Anyone studying biological chemistry (biochemistry) is interested in covalent bonding because carbon, the element that is the basis of organic chemistry, forms covalent bonds with a wide variety of different elements. Thus, the substances that are characteristic of living things are covalently bonded. For a description of another type of bond, see Box 2-1.

MOLECULES AND COMPOUNDS

When two or more atoms unite covalently, they form a **molecule** (MOL-eh-kule). A molecule is thus the smallest unit of a covalently bonded substance that retains all the properties of that substance. A molecule can be made of like atoms—the oxygen molecule is made of two identical atoms, for example—but more often a molecule is made of atoms of two or more different elements. For example, a water molecule (H_2O) contains one atom of oxygen (O) and two atoms of hydrogen (H) (see Fig. 2-5). Note that chemists do not consider ionically bonded substances to be composed of molecules, as their atoms are held together by electrical attraction only. The bonds that hold these atoms together are weak, and the components separate easily in solution into ions, as already described.

Any substance composed of two or more different elements is called a **compound.** This definition includes both ionically and covalently bonded substances. The formula for a compound shows all the elements that make up that compound in their proper ratio, such as NaCl, H_2O, and CO_2. Some compounds are made of a few elements in a

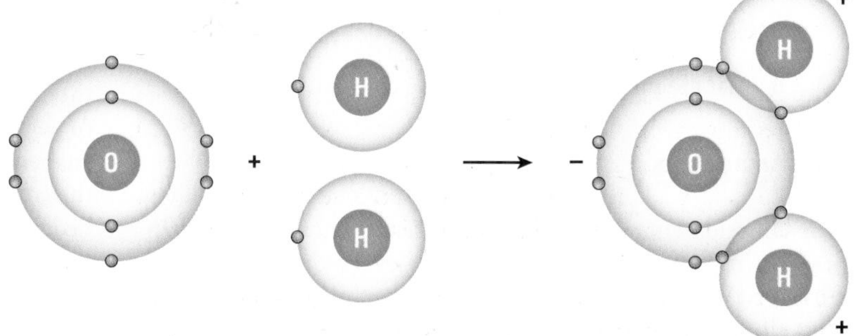

Figure 2-5 Formation of water. KEY POINT Water is formed by polar covalent bonds. The unequal sharing of electrons makes the region near the oxygen nucleus more negative and the region near the hydrogen nucleus more positive. ZOOMING IN How many hydrogen atoms bond with an oxygen atom to form water?

Box 2-1 *A Closer Look*

Hydrogen Bonds: Strength in Numbers

In contrast to ionic and covalent bonds, which hold atoms together, hydrogen bonds hold molecules together. Hydrogen bonds are much weaker than ionic or covalent bonds—in fact, they are more like "attractions" between molecules. While ionic and covalent bonds rely on electron transfer or sharing, hydrogen bonds form bridges between two molecules. A hydrogen bond forms when a slightly positive hydrogen atom in one molecule is attracted to a slightly negative atom in another molecule. Even though a single hydrogen bond is weak, many hydrogen bonds between two molecules can be strong.

Hydrogen bonds hold water molecules together, with the slightly positive hydrogen atom in one molecule attracted to a slightly negative oxygen atom in another. Many of water's unique properties come from its ability to form hydrogen bonds. For example, hydrogen bonds keep water liquid over a wide range of temperatures, which provides a constant environment for body cells.

Hydrogen bonds form not only between molecules but also within large molecules. Hydrogen bonds between regions of the same molecule cause it to fold and coil into a specific shape, as in the process that creates the precise three-dimensional structure of proteins. Because a protein's structure determines its function in the body, hydrogen bonds are essential to protein activity.

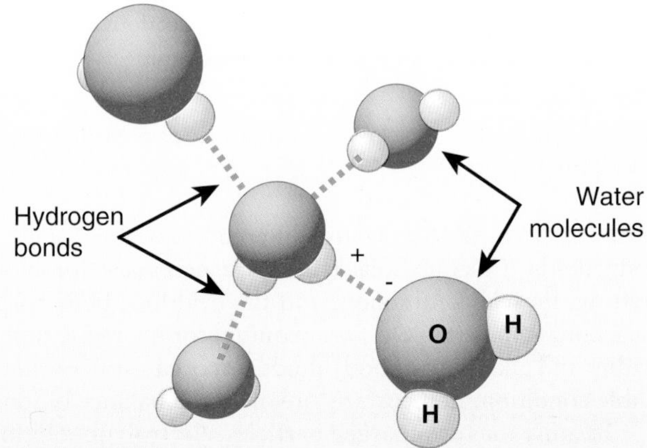

Hydrogen bonds. The bonds shown here are holding water molecules together.

simple combination. For example, molecules of the gas carbon monoxide (CO) contain one atom of carbon (C) and one atom of oxygen (O). Other compounds have very large and complex molecules. Such complexity characterizes many of the compounds found in living organisms. Some protein molecules, for example, have thousands of atoms.

It is interesting to observe how different a compound is from any of its constituents. For example, a molecule of liquid water is formed from oxygen and hydrogen, both of which are gases. Another example is the sugar glucose ($C_6H_{12}O_6$). Its constituents include 12 atoms of the gas hydrogen, 6 atoms of the gas oxygen, and 6 atoms of the solid element carbon. The component gases and the solid carbon do not in any way resemble the glucose.

CHECKPOINTS 

- 2-3 What are the two main types of chemical bonds and how are they formed?
- 2-4 What happens when an electrolyte goes into solution?
- 2-5 What are molecules and what are compounds?

Mixtures

Not all elements or compounds react chemically when brought together. The air we breathe every day is a combination of gases, largely nitrogen, oxygen, and carbon dioxide, along with smaller percentages of other substances. The constituents in the air maintain their identity, although the proportions of each may vary. Blood plasma—the fluid portion of blood—is also a combination in which the various components maintain their identity. The many valuable compounds in the plasma remain separate entities with their own properties. Such combinations are called **mixtures**—blends of two or more substances **(Table 2-2)**.

SOLUTIONS AND SUSPENSIONS

A mixture formed when one substance dissolves in another is called a **solution.** One example is salt water. In a solution, the component substances cannot be distinguished from each other and remain evenly distributed throughout; that is, the mixture is homogeneous (ho-mo-JE-ne-us). The dissolving substance, which in the body is water, is the **solvent.** The substance dissolved, table salt in the case of salt water, is the **solute.** An **aqueous** (A-kwe-us) **solution** is one in which water is the solvent. Aqueous solutions of glucose, salts, or both of these together are used for intravenous fluid treatments.

In some mixtures, the substance distributed in the background material is not dissolved and will settle out unless the mixture is constantly shaken. This type of nonuniform, or heterogeneous (het-er-o-JE-ne-us), mixture is called a **suspension.** The particles in a suspension are separate from the material in which they are dispersed, and they settle out because they are large and heavy. Examples of suspensions are milk of magnesia, finger paints, and in the body, red blood cells suspended in blood plasma.

One other type of mixture is important in body function. Some organic compounds form **colloids,** in which the

Table 2-2 Mixtures

Type	Definition	Example
Solution	Homogeneous mixture formed when one substance (solute) dissolves in another (solvent)	Table salt (NaCl) dissolved in water; table sugar (sucrose) dissolved in water
Suspension	Heterogeneous mixture in which one substance is dispersed in another but will settle out unless constantly mixed	Red blood cells in blood plasma; milk of magnesia
Colloid	Heterogeneous mixture in which the suspended particles remain evenly distributed based on the small size and opposing charges of the particles	Blood plasma; cytosol

molecules do not dissolve yet remain evenly distributed in the suspending material. The particles have electric charges that repel each other, and the molecules are small enough to stay in suspension. The fluid that fills the cells (cytosol) is a colloidal suspension, as is blood plasma.

Many mixtures are complex, with properties of solutions, suspensions, and colloidal suspensions. For instance, blood plasma has dissolved compounds, making it a solution. The red blood cells and other formed elements give blood the property of a suspension. The proteins in the plasma give it the property of a colloidal suspension. Chocolate milk also has all three properties.

THE IMPORTANCE OF WATER

Water is the most abundant compound in the body. No plant or animal can live very long without it. Water is of critical importance in all physiological processes in body tissues. A deficiency of water, or dehydration (de-hi-DRA-shun), can be a serious threat to health, as illustrated by Margaret's case study. Water carries substances to and from the cells and makes possible the essential processes of absorption, exchange, secretion, and excretion. What are some of the properties of water that make it such an ideal medium for living cells?

- Water can dissolve many different substances in large amounts. For this reason, it is called the *universal solvent*. Many of the body's necessary materials, such as gases and nutrients, dissolve in water to be carried from place to place. Substances, such as salt, that mix with or dissolve in water are described as *hydrophilic* ("water loving"); substances such as fats that do not dissolve in water are described as *hydrophobic* ("water fearing").
- Water is stable as a liquid at ordinary temperatures. It does not freeze until the temperature drops to 0°C (32°F) and does not boil until the temperature reaches 100°C (212°F). This stability provides a constant environment for living cells. Water can also be used to distribute heat throughout the body and to cool the body by evaporation of sweat from the body surface.
- Water participates in the body's chemical reactions. It is needed directly in the digestive process and in many of the metabolic reactions that occur in the cells.

CHECKPOINTS 

- ☐ 2-6 What is the difference between solutions and suspensions?
- ☐ 2-7 What is the most abundant compound in the body?

Acids, Bases, and Salts

An **acid** (AH-sid) is a chemical substance capable of donating a hydrogen ion (H^+) to another substance. A common example is hydrochloric acid (HCl), the acid found in stomach juices. HCl releases hydrogen ions in solution as follows:

HCl	→	H^+	+	Cl^-
(hydrochloric acid)		(hydrogen ion)		(chloride ion)

A **base** is a chemical substance, usually containing a hydroxide ion (OH^-), that can accept a hydrogen ion. A base is also called an alkali (AL-kah-li), and bases are described as alkaline. Sodium hydroxide, which releases hydroxide ions in solution, is an example of a base:

NaOH	→	Na^+	+	OH^-
(sodium hydroxide)		(sodium ion)		(hydroxide ion)

A reaction between an acid and a base produces a **salt** and also water. In the reaction, the hydrogen of the acid is replaced by the positive ion of the base. A common example of a salt is sodium chloride (NaCl), or table salt, produced by the reaction:

$$HCl + NaOH \rightarrow NaCl + H_2O$$

THE pH SCALE

The greater the concentration of hydrogen ions in a solution, the greater the acidity of that solution. The greater the concentration of hydroxide ion (OH^-), the greater the alkalinity of the solution. Based on changes in the balance of ions in solution, as the concentration of hydrogen ions increases, the concentration of hydroxide ions decreases. Conversely, as the concentration of hydroxide ions increases, the concentration of hydrogen ions decreases.

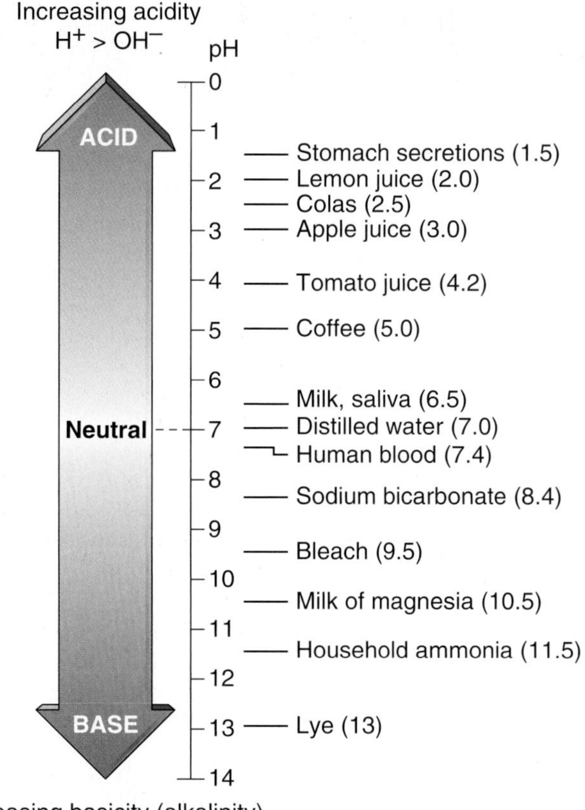

Figure 2-6 **The pH scale.** Degree of acidity or alkalinity is shown in pH units. This scale also shows the pH of some common substances. **ZOOMING IN** What happens to the amount of hydroxide ion (OH^-) present in a solution when the amount of hydrogen ion (H^+) increases?

Acidity and alkalinity are indicated by **pH** units, which represent the relative concentrations of hydrogen and hydroxide ions in a solution. The pH units are listed on a scale from 0 to 14, with 0 being the most acidic and 14 being the most basic **(Fig. 2-6)**. A pH of 7.0 is neutral. At pH 7.0, the solution has an equal number of hydrogen and hydroxide ions. Pure water has a pH of 7.0. Solutions that measure less than 7.0 are acidic; those that measure above 7.0 are alkaline (basic).

Because the pH scale is based on multiples of 10, each pH unit on the scale represents a 10-fold change in the number of hydrogen and hydroxide ions present. A solution registering 5.0 on the scale has 10 times the number of hydrogen ions as a solution that registers 6.0. The pH 5.0 solution also has one-tenth the number of hydroxide ions as the solution of pH 6.0. A solution registering 9.0 has one-tenth the number of hydrogen ions and 10 times the number of hydroxide ions as one registering 8.0. Thus, the lower the pH reading, the greater is the acidity, and the higher the pH, the greater is the alkalinity.

Blood and other body fluids are close to neutral but are slightly on the alkaline side, with a pH range of 7.35 to 7.45. Urine averages pH 6.0 but may range from 4.6 to 8.0 depending on body conditions and diet. **Figure 2-6** shows the pH of some other common substances.

Because body fluids are on the alkaline side of neutral, the body may be in a relatively acidic state even if the pH does not drop below 7.0. For example, if a patient's pH falls below 7.35 but is still greater than 7.0, the patient is described as being in an acidic state known as *acidosis*. Thus, within this narrow range, physiologic acidity differs from acidity as defined by the pH scale.

An increase in pH to readings greater than 7.45 is termed *alkalosis*. Any shifts in pH to readings above or below the normal range can be dangerous, even fatal.

BUFFERS

In a healthy person, body fluids are delicately balanced within narrow limits of acidity and alkalinity. This balanced chemical state is maintained in large part by **buffers**. Chemical buffers form a system that prevents sharp changes in hydrogen ion concentration and thus maintains a relatively constant pH. Buffers are important in maintaining stability in the pH of body fluids. More information about body fluids, pH, and buffers can be found in Chapter 19.

CHECKPOINTS 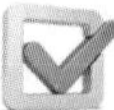

- 2-8 What number is neutral on the pH scale? What kind of compound measures lower than this number? Higher?
- 2-9 What is a buffer?

Isotopes and Radioactivity

Elements may exist in several forms, each of which is called an **isotope** (I-so-tope). These forms are alike in their numbers of protons and electrons, but differ in their atomic weights because of differing numbers of neutrons in the nucleus. The most common form of oxygen, for example, has eight protons and eight neutrons in the nucleus, giving the atom an atomic weight of 16 atomic mass units (amu). But there are some isotopes of oxygen with only 6 or 7 neutrons in the nucleus and others with 9 to 11 neutrons. The isotopes of oxygen thus range in atomic weight from 14 to 19 amu.

Some isotopes are stable and maintain constant characteristics. Others disintegrate (fall apart) and give off rays of atomic particles. Such isotopes are said to be **radioactive**. Radioactive elements, also called *radioisotopes*, may occur naturally, as is the case with isotopes of the very heavy elements radium and uranium. Others may be produced artificially by placing the atoms of lighter, nonradioactive elements in accelerators that smash their nuclei together.

The rays given off by some radioisotopes are used in the treatment of cancer because they have the ability to penetrate and destroy tumor cells. Radiation therapy is often given by means of machines that are able to release tumor-destroying atomic particles. A growing tumor contains immature, dividing cancer cells, which are more sensitive to the effects of radiation than are mature body cells. The

Box 2-2 Hot Topics

Radioactive Tracers: Medicine Goes Nuclear

Like radiography, computed tomography (CT), and magnetic resonance imaging, **nuclear medicine imaging** (NMI) offers a noninvasive way to look inside the body. An excellent diagnostic tool, NMI shows not only structural details but also provides information about body function. NMI can help diagnose cancer, stroke, and heart disease earlier than techniques that provide only structural information.

NMI uses **radiotracers**, radioactive substances that specific organs absorb. For example, radioactive iodine is used to image the thyroid gland, which absorbs more iodine than any other organ. After a patient ingests, inhales, or is injected with a radiotracer, a device called a gamma camera detects the radiotracer in the organ under study and produces a picture, which is used in making a diagnosis. Radiotracers are broken down and eliminated through urine or feces, so they leave the body quickly. A patient's exposure to radiation in NMI is usually considerably lower than with x-ray or CT scan.

Three NMI techniques are **positron emission tomography** (PET), **bone scanning**, and the **thallium stress test**. PET is often used to evaluate brain activity by measuring the brain's use of radioactive glucose. PET scans can reveal brain tumors because tumor cells are often more metabolically active than normal cells and thus absorb more radiotracer. Bone scanning detects radiation from a radiotracer absorbed by bone tissue with an abnormally high metabolic rate, such as a bone tumor. The thallium stress test is used to diagnose heart disease. A nuclear medicine technologist injects the patient with radioactive thallium, and a gamma camera images the heart during exercise and then rest. When compared, the two sets of images help to evaluate blood flow to the working, or "stressed," heart.

greater sensitivity of these younger cells allows radiation therapy to selectively destroy them with minimal damage to normal tissues. Modern radiation instruments produce tremendous amounts of energy (in the multimillion electron-volt range) that can destroy deep-seated cancers without causing serious skin reactions.

In radiation treatment, a radioisotope, such as cobalt 60, is sealed in a stainless steel cylinder and mounted on an arm or crane. Beams of radioactivity are then directed through a porthole to the area to be treated. Implants containing radioisotopes in the form of needles, seeds, or tubes also are widely used in the treatment of different types of cancer.

In addition to its therapeutic values, irradiation is extensively used in diagnosis. X-rays penetrate tissues and produce an image of their interior on a photographic plate. Radioactive iodine and other "tracers" taken orally or injected into the bloodstream are used to diagnose abnormalities of certain body organs, such as the thyroid gland (see Box 2-2). When using radiation in diagnosis or therapy, healthcare personnel must follow strict precautions to protect themselves and the patient, because the rays can destroy healthy as well as diseased tissues.

CHECKPOINT

2-10 What word is used to describe isotopes that give off radiation?

Organic Compounds

Of the 92 elements that exist in nature, only 26 have been found in living organisms. Most of these are light in weight, and not all are present in large quantities. Hydrogen, oxygen, carbon, and nitrogen make up about 96% of body weight (Fig. 2-7). Nine additional elements—calcium, sodium, potassium, phosphorus, sulfur, chlorine, magnesium, iron, and iodine—make up most of the remaining 4% of the body's elements. The remaining 13, including zinc, selenium, copper, cobalt, chromium, and others, are present in extremely small (trace) amounts totaling about 0.1% of body weight.

The chemical compounds that characterize living things are called **organic compounds**. All of these are built on the element **carbon**. Because carbon atoms can combine with

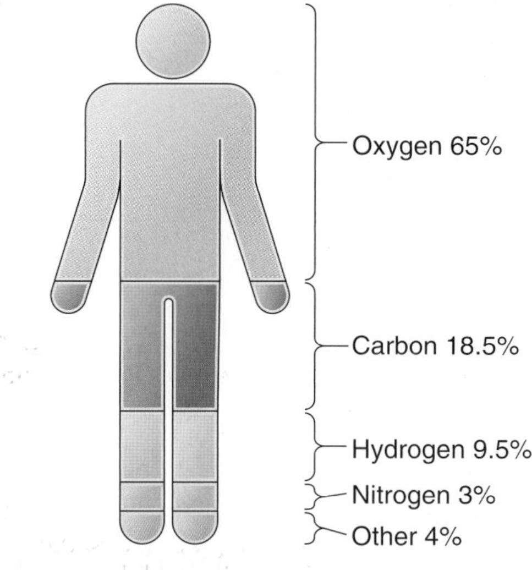

Figure 2-7 The body's chemical composition by weight. KEY POINT Oxygen, carbon, hydrogen, and nitrogen make up about 96% of body weight.

a variety of different elements and can even bond to other carbon atoms to form long chains, most organic compounds consist of large, complex molecules. The starch found in potatoes, the fat and protein in tissues, hormones, and many drugs are examples of organic compounds. These large molecules are often formed from simpler molecules called *building blocks*, or *monomers (mono-* means "one"), which bond together in long chains.

The main types of organic compounds are carbohydrates, lipids, and proteins. All of these organic compounds contain carbon, hydrogen, and oxygen as their main ingredients. Carbohydrates, lipids, and proteins (in addition to minerals, vitamins, and water) must be taken in as part of a normal diet. These nutrients are discussed further in Chapters 17 and 18.

CARBOHYDRATES

The building blocks of **carbohydrates** (kar-bo-HI-drates) are simple sugars, or **monosaccharides** (mon-o-SAK-ah-rides) (Fig. 2-8). (The word root *sacchar/o* means "sugar.") **Glucose** (GLU-kose), a simple sugar that circulates in the blood as a cellular nutrient, is an example of a monosaccharide. Two simple sugars may be linked together to form a **disaccharide** (see Fig. 2-8B), as represented by sucrose, or table sugar. More complex carbohydrates, or **polysaccharides**, consist of many simple sugars linked together with multiple side chains (see Fig. 2-8C). (The prefix *di-* means "two" and *poly-* means "many.") Examples of polysaccharides are starch, which is manufactured in plant cells, and **glycogen** (GLI-ko-jen), a storage form of glucose found in liver cells and skeletal muscle cells. Carbohydrates in the form of sugars and starches are important dietary sources of energy.

LIPIDS

Lipids are a class of organic compounds that are not soluble in water. They are mainly found in the body as **fat**. Simple fats are made from a substance called glycerol (GLIS-er-ol), commonly known as glycerin, in combination with three fatty acids (Fig. 2-9). One fatty acid is attached to each of the three carbon atoms in glycerol, so simple fats are described as triglycerides (tri-GLIS-er-ides) (the prefix *tri-* means "three"). Fats insulate the body and protect internal organs. In addition, fats are the main form in which energy is stored.

Two other types of lipids are important in the body. Phospholipids (fos-fo-LIP-ids) are complex lipids containing the element phosphorus. Among other functions, phospholipids make up a major part of the membrane around living cells. **Steroids** are lipids that contain rings of carbon

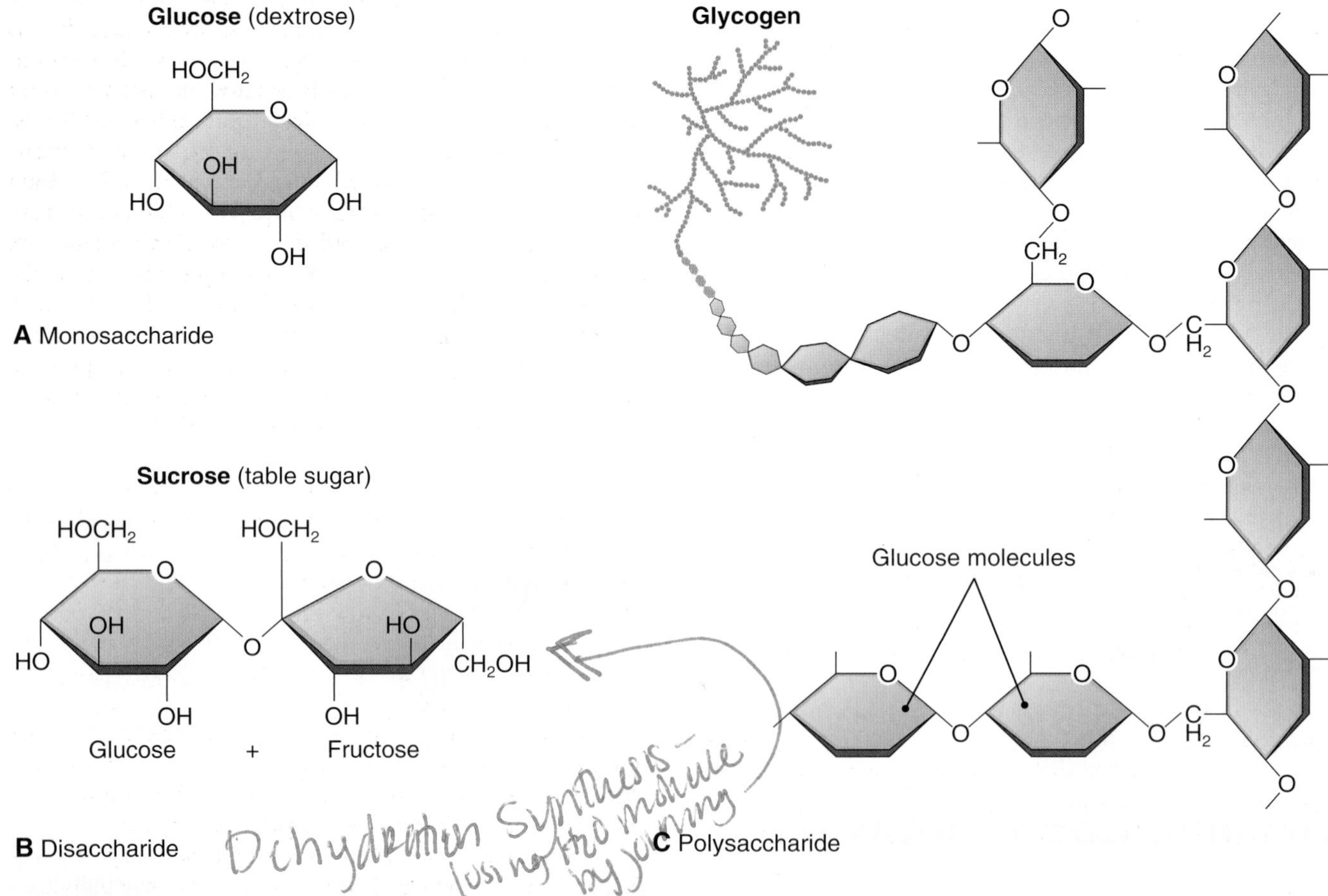

Figure 2-8 **Examples of carbohydrates.** KEY POINT A monosaccharide **(A)** is a simple sugar. A disaccharide **(B)** consists of two simple sugars linked together, whereas a polysaccharide **(C)** consists of many simple sugars linked together in chains. ZOOMING IN What are the building blocks (monomers) of disaccharides and polysaccharides?

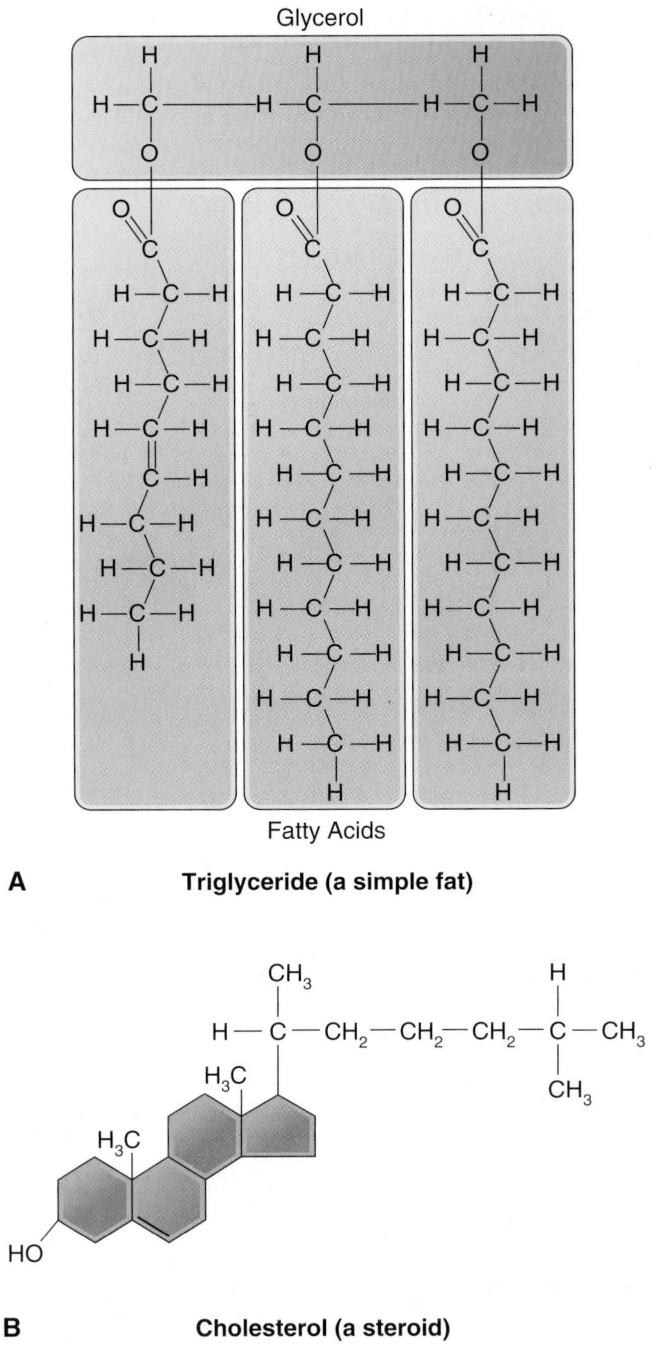

Glycerol

Fatty Acids

A **Triglyceride (a simple fat)**

B **Cholesterol (a steroid)**

Figure 2-9 **Lipids.** KEY POINT **A.** A triglyceride, a simple fat, contains glycerol combined with three fatty acids. **B.** Cholesterol is a type of steroid, a lipid that contains rings of carbon atoms. ZOOMING IN How many carbon atoms are in glycerol?

atoms. They include **cholesterol** (ko-LES-ter-ol), another component of cellular membranes **(see Fig. 2-9B)**, and certain hormones, such as cortisol, produced by the adrenal glands and the sex hormones produced by the ovaries and testes.

PROTEINS

All **proteins** (PRO-tenes) contain, in addition to carbon, hydrogen, and oxygen, the element **nitrogen** (NI-tro-jen). They may also contain sulfur or phosphorus. Proteins are the body's structural materials, found in muscle, bone, and connective tissue. They also make up the pigments that give hair, eyes, and skin their color. It is proteins that make each individual physically distinct from others. Aside from their structural importance, various proteins are essential for body functions. They regulate metabolic reactions and participate in the activities of all systems.

Proteins are composed of monomers called **amino** (ah-ME-no) **acids (Fig. 2-10)**. Although only about 20 different amino acids exist in the body, a vast number of proteins can be made by linking them together in different-sized molecules and in different combinations.

Each amino acid contains an acid group (COOH) and an amino group (NH_2), the part of the molecule that has the nitrogen. These groups are attached to either side of a carbon atom linked to a hydrogen atom. The remainder of the molecule, symbolized by R in **Figure 2-10A**, is different in each amino acid, ranging from a single hydrogen atom to a complex chain or ring of carbon and other elements. It is variations in the R region of the molecule that accounts for the differences in the amino acids.

In forming proteins, the acid group of one amino acid can form a covalent bond with the amino group of another amino acid. This bond is called a *peptide bond*. Many amino acids linked together in this way form a *polypeptide*, which is essentially a chain of amino acids. Proteins are long polypeptides formed into different three-dimensional shapes. The various shapes are created by other types of chemical bonds within the polypeptide. These bonds may cause the chain to fold into a pleated sheet, or β-sheet **(see Fig. 2-10C)**. Other polypeptides coil into a helix (spiral). Such coiled, or fibrous, proteins are important in body structure, as in muscle tissue and bone. Internal bonds may then cause the coiled chain to fold back on itself. Several polypeptide chains also may be folded together. These folded, or globular, proteins are important in body functions. For example, they form the oxygen-carrying hemoglobin in red blood cells, some hormones, antibodies needed for immunity, enzymes (described below), and many other metabolically active compounds. The overall three-dimensional shape of a protein is important to its function, as can be seen in the activity of enzymes.

Enzymes **Enzymes** (EN-zimes) are proteins that are essential for metabolism. They are **catalysts** (KAT-ah-lists) in the hundreds of reactions that take place within cells. Without these catalysts, which increase the speed of chemical reactions, metabolism would not occur at a fast enough rate to sustain life. Because each enzyme works only on a specific substance, or **substrate**, and does only one specific chemical job, many different enzymes are needed. Like all catalysts, enzymes take part in reactions only temporarily; they are not used up or changed by the reaction. Therefore, they are needed in very small amounts. Many of the vitamins and minerals required in the diet are parts of enzymes.

An enzyme's shape is important in its action. Just as the shape of a key must fit that of its lock, an enzyme's shape must match the shape of the substrate it acts on. This so-called "lock-and-key" mechanism is illustrated in **Figure 2-11**. Harsh conditions, such as extremes of temperature or pH,

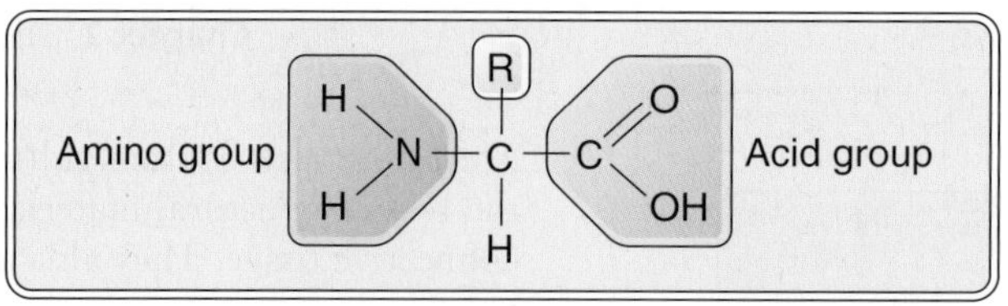

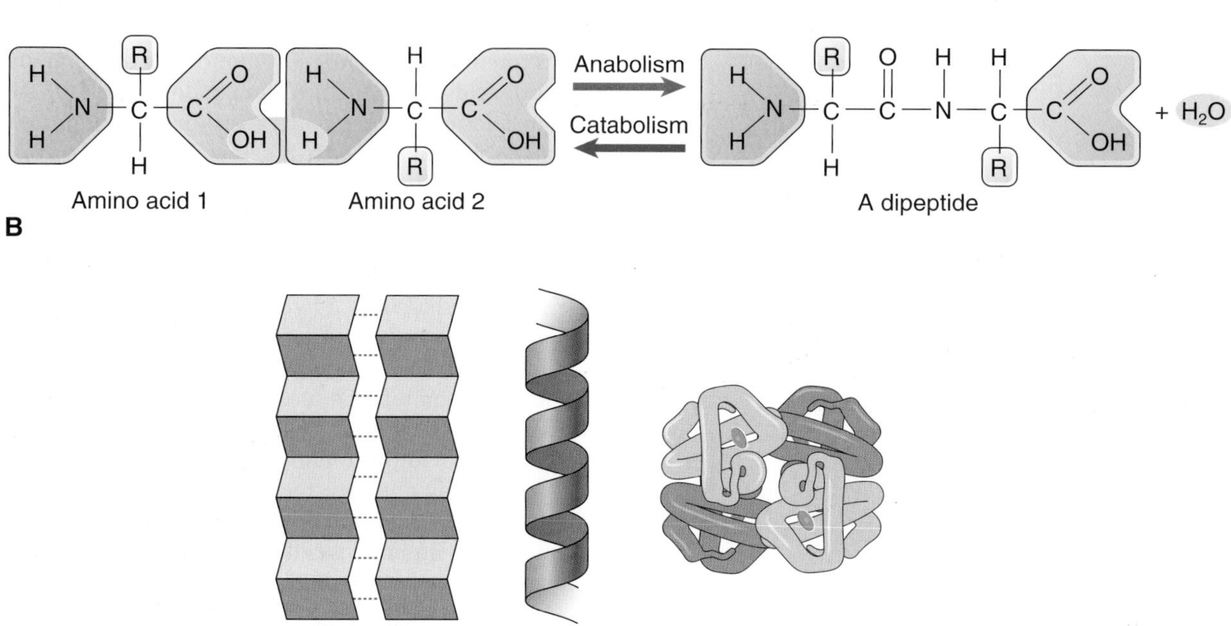

Figure 2-10 Proteins. KEY POINT **A.** Amino acids are the building blocks of proteins. Each amino acid contains an amino group and an acid group attached to a carbon atom. The remainder of the molecule (shown by R) can vary in 20 different ways. **B.** The acid group of one amino acid can react with the amino group of another forming a peptide bond. Further additions of amino acids result in formation of a polypeptide chain. **C.** Proteins have characteristic shapes, which are critical to their function. ZOOMING IN What part of an amino acid contains nitrogen?

can alter the shape of any protein, such as an enzyme, and destroy its ability to function. The alteration of a protein so that it can no longer function is termed **denaturation**. Such an event is always harmful to the cells.

You can usually recognize the names of enzymes because, with few exceptions, they end with the suffix *ase*. Examples are lipase, protease, and oxidase. The first part of the name usually refers to the substance acted on or the type of reaction in which the enzyme is involved.

NUCLEOTIDES

One additional class of organic compounds is composed of building blocks called **nucleotides** (NU-kle-o-tides) **(Fig. 2-12)**. A nucleotide contains:

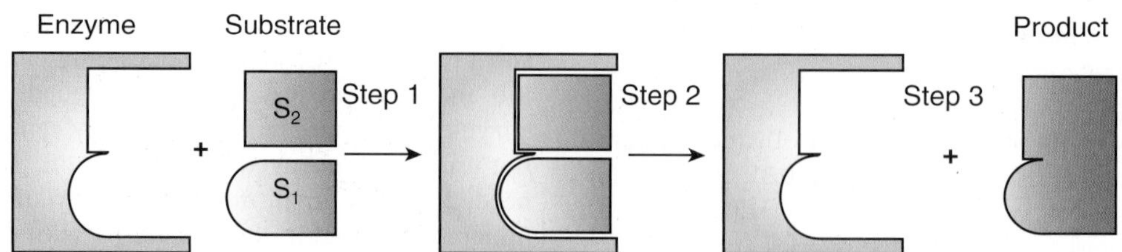

Figure 2-11 Diagram of enzyme action. KEY POINT An enzyme joins with substrate 1 (S_1) and substrate 2 (S_2) and speeds up the chemical reaction in which the two substrates bond. Once a new product is formed from the substrates, the enzyme is released unchanged. ZOOMING IN How does the shape of the enzyme before the reaction compare with its shape after the reaction?

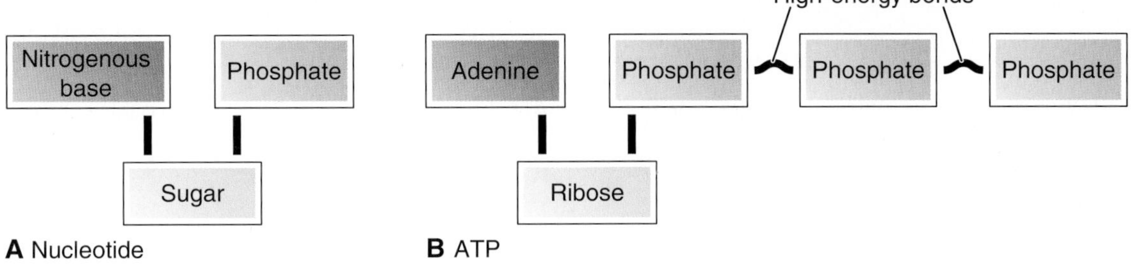

2

Figure 2-12 Nucleotides. KEY POINT **A.** A nucleotide consists of a nitrogenous base, a sugar, and one or more phosphate groups. **B.** ATP has high energy bonds between the phosphates. When these bonds are broken, energy is released. **ZOOMING IN** What does the prefix *tri* in adenosine triphosphate mean?

- A nitrogenous (nitrogen-containing) base.
- A sugar, usually a sugar called ribose or a related sugar called deoxyribose, which has one less oxygen atom.
- A phosphate group, which contains phosphorus. There may be more than one phosphate group in the nucleotide.

The nucleic acids DNA and RNA involved in the transmission of genetic traits and their expression in the cell are composed of nucleotides. These are discussed in further detail in Chapter 3. ATP, the cell's high energy compound, is a nucleotide. The extra energy in ATP is stored in special bonds between the nucleotide's three phosphates **(see Fig. 2-12B)**. When these bonds are broken catabolically, energy is released for cellular activities. Learn more about ATP and its role in metabolism in Chapter 18.

CHECKPOINTS 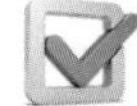

- **2-11** What element is the basis of organic chemistry?
- **2-12** What are the three main categories of organic compounds?
- **2-13** What is an enzyme?
- **2-14** What is in a nucleotide and what compounds are made of nucleotides?

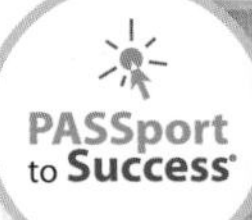

See the Student Resources on *thePoint* to view an animation on enzymes. In addition, the Health Professions box, Pharmacists and Pharmacy Technicians, describes some professions that require knowledge of chemistry.

A&P in Action Revisited

Margaret: Back in Balance

"Good morning, Mrs. Ringland. How are you feeling today?" asked Angela.

"Much better, thank you," replied Margaret. "I'm so grateful that my niece found me when she did."

"I'm glad, too," said Angela. "With the heat wave we're having, dehydration can become a very serious problem. Older adults are particularly at risk of dehydration because with age there usually is a decrease in muscle tissue, which contains a lot of water, and a relative increase in body fat, which does not. So, older adults don't have as much water reserve as younger adults. But," Angela continued as she flipped through Margaret's chart, "It looks like you're well on your way to a full recovery. Your electrolytes are back in balance. Your blood pressure is back to normal and your heart rate is good too. Your increased urine output tells me that your other organs are recovering as well."

"Does that mean I can get rid of this IV?" asked Margaret.

"Well, I'll check with your doctor first," replied Angela, "But, when you do have the IV removed, you will need to make sure that you drink plenty of fluids."

It was the end of another long shift and Angela was at her locker, changing into a pair of shorts and a T-shirt. As she closed her locker, she thought of Margaret once again. It always amazed her that chemistry could have such a huge impact on the body as a whole. She grabbed her water bottle, took a long drink, and headed out into the scorching heat.

In this case, we see that health professionals require a background in chemistry to understand how the body works—when healthy and when not. As you learn more about the human body, consider referring back to this chapter when necessary. For more information about the elements that make up every single substance within the body, see Appendix 1: Periodic Table of the Elements at the back of this book.

Chapter Wrap-Up

Summary Overview

A detailed chapter outline with space for note taking is on *thePoint*. The figure below illustrates the main topics covered in this chapter.

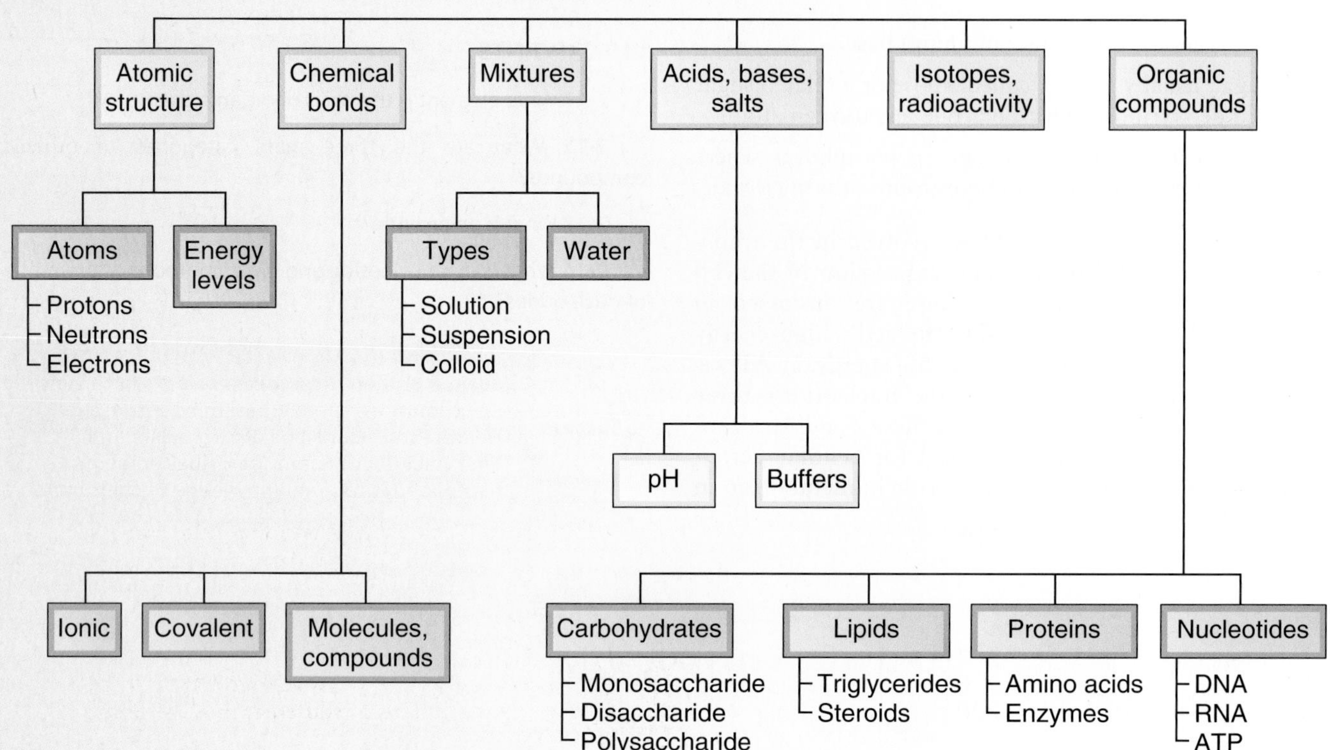

Key Terms

The terms listed below are emphasized in this chapter. Knowing them will help you organize and prioritize your learning. These and other boldface terms are defined in the Glossary with phonetic pronunciations.

acid
amino acid
anion
aqueous
atom
base
buffer
carbohydrate
catalyst
cation
chemistry
colloid
compound
denaturation
electrolyte
electron
element
enzyme
glucose
glycogen
ion
isotope
lipid
molecule
nucleotide
neutron
pH
protein
proton
radioactive
salt
solute
solution
solvent
steroid
substrate
suspension
valence

Word Anatomy

Scientific terms are built from standardized word parts (prefixes, roots, and suffixes). Learning the meanings of these parts can help you remember words and interpret unfamiliar terms.

WORD PART	MEANING	EXAMPLE
Chemical Bonds		
co-	together	*Covalent* bonds form when atoms share electrons.
Solutions and Suspensions		
aqu/e	water	In an *aqueous* solution, water is the solvent.
hom/o-	same	*Homogeneous* mixtures are the same throughout.
heter/o-	different	*Heterogeneous* solutions are different (not uniform) throughout.
hydr/o	water	*Dehydration* is a deficiency of water.
-phil	to like	*Hydrophilic* substances "like" water—they mix with or dissolve in it.
-phobia	fear	*Hydrophobic* substances "fear" water—they repel and do not dissolve in it.
Organic Compounds		
sacchar/o	sugar	A *monosaccharide* consists of one simple sugar.
mon/o-	one	In *monosaccharide*, "mono-" refers to one.
di-	twice, double	A *disaccharide* consists of two simple sugars.
poly-	many	A *polysaccharide* consists of many simple sugars.
glyc/o	sugar, glucose, sweet	*Glycogen* is a storage form of glucose. It breaks down to release glucose.
tri-	three	*Triglycerides* have one fatty acid attached to each of three carbon atoms.
de-	remove	*Denaturation* of a protein removes its ability to function (changes its nature).
-ase	suffix used in naming enzymes	*A lipase* is an enzyme that acts on lipids.

Questions for Study and Review

BUILDING UNDERSTANDING

Fill in the blanks

1. The subunits of elements are atoms.
2. The atomic number is the number of protons in an atom's nucleus.
3. A mixture of solute dissolved in solvent is called a(n) solution.
4. Blood has a pH of 7.35 to 7.45. Gastric juice has a pH of about 2.0. The more alkaline fluid is blood.
5. Proteins that catalyze metabolic reactions are called enzymes

Matching > Match each numbered item with the most closely related lettered item.

E **6.** A simple carbohydrate such as glucose
A **7.** A complex carbohydrate such as glycogen
B **8.** An important component of cell membranes
C **9.** Examples include DNA, RNA, and ATP
D **10.** The basic building block of protein

a. polysaccharide
b. phospholipid
c. nucleotide
d. amino acid
e. monosaccharide

Multiple Choice

B **11.** What type of mixture is red blood cells "floating" in plasma?
a. compound
b. suspension
c. colloid
d. solution

D **12.** What is the most abundant compound in the body?
a. carbohydrate
b. protein
c. lipid
d. water

B **13.** Which compound releases ions when in solution?
a. solvent
b. electrolyte
c. anion
d. colloid

____ **14.** Which chemical can donate hydrogen ions to other substances?
a. acid
b. base
c. salt
d. catalyst

____ **15.** Which element is always found in organic compounds?
a. oxygen
b. carbon
c. nitrogen
d. phosphorus

UNDERSTANDING CONCEPTS

____ **16.** Compare and contrast the following terms:
a. element and atom
b. molecule and compound
c. proton, neutron, and electron
d. anion and cation
e. ionic bond and covalent bond
f. acid and base

17. What are some of the properties of water that make it an ideal medium for living cells?

18. What is pH? Discuss the role of buffers in maintaining pH homeostasis in the body.

19. What are the characteristics of organic compounds?

20. Compare and contrast carbohydrates, proteins, and nucleotides.

21. Describe three different types of lipids.

22. Define the term *enzyme* and discuss the relationship between enzyme structure and enzyme function.

CONCEPTUAL THINKING

23. Based on your understanding of strong acids and bases, why does the body have to be kept at a close-to-neutral pH?

24. In Margaret's case, she was hypotensive when she arrived at the hospital. Explain the link between dehydration and low blood pressure.

25. In Margaret's case, an aqueous solution of 5% dextrose was used to rehydrate her. Name the solution's solute and solvent.

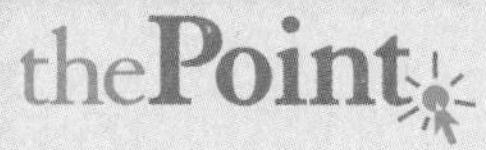

For more questions, see the learning activities on *thePoint*.

CHAPTER 3

Cells and Their Functions

A&P in Action

Jim's Case: How Cellular Events Affect the Whole Body

The buzzer sounded, signaling the end of the third quarter, and the Legal Eagles trailed by 10 points. Jim slammed the basketball down with disgust—he wasn't about to lose to a bunch of accountants. As usual, he'd have to step up his game to make up for the rest of the team.

Jim's attitude on the basketball court reflected his approach off the court. He worked long hours and had little patience for anyone who did not keep up with his grueling pace. By some accounts, Jim was a success—he was a partner in a large downtown law firm, he owned a big house, and he drove a fast car. However, his success came at a heavy cost. Jim's body wasn't keeping up with his lifestyle. He was overweight, out of shape, and had high blood pressure. The extra blood vessels needed to feed Jim's fat cells (called adipocytes) required his heart to pump harder to force blood through them. Since most cardiac muscle cells lack the ability to replicate themselves (a process called mitosis), they responded by synthesizing more contractile proteins. This allowed his cardiac muscle to contract with more force, but also resulted in thickening of the heart walls, which, in the long run, had actually decreased his heart's efficiency.

Hypertension wasn't the only problem with Jim's cardiovascular system. Cholesterol from Jim's lipid-rich diet formed growths, called plaques, in the walls of many of his blood vessels. In his heart, fatty plaques bulged into the lumens of the coronary arteries, obstructing blood flow to his cardiac muscle cells. Over the years, Jim's coronary arteries compensated for his heart's lack of oxygen and nutrients by growing new vessel branches around the blockages—natural bypasses, made possible by mitosis, which reestablished blood flow to the muscle cells. At the best of times, Jim's heart received just enough oxygen and nutrients to pump adequate amounts of blood to his cells. Playing in the basketball game today, Jim had placed an unusually high demand on his heart, and it was having a difficult time keeping up.

The buzzer sounded again, signaling the start of the fourth quarter. With great effort, Jim won the jump ball, and his team began to move toward their opponents' basket. Jim was left behind at center court when he crumpled to the ground, clutching his chest, his cardiovascular system unable to meet the demands of his cardiac muscle. Jim was having a heart attack.

As we will see later, oxygen deficiency caused irreparable damage to Jim's cardiac muscle cells. When reading Chapter 3, keep in mind that events at the cellular level have ramifications for the structure and function of tissues, organs, and even the whole body.

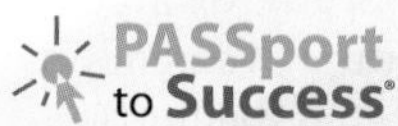

Ancillaries *At-A-Glance*

Visit *thePoint* to access the PASSport to Success and the following resources. For guidance in using these resources most effectively, see pp. ix–xviii.

Learning TOOLS

- Learning Style Self-Assessment
- Live Advise Online Student Tutoring
- Tips for Effective Studying

Learning RESOURCES

- E-book: Chapter 3
- Web Figure: Electron micrograph of an animal cell magnified over 48,000 times
- Web Figure: Electron micrograph of an animal cell magnified over 20,000 times
- Web Figure: Electron micrograph of a replicated chromosome
- Animation: Osmosis
- Animation: Function of Proteins in the Plasma Membrane
- Animation: The Cell Cycle and Mitosis
- Health Professions: Cytotechnologist
- Detailed Chapter Outline
- Answers to Questions for Study and Review
- Audio Pronunciation Glossary

Learning ACTIVITIES

- Pre-Quiz
- Visual Activities
- Kinesthetic Activities
- Auditory Activities

Learning Outcomes

After careful study of this chapter, you should be able to:

1 List three types of microscopes used to study cells, ***p. 38***

2 Describe the composition and functions of the plasma membrane, ***p. 39***

3 Describe the cytoplasm of the cell, including the name and function of the main organelles, ***p. 42***

4 Describe methods by which substances enter and leave cells that do not require cellular energy, ***p. 44***

5 Describe methods by which substances enter and leave cells that require cellular energy, ***p. 47***

6 Explain what will happen if cells are placed in solutions with concentrations the same as or different from those of the cell fluids, ***p. 47***

7 Describe the composition, location, and function of the DNA in the cell, ***p. 48***

8 Compare the function of three types of RNA in cells, ***p. 51***

9 Explain briefly how cells make proteins, ***p. 51***

10 Name and briefly describe the stages in mitosis, ***p. 53***

11 Use the case study to discuss the importance of cells to the functioning of the body as a whole, ***pp. 36, 55***

12 Show how word parts are used to build words related to cells and their functions (see Word Anatomy at the end of the chapter), ***p. 57***

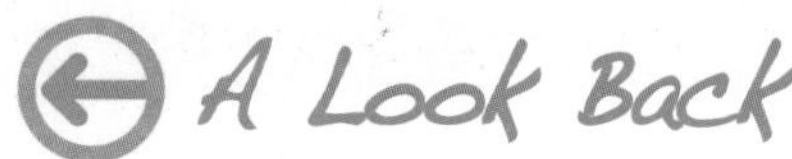

The chemicals we learned about in Chapter 2 are the building blocks of cells, the fundamental structures of all organisms. In this chapter, we will also learn more about the nucleotides, first introduced in Chapter 2.

The cell is the basic unit of all life. It is the simplest structure that shows all the characteristics of life, including organization, metabolism, responsiveness, homeostasis, growth, and reproduction. In fact, it is possible for a single cell to live independently of other cells. Examples of some free-living cells are microscopic organisms such as protozoa and bacteria, some of which produce disease. As we saw in Chapter 1, cells make up all tissues in a multicellular organism. All the activities of the human body, which is composed of trillions of cells, result from the activities of individual cells. Cells produce all the materials manufactured within the body.

Microscopes

The study of cells is **cytology** (si-TOL-o-je). Scientists first saw the outlines of cells in dried plant tissue almost 350 years ago. They were using a **microscope**, a magnifying instrument that allowed them for the first time to examine structures not visible with the naked eye. Study of a cell's internal structure, however, depended on improvements in the design of the single-lens microscope used in the late seventeenth century. The following three microscopes, among others, are used today:

- The **compound light microscope** is the microscope most commonly used in laboratories. This instrument, which can magnify an object up to 1,000 times, has two lenses and uses visible light for illumination.
- The **transmission electron microscope** (**TEM**) uses an electron beam in place of visible light and can magnify an image up to 1 million times.
- The **scanning electron microscope** (**SEM**) does not magnify as much as the TEM (100,000×) and shows only surface features; however, it provides a three-dimensional view of an object.

Figure 3-1 shows some cell structures viewed with each of these types of microscopes. The structures are cilia—short, hairlike projections from the cell that move nearby fluids. The metric unit used for microscopic measurements is the **micrometer** (MI-kro-me-ter). This unit is 1/1,000 of a millimeter and is abbreviated as mcm.

Before scientists can examine cells and tissues under a microscope, they must usually color them with special dyes called *stains* to aid in viewing. These stains produce the

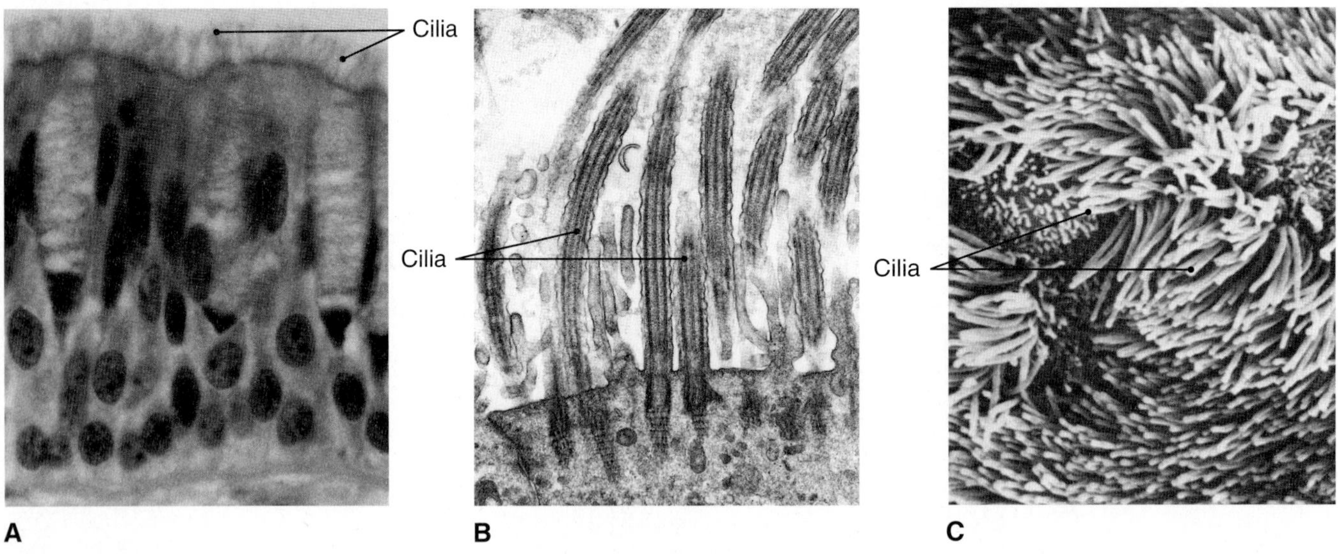

Figure 3-1 Cilia photographed under three different microscopes. KEY POINT Each type of microscope produces a different type of image that reveals different aspects of structure. **A.** Cilia (hairlike projections) in cells lining the trachea under the highest magnification of a compound light microscope (1,000×). **B.** Cilia in the bronchial lining viewed with a transmission electron microscope (TEM). Internal components are visible at this much higher magnification. **C.** Cilia on cells lining an oviduct as seen with a scanning electron microscope (SEM) (7,000×). A three-dimensional view can be seen. (A, Reprinted with permission from Cormack DH. *Essential Histology*, 2nd ed. Philadelphia, PA: Lippincott Williams & Wilkins, 2001; B, Reprinted with permission from Quinton P, Martinez R, eds. *Fluid and Electrolyte Transport in Exocrine Glands in Cystic Fibrosis*. San Francisco, CA: San Francisco Press, 1982; C, Reprinted with permission from Hafez ESE. *Scanning Electron Microscopic Atlas of Mammalian Reproduction*. Tokyo, Japan: Igaku Shoin, 1975.) ZOOMING IN Which microscope shows the most internal structure of the cilia? Which shows the cilia in three dimensions?

variety of colors seen in photographs (micrographs) of cells and tissues taken under a microscope.

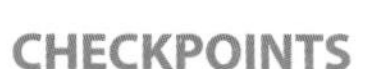
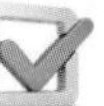

CHECKPOINTS

- 3-1 What characteristics of life does a cell show?
- 3-2 Name three types of microscopes.

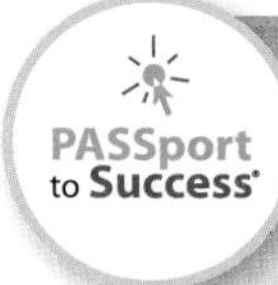

PASSport to Success

See the student resources on *thePoint* for information on careers in cytotechnology, the clinical laboratory study of cells, as well as to view electron micrographs of the cell.

Cell Structure

Just as people may look different but still have certain features in common—two eyes, a nose, and a mouth, for example—all cells share certain characteristics. Refer to **Figure 3-2** as we describe some of the structures that are common to most animal cells. A summary table follows the descriptions.

PLASMA MEMBRANE

The outer layer of the cell is the **plasma membrane** (**Fig. 3-3**). (This cell part is still often called the *cell membrane*, although this older term fails to distinguish between the cell's outer membrane and other internal cellular membranes.) The plasma membrane not only encloses the cell contents but also participates in many cellular activities, such as growth, reproduction, and communication between cells, and is especially important in regulating what can enter and leave the cell.

The plasma membrane may also function in absorption of materials from the cell's environment. For this purpose, the membrane of some cells is folded out into multiple small projections called *microvilli* (mi-kro-VIL-li; **see Fig. 3-2**). These projections increase the membrane's surface area, allowing for greater absorption, much as a sponge's many holes provide increased surface for absorption. Microvilli are found on cells that line the small intestine, where they promote absorption of digested foods into the circulation. They are also found on kidney cells, where they reabsorb materials that have been filtered out of the blood.

Components of the Plasma Membrane The main substance of the plasma membrane is a double layer—or bilayer—of lipid molecules. Because these lipids contain the element phosphorus, they are called *phospholipids*. We introduced these lipids in Chapter 2, along with cholesterol, another type of lipid found in the plasma membrane. Molecules of cholesterol are located between the phospholipids, and strengthen the membrane.

Carbohydrates are present in small amounts in the membrane, combined either with proteins (glycoproteins) or with lipids (glycolipids). These carbohydrates help cells

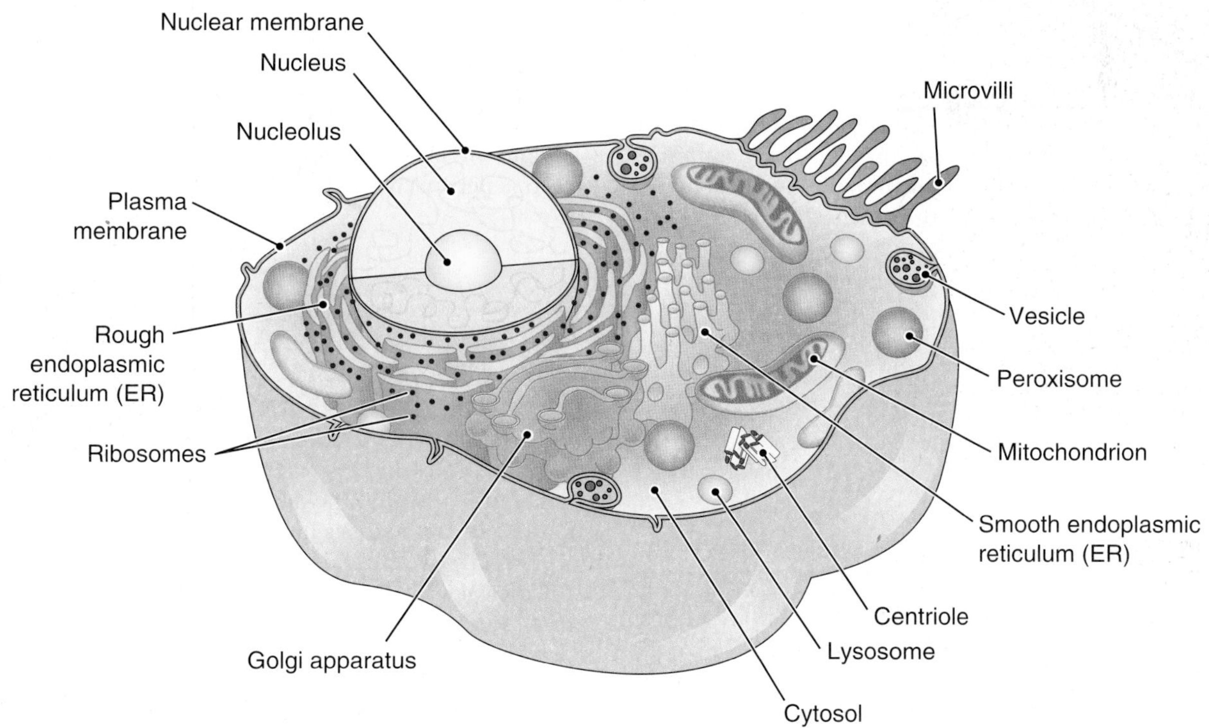

Figure 3-2 A generalized animal cell, sectional view. ZOOMING IN What is attached to the ER to make it look rough? What is the liquid part of the cytoplasm called?

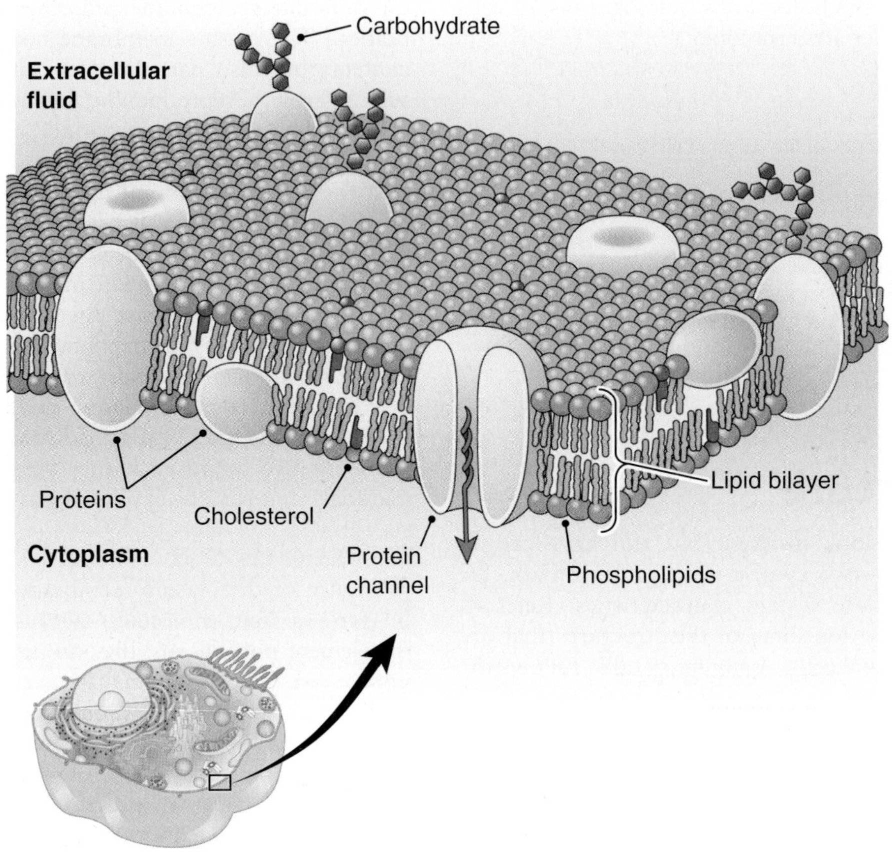

Figure 3-3 The plasma membrane. This drawing shows the current concept of its structure. KEY POINT The membrane is composed of a double layer of phospholipids with proteins and other materials imbedded in it. ZOOMING IN Why is the plasma membrane described as a bilayer?

to recognize each other and to stick together. A variety of different proteins float within the lipid bilayer. Some of these proteins extend all the way through the membrane, and some are located near the membrane's inner or outer surface. The importance of these proteins will be revealed in later chapters, but they are listed here along with their function, as well as summarized and illustrated in Table 3-1.

- Channels—pores in the membrane that allow specific substances to enter or leave. Certain ions travel through channels in the membrane.
- Transporters—shuttle substances from one side of the membrane to the other. Glucose, for example, is carried into cells using transporters.
- Receptors—points of attachment for materials coming to the cell in the blood or tissue fluid. Some hormones, for example, must attach to receptors on the cell surface before they can act upon the cell, as described in Chapter 11 on the endocrine system.
- Enzymes—participate in reactions occurring at the plasma membrane.
- Linkers—give shape to the membrane and help cells attach to each other.
- Cell identity markers—proteins unique to an individual's cells. These are important in the immune system and are also a factor in transplantation of tissue from one person to another.

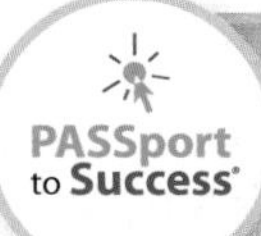

See the student resources on *thePoint* to view an animation on the functions of proteins in the plasma membrane.

The Membrane Potential The plasma membrane of a living cell carries a difference in electric charge (voltage) on either side which is known as a **membrane** (or transmembrane) **potential** (po-TEN-shal). This difference is created by positive and negative ions, mainly Na^+ (sodium), K^+ (potassium), Cl^- (chloride), and Ca^{2+} (calcium), concentrated on either side of the membrane and by negatively charged proteins held inside (Fig. 3-4). Ion concentrations are determined by:

- Channels in the plasma membrane, which may be opened or closed to the ions at any given time
- Specific ion transporters, or pumps, that can move the ions across the membrane

Table 3-1 Proteins in the Plasma Membrane and Their Functions

Type of Protein	Function	Illustration
Channels	Pores in the membrane that allow passage of specific substances, such as ions	
Transporters	Shuttle substances, such as glucose, across the membrane	
Receptors	Allow for attachment of substances, such as hormones, to the membrane	
Enzymes	Participate in reactions at the surface of the membrane	
Linkers	Give structure to the membrane and attach cells to other cells	
Cell identity markers	Proteins unique to a person's cells; important in the immune system and in transplantation of tissue from one person to another	

In a resting state, the inside of the membrane is negative by about 70 mV as compared to the outside. This electric charge can provide power, much like a battery, for driving membrane functions. In mitochondria, it is used to generate ATP. The membrane potential is also important in cellular communication.

Change in the potential can also be used to transmit signals from one part of the membrane to another, as it does in nerve cells. A reversal of the potential at one point creates a reversal of charge along the membrane (outside more negative; inside more positive), much like an electric current. Such reversals can be initiated by several forces, including chemicals, electric energy (voltage), and various other physical stimuli, such as light and pressure. We will learn more about the value of the membrane potential when we discuss the nervous, muscular, and cardiovascular systems.

THE NUCLEUS

Just as the body has different organs to carry out special functions, the cell contains specialized structures that perform different tasks **(Table 3-2)**. These structures are called **organelles,** which means "little organs." The largest of the organelles is the **nucleus** (NU-kle-us), which is surrounded by a membrane, the *nuclear membrane*, that encloses its contents.

The nucleus is often called the *control center* of the cell because it contains the **chromosomes** (KRO-mo-somes), the threadlike units of heredity that are passed on from parents to their children. It is information contained in the chromosomes that governs all cellular activities, as described later in this chapter. Most of the time, the chromosomes are loosely distributed throughout the nucleus, giving it a uniform, dark appearance when stained and examined under a microscope

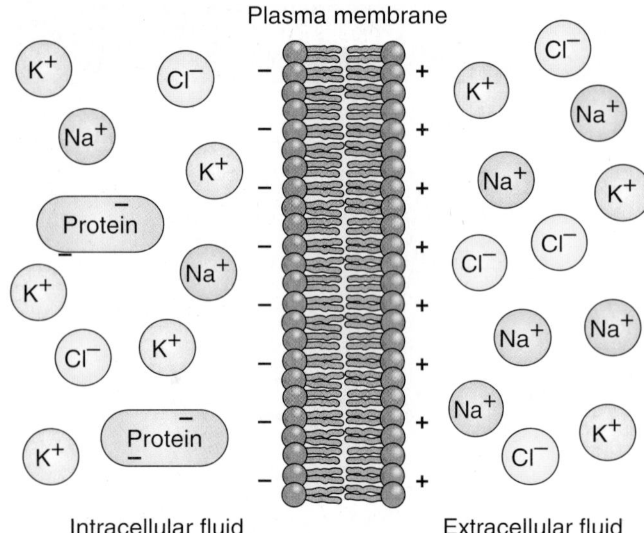

Figure 3-4 The membrane potential. KEY POINT The plasma membrane carries an electric charge created by ions on either side of the membrane. Sodium (Na^+) and chloride (Cl^-) ions predominate in the extracellular fluid; potassium (K^+) ions predominate in the intracellular fluid. Calcium (Ca^{2+}) ions also may be important, but are not shown on this diagram. ZOOMING IN What large, negatively charged ions contribute to the negative charge along the intracellular plasma membrane?

(see Fig. 3-2). When the cell is dividing, however, the chromosomes tighten into their visible threadlike forms.

Within the nucleus is a smaller globule called the **nucleolus** (nu-KLE-o-lus), which means "little nucleus." The job of the nucleolus is to assemble ribosomes, small bodies outside the nucleus that are involved in the manufacture of proteins.

THE CYTOPLASM

The remaining organelles are part of the **cytoplasm** (SI-to-plazm), the material that fills the cell from the nuclear membrane to the plasma membrane. The liquid part of the cytoplasm is the **cytosol**, a suspension of nutrients, electrolytes, enzymes, and other specialized materials in water. The main organelles are described here (see Table 3-2).

The **endoplasmic reticulum** (en-do-PLAS-mik re-TIK-u-lum) is a membranous network located between the nuclear membrane and the plasma membrane. Its name literally means "network" (reticulum) "within the cytoplasm" (endoplasmic), but for ease, it is almost always called simply the **ER**. In some areas, the ER appears to have an even surface and is described as *smooth ER*. This type of ER is involved with the synthesis of lipids. In other areas, the ER has a gritty, uneven surface, causing it to be described as *rough ER*. The rough ER's texture comes from small bodies, called **ribosomes** (RI-bo-somz), attached to its surface. Ribosomes are necessary for the manufacture of proteins, as described later. Recall that ribosomes are assembled in the nucleolus. They may then become attached to the ER or be free in the cytoplasm.

The **mitochondria** (mi-to-KON-dre-ah) are large, round or bean-shaped organelles with folded membranes on the inside. Within the mitochondria, the energy from nutrients is converted to cellular energy in the form of ATP. Mitochondria are the cell's "power plants." Active cells,

Box 3-1 *Clinical Perspectives*

Lysosomes and Peroxisomes: Cellular Recycling

Two organelles that play a vital role in cellular disposal and recycling are lysosomes and peroxisomes. **Lysosomes** contain enzymes that break down carbohydrates, lipids, proteins, and nucleic acids. These powerful enzymes must be kept within the lysosome because they would digest the cell if they escaped. In a process called **autophagy** (aw-TOF-ah-je), the cell uses lysosomes to safely recycle cellular structures, fusing with and digesting worn-out organelles. The digested components then return to the cytoplasm for reuse. Lysosomes also break down foreign material, as when cells known as **phagocytes** (FAG-o-sites) engulf bacteria and then use lysosomes to destroy them. The cell may also use lysosomes to digest itself during **autolysis** (aw-TOL-ih-sis), a normal part of development. *Auto-* means "self," and cells that are no longer needed "self-destruct" by releasing lysosomal enzymes into their own cytoplasm.

Peroxisomes are small membranous sacs that resemble lysosomes but contain different kinds of enzymes. They break down toxic substances that may enter the cell, such as drugs and alcohol, but their most important function is to break down free radicals. These substances are by-products of normal metabolic reactions but can kill the cell if not neutralized by peroxisomes.

Disease may result if either lysosomes or peroxisomes are unable to function. In Tay–Sachs disease, nerve cells' lysosomes lack an enzyme that breaks down certain kinds of lipids. These lipids build up inside the cells, causing malfunction that leads to brain injury, blindness, and death. Disease may also result if lysosomes or peroxisomes function when they should not. Some investigators believe this is the case in autoimmune diseases, in which the body develops an immune response to its own cells. Phagocytes engulf the cells and lysosomes destroy them. In addition, body cells themselves may self-destruct through autolysis. The joint disease rheumatoid arthritis is one such example.

Table 3-2 Cell Parts

Name	Description	Function
PLASMA MEMBRANE	Outer layer of the cell; composed mainly of lipids and proteins	Encloses the cell contents; regulates what enters and leaves the cell; participates in many activities, such as growth, reproduction, and interactions between cells
Microvilli	Short extensions of the plasma membrane	Absorb materials into the cell
NUCLEUS	Large, dark-staining organelle near the center of the cell, composed of DNA and proteins	Contains the chromosomes, the hereditary direct all cellular activities
Nucleolus	Small body in the nucleus; composed of RNA, DNA, and protein	Makes ribosomes
CYTOPLASM	Colloidal suspension that fills the cell from the nuclear membrane to the plasma membrane	Site of many cellular activities; consists of cytosol and organelles
Cytosol	The fluid portion of the cytoplasm	Surrounds the organelles
Endoplasmic reticulum (ER)	Network of membranes within the cytoplasm. Rough ER has ribosomes attached to it; smooth ER does not	Rough ER sorts proteins and forms them into more complex compounds; smooth ER is involved with lipid synthesis
Ribosomes	Small bodies free in the cytoplasm or attached to the ER; composed of RNA and protein	Manufacture proteins
Mitochondria	Large organelles with internal folded membranes	Convert energy from nutrients into ATP
Golgi apparatus	Layers of membranes	Makes compounds containing proteins; sorts and prepares these compounds for transport to other parts of the cell or out of the cell
Lysosomes	Small sacs of digestive enzymes	Digest substances within the cell
Peroxisomes	Membrane-enclosed organelles containing enzymes	Break down harmful substances
Vesicles	Small membrane-bound sacs in the cytoplasm	Store materials and move materials into or out of the cell in bulk
Centrioles	Rod-shaped bodies (usually two) near the nucleus	Help separate the chromosomes during cell division
SURFACE PROJECTIONS	Structures that extend from the cell	Move the cell or the fluids around the cell
Cilia	Short, hairlike projections from the cell	Move the fluids around the cell
Flagellum	Long, whiplike extension from the cell	Moves the cell

such as muscle cells or sperm cells, need lots of energy and thus have large numbers of mitochondria.

Another organelle in a typical cell is the **Golgi** (GOL-je) **apparatus** (also called Golgi complex), a stack of membranous sacs involved in sorting and modifying proteins and then packaging them for export from the cell.

Several types of organelles appear as small sacs in the cytoplasm. These include **lysosomes** (LI-so-somz), which contain digestive enzymes. (The root *lys/o* means "dissolving" or "separating.") Lysosomes remove waste and foreign materials from the cell. They are also involved in destroying old and damaged cells as needed for repair and remodeling of tissue. **Peroxisomes** (per-OK-sih-somz) have enzymes that destroy harmful substances produced in metabolism (see Box 3-1). **Vesicles** (VES-ih-klz) are small, membrane-bound storage sacs. They can be used to move materials into or out of the cell, as described later.

Centrioles (SEN-tre-olz) are rod-shaped bodies near the nucleus that function in cell division. They help to organize the cell and divide the cell contents during this process.

SURFACE ORGANELLES

Some cells have structures projecting from their surface that are used for motion. **Cilia** (SIL-e-ah) are small, hairlike projections that wave, creating movement of the fluids around the cell (see Fig. 3-1). For example, cells that line the passageways of the respiratory tract have cilia that move impurities out of the system. Ciliated cells move the egg cell from the ovary to the uterus in the female reproductive tract.

A long, whiplike extension from a cell is a **flagellum** (flah-JEL-lum). The only type of cell in the human body that has a flagellum is the male sperm cell. Each human sperm cell has a flagellum that propels it toward the egg in the female reproductive tract.

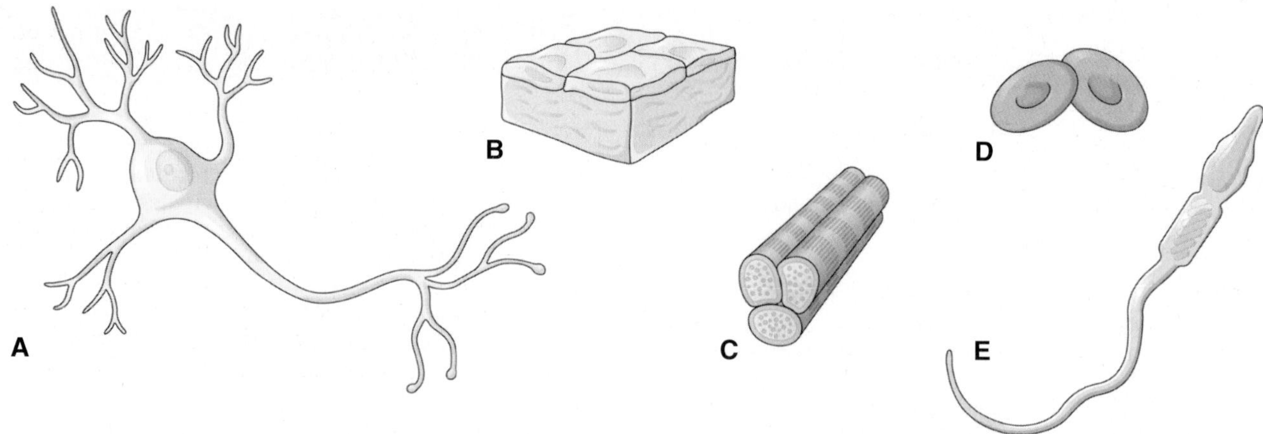

Figure 3-5 Cellular diversity. KEY POINT Cells vary in structure according to their functions. **A.** A neuron has long extensions that pick up and transmit electric impulses. **B.** Epithelial cells cover and protect underlying tissue. **C.** Muscle cells have fibers that produce contraction. **D.** Red blood cells lose most organelles, which maximize their oxygen-carrying capacity, and have a small, round shape that lets them slide through blood vessels. **E.** A sperm cell is small and light and swims with a flagellum. ZOOMING IN Which of the cells shown would best cover a large surface area?

CELLULAR DIVERSITY

Although all cells have some fundamental similarities, individual cells may vary widely in size, shape, and composition according to their function. The average cell size is 10 to 15 mcm, but cells may range in size from the 7 mcm of a red blood cell to the 200 mcm or more in the length of a muscle cell.

Cell shape is related to cell function **(Fig. 3-5)**. A neuron (nerve cell) has long fibers that transmit electric energy from place to place in the nervous system. Cells in surface layers have a modified shape that covers and protects the tissue beneath. Red blood cells are small and round, which lets them slide through tiny blood vessels. They also have an indented shape to provide more surface area for gas exchange. As red blood cells mature, they lose the nucleus and most other organelles, making the greatest possible amount of space available to carry oxygen.

Aside from cilia and flagella, all the organelles described above are present in most human cells. They may vary in number, however. For example, cells producing lipids have lots of smooth ER. Cells that secrete proteins have lots of ribosomes and a prominent Golgi apparatus. All active cells have lots of mitochondria to manufacture the ATP needed for energy.

CHECKPOINTS 

☐ 3-3 What is the main substance of the plasma membrane, and what are the three types of materials found within the membrane?

☐ 3-4 What is the membrane potential, and what types of substances maintain the membrane potential?

☐ 3-5 What are cell organelles?

☐ 3-6 Why is the nucleus called the cell's control center?

☐ 3-7 What are the two types of organelles used for movement, and what do they look like?

Movement of Substances across the Plasma Membrane

The plasma membrane serves as a barrier between the cell and its environment. Nevertheless, nutrients, oxygen, and many other substances needed by the cell must be taken in and waste products must be eliminated. Clearly, some substances can be exchanged between the cell and its environment through the plasma membrane. For this reason, the plasma membrane is described at a simple level as **semipermeable** (sem-e-PER-me-ah-bl). It is permeable, or passable, to some molecules but impassable to others.

The ability of a substance to travel through the membrane is based on several factors. Molecular size is one factor that determines passage. Nutrients, for example, must be split into small molecules by digestion in order to enter a cell. Solubility and electric charge are also considerations. In many cases, protein channels and transporters in the membrane help to move specific materials through.

Because size is not the only limiting factor in membrane transport, and because the plasma membrane also can select what will go through in either direction, the membrane is most accurately described, not as simply semipermeable, but as **selectively permeable**. It regulates what can enter and leave based on the cell's needs. Various physical processes are involved in exchanges through the plasma membrane. One way of grouping these processes is according to whether they do or do not require cellular energy.

MOVEMENT THAT DOES NOT REQUIRE CELLULAR ENERGY

The adjective *passive* describes movement through the plasma membrane that does not require energy output by the cell.

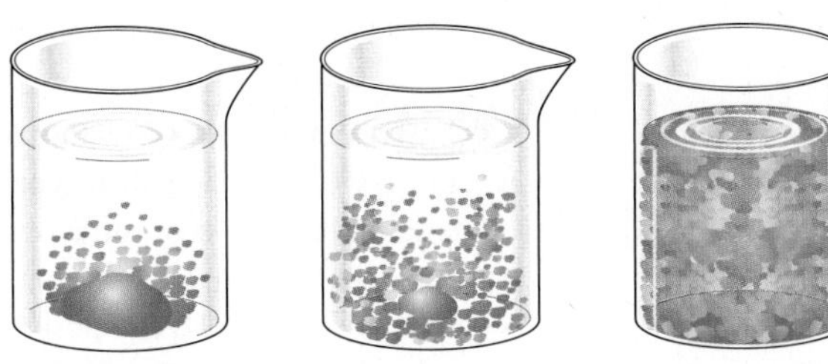

Figure 3-6 Diffusion of a solid in a liquid. KEY POINT The molecules of the solid tend to spread evenly throughout the liquid as they dissolve.

Passive mechanisms depend on the internal energy of the moving particles or the application of some outside source of energy. These methods include diffusion, facilitated diffusion, osmosis, and filtration.

Diffusion Diffusion is the constant movement of particles from a region of relatively higher concentration to one of lower concentration. Just as couples on a crowded dance floor spread out into all the available space to avoid hitting other dancers, diffusing substances spread throughout their available space until their concentration everywhere is the same—that is, they reach equilibrium (Fig. 3-6). This movement from higher to lower concentrations uses the particles' internal energy and does not require cellular energy, just as a sled will move from the top to the bottom of a snowy hill. The particles are said to follow their *concentration gradient* from higher concentration to lower concentration.

Simple diffusion through the plasma membrane is mostly limited to lipid-soluble substances that can dissolve in the membrane. Gases and lipids, for example, can diffuse freely into and out of the cells. Other substances, including water-soluble electrolytes and nutrients, require a modified form of diffusion called **facilitated diffusion**. In this process, water-soluble materials move across the plasma membrane in the direction of the concentration gradient (from higher to lower concentration), but transporters are used to move the material at a faster rate (Fig. 3-7). For example, glucose, the sugar that is the main energy source for cells, moves through the plasma membrane by means of facilitated diffusion.

Osmosis Osmosis (os-MO-sis) is a special type of diffusion. The term applies specifically to the diffusion of water through a semipermeable membrane. Water moves rapidly through the plasma membrane of most cells with the help of channels called *aquaporins* (a-kwa-POR-ins). The water molecules move, as expected, from an area where there are more of them to an area where there are fewer of them. That is, the solvent (the water molecules) moves from an area of lower *solute* concentration to an area of higher *solute* concentration, as demonstrated in Figure 3-8.

For a physiologist studying water's flow across membranes, as in exchange of fluids through capillaries in the circulation, it is helpful to know the direction in which water will flow and at what rate it will move. A measure of the force driving osmosis is called the *osmotic pressure*.

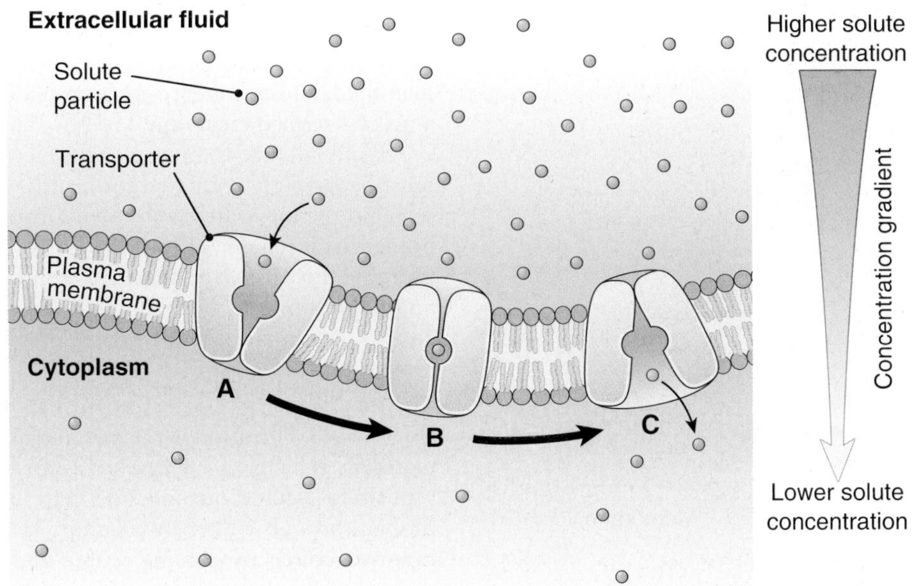

Figure 3-7 Facilitated diffusion. KEY POINT Protein transporters in the plasma membrane move solute particles through a membrane from an area of higher concentration to an area of lower concentration. **A.** A solute particle enters the transporter. **B.** The transporter changes shape. **C.** The transporter releases the solute particle on the other side of the membrane. ZOOMING IN How would a change in the number of transporters affect a solute's movement by facilitated diffusion?

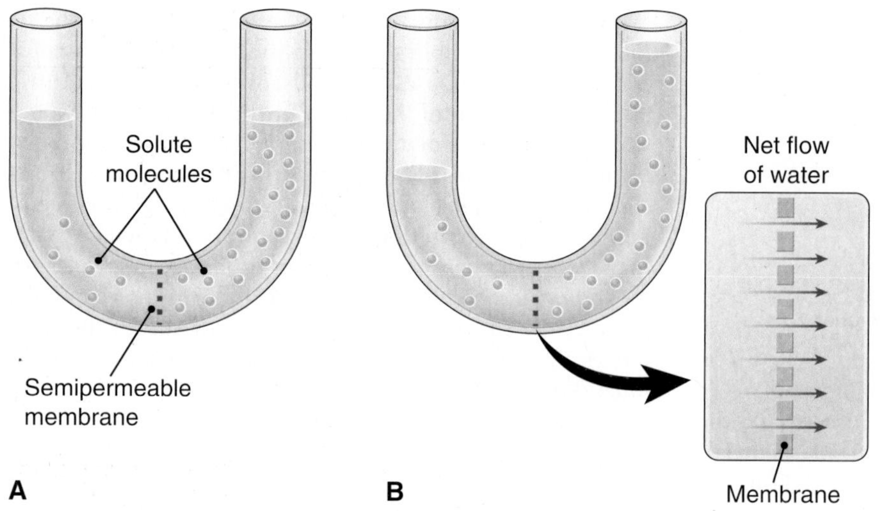

Figure 3-8 A simple demonstration of osmosis. KEY POINT The direction of water flow tends to equalize concentrations of solutions. Solute molecules are shown in *yellow*. All of the solvent (*blue*) is composed of water molecules. **A.** Two solutions with different concentrations of solute are separated by a semipermeable membrane. Water can flow through the membrane, but the solute cannot. **B.** Water flows into the more concentrated solution, raising the level of the liquid in that side. ZOOMING IN What would happen in this system if the solute could pass through the membrane?

This force can be measured, as illustrated in **Figure 3-9**, by applying enough pressure to the surface of a liquid to stop the inward flow of water by osmosis. The pressure needed to counteract osmosis is the osmotic pressure. In practice, the term *osmotic pressure* is used to describe a solution's tendency to draw water in. This force is directly related to concentration: the higher a solution's concentration, the greater is its tendency to draw water in.

How Osmosis Affects Cells Because water can move easily through the cell membrane, the fluid outside all cells must have the same concentration of dissolved substances (solutes) as the fluids inside the cells for maintenance of a normal fluid balance. If this balance is altered, water will move rapidly into or out of the cell by osmosis **(Fig. 3-10)**. Solutions with concentrations equal to the concentration of the cytoplasm are described as isotonic (i-so-TON-ik). Tissue fluids and blood plasma are isotonic for body cells. Manufactured solutions that are isotonic for the cells and can thus be used intravenously (IV) to replace body fluids include 0.9% salt, or normal saline, and 5% dextrose (glucose).

A solution that is less concentrated than the intracellular fluid is described as **hypotonic.** Based on the principles of osmosis already explained, a cell placed in a hypotonic solution draws water in, swells, and may burst, as happens to Jim's cardiac muscle cells in the case study. When a red blood cell draws in water and bursts in this way, the cell is said to undergo **hemolysis** (he-MOL-ih-sis). If a cell is placed in a **hypertonic** solution, which is more concentrated than the cellular fluid, it loses water to the surrounding fluids and shrinks, a process termed **crenation** (kre-NA-shun) **(see Fig. 3-10)**.

Fluid balance is an important facet of homeostasis and must be properly regulated for health. You can figure out in which direction water will move through the plasma membrane if you remember the saying "water follows salt," salt meaning any dissolved material (solute). The total amount and distribution of body fluids is discussed in Chapter 19. **Table 3-3** summarizes the effects of different solution concentrations on cells.

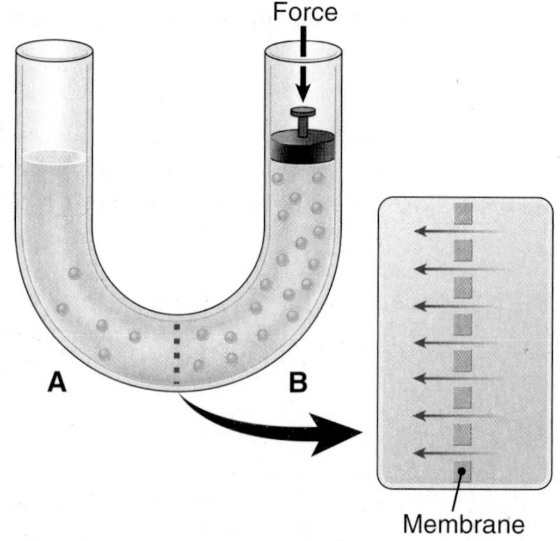

Figure 3-9 Osmotic pressure. KEY POINT Osmotic pressure is the force needed to stop the flow of water by osmosis. Pressure on the surface of the fluid in side B counteracts the osmotic flow of water from side A to side B. ZOOMING IN What would happen to osmotic pressure if the concentration of solute were increased on side B of this system?

Filtration Filtration is the passage of water and dissolved materials through a membrane as a result of a mechanical ("pushing") force on one side **(Fig. 3-11)**. In a car, oil is pushed through a filter by a pump. At home, one can make espresso coffee by forcing water and dissolved materials through a filter under pressure. An example of physiologic filtration is the movement of materials out of the capillaries and into the tissues under the force of blood pressure, created by heart contractions (see Chapter 14). Another example occurs in the kidneys as materials are filtered out of the blood in the first step of urine formation (see Chapter 19).

3

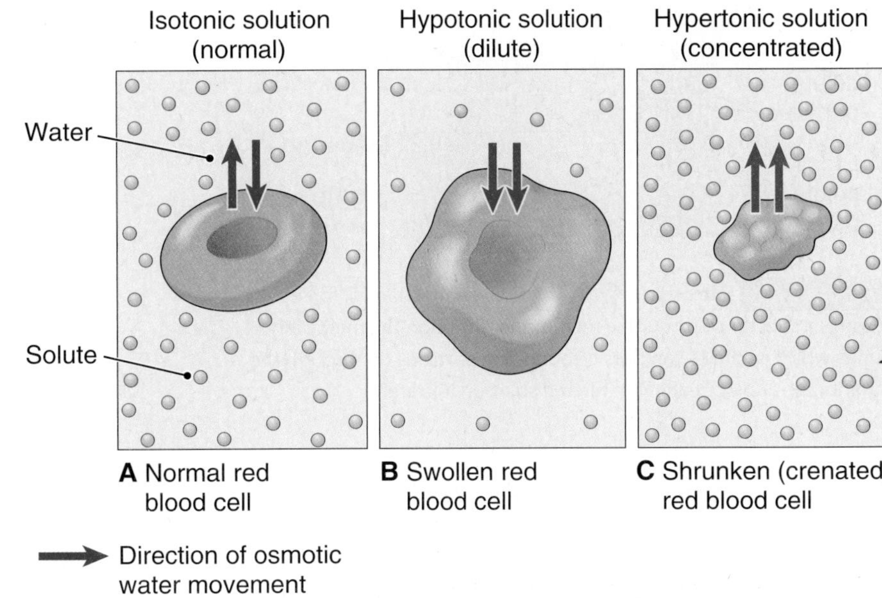

Figure 3-10 The effect of osmosis on cells. KEY POINT Cells must be kept in fluids that are compatible with the concentration of their intracellular fluid. This figure shows how water moves through a red blood cell membrane in solutions with three different concentrations of solute. **A.** The isotonic (normal) solution has the same concentration as the cellular fluid, and water moves into and out of the cell at the same rate. **B.** A cell placed in a hypotonic (more dilute) solution draws water in, causing the cell to swell and perhaps undergo hemolysis (bursting). **C.** The hypertonic (more concentrated) solution draws water out of the cell, causing it to shrink, an effect known as crenation. ZOOMING IN What would happen to red blood cells in the body if blood lost through injury were replaced with pure water?

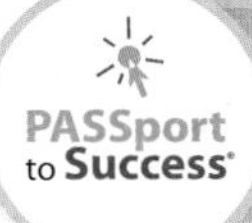

See the student resources on *thePoint* to view an animation on osmosis and osmotic pressure.

MOVEMENT THAT REQUIRES CELLULAR ENERGY

Movement across the membrane that requires energy is described as *active*. These methods include active transport and bulk transport.

Active Transport The plasma membrane has the ability to move small solute particles into or out of the cell opposite to the direction in which they would normally flow by diffusion. That is, the membrane moves them against the concentration gradient from an area where they are in relatively lower concentration to an area where they are in higher concentration. Because this movement goes against the natural flow of particles, it requires energy just as getting a sled to the top of a hill requires energy. For this reason, it is called **active transport**. It also requires transporters for the particles in the plasma membrane.

This process of active transport is one important function of the living cellular membrane. The nervous system and muscular system, for example, depend on the active transport of sodium, potassium, and calcium ions for proper function. The kidneys also carry out active transport in regulating the composition of urine. By means of active transport, the cell can take in what it needs from the surrounding fluids and remove materials from the cell.

Bulk Transport There are several active methods for moving large quantities of material into or out of the cell. These methods are grouped together as **bulk transport**,

Table 3-3 Solutions and Their Effects on Cells

Type of Solution	Description	Examples	Effect on Cells
Isotonic	Has the same concentration of dissolved substances as the fluid in the cell	0.9% salt (normal saline); 5% glucose (dextrose)	None; cell in equilibrium with its environment
Hypotonic	Has a lower concentration of dissolved substances than the fluid in the cell	Less than 0.9% salt or 5%	Cell takes in water, swells, and may burst; red blood cell undergoes hemolysis
Hypertonic	Has a higher concentration of dissolved substances than the fluid in the cell	Higher than 0.9% salt or 5% dextrose	Cell will lose water and shrink; cell undergoes crenation

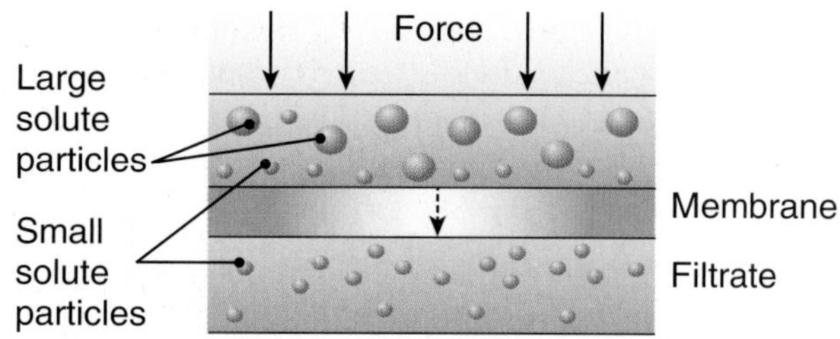

Figure 3-11 Filtration. KEY POINT A mechanical force pushes a substance through a membrane, although the membrane limits which particles can pass through. The particles go through the membrane and appear in the filtered solution (filtrate).

because of the amounts of material moved. They are also referred to as **vesicular transport**, because small sacs, or vesicles, are needed for the processes. These processes are grouped according to whether materials are moved into or out of the cells, as follows:

- **Endocytosis** (en-do-si-TO-sis) is a term that describes the bulk movement of materials into the cell. Some examples are
  - **Phagocytosis** (fag-o-si-TO-sis), in which relatively large particles are engulfed by the plasma membrane and moved into the cell **(Fig. 3-12)**. (The root *phag/o* means "to eat.") Certain white blood cells carry out phagocytosis to rid the body of foreign material and dead cells. Material taken into a cell by phagocytosis is first enclosed in a vesicle made from the plasma membrane and is later destroyed by lysosomes.
  - **Pinocytosis** (pi-no-si-TO-sis), in which the plasma membrane engulfs droplets of fluid. This is a way for large protein molecules in suspension to travel into the cell. The word *pinocytosis* means "cell drinking."
  - **Receptor-mediated endocytosis**, which involves the intake of substances using specific binding sites, or receptors, in the plasma membrane. The bound material, or *ligand* (LIG-and), is then drawn into the cell by endocytosis. Some examples of ligands are certain lipoproteins involved in cholesterol metabolism, some hormones, and certain vitamins. Cholesterol metabolism is mentioned in Jim's case study as it affects cardiovascular health.
- In **exocytosis**, the cell moves materials out in vesicles **(Fig. 3-13)**. One example of exocytosis is the export of neurotransmitters from neurons (neurotransmitters are chemicals that control the activity of the nervous system).

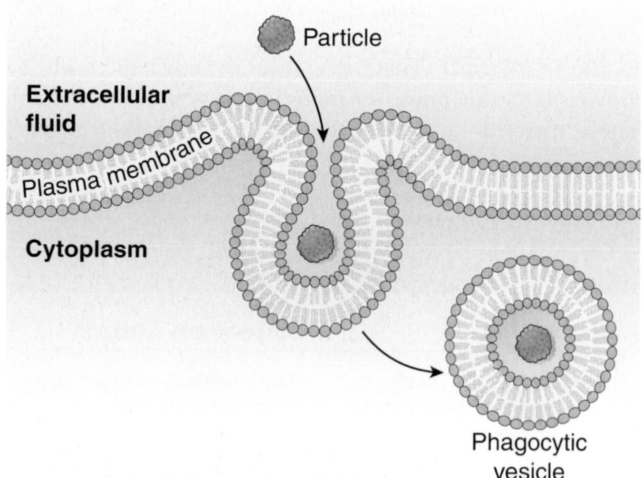

Figure 3-12 Phagocytosis. KEY POINT The plasma membrane encloses a particle from the extracellular fluid. The membrane then pinches off, forming a vesicle that carries the particle into the cytoplasm. ZOOMING IN What organelle would likely help to destroy a particle taken in by phagocytosis?

All the transport methods described above are summarized in **Table 3-4**.

CHECKPOINTS 

3-8 What types of movement through the plasma membrane do not require cellular energy, and what types of movement do require cellular energy?

3-9 What term describes a fluid that is the same concentration as the intracellular fluid? What type of fluid is less concentrated? More concentrated?

Protein Synthesis

Because proteins play an indispensable part in the body's structure and function, we need to identify the cellular substances that direct protein production. As noted earlier, the hereditary units that govern the cell are the chromosomes in the nucleus. Each chromosome in turn is divided into multiple subunits, called **genes (Fig. 3-14)**. It is the genes that carry the messages for the development of particular inherited characteristics, such as brown eyes, curly hair, or blood type, and they do so by directing protein manufacture in the cell.

STRUCTURE OF DNA AND RNA

Genes are distinct segments of the complex organic chemical that makes up the chromosomes, a substance called **deoxyribonucleic** (de-ok-se-RI-bo-nu-kle-ik) **acid**, or **DNA**. DNA is composed of subunits called nucleotides, introduced in Chapter 2 **(see Fig. 3-14)**. A related compound, **ribonucleic**

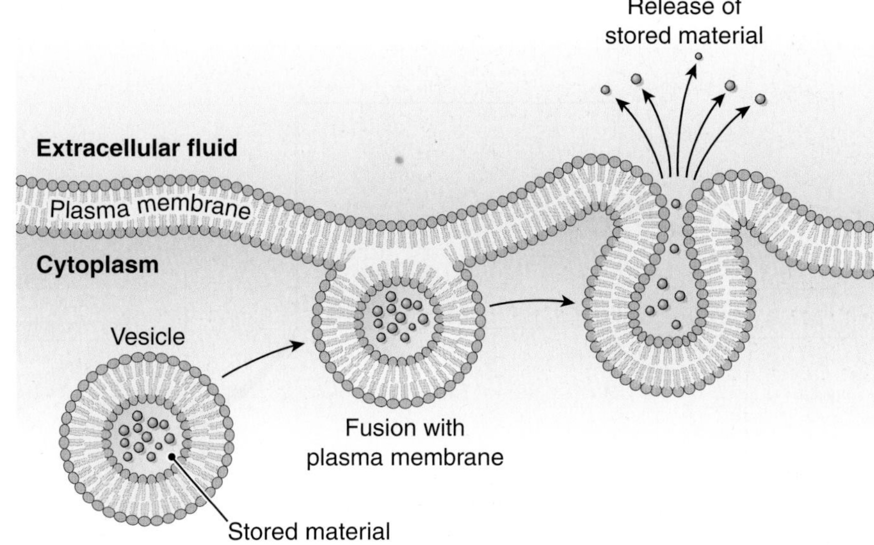

Figure 3-13 Exocytosis. KEY POINT A vesicle fuses with the plasma membrane then ruptures and releases its contents.

Table 3-4 Membrane Transport

Process	Definition	Example
Do not require cellular energy (passive)		
Diffusion	Random movement of particles with the concentration gradient (from higher concentration to lower concentration) until they reach equilibrium	Movement of lipid-soluble materials into and out of the cell
Facilitated diffusion	Movement of materials across the plasma membrane along the concentration gradient using transporters to speed the process	Movement of glucose into the cells
Osmosis	Diffusion of water through a semipermeable membrane	Movement of water across the plasma membrane
Filtration	Movement of materials through a membrane under mechanical force	Movement of materials out of the blood under the force of blood pressure
Require cellular energy		
Active transport	Movement of materials through the plasma membrane against the concentration gradient using transporters	Transport of ions (e.g., Na^+, K^+, and Ca^{2+}) in the nervous system and muscular system
Bulk transport	Movement of large amounts of material through the plasma membrane using vesicles; also called vesicular transport	
Endocytosis	Transport of bulk amounts of materials into the cell using vesicles	Phagocytosis—intake of large particles, as when white blood cells take in waste materials; also pinocytosis (intake of fluid), and receptor-mediated endocytosis, requiring binding sites in the plasma membrane
Exocytosis	Transport of bulk materials out of the cell using vesicles	Release of neurotransmitters from neurons

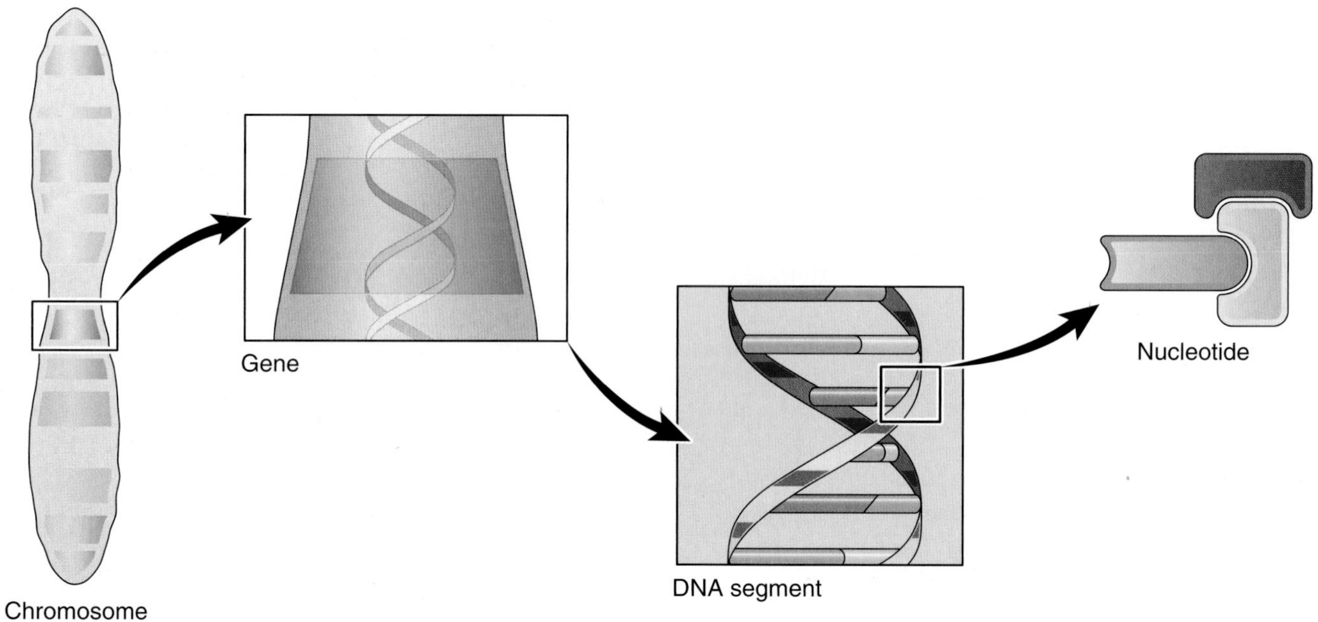

Figure 3-14 Subdivisions of a chromosome. KEY POINT A gene is a distinct region of a chromosome. The entire chromosome is made of DNA. Nucleotides are the building blocks of DNA.

(RI-bo-nu-kle-ik) **acid**, or **RNA**, which participates in protein synthesis but is not part of the chromosomes, is also composed of nucleotides. As noted, a nucleotide contains a sugar, a phosphate, and a nitrogen-containing base. The sugar and phosphate are constant in each nucleotide, although DNA has the sugar deoxyribose and RNA has the sugar ribose. The sugars and phosphates alternate to form a long chain to which the nitrogen bases are attached. The five different nucleotides that appear in DNA and RNA thus differ in the nature of their nitrogen base. Three of the five nucleotides are common to both DNA and RNA. These are the nucleotides containing the nitrogen bases adenine (A), guanine (G), and cytosine (C). However, DNA has one nucleotide containing thymine (T), whereas RNA has one containing uracil (U). Table 3-5 compares the structure and function of DNA and RNA.

DNA AND PROTEIN SYNTHESIS

Most of the DNA in the cell is organized into chromosomes within the nucleus (a small amount of DNA is in the mitochondria located in the cytoplasm). Figure 3-15 shows a section of a chromosome and illustrates that the DNA exists as a double strand. Visualizing the complete molecule as a ladder, the sugar and phosphate units of the nucleotides make up the "side rails" of the ladder, and the nitrogen bases project from the side rails to make up the ladder's "steps." The two DNA strands are paired very specifically according to

Table 3-5 Comparison of DNA and RNA

	DNA	RNA
Location	Almost entirely in the nucleus	Almost entirely in the cytoplasm
Composition	Nucleotides contain adenine (A), guanine (G), cytosine (C), or thymine (T) Sugar: deoxyribose	Nucleotides contain adenine (A), guanine (G), cytosine (C), or uracil (U) Sugar: ribose
Structure	Double-stranded helix formed by nucleotide pairing A–T; G–C	Single strand
Function	Makes up the chromosomes, hereditary units that control all cellular activities; divided into genes that carry the nucleotide codes for the manufacture of proteins	Manufacture proteins according to the codes carried in the DNA; three main types: messenger RNA(mRNA), ribosomal RNA (rRNA), and transfer RNA (tRNA)

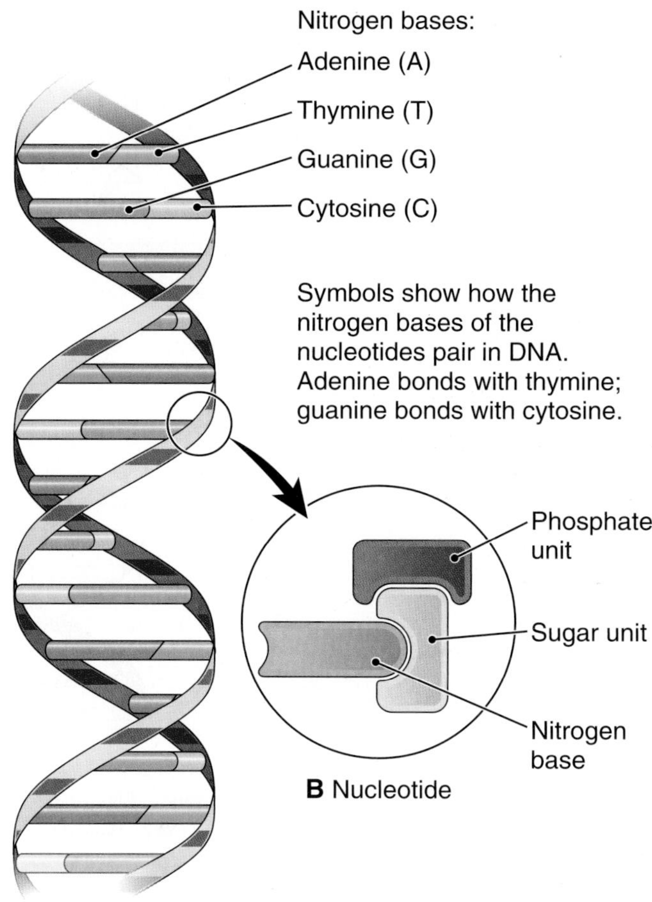

Figure 3-15 Structure of DNA. A. This schematic representation of a chromosomal segment shows the paired nucleic acid strands twisted into a double helix. **B.** Each structural unit, or nucleotide, consists of a phosphate unit and a sugar unit attached to a nitrogen base. The sugar unit in DNA is deoxyribose. KEY POINT There are four different nucleotides in DNA. Their arrangement "spells out" the genetic instructions that control all activities of the cell. ZOOMING IN Two of the DNA nucleotides (A and G) are larger in size than the other two (T and C). How do the nucleotides pair up with regard to size?

the identity of the nitrogen bases in the nucleotides. Adenine (A) always pairs with thymine (T); guanine (G) always pairs with cytosine (C). The two strands of DNA are held together by weak bonds (hydrogen bonds; see Box 2-1). The doubled strands then coil into a spiral, giving DNA the descriptive name *double helix*.

The message of the DNA that makes up the individual genes is actually contained in the varying pattern of the four nucleotides along the strand. The nucleotides are like four letters in an alphabet that can be combined in different ways to make a variety of words. The words represent the amino acids used to make proteins, and a long string of words makes up a gene. Each gene thus codes for the building of amino acids into a specific cellular protein. Remember that all enzymes are proteins, and enzymes are essential for all cellular reactions. DNA is thus the cell's master blueprint.

In light of observations on cellular diversity, you may wonder how different cells in the body can vary in appearance and function if they all have the same amount and same kind of DNA. The answer to this question is that only portions of the DNA in a given cell are active at any one time. In some cells, regions of the DNA can be switched on and off, under the influence of hormones, for example. However, as cells differentiate during development and become more specialized, regions of the DNA are permanently shut down, leading to the variations in the different cell types. Scientists now realize that the control of DNA action throughout a cell's life span is a very complex matter involving not only the DNA itself but proteins as well.

ROLE OF RNA IN PROTEIN SYNTHESIS

A blueprint is only a guide. The information it contains must be interpreted and acted upon, and RNA is the substance needed for these steps. RNA is much like DNA except that it exists as a single strand of nucleotides and has uracil (U) instead of thymine (T). Thus, when RNA pairs up with another molecule of nucleic acid to manufacture proteins, as explained below, adenine (A) bonds with uracil (U) instead of thymine (T).

A detailed account of protein synthesis is beyond the scope of this book, but a highly simplified description and illustrations of the process are presented. The process begins with the transfer of information from DNA to RNA in the nucleus, a process known as *transcription* (Fig. 3-16). Before transcription begins, the DNA breaks its weak bonds and uncoils into single strands. Then a matching strand of RNA forms along one of the DNA strands by the process of nucleotide pairing. For example, if the DNA strand reads CGAT, the corresponding mRNA will read GCUA. (Remember that RNA has U instead of T to bond with A.) When complete, this messenger RNA (mRNA) leaves the nucleus and travels to a ribosome in the cytoplasm (Fig. 3-17). Recall that ribosomes are the site of protein synthesis in the cell.

Ribosomes are composed of an RNA type called ribosomal RNA (rRNA) and also protein. At the ribosomes, the genetic message now contained within mRNA is decoded to build amino acids into the long chains that form proteins, a process termed *translation*. This final step requires a third RNA type, transfer RNA (tRNA), small molecules present in the cytoplasm (see Fig. 3-17). Note that both rRNA and tRNA are formed by the transcription process illustrated in Figure 3-16.

Each transfer RNA carries a specific amino acid that can be added to a protein chain. A nucleotide code on each tRNA determines whether or not its amino acid will be added. After the amino acid chain is formed, it must be coiled and folded into the proper shape for that protein, as noted in Chapter 2. Table 3-6 summarizes information on the different types of RNA. Also see Box 3-2, Proteomics: So Many Proteins, So Few Genes.

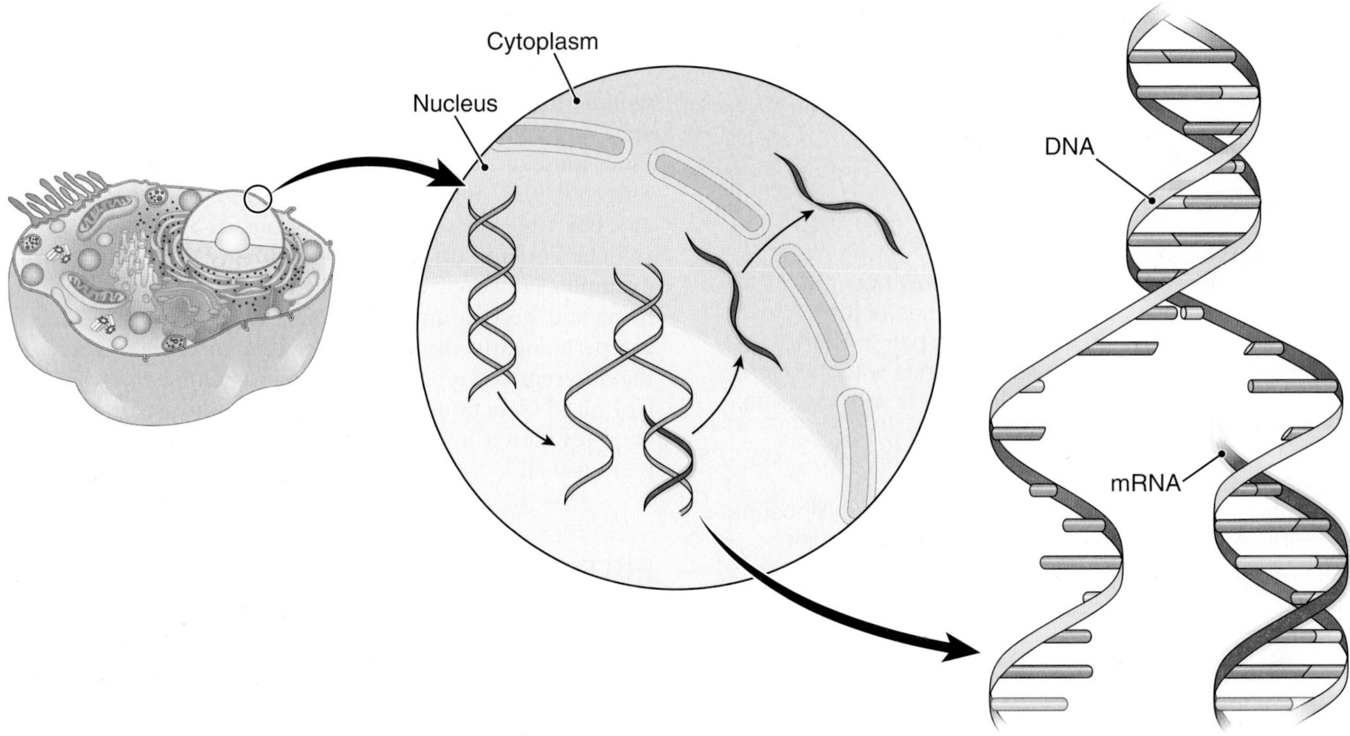

Figure 3-16 Transcription. KEY POINT In the first step of protein synthesis, the DNA code is transcribed into messenger RNA (mRNA) by nucleotide base pairing. An enlarged view of the nucleic acids during transcription shows how mRNA forms according to the nucleotide pattern of the DNA. Note that adenine (A, *red*) in DNA bonds with uracil (U, *brown*) in RNA.

CHECKPOINTS 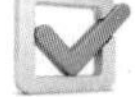

- 3-10 What are the building blocks of nucleic acids?
- 3-11 What category of compounds does DNA code for in the cell?
- 3-12 What three types of RNA are active in protein synthesis?

Cell Division

For growth, repair, and reproduction, cells must multiply to increase their numbers. The cells that form the sex cells (egg and sperm) divide by the process of *meiosis* (mi-O-sis), which cuts the chromosome number in half to prepare for union of the egg and sperm in fertilization. If not for this preliminary reduction, the number of chromosomes in the

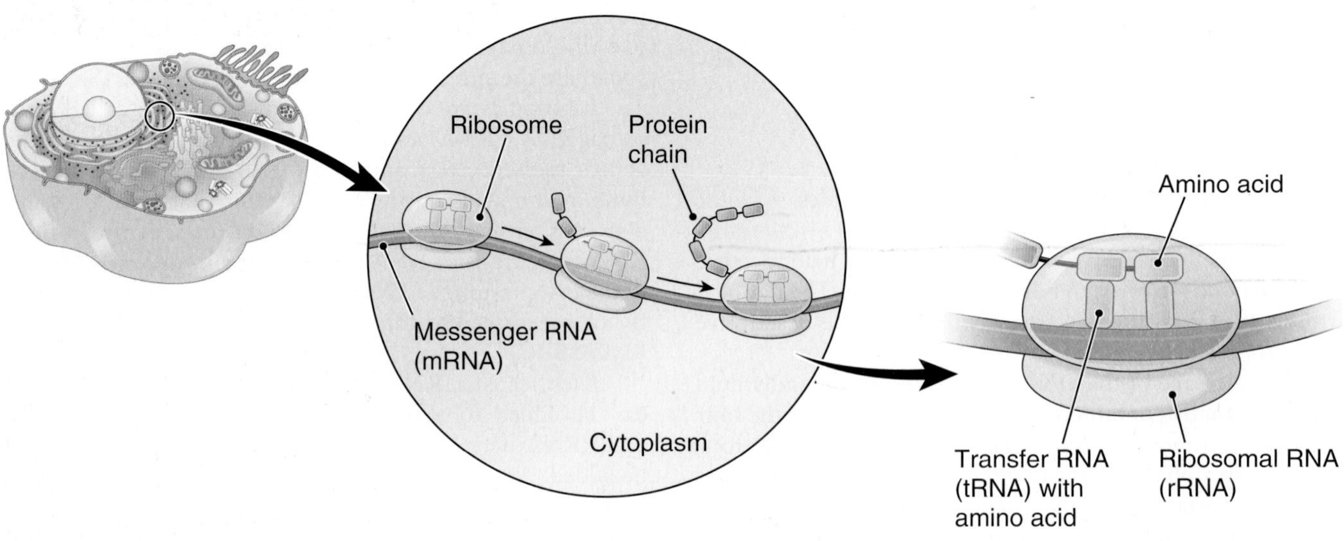

Figure 3-17 Translation. KEY POINT In protein synthesis, messenger RNA (mRNA) travels to the ribosomes in the cytoplasm. The information in the mRNA codes for the building of proteins from amino acids. Transfer RNA (tRNA) molecules bring amino acids to the ribosomes to build each protein.

Table 3-6 RNA

Types	Function
Messenger RNA (mRNA)	Is built on a strand of DNA in the nucleus and transcribes the nucleotide code; moves to cytoplasm and attaches to a ribosome
Ribosomal RNA (rRNA)	With protein makes up the ribosomes, the sites of protein synthesis in the cytoplasm; involved in the process of translating the genetic message into a protein
Transfer RNA (tRNA)	Works with other forms of RNA to translate the genetic code into protein; each molecule of tRNA carries an amino acid that can be used to build a protein at the ribosome

offspring would constantly double. The process of meiosis is discussed in Chapter 20. All other body cells, known as *somatic cells*, are formed by a process called **mitosis** (mi-TO-sis). In this process, each original parent cell becomes two identical daughter cells. Somatic cells develop from actively dividing cells called *stem cells*, which we will discuss in more detail in Chapter 4 with relation to tissues.

PREPARATION FOR MITOSIS

Before mitosis can occur, the genetic information (DNA) in the parent cell must be replicated (doubled), so that each of the two new daughter cells will receive a complete set of chromosomes. For example, a human cell that divides by mitosis must produce two cells with 46 chromosomes each, the same number of chromosomes that are present in the original parent cell. DNA replicates during **interphase**, the stage in the cell's life cycle between one mitosis and the next. During this phase, DNA uncoils from its double-stranded form, and each strand takes on a matching strand of nucleotides according to the pattern of A–T, G–C pairing. There are now two strands, each identical to the original double helix. The strands are held together at a region called the *centromere* (SEN-tro-mere) until they separate during mitosis. A typical cell lives in interphase for most of its life cycle and spends only a relatively short period in mitosis. For example, a cell reproducing every 20 hours spends only about one hour in mitosis and the remaining time in interphase.

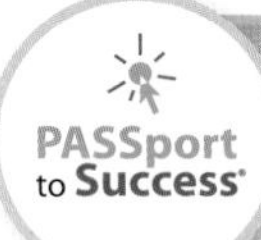

See the student resources on *thePoint* for a photomicrograph of a replicated chromosome.

STAGES OF MITOSIS

Although mitosis is a continuous process, distinct changes can be seen in the dividing cell at four stages **(Fig. 3-18)**.

- In **prophase** (PRO-faze), the doubled strands of DNA return to their tightly wound spiral organization and

Box 3-2 Hot Topics

Proteomics: So Many Proteins, So Few Genes

To build the many different proteins that make up the body, cells rely on instructions encoded in the genes. Collectively, all the different genes on all the chromosomes make up the **genome**. Genes contain the instructions for making proteins, and proteins perform the body's functions.

Scientists are now studying the human **proteome**—all the proteins that can be expressed in a cell—to help them understand protein structure and function. Unlike the genome, the proteome changes as the cell's activities and needs change. In 2003, after a decade of intense scientific activity, investigators mapped the entire human genome. We now realize that it probably contains no more than 25,000 genes, far fewer than initially expected. How could this relatively small number of genes code for several million proteins? They concluded that genes were not the whole story.

Gene transcription is only the beginning of protein synthesis. In response to cellular conditions, enzymes can snip newly transcribed mRNA into several pieces, each of which a ribosome can use to build a different protein. After each protein is built, enzymes can further modify the amino acid strands to produce several more different proteins. Other molecules help the newly formed proteins to fold into precise shapes and interact with each other, resulting in even more variations. Thus, while a gene may code for a specific protein, modifications after gene transcription can produce many more unique proteins. There is much left to discover about the proteome, but scientists hope that future research will lead to new techniques for detecting and treating disease.

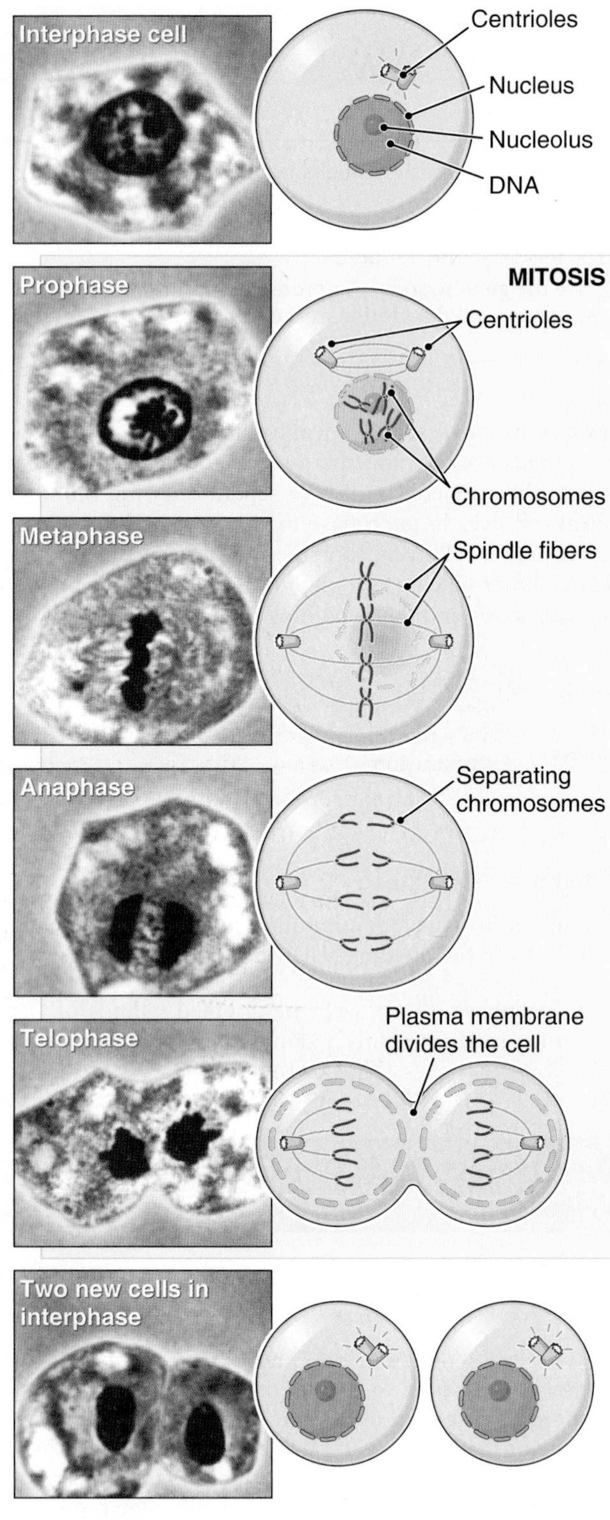

Figure 3-18 The stages of mitosis. KEY POINT Although it is a continuous process, mitosis can be seen in four stages. When it is not dividing, the cell is in interphase. The cell shown is for illustration only. It is not a human cell, which has 46 chromosomes. (Photomicrographs reprinted with permission from Cormack DH. *Essential Histology*, 2nd ed. Philadelphia, PA: Lippincott Williams & Wilkins, 2001.) ZOOMING IN If the original cell shown has 46 chromosomes, how many chromosomes will each new daughter cell have?

become visible under the microscope as dark, thread-like chromosomes. The nucleolus and the nuclear membrane begin to disappear. In the cytoplasm, the two centrioles move toward opposite ends of the cell, and a spindle-shaped structure made of thin fibers begins to form between them.

- In **metaphase** (MET-ah-faze), the chromosomes line up across the center (equator) of the cell attached to the spindle fibers.
- In **anaphase** (AN-ah-faze), the centromere splits and the duplicated chromosomes separate and begin to move toward opposite ends of the cell.
- As mitosis continues into **telophase** (TEL-o-faze), a membrane appears around each group of separated chromosomes, forming two new nuclei.

Also during telophase, the plasma membrane pinches off to divide the cell. The midsection between the two areas becomes progressively smaller until, finally, the cell splits into two. There are now two new cells, or daughter cells, each with exactly the same kind and amount of DNA as was present in the parent cell. In just a few types of cells, skeletal muscle cells for example, the cell itself does not divide following nuclear division. The result, after multiple mitoses, is a giant single cell with multiple nuclei. This pattern is extremely rare in human cells.

CHECKPOINTS 

☐ 3-13 What must happen to the DNA in a cell before mitosis can occur? During what stage in the cell life cycle does this occur?

☐ 3-14 What are the four stages of mitosis?

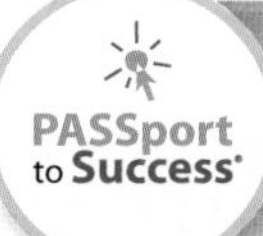

See the student resources on *thePoint* to view the animation *The Cell Cycle and Mitosis.*

Cell Aging

As cells multiply throughout life, changes occur that may lead to their damage and death. Harmful substances, produced in the course of normal metabolism, can injure cells unless they are destroyed. Lysosomes may deteriorate as they age, releasing enzymes that can harm the cell. Alteration of the genes, or **mutation**, is a natural occurrence in the process of cell division and is increased by exposure to harmful substances and radiation in the environment. Mutations usually harm cells and may lead to damage and death.

As a person ages, the overall activity of the body cells slows. One example of this change is the slowing down of repair processes. A bone fracture, for example, takes considerably longer to heal in an old person than in a young person.

One theory on aging holds that cells are preprogrammed to divide only a certain number of times before they die.

Support for this idea comes from the fact that cells taken from a young person divide more times when grown in the laboratory than similar cells taken from an older individual. This programmed cell death, known as *apoptosis* (ah-pop-TO-sis), is a natural part of growth and remodeling before birth in the developing embryo. For example, apoptosis removes cells from the embryonic limb buds in the development of fingers and toes. Apoptosis also is needed in repair and remodeling of tissue throughout life. Cells subject to wear and tear regularly undergo apoptosis and are replaced. For example, the cells lining the digestive tract are removed and replaced every 2 to 3 days. This "cellular suicide" is an orderly, genetically programmed process. The "suicide" genes code for enzymes that destroy the cell quickly without damaging nearby cells. Phagocytes then eliminate the dead cells.

A&P in Action Revisited

Jim's Homeostatic Imbalance Gets Worse

Let's consider what was happening in Jim's body when he overexerted himself on the basketball court: his rapidly beating heart forced blood around a fatty plaque that bulged into the central opening (lumen) of a coronary artery. Unable to resist the high pressure within the artery, the plaque ruptured and stimulated blood platelets to form a clot in the damaged vessel. Unfortunately for Jim, the clot prevented millions of cardiac muscle cells from receiving oxygen-rich blood. Without oxygen, the cells' mitochondria could not manufacture ATP; without ATP, the contractile proteins in the cells could not shorten. Within minutes, the cardiac muscle cells downstream from the clot stopped contracting, forcing Jim's heart into an irregular rhythm. This alteration dramatically decreased the volume of blood leaving his heart. Brain cells, called neurons, also depend on oxygen to manufacture ATP, and without adequate blood flow, they too began to shut down, causing Jim to lose consciousness.

Inside Jim's oxygen-starved cardiac muscle cells, lack of ATP had other serious consequences. Transporter proteins embedded in the cells' plasma membranes began to shut down. Without these transporters, the cells could not regulate their solute concentration. Quickly, the cells' cytoplasm became hypertonic to the surrounding tissue fluid. Following its osmotic gradient, extracellular water entered the affected cardiac muscle cells, causing them to burst and die. Jim is in big trouble.

In this case, we saw that events within Jim's cardiac muscle cells affected his whole body. Your understanding of cellular structure and function will help you to make sense of the structure and function of tissues, organs, and, ultimately, the entire body. Without immediate help, Jim's chances of survival are low. The case study in Chapter 13, The Heart will introduce you to some of the medical techniques that will return Jim to a state of homeostasis and save his life.

Chapter Wrap-Up

Summary Overview

A detailed chapter outline with space for note-taking is on *thePoint*. The figure below illustrates the main topics covered in this chapter.

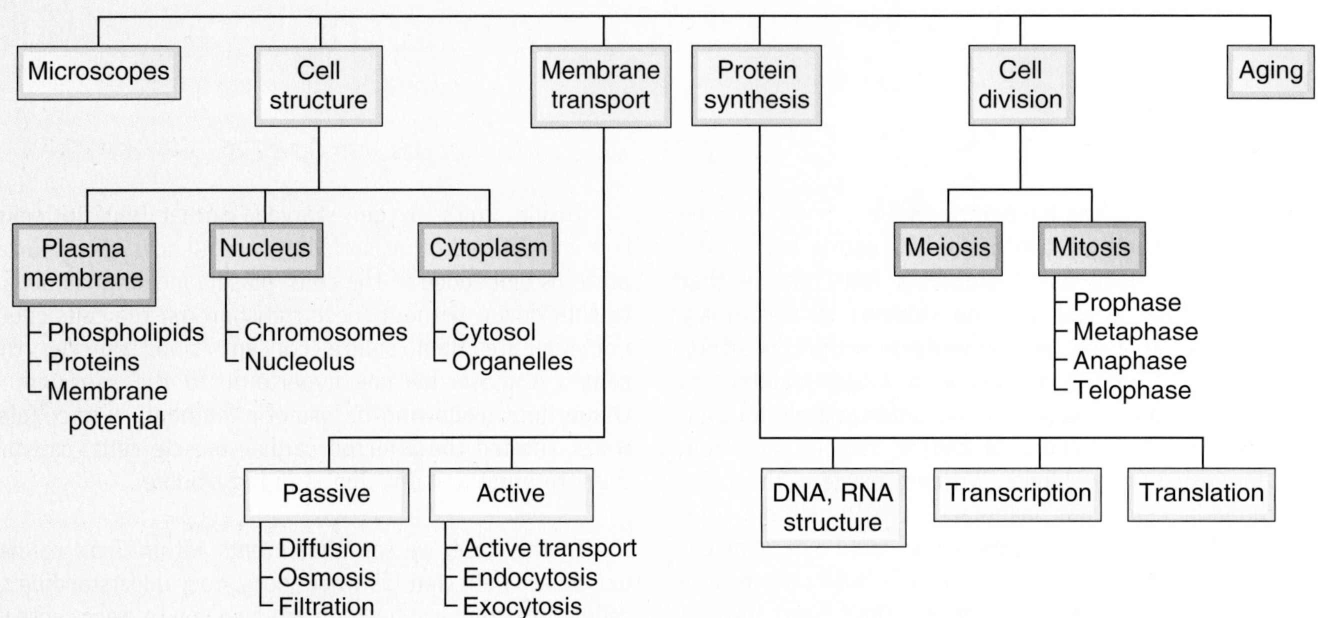

Key Terms

The terms listed below are emphasized in this chapter. Knowing them will help you organize and prioritize your learning. These and other boldface terms are defined in the Glossary with phonetic pronunciations.

active transport
chromosome
cytology
cytoplasm
diffusion
DNA
endocytosis
exocytosis
filtration
gene
hemolysis
hypertonic
hypotonic
interphase
isotonic
membrane potential
micrometer
microscope
mitochondria
mitosis
nucleus
organelle
osmosis
phagocytosis
plasma membrane
ribosome
RNA

Word Anatomy

Scientific terms are built from standardized word parts (prefixes, roots, and suffixes). Learning the meanings of these parts can help you remember words and interpret unfamiliar terms.

WORD PART	MEANING	EXAMPLE
Microscopes		
cyt/o	cell	*Cytology* is the study of cells.
micr/o	small	*Microscopes* are used to view structures too small to see with the naked eye.
Cell Structure		
bi-	two	The lipid *bilayer* is a double layer of lipid molecules.
-some	body	*Ribosomes* are small bodies in the cytoplasm that help make proteins.
chrom/o-	color	*Chromosomes* are small, threadlike bodies that stain darkly with basic dyes.
end/o-	in, within	The *endoplasmic* reticulum is a membranous network within the cytoplasm.
lys/o	loosening, dissolving, separating	*Lysosomes* are small bodies (organelles) with enzymes that dissolve materials (*see also hemolysis*).
Movement Across the Plasma Membrane		
semi-	partial, half	A *semipermeable* membrane lets some molecules pass through but not others.
iso-	same, equal	An *isotonic* solution has the same concentration as that of the cytoplasm.
hypo-	deficient, below, beneath	A *hypotonic* solution's concentration is lower than that of the cytoplasm.
hem/o	blood	*Hemolysis* is the destruction of red blood cells.
hyper-	above, over, excessive	A *hypertonic* solution's concentration is higher than that of the cytoplasm.
phag/o	to eat, ingest	In *phagocytosis*, the plasma membrane engulfs large particles and moves them into the cell.
pin/o	to drink	In *pinocytosis*, the plasma membrane "drinks" (engulfs) droplets of fluid.
ex/o-	outside, out of, away	In *exocytosis*, the cell moves material out from vesicles.
Cell Division		
inter-	between	*Interphase* is the stage between one cell division (mitosis) and the next
pro-	before, in front of	*Prophase* is the first stage of mitosis.
meta-	change	*Metaphase* is the second stage of mitosis when the chromosomes change position and line up across the equator.
ana-	upward, back, again	In the *anaphase* stage of mitosis, chromosomes move to opposite sides of the cell.
tel/o-	end	*Telophase* is the last stage of mitosis.

Questions for Study and Review

BUILDING UNDERSTANDING

Fill in the blanks

1. The part of the cell that regulates what can enter or leave is the _____.
2. The cytosol and organelles make up the _____.
3. If Solution A has more solute and less water than Solution B, then Solution A is _____ to Solution B.
4. Mechanisms that require energy to move substances across the plasma membrane are called _____ transport mechanisms.
5. Distinct segments of DNA that code for specific proteins are called _____.

Matching > Match each numbered item with the most closely related lettered item.

___ 6. DNA duplication takes place
___ 7. DNA is tightly wound into chromosomes
___ 8. Chromosomes line up along the cell's equator
___ 9. Chromosomes separate and move toward opposite ends of the cell
___ 10. Cell membrane pinches off, dividing the cell into two new daughter cells

a. metaphase
b. anaphase
c. telophase
d. interphase
e. prophase

Multiple Choice

___ 11. What is the voltage difference on either side of the plasma membrane called?
- a. interphase
- b. membrane potential
- c. selective permeability
- d. transcription

___ 12. Where does ATP synthesis occur?
- a. endoplasmic reticulum
- b. Golgi apparatus
- c. mitochondria
- d. nucleus

___ 13. What is movement of solute from a region of high concentration to one of lower concentration called?
- a. diffusion
- b. endocytosis
- c. exocytosis
- d. osmosis

___ 14. A DNA sequence reads: TGAAC. What is its mRNA sequence?
- a. ACTTG
- b. ACUUG
- c. CAGGT
- d. CAGGU

___ 15. Which process produces new somatic cells?
- a. crenation
- b. hemolysis
- c. meiosis
- d. mitosis

UNDERSTANDING CONCEPTS

16. List the components of the plasma membrane and state a function for each.
17. Compare and contrast the following cellular components:
    - a. microvilli and cilia
    - b. nucleus and nucleolus
    - c. rough ER and smooth ER
    - d. lysosome and peroxisome
    - e. DNA and RNA
    - f. chromosome and gene
18. List and define six methods by which materials cross the plasma membrane. Which of these requires cellular energy?
19. Why is the plasma membrane described as selectively permeable?
20. What will happen to a red blood cell placed in a 5.0% salt solution? In distilled water?
21. Describe the role of each of the following in protein synthesis: DNA, nucleotide, RNA, ribosomes, rough ER, and Golgi apparatus.

CONCEPTUAL THINKING

22. Making pickles is a good example of osmosis and diffusion. To make pickles you submerge cucumbers in a vinegar and salt solution. Assuming that the cucumber is only permeable to vinegar and water, in which direction will the vinegar diffuse? In which direction will water osmose? Where is the highest osmotic pressure—in the cucumber or in the surrounding vinegar-salt solution?

23. In Jim's case, his cardiac muscle cells adapted to his unhealthy lifestyle by synthesizing more contractile proteins. Beginning with events in the nucleus, describe the process of manufacturing a contractile protein.

24. In Jim's case, we saw that changes at the cellular level can ultimately affect the entire organism. Explain why this is so.

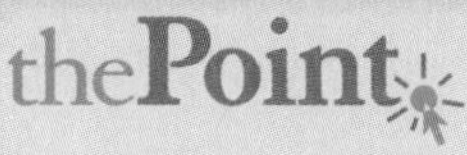

For more questions, see the learning activities on *thePoint*.

CHAPTER

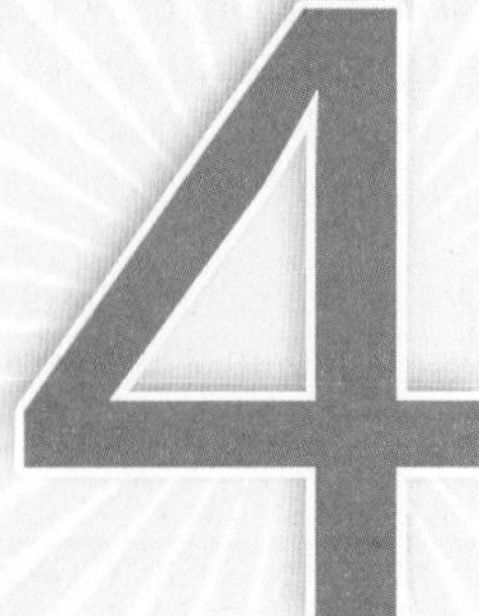

Tissues, Glands, and Membranes

A&P in Action

Ben's Case: How Tissue Damage Affects the Entire Body

"Cough. Cough. Cough." Alison awoke with a start. Not again, she thought as she stumbled out of bed toward the baby's room. For the last few days, Alison's 2-year-old was sick with what appeared to be a nasty chest infection. This wasn't unusual for Ben—he had come down with several lung infections in the past and often seemed congested, but Alison had chalked this up to normal childhood illnesses. Lately though, Alison had become more worried, especially after taking Ben to their community center, where she noticed that he seemed smaller than the rest of the children of his age and had trouble keeping up with them as they played in the gym. I'll take him in to see the doctor tomorrow, Alison thought as she sat down in the rocking chair beside Ben's crib and began patting his back.

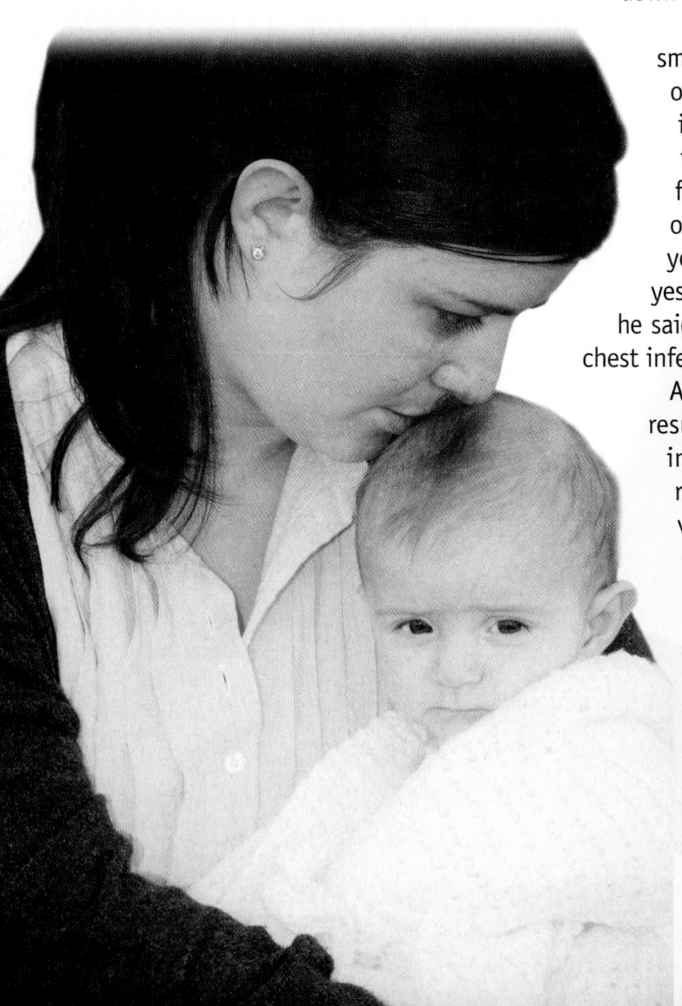

At the medical center, Ben's doctor examined him carefully. Ben was smaller and weighed less than most boys of his age, despite his mom's observation that he had a good appetite. His recurrent respiratory infections were also cause for worry. In addition, Alison reported that Ben had frequent bowel movements with stools that were often foul smelling and greasy. The doctor's next question caught Alison off guard. "When you kiss your son, does he taste saltier than what you might expect?" The doctor wasn't surprised when Alison answered yes. "I need to run a few more tests before I can make a diagnosis," he said. "In the meantime, let's start Ben on some oral antibiotics for his chest infection."

A few days later, Ben's doctor reviewed his chart and the lab test results. Chest and sinus radiography showed evidence of bacterial infection and thickening of the epithelial membrane lining Ben's respiratory passages. The blood test indicated that Ben had elevated levels of the pancreatic enzyme immunoreactive trypsinogen. Genetic testing revealed mutations in a specific gene called CFTR. The sweat test revealed that Ben's sweat glands excreted abnormally high concentrations of sodium chloride. With the evidence he had, the doctor was ready to make his diagnosis. Ben had cystic fibrosis.

Cystic fibrosis is caused by a mutation in a gene that codes for a channel protein in the plasma membrane of certain types of cells. Although the disease affects certain cells of only one of the four types of tissue (epithelial tissue), its consequences are seen in many different organs and systems—especially the respiratory and digestive systems. We will learn more about the implications of this tissue disease later in the chapter.

PASSport to Success®

Ancillaries At-A-Glance

Visit thePoint to access the PASSport to Success and the following resources. For guidance in using these resources most effectively, see pp. ix–xviii.

Learning TOOLS

- Learning Style Self-Assessment
- Live Advise Online Student Tutoring
- Tips for Effective Studying

Learning RESOURCES

- E-book: Chapter 4
- Web Chart: Epithelial Tissue
- Web Chart: Connective Tissue
- Health Professions: Histotechnologist
- Detailed Chapter Outline
- Answers to Questions for Study and Review
- Audio Pronunciation Glossary

Learning ACTIVITIES

- Pre-Quiz
- Kinesthetic Activities
- Auditory Activities

Learning Outcomes

After careful study of this chapter, you should be able to:

1. Name the four main groups of tissues and give the location and general characteristics of each, ***p. 62***
2. Describe the difference between exocrine and endocrine glands and give examples of each, ***p. 64***
3. Give examples of circulating, generalized, and structural connective tissues, ***p. 65***
4. Describe three types of epithelial membranes, ***p. 70***
5. List several types of connective tissue membranes, ***p. 72***
6. Using the case study, describe the consequence of tissue changes on organs and systems, ***pp. 60, 73***
7. Show how word parts are used to build words related to tissues, glands, and membranes (see Word Anatomy at the end of the chapter), ***p. 75***

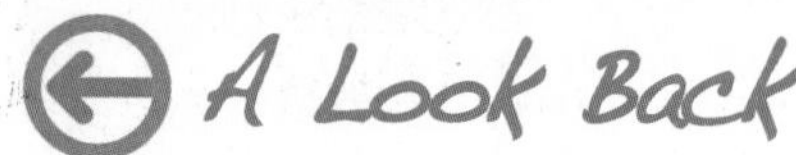

In Chapter 3, we learned about cells, their structure, and function. Cells work together to form tissues, which are the subject of this chapter.

Tissues are groups of cells similar in structure, arranged in a characteristic pattern, and specialized for the performance of specific tasks. The study of tissues is known as **histology** (his-TOL-o-je). This study shows that the form, arrangement, and composition of cells in different tissues account for their properties. The tissues in our bodies might be compared with the different materials used to construct a building. Think for a moment of the great variety of building materials used according to need—wood, stone, steel, plaster, insulation, and others. Each of these has different properties, but together they contribute to the building as a whole. The same may be said of tissues.

Tissue Origins

During development, all tissues derive from young, actively dividing cells known as **stem cells** (Box 4-1). These active cells gradually differentiate into all the different body tissues. Throughout life, the rate at which these cells multiply varies. Tissues subject to wear and tear, such as skin and the lining of the digestive and respiratory tracts, maintain a large population of stem cells that continue to divide in order to replace lost or damaged cells. Once we reach maturity, however, few stem cells remain in highly specialized tissues, including nervous tissue and muscle tissue. The cells in these tissues do not continue to divide, but remain in interphase, as described in Chapter 3. Between these two extremes are cells, such as those in the liver and kidney, that live for a few years and are then replaced.

Regardless of their turnover rate, all tissues maintain at least a small stem cell population that can go into action in response to injury. Because of having few stem cells, nervous tissue and muscle tissue repair themselves slowly, if at all. Brain tissue injured by a stroke or heart muscle tissue injured by a heart attack has very limited ability to recover. The liver, however, can regenerate in a few months, even if up to one-half of it is removed. For this reason, a portion of the liver can be transplanted from one person to another, and the donor's organ will be restored.

Stem cells give rise to four main tissue groups, as follows:

- **Epithelial** (ep-ih-THE-le-al) **tissue** covers surfaces, lines cavities, and forms glands.
- **Connective tissue** supports and forms the framework of all parts of the body.
- **Muscle tissue** contracts and produces movement.
- **Nervous tissue** conducts nerve impulses.

Box 4-1 *Hot Topics*

Stem Cells: So Much Potential

At least 200 different types of cells are found in the human body, each with its own unique structure and function. All originate from unspecialized precursors called **stem cells**, which exhibit two important characteristics: they can divide repeatedly and have the potential to become specialized cells.

Stem cells come in two types. **Embryonic stem cells**, found in early embryos, are the source of all body cells and potentially can differentiate into any cell type. **Adult stem cells**, found in babies and children as well as adults, are stem cells that remain in the body after birth and can differentiate into different cell types. They assist with tissue growth and repair. For example, in red bone marrow, these cells differentiate into blood cells, whereas in the skin, they differentiate into new skin cells to replace cells in surface layers that are shed continually or cells that are damaged by a cut, scrape, or other injury.

The potential healthcare applications of stem cell research are numerous. In the near future, stem cell transplants may be used to repair damaged tissues in treating illnesses such as diabetes, cancer, heart disease, Parkinson disease, and spinal cord injury. This research may also help explain how cells develop and why some cells develop abnormally, causing birth defects and cancer. Scientists may also use stem cells to test drugs before trying them on animals and humans.

But stem cell research is controversial. Some argue that it is unethical to use embryonic stem cells because they are obtained from aborted fetuses or fertilized eggs left over from in vitro fertilization. Others argue that these cells would be discarded anyway and have the potential to improve lives. A possible solution is the use of adult stem cells. However, adult stem cells are less abundant than embryonic stem cells and lack their potential to differentiate, so more research is needed to make this a viable option.

This chapter concentrates mainly on epithelial and connective tissues, the less specialized of the four types. Muscle and nervous tissues receive more attention in later chapters.

Epithelial Tissue

Epithelial tissue, or **epithelium** (ep-ih-THE-le-um), forms a protective covering for the body. It is the main tissue of the skin's outer layer. It also forms membranes, ducts, and the lining of body cavities and hollow organs, such as the organs of the digestive, respiratory, and urinary tracts.

STRUCTURE OF EPITHELIAL TISSUE

Epithelial cells are tightly packed to better protect underlying tissue or form barriers between systems. The cells vary in shape and arrangement according to their function. In shape, the cells may be described as follows:

- **Squamous** (SKWA-mus)—flat and irregular
- **Cuboidal**—square
- **Columnar**—long and narrow

The cells may be arranged in a single layer, in which case it is described as **simple** (Fig. 4-1). Simple epithelium functions as a thin barrier through which materials can pass fairly easily. For example, simple epithelium allows for absorption of materials from the lining of the digestive tract into the blood and allows for passage of oxygen from the blood to body tissues. Areas subject to wear and tear that require protection are covered with epithelial cells in multiple layers, an arrangement described as **stratified** (Fig. 4-2). If the cells are staggered so that they appear to be in multiple layers but really are not, they are termed *pseudostratified.*

Terms for both shape and arrangement are used to describe epithelial tissue. Thus, a single layer of flat, irregular cells would be described as *simple squamous epithelium*, whereas tissue with many layers of these same cells would be described as *stratified squamous epithelium.*

Some organs, such as the urinary bladder, must vary a great deal in size as they work. These organs are lined with **transitional epithelium**, which is capable of great expansion but returns to its original form once tension is relaxed—as when, in this case, the urinary bladder is emptied.

SPECIAL FUNCTIONS OF EPITHELIAL TISSUE

Some epithelial tissues produce secretions, including **mucus** (MU-kus) (a clear, sticky fluid), digestive juices, sweat, and other substances. The air that we breathe passes over epithelium that lines the respiratory passageways. Mucus-secreting **goblet cells**, named for their shape, are scattered among the pseudostratified epithelial cells (Fig. 4-3A). The epithelial cells also have cilia (see Chapter 3). Together, the

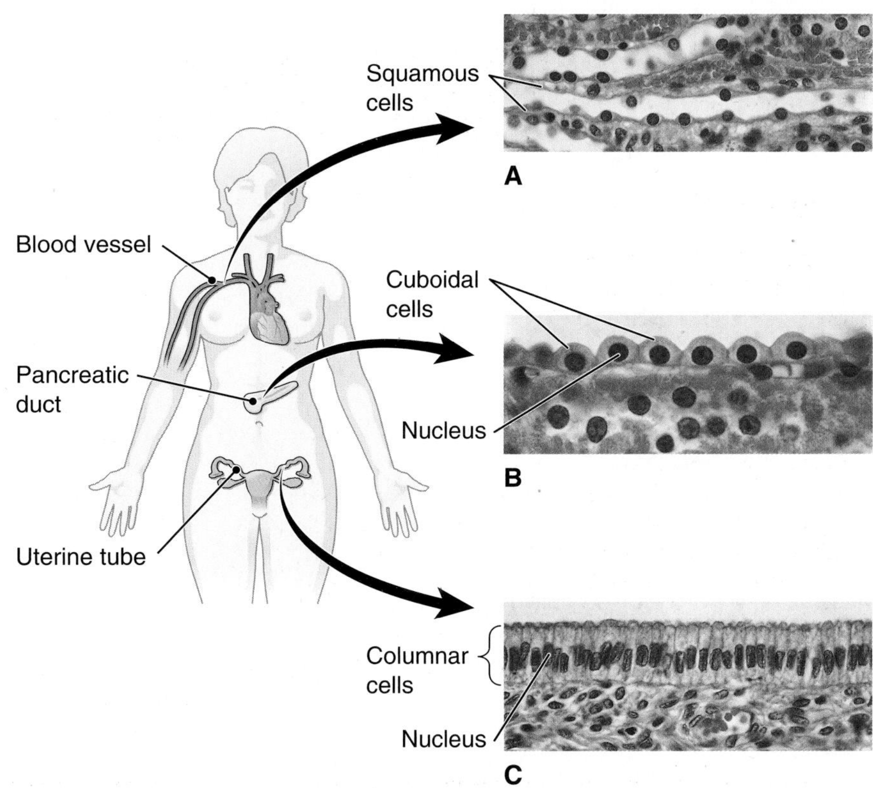

Figure 4-1 Simple epithelial tissues. KEY POINT Epithelial tissue can be described by the shape of its cells. **A.** Simple squamous epithelium has flat, irregular cells with flat nuclei. **B.** Cuboidal epithelial cells are square in shape with round nuclei. **C.** Columnar epithelial cells are long and narrow with ovoid nuclei. (Reprinted with permission from Cormack DH. *Essential Histology*, 2nd ed. Philadelphia, PA: Lippincott Williams & Wilkins, 2001.) ZOOMING IN In how many layers are these epithelial cells?

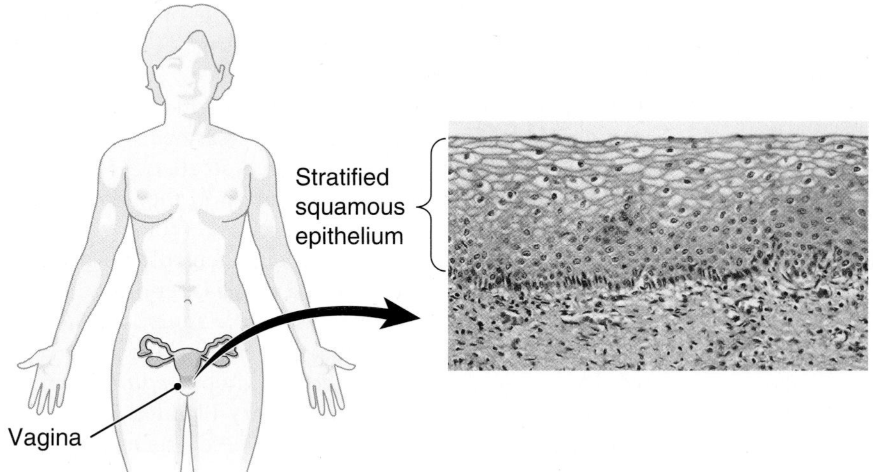

Figure 4-2 **Stratified squamous epithelium.** KEY POINT Stratified epithelium has multiple layers of cells. (Reprinted with permission from Cormack DH. *Essential Histology*, 2nd ed. Philadelphia, PA: Lippincott Williams & Wilkins, 2001.) ZOOMING IN What is the function of stratified epithelium?

mucus and the cilia help trap bits of dust and other foreign particles that could otherwise reach and damage the lungs. The digestive tract is lined with simple columnar epithelium that also contains goblet cells. They secrete mucus that protects the lining of the digestive organs **(see Fig. 4.3B)**.

PASSport to Success: See the student resources on *thePoint* for a summary chart on epithelial tissue.

Epithelium repairs itself quickly after it is injured. In areas of the body subject to normal wear and tear, such as the skin, the inside of the mouth, and the lining of the intestinal tract, epithelial stem cells reproduce frequently, replacing dead or damaged cells. Certain areas of the epithelium that form the outer layer of the skin are capable of modifying themselves for greater strength whenever they are subjected to unusual wear and tear; the growth of calluses is a good example of this response.

GLANDS

The active cells of many glands are epithelial cells. A gland is an organ specialized to produce a substance that is sent out to other parts of the body. The gland manufactures these secretions from materials removed from the blood. Glands are divided into two categories based on how they release their secretions:

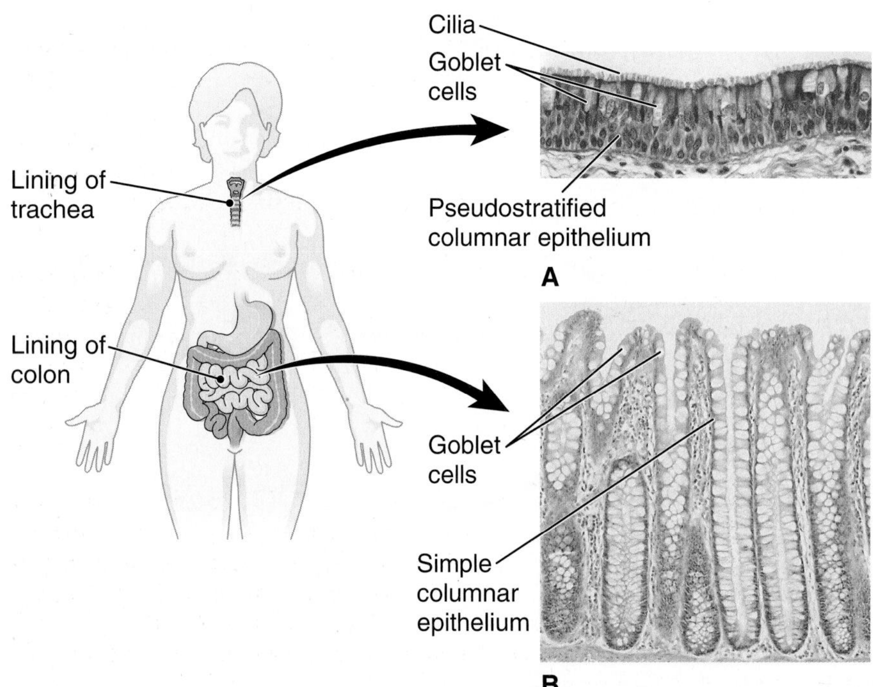

Figure 4-3 **Special features of epithelial tissues.** KEY POINT Tissues are modified for special functions. **A.** The lining of the trachea showing cilia and goblet cells that secrete mucus. **B.** The lining of the intestine showing goblet cells. (Reprinted with permission from Cormack DH. *Essential Histology*, 2nd ed. Philadelphia, PA: Lippincott Williams & Wilkins, 2001.)

- **Exocrine** (EK-so-krin) **glands** produce secretions that are carried out of the body (recall that *ex/o* means "outside" or "away from.") The exocrine glands have ducts or tubes to carry their secretions away from the gland (except for the single goblet cells that secrete mucus). Their secretions are delivered into an organ, a cavity, or to the body surface and act in a limited area near their source. Examples of exocrine glands include the glands in the stomach and intestine that secrete digestive juices, the salivary glands, the sweat and sebaceous (oil) glands of the skin, and the lacrimal glands that produce tears. Exocrine glands are involved in Ben's case of cystic fibrosis. The exocrine glands are discussed in greater detail in the chapters on specific systems. In structure, an exocrine gland may consist of a single cell, such as a goblet cell. Most, however, are composed of multiple cells in various arrangements, including tubular, coiled, or saclike formations.
- **Endocrine** (EN-do-krin) **glands** secrete not through ducts, but directly into surrounding tissue fluid. Most often the secretions are then absorbed into the bloodstream, which distributes them internally, as indicated by the prefix *end/o,* meaning "within." These secretions, called **hormones**, have effects on specific tissues known as the *target tissues*. Endocrine glands have an extensive network of blood vessels. These so-called ductless glands include the pituitary, thyroid, adrenal glands, and others described in greater detail in Chapter 11.

CHECKPOINTS 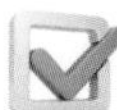

☐ **4-1** What are the three basic shapes of epithelial cells?

☐ **4-2** What are the two categories of glands based on their method of secretion?

Connective Tissue

The supporting fabric everywhere in the body is connective tissue. This is so extensive and widely distributed that if we were able to dissolve all the tissues except connective tissue, we would still be able to recognize the entire body. Connective tissue has large amounts of nonliving material between the cells. This intercellular background material or **matrix** (MA-trix) contains varying amounts of water, fibers, and hard minerals.

Histologists, specialists in the study of tissues, have numerous ways of classifying connective tissues based on their structure or function. Here we describe the different types according to their distribution and function, while listing them in order of increasing hardness.

- Circulating connective tissue has a fluid consistency; its cells are suspended in a liquid matrix. The two types are blood, which circulates in blood vessels **(Fig. 4-4)**, and lymph, a fluid derived from blood that circulates in lymphatic vessels. Chapters 12 and 15 have more information on circulating connective tissue.
- Generalized connective tissue is widely distributed. It supports and protects structures. Some is loosely held together in a semiliquid matrix. Some is denser and contains many fibers. Cells called **fibroblasts** produce the various fibers in all connective tissue. (The word ending *-blast* refers to a young and active cell.) Examples of structures composed of this denser connective tissue are tendons, ligaments, and the capsules (coverings) around some organs.
- Structural connective tissue is mainly associated with the skeleton. Examples are cartilage, which has a very firm consistency, and bone tissue, which is hardened by minerals in the matrix.

The generalized and structural connective tissues are described in greater detail below.

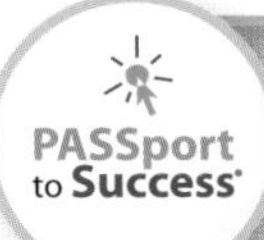

See the student resources on *thePoint* for a summary chart of the connective tissue types.

GENERALIZED CONNECTIVE TISSUE

This tissue is found throughout the body and is less specific in function than other types. There are two forms: loose and dense.

Loose Connective Tissue As the name implies, loose connective tissue has a soft or semiliquid consistency. There are two types:

- **Areolar** (ah-RE-o-lar) **tissue** is named from a word that means "space" because of its open composition **(see Fig. 4-4B)**. It contains cells and fibers in a soft, jellylike matrix. This tissue is found in thin layers (membranes), around vessels and organs, between muscles, and under the skin. It is the most common type of connective tissue.
- **Adipose** (AD-ih-pose) **tissue** contains cells (adipocytes) that are able to store large amounts of fat **(see Fig. 4-4C)**. The fat in this tissue is a reserve energy supply for the body. Adipose tissue is also a heat insulator, as in the underlying layers of the skin, and is protective padding for organs and joints.

Dense Connective Tissue The presence of many fibers gives dense connective tissue its firmness, strength, and flexibility. The main type of fiber in this and other connective tissue is **collagen** (KOL-ah-jen), a flexible white protein **(see Box 4-2)**. The different types vary in the main fibers they contain and how they are arranged:

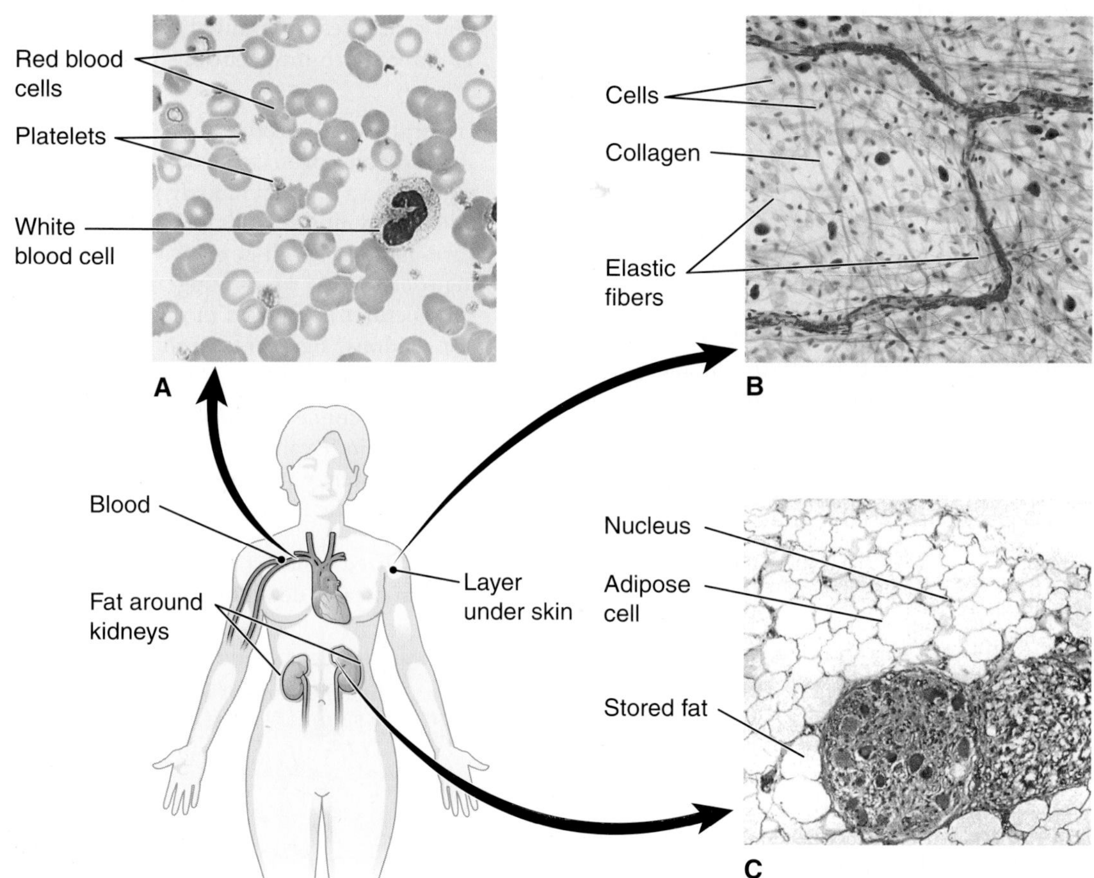

Figure 4-4 **Circulating and generalized (loose) connective tissue.** KEY POINT Connective tissue is classified according to its distribution and the consistency of its matrix. **A.** Blood smear showing various blood cells in a liquid matrix. **B.** Areolar connective tissue, a mixture of cells and fibers in a jelly-like matrix. **C.** Adipose tissue shown here surrounding dark-staining glandular tissue. The slide shows areas where fat is stored and nuclei at the edge of the cells. (A, Reprinted with permission from McClatchey KD. *Clinical Laboratory Medicine*, 2nd ed. Baltimore, MD: Lippincott Williams & Wilkins, 2001; B, Reprinted with permission from Cormack DH. *Essential Histology*, 2nd ed. Philadelphia, PA: Lippincott Williams & Wilkins, 2001; C, Reprinted with permission from Mills SE. *Histology for Pathologists*, 3rd ed. Philadelphia, PA: Lippincott Williams & Wilkins, 2006.) ZOOMING IN Which of these tissues has the most fibers? Which of these tissues is modified for storage?

- **Irregular dense connective tissue** has mostly collagenous fibers in random arrangement. This tissue makes up the fibrous membranes that cover various organs, as described later in this chapter. Particularly strong forms make up the tough capsules around certain organs, such as the kidney, the liver, and some glands.
- **Regular dense connective tissue** also has mostly collagenous fibers, but they are in a regular, parallel alignment like the strands of a cable. This tissue can pull in one direction. Examples are the cordlike **tendons**, which connect muscles to bones, and the **ligaments**, which connect bones to other bones **(Fig. 4-5A)**.
- **Elastic connective tissue** has many elastic fibers that allow it to stretch and then return to its original length. This tissue appears in the vocal cords, the respiratory passageways, and the walls of blood vessels.

STRUCTURAL CONNECTIVE TISSUE

The structural connective tissues are mainly associated with the skeleton and are stronger and more solid than all the other groups.

Cartilage Because of its strength and flexibility, cartilage is a structural material and provides reinforcement. It is also a shock absorber and a bearing surface that reduces friction between moving parts, as at joints. The cells that produce cartilage are **chondrocytes** (KON-dro-sites), a name derived from the word root *chondro*, meaning "cartilage" and the root *cyto*, meaning "cell." There are three forms of cartilage:

- **Hyaline** (HI-ah-lin) **cartilage** is the tough translucent material, popularly called gristle, that covers the ends of the long bones **(see Fig. 4-5B)**. You can feel hyaline cartilage at the tip of your nose and along the front of

4

Box 4-2 *A Closer Look*

Collagen: The Body's Scaffolding

The most abundant protein in the body, making up about 25% of total protein, is collagen. Its name, derived from a Greek word meaning "glue," reveals its role as the main structural protein in connective tissue.

Fibroblasts secrete collagen molecules into the surrounding matrix, where the molecules are then assembled into fibers. These fibers give the matrix its strength and its flexibility. Collagen fibers' high tensile strength makes them stronger than steel fibers of the same size, and their flexibility confers resilience on the tissues that contain them. For example, collagen in skin, bone, tendons, and ligaments resists pulling forces, whereas collagen found in joint cartilage and between vertebrae resists compression. Based on amino acid structure, there are at least 19 types of collagen, each of which imparts a different property to the connective tissue containing it.

The arrangement of collagen fibers in the matrix reveals much about the tissue's function. In the skin and membranes covering muscles and organs, collagen fibers are arranged irregularly, with fibers running in all directions. The result is a tissue that can resist stretching forces in many different directions. In tendons and ligaments, collagen fibers have a parallel arrangement, forming strong ropelike cords that can resist longitudinal pulling forces. In bone tissue, collagen fibers' meshlike arrangement promotes deposition of calcium salts into the tissue, which gives bone strength while also providing flexibility.

Collagen's varied properties are also evident in the preparation of a gelatin dessert. Gelatin is a collagen extract made by boiling animal bones and other connective tissue. It is a viscous liquid in hot water but forms a semisolid gel on cooling.

your throat, where rings of this tissue reinforce the trachea ("windpipe.") Hyaline cartilage also reinforces the larynx ("voicebox") at the top of the trachea, and can be felt anteriorly at the top of the throat as the "Adam's apple."

- **Fibrocartilage** (fi-bro-KAR-tih-laj) is firm and rigid, and is found between vertebrae (segments) of the spine, at the anterior joint between the pubic bones of the hip, and in the knee joint.

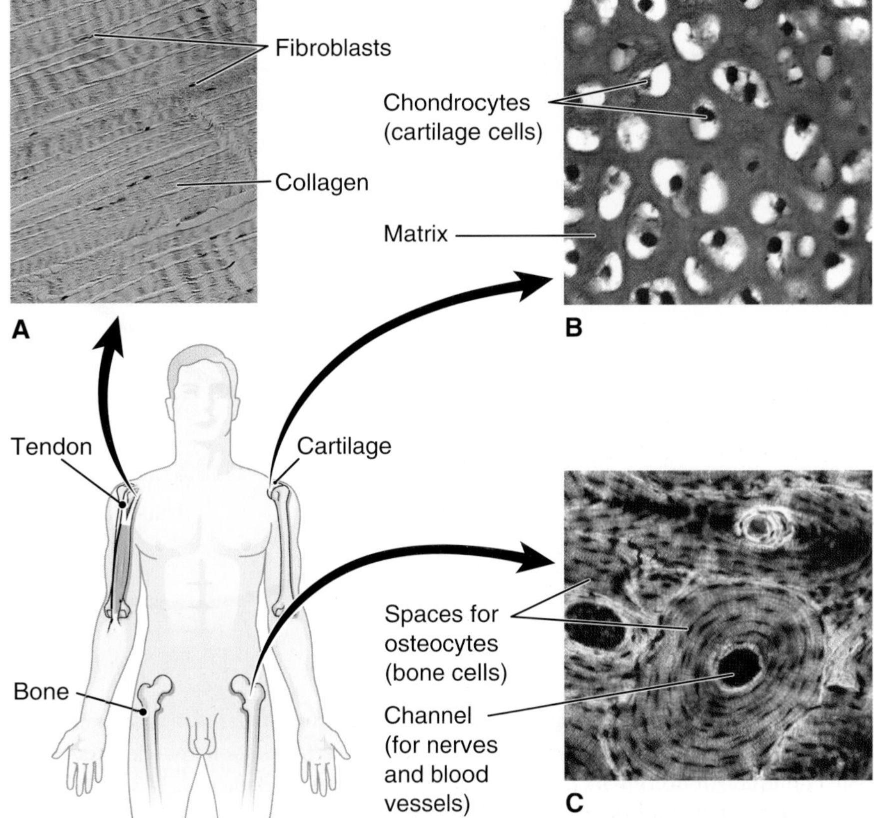

Figure 4-5 Generalized (dense) and structural connective tissue. KEY POINT Fibers are a key component of connective tissue. **A.** Fibrous connective tissue. In tendons and ligaments, collagenous fibers are arranged in the same direction. **B.** In cartilage, the cells (chondrocytes) are enclosed in a firm matrix. **C.** Bone is the hardest connective tissue. The cells (osteocytes) are within the hard matrix. (A and B, Reprinted with permission from Mills SE. *Histology for Pathologists*, 3rd ed. Philadelphia, PA: Lippincott Williams & Wilkins, 2006; C, Reprinted with permission from Gartner LP, Hiatt JL. *Color Atlas of Histology*, 4th ed. Baltimore, MD: Lippincott Williams & Wilkins, 2005.)

- **Elastic cartilage** can spring back into shape after it is bent. An easy place to feel the properties of elastic cartilage is in the outer portion of the ear. It is also located in the larynx.

Bone The tissue that composes bones, called **osseous** (OS-e-us) **tissue**, is much like cartilage in its cellular structure **(see Fig. 4-5C)**. In fact, the fetal skeleton in the early stages of development is made almost entirely of cartilage. This tissue gradually becomes impregnated with salts of calcium and phosphorus that make bone characteristically solid and hard. The cells that form bone are called **osteoblasts** (OS-te-o-blasts), a name that combines the root for bone (*osteo*) with the ending *-blast*. As these cells mature, they are referred to as **osteocytes** (OS-te-o-sites). Within the osseous tissue are nerves and blood vessels. A specialized type of tissue, the bone marrow, is enclosed within bones. The red bone marrow contained in certain regions produces blood cells. Chapter 6 has more information on bones.

CHECKPOINTS 

4-3 What is the general name for the intercellular material in connective tissue?

4-4 What protein makes up the main fibers in connective tissue?

4-5 Give some examples of circulating, generalized, and structural connective tissue.

Muscle Tissue

Muscle tissue is capable of producing movement by contraction of its cells, which are called *muscle fibers* because most of them are long and threadlike. If you were to pull apart a piece of well-cooked meat, you would see small groups of these muscle fibers. Muscle tissue is usually classified as follows:

- **Skeletal muscle**, which works with tendons and bones to move the body **(Fig. 4-6A)**. This type of tissue is described as **voluntary muscle** because we make it contract by conscious thought. The cells in skeletal muscle are very large and are remarkable in having multiple nuclei and a pattern of dark and light banding described as **striations**. For this reason, skeletal muscle is also called *striated muscle*. Chapter 7 has more details on skeletal muscles.

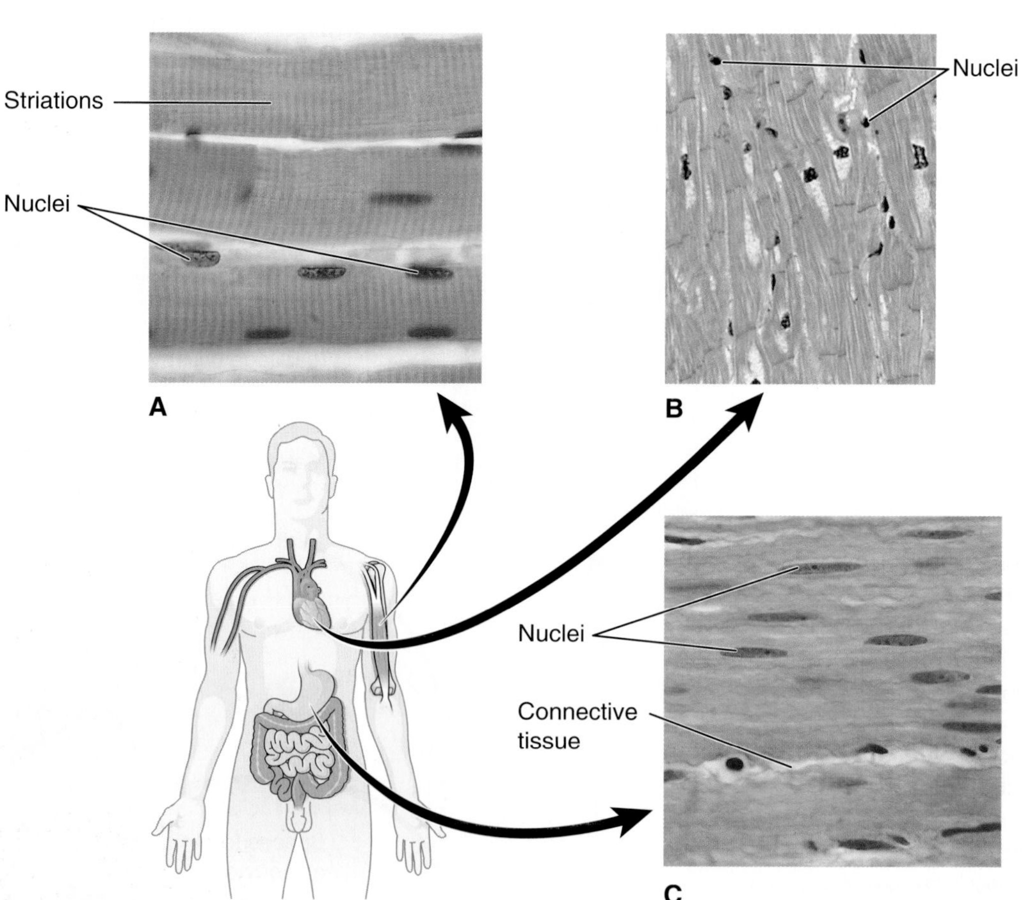

Figure 4-6 Muscle tissue. KEY POINT There are three types of muscle tissue. **A.** Skeletal muscle cells have bands (striations) and multiple nuclei. **B.** Cardiac muscle makes up the wall of the heart. **C.** Smooth muscle is found in soft body organs and in vessels. (A and C, Reprinted with permission from Cormack DH. *Essential Histology*, 2nd ed. Philadelphia, PA: Lippincott Williams & Wilkins, 2001; B, Reprinted with permission from Gartner LP, Hiatt JL. *Color Atlas of Histology*, 4th ed. Baltimore, MD: Lippincott Williams & Wilkins, 2005.)

- **Cardiac muscle**, which forms the bulk of the heart wall and is known also as **myocardium** (mi-o-KAR-de-um) (see Fig. 4-6B). This muscle produces the regular contractions known as *heartbeats*. Cardiac muscle is described as **involuntary muscle** because it typically contracts independently of thought. Most of the time we are not aware of its actions at all. Cardiac muscle has branching cells that form networks. The heart and cardiac muscle are discussed in Chapter 13.
- **Smooth muscle** is also involuntary muscle (see Fig. 4-6C). It forms the walls of the hollow organs in the ventral body cavities, including the stomach, intestines, gallbladder, and urinary bladder. Together these organs are known as viscera (VIS-eh-rah), so smooth muscle is sometimes referred to as *visceral muscle*. Smooth muscle is also found in the walls of many tubular structures, such as the blood vessels and the tubes that carry urine from the kidneys to the bladder. A smooth muscle is also attached to the base of each body hair. Contraction of these muscles causes the condition of the skin that we call *gooseflesh*. Smooth muscle cells are of a typical size and taper at each end. They are not striated and have only one nucleus per cell. Structures containing smooth muscle are discussed in the chapters on the various body systems.

Muscle tissue, like nervous tissue, repairs itself only with difficulty or not at all once an injury has been sustained. When injured, muscle tissue is frequently replaced with connective tissue.

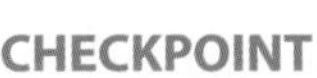

CHECKPOINT

- [ ] 4-6 What are the three types of muscle tissue?

Nervous Tissue

The human body is made up of countless structures, each of which contributes to the action of the whole organism. This aggregation of structures might be compared to a large corporation. For all the workers in the corporation to coordinate their efforts, there must be some central control, such as the president or CEO. In the body, this central agent is the **brain** (Fig. 4-7A). Each body structure is in direct communication with the brain by means of its own set of "wires," called **nerves** (see Fig. 4-7B). Nerves from even the most remote parts of the body come together and feed into a great trunk cable called the **spinal cord**, which in turn leads into the central switchboard of the brain. Here, messages come in and orders go out 24 hours a day. Some nerves, the cranial nerves, connect directly with the brain and do not communicate with the spinal cord. This entire control system, including the brain, is made of nervous tissue.

THE NEURON

The basic unit of nervous tissue is the **neuron** (NU-ron), or nerve cell (see Fig. 4-7C). A neuron consists of a nerve cell body plus small branches from the cell called *fibers*. These fibers carry nerve impulses to and from the cell body.

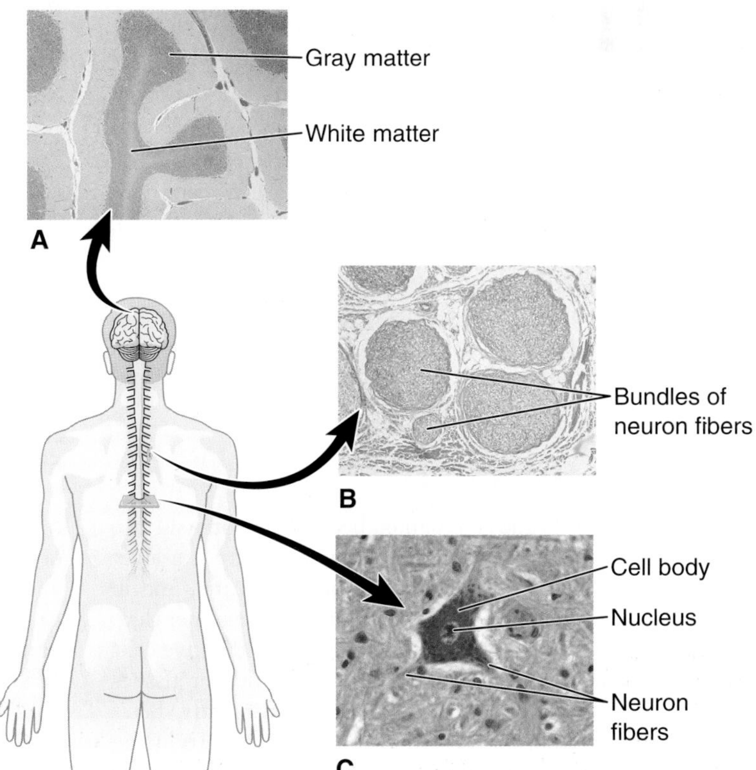

Figure 4-7 **Nervous tissue. A.** Brain tissue. **B.** Cross section of a nerve. **C.** A neuron, or nerve cell. (Reprinted with permission from Cormack DH. *Essential Histology*, 2nd ed. Philadelphia, PA: Lippincott Williams & Wilkins, 2001.)

Neurons may be quite long; their fibers can extend for several feet. A **nerve** is a bundle of such nerve cell fibers held together with connective tissue **(see Fig. 4-7B)**.

Just as wires are insulated to keep them from being short-circuited, some neuron fibers are insulated and protected by a coating of material called **myelin** (MI-eh-lin). Groups of myelinated fibers form "white matter," named for the color of the myelin, which is much like fat in appearance and consistency.

Some neuron fibers are unmyelinated, as are all cell bodies. These areas appear gray in color. Because the outer layer of the brain has large collections of cell bodies and unmyelinated fibers, the brain is popularly termed *gray matter*, even though its interior is composed of white matter **(see Fig. 4-7A)**.

NEUROGLIA

Nervous tissue is supported and protected by specialized cells known as **neuroglia** (nu-ROG-le-ah) or *glial* (GLI-al) *cells*, which are named from the Greek word *glia* meaning "glue." Some of these cells protect the brain from harmful substances; others get rid of foreign organisms and cellular debris; still others form the myelin sheath around axons. They do not, however, transmit nerve impulses.

A more detailed discussion of nervous tissue and the nervous system appears in Chapters 8 and 9.

CHECKPOINTS 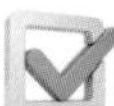

☐ **4-7** What is the basic cell of the nervous system and what is its function?

☐ **4-8** What are the nonconducting support cells of the nervous system called?

Membranes

Membranes are thin sheets of tissue. Their properties vary: some are fragile, and others tough; some are transparent, and others opaque (i.e., you cannot see through them). Membranes may cover a surface, may be a dividing partition, may line a hollow organ or body cavity, or may anchor an organ. They may contain cells that secrete lubricants to ease the movement of organs, such as the heart and lung, and the movement of joints. Epithelial membranes and connective tissue membranes are described below.

EPITHELIAL MEMBRANES

An **epithelial membrane** is so named because its outer surface is made of epithelium. Underneath, however, there is a layer of connective tissue that strengthens the membrane, and in some cases, there is a thin layer of smooth muscle under that. Epithelial membranes are made of closely packed active cells that manufacture lubricants and protect the deeper tissues from invasion by microorganisms. In the case study, Ben's epithelial membranes are involved in his disease, producing widespread effects. Epithelial membranes are of several types:

- **Serous** (SE-rus) **membranes** line the walls of body cavities and are folded back onto the surface of internal organs, forming their outermost layer.
- **Mucous** (MU-kus) **membranes** line tubes and other spaces that open to the outside of the body.
- The **cutaneous** (ku-TA-ne-us) **membrane**, commonly known as the skin, has an outer layer of epithelium. This membrane is complex and is discussed in detail in Chapter 5.

Serous Membranes Serous membranes line the closed ventral body cavities and do not connect with the outside of the body. They secrete a thin, watery lubricant, known as serous fluid, that allows organs to move with a minimum of friction. The thin epithelium of serous membranes is a smooth, glistening kind of tissue called **mesothelium** (meso-THE-le-um). The membrane itself may be referred to as the **serosa** (se-RO-sah).

There are three serous membranes:

- **The pleurae** (PLU-re), or **pleuras** (PLU-rahs), line the thoracic cavity and cover each lung.
- The **serous pericardium** (per-ih-KAR-de-um) forms part of a sac that encloses the heart, which is located in the chest between the lungs.
- The **peritoneum** (per-ih-to-NE-um) is the largest serous membrane. It lines the walls of the abdominal cavity, covers the abdominal organs, and forms supporting and protective structures within the abdomen (see Fig. 17-2 in Chapter 17).

Serous membranes are arranged so that one portion forms the lining of a closed cavity, while another part folds back to cover the surface of the organ contained in that cavity. The relationship between an organ and the serous membrane around it can be visualized by imagining your fist punching into a large, soft balloon **(Fig. 4-8)**. Your fist is the organ and the serous membrane around it is in two layers, one against your fist and one folded back to form an outer layer. Although in two layers, each serous membrane is continuous.

The portion of the serous membrane attached to the wall of a cavity or sac is known as the **parietal** (pah-RI-eh-tal) **layer**; the word *parietal* refers to a wall. In the example above, the parietal layer is represented by the outermost layer of the balloon. Parietal pleura lines the thoracic (chest) cavity, and parietal pericardium lines the fibrous sac (the fibrous pericardium) that encloses the heart **(see Fig. 4-8B)**.

Because internal organs are called *viscera*, the portion of the serous membrane attached to an organ is the **visceral layer**. Visceral pericardium is on the surface of the heart, and each lung surface is covered by visceral pleura. Portions of the peritoneum that cover organs in the abdomen are named according to the particular organ involved. The visceral layer in our balloon example is in direct contact with your fist.

A serous membrane's visceral and parietal layers normally are in direct contact with a minimal amount of

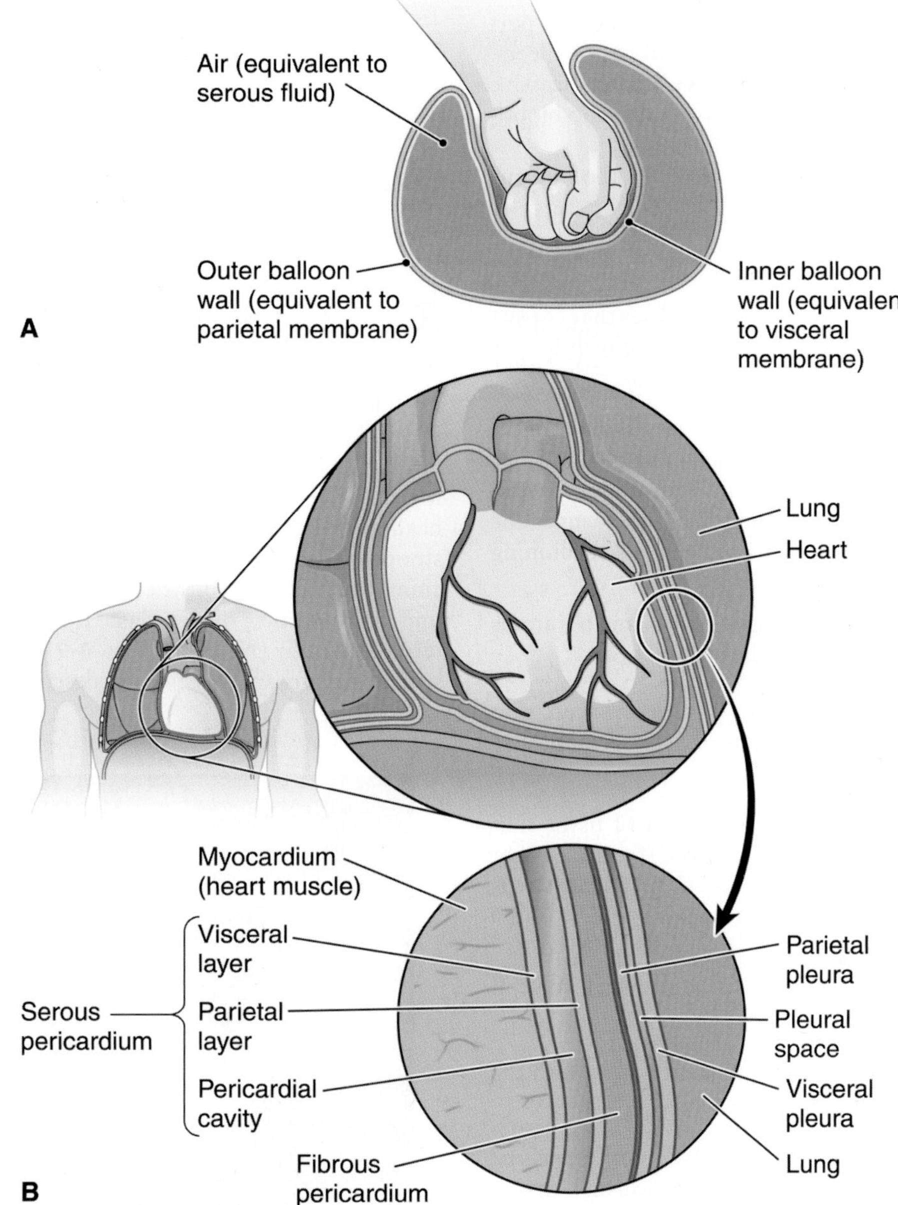

Figure 4-8 **Organization of serous membranes.** KEY POINT A serous membrane that encloses an organ has a visceral and a parietal layer. **A.** An organ fits into a serous membrane like a fist punching into a soft balloon. **B.** The outer layer of a serous membrane is the parietal layer. The inner layer is the visceral layer. The fibrous pericardium reinforces the serous pericardium around the heart. The pleura is the serous membrane around the lungs.

lubricant between them. The area between the two layers forms a potential space. That is, it is *possible* for a space to exist there, although normally one does not. Only if substances accumulate between the layers, as when inflammation causes the production of excessive amounts of fluid, is there an actual space.

Mucous Membranes Mucous membranes are so named because they produce mucus. (Note that the adjective *mucous* contains an "o," whereas the noun *mucus* does not). These membranes form extensive continuous linings in the digestive, respiratory, urinary, and reproductive systems, all of which are connected with the outside of the body. These membranes vary somewhat in both structure and function. The cells that line the nasal cavities and the respiratory passageways have cilia. The microscopic cilia move in waves that force secretions outward. In this way, foreign particles, such as bacteria, dust, and other impurities trapped in the sticky mucus, are prevented from entering the lungs and causing harm. Ciliated epithelium is also found in certain tubes of both the male and the female reproductive systems.

The mucous membranes that line the digestive tract have special functions. For example, the stomach's mucous membrane protects its deeper tissues from the action of powerful digestive juices. If for some reason a portion of this membrane is injured, these juices begin to digest a part of the stomach itself—as happens in cases of peptic ulcers. Mucous membranes located farther along in the digestive system are designed to absorb nutrients, which the bloodstream then transports to all cells.

The noun **mucosa** (mu-KO-sah) refers to the mucous membrane of an organ.

CONNECTIVE TISSUE MEMBRANES

The following list is an overview of membranes that consist of connective tissue with no epithelium. These membranes are described in greater detail in later chapters.

- **Synovial** (sin-O-ve-al) **membranes** are thin connective tissue membranes that line the joint cavities. They secrete a lubricating fluid that reduces friction between the ends of bones, thus permitting free movement of the joints. Synovial membranes also line small cushioning sacs near the joints called **bursae** (BUR-se).
- The **meninges** (men-IN-jeze) are several membranous layers covering the brain and the spinal cord.

Fascia (FASH-e-ah) refers to fibrous bands or sheets that support organs and hold them in place. Fascia is found in two regions:

- **Superficial fascia** is the continuous sheet of tissue that underlies the skin and contains adipose (fat) tissue that insulates the body and protects the skin. This tissue is also called *subcutaneous fascia* because it is located beneath the skin.
- **Deep fascia** covers, separates, and protects skeletal muscles.

Finally, there are membranes whose names all start with the prefix *peri* because they are around organs:

- The **fibrous pericardium** (per-e-KAR-de-um) forms the cavity that encloses the heart, the pericardial cavity. This fibrous sac and the serous pericardial membranes described above are often described together as the pericardium **(see Fig. 4-8B)**.
- The **periosteum** (per-e-OS-te-um) is the membrane around a bone.
- The **perichondrium** (per-e-KON-dre-um) is the membrane around cartilage.

CHECKPOINT 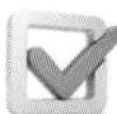

☐ 4-9 What are the three types of epithelial membranes?

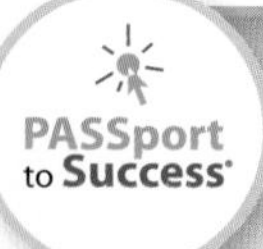

See the student resources on *thePoint* for information on careers in histotechnology—the laboratory study of tissues.

Tissues and Aging

With aging, tissues lose elasticity and collagen becomes less flexible. These changes affect the skin most noticeably, but internal changes occur as well. The blood vessels, for example, have a reduced capacity to expand. Less blood supply, lower metabolism, and decline in hormone levels slow the healing process. Tendons and ligaments stretch, causing a stooped posture and joint instability. Bones may lose calcium salts, becoming brittle and prone to fracture. With age, muscles and other tissues waste from loss of cells, a process termed *atrophy* (AT-ro-fe) **(Fig. 4-9)**. Changes that apply to specific organs and systems are described in later chapters.

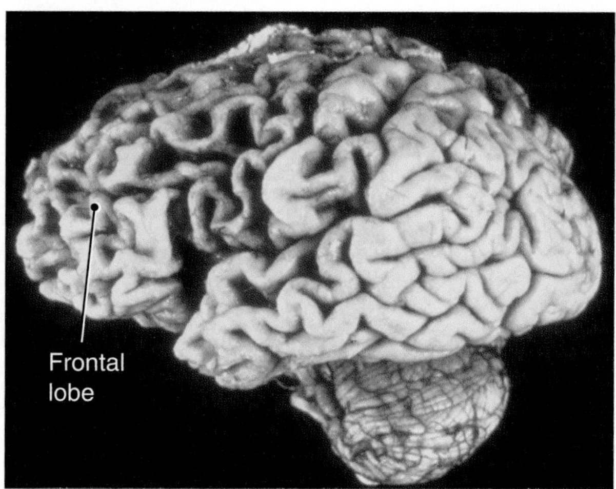

Figure 4-9 Atrophy of the brain. KEY POINT Brain tissue has thinned and large spaces appear between sections of tissue, especially in the frontal lobe. (Reprinted with permission from Okazaki H, Scheithauer BW. *Atlas of Neuropathology*. New York, NY: Gower Medical Publishing, 1988.)

A&P in Action Revisited

Ben's Defective Plasma Membrane Channel

Ben's parents were shocked when the doctor diagnosed their 2-year-old with cystic fibrosis. Their immediate concern was, of course, for their son. The doctor reassured them that with proper treatment their son could lead a relatively normal life for the present and that, in the future, new therapies might extend the lifespan of those with CF and even offer a cure. He asserted that they were not to blame for Ben's condition. Cystic fibrosis is an inherited disease—Ben's parents each carried a defective gene in their DNA and both had, by chance, passed copies to Ben. As a result, Ben was unable to synthesize a channel protein found in the plasma membranes of exocrine gland cells. Normally, this channel regulates the movement of chloride into the cell. Because the channels did not work in Ben's epithelial cells, chloride was trapped outside the cells. The negatively charged chloride ions attract positively charged sodium ions normally found in extracellular fluid. These two ions form the salt, sodium chloride, which is lost in high amounts in the sweat of individuals with cystic fibrosis.

Abnormal chloride channel function causes epithelial glands in many organs to produce thick, sticky mucus. In the lungs, this mucus causes difficulty breathing, inflammation, and bacterial infection. The thick mucus also decreases the ability of the large and small intestines to absorb nutrients, resulting in low weight gain, poor growth, and vitamin deficiencies. This problem is compounded by damage to the pancreas, preventing production of essential digestive enzymes.

In this case, we saw that a defective plasma membrane channel in Ben's epithelial cells had widespread effects on his whole body. In later chapters, as you learn about the body's organs, remember that their structure and function are closely related to the condition of their constituent tissues. Cystic fibrosis is an inherited disease. The case study in Chapter 21, Development and Heredity will follow Alison as she learns more about Ben's condition.

Chapter Wrap-Up

Summary Overview

A detailed chapter outline with space for note-taking is on *thePoint*. The figure below illustrates the main topics covered in this chapter.

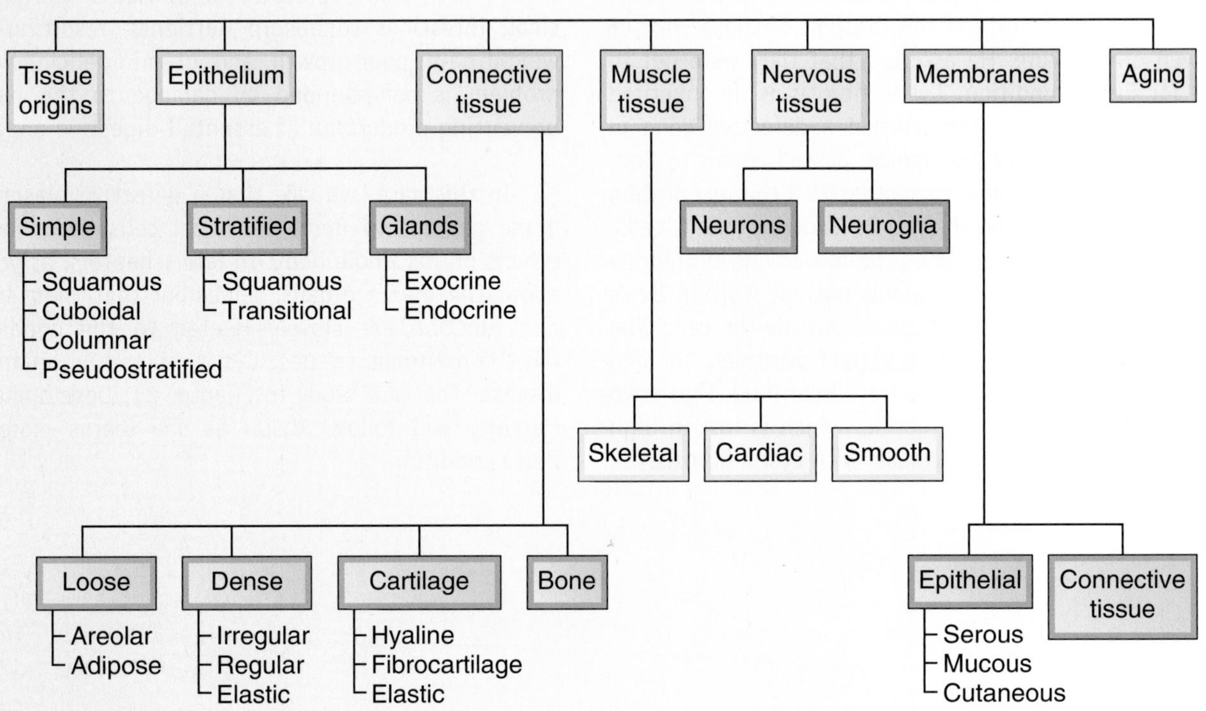

Key Terms

The terms listed below are emphasized in this chapter. Knowing them will help you organize and prioritize your learning. These and other boldface terms are defined in the Glossary with phonetic pronunciations.

adipose
areolar
cartilage
chondrocyte
collagen
endocrine
epithelium
exocrine
fascia
fibroblast
histology
matrix
membrane
mucosa
mucus
myelin
neuroglia
neuron
osteocyte
parietal
serosa
stem cell
visceral

Word Anatomy

Scientific terms are built from standardized word parts (prefixes, roots, and suffixes). Learning the meanings of these parts can help you remember words and interpret unfamiliar terms.

WORD PART	MEANING	EXAMPLE
hist/o	tissue	*Histology* is the study of tissues.
Epithelial Tissue		
epi-	on, upon	*Epithelial* tissue covers body surfaces.
pseud/o-	false	*Pseudostratified* epithelium appears to be in multiple layers but is not.
Connective Tissue		
blast/o	immature cell, early stage of cell	A *fibroblast* is a cell that produces fibers.
chondr/o	cartilage	A *chondrocyte* is a cartilage cell.
oss, osse/o	bone, bone tissue	*Osseous* tissue is bone tissue.
oste/o	bone, bone tissue	An *osteocyte* is a mature bone cell.
Muscle Tissue		
my/o	muscle	The *myocardium* is the heart muscle.
cardi/o	heart	See preceding example.
Nervous Tissue		
neur/o	nerve, nervous system	A *neuron* is a nerve cell.
Membranes		
pleur/o	side, rib	The *pleurae* are membranes that line the chest cavity.
peri-	around	The *peritoneum* wraps around the abdominal organs.
arthr/o	joint	An *arthroscope* is used to examine the interior of a joint.

Questions for Study and Review

BUILDING UNDERSTANDING

Fill in the blanks

1. A group of similar cells arranged in a characteristic pattern is called a(n) _____.
2. Glands that secrete their products directly into the blood are called _____ glands.
3. Tissue that supports and forms the framework of the body is called _____ tissue.
4. Skeletal muscle is also described as _____ muscle.
5. Nerve tissue is supported by specialized cells known as _____.

Matching > Match each numbered item with the most closely related lettered item.

___ 6. Membrane around the heart
___ 7. Membrane around each lung
___ 8. Membrane around bone
___ 9. Membrane around cartilage
___ 10. Membrane around abdominal organs

a. perichondrium
b. pericardium
c. peritoneum
d. periosteum
e. pleura

Multiple Choice

___ 11. You look under the microscope and see tissue composed of a single layer of long and narrow cells. What is it?

a. simple cuboidal epithelium
b. simple columnar epithelium
c. stratified cuboidal epithelium
d. stratified columnar epithelium

___ 12. What tissue forms tendons and ligaments?

a. areolar connective tissue
b. loose connective tissue
c. regular, dense connective tissue
d. cartilage

___ 13. Which tissue is composed of long striated cells with multiple nuclei?

a. smooth muscle
b. cardiac muscle
c. skeletal muscle
d. nervous

___ 14. What is a bundle of nerve cell fibers held together with connective tissue?

a. dendrite
b. axon
c. nerve
d. myelin

___ 15. Which membrane is formed from connective tissue?

a. cutaneous
b. mucous
c. serous
d. synovial

UNDERSTANDING CONCEPTS

16. Explain how epithelium is classified and discuss at least three functions of this tissue type.
17. Compare the structure and function of exocrine and endocrine glands and give two examples of each type.
18. Describe the functions of connective tissue. Name two kinds of fibers found in connective tissue and discuss how their presence affects tissue function.
19. Compare and contrast the three different types of muscle tissue.
20. Compare serous and mucous membranes.

CONCEPTUAL THINKING

21. Use the structural descriptions to identify the tissues:

a. Tightly packed cuboidal cells arranged in a single layer.

b. Abundant extracellular matrix containing parallel collagen fibers.

c. Tightly packed short, branched, and striated cells.

22. The middle ear is connected to the pharynx (throat) by the auditory tube. All are lined by a continuous mucous membrane. Using this information, describe why a throat infection (pharyngitis) may lead to an ear infection (otitis media).

23. In Ben's case, the production of abnormally thick sticky mucus resulted in lung and digestive disorders. What are some of the normal functions of mucus in the body?

24. In Ben's case, an abnormal epithelial channel protein had widespread effects. Another hereditary disease, osteogenesis imperfecta, is characterized by abnormal collagen fiber synthesis. Which tissue type would be most affected by this disorder? List some possible symptoms of this disease.

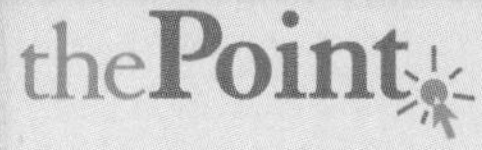

For more questions, see the learning activities on *thePoint*.

CHAPTER 5

The Integumentary System

A&P in Action

Paul's Case: Sun-Damaged Skin

"Wait a minute," Paul said to his reflection in the mirror as he examined his face after shaving. He had noticed a small nodule to the side of his left nostril. The lump was mostly pink with a pearly-white border, and painless to the touch. *I haven't seen that before. Probably just a pimple, or maybe a small cyst*, Paul thought, although he couldn't help thinking back to the many hours he had spent as a kid sailing competitively at the seashore. *I know sun exposure isn't great for your skin, even dangerous, and I wasn't real careful about wearing sunscreen. Even if I did, it would have washed off anyway while I was sailing*, he rationalized. Paul finished his trimming and decided the lump was probably nothing.

Despite his attempts to forget about the lump, Paul was concerned. Over the next several days, he showed the small, rounded mass to several people to get their opinions. No one had an answer when he asked, "What do you think this is?" When several weeks produced no change, except maybe a little depression in the center of the mass, worry led him to make an appointment with a dermatologist.

"Well Paul, I'm not sure. It could be nothing, but we'd better look a little closer," said Dr. Nielsen. "It could be benign, but we have to be sure that it's not a small skin cancer. This is a very common site for such a lesion. Basal cell and squamous cell carcinomas arise from the top layer of skin cells, especially in sun-exposed areas. UV rays from the sun can damage DNA, causing the cells to divide more rapidly than normal, resulting in an abnormal growth. Basal cell and squamous cell carcinomas are the most common forms of cancer but are usually completely treatable. We'll remove this and send it to the pathology lab to see what's going on." Paul left Dr. Nielsen's office with a small bandage over the site of excision, some ointment to apply, and instructions to call the office in 3 days.

Paul's dermatologist suspects that he may have skin cancer—a disease affecting the integumentary system. In this chapter, we learn that skin is just one part of the system. Later in the chapter, we revisit Paul and learn the final diagnosis of that lump on his nose.

PASSport to Success®

Ancillaries *At-A-Glance*

Visit *thePoint* to access the PASSport to Success and the following resources. For guidance in using these resources most effectively, see pp. ix–xviii.

Learning TOOLS

- Learning Style Self-Assessment
- Live Advise Online Student Tutoring
- Tips for Effective Studying

Learning RESOURCES

- E-book: Chapter 5
- Web Chart: Skin Structure
- Web Chart: Accessory Skin Structures
- Animation: Wound Healing
- Health Professions: Registered Nurse

Learning ACTIVITIES

- Pre-Quiz
- Visual Activities
- Kinesthetic Activities
- Auditory Activities

Learning Outcomes

After careful study of this chapter, you should be able to:

1. Name and describe the layers of the skin, ***p. 80***
2. Describe the subcutaneous layer, ***p. 82***
3. Give the location and function of the accessory structures of the integumentary system, ***p. 82***
4. List the main functions of the integumentary system, ***p. 84***
5. Discuss the factors that contribute to skin color, ***p. 85***
6. Using information in the case study and the text, describe the specific layer of the integumentary system that was sun-damaged, ***pp. 78, 87***
7. Show how word parts are used to build words related to the integumentary system (see Word Anatomy at the end of the chapter), ***p. 89***

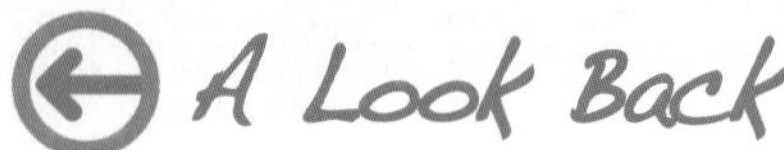

The skin is introduced in Chapter 4 as one of the epithelial membranes, the cutaneous membrane. In this chapter, we describe the skin in much greater detail, as it forms the major portion of the integumentary system. This system provides a first line of defense against infectious microorganisms as well as other harmful agents.

Although the skin may be viewed simply as a membrane enveloping the body, it is far more complex than the other epithelial membranes previously described. The skin is associated with accessory structures, also known as appendages, which include glands, hair, and nails. Together with blood vessels, nerves, and sensory organs, the skin and its associated structures form the **integumentary** (in-teg-u-MEN-tar-e) **system.** This name is from the word integument (in-TEG-u-ment), which means "covering." The term *cutaneous* (ku-TA-ne-us) also refers to the skin. The functions of this system are discussed later in the chapter after a description of its structure.

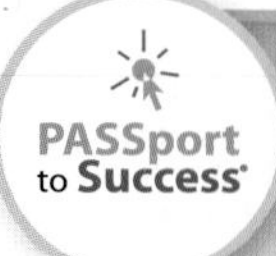

See the student resources on *thePoint* for a summary chart of skin structure.

Structure of the Skin

The skin consists of two layers **(Fig. 5-1)**:

- The **epidermis** (ep-ih-DER-mis), the outermost portion, which itself is subdivided into thin layers called **strata** (STRA-tah) (sing. stratum). The epidermis is composed entirely of epithelial cells and contains no blood vessels.

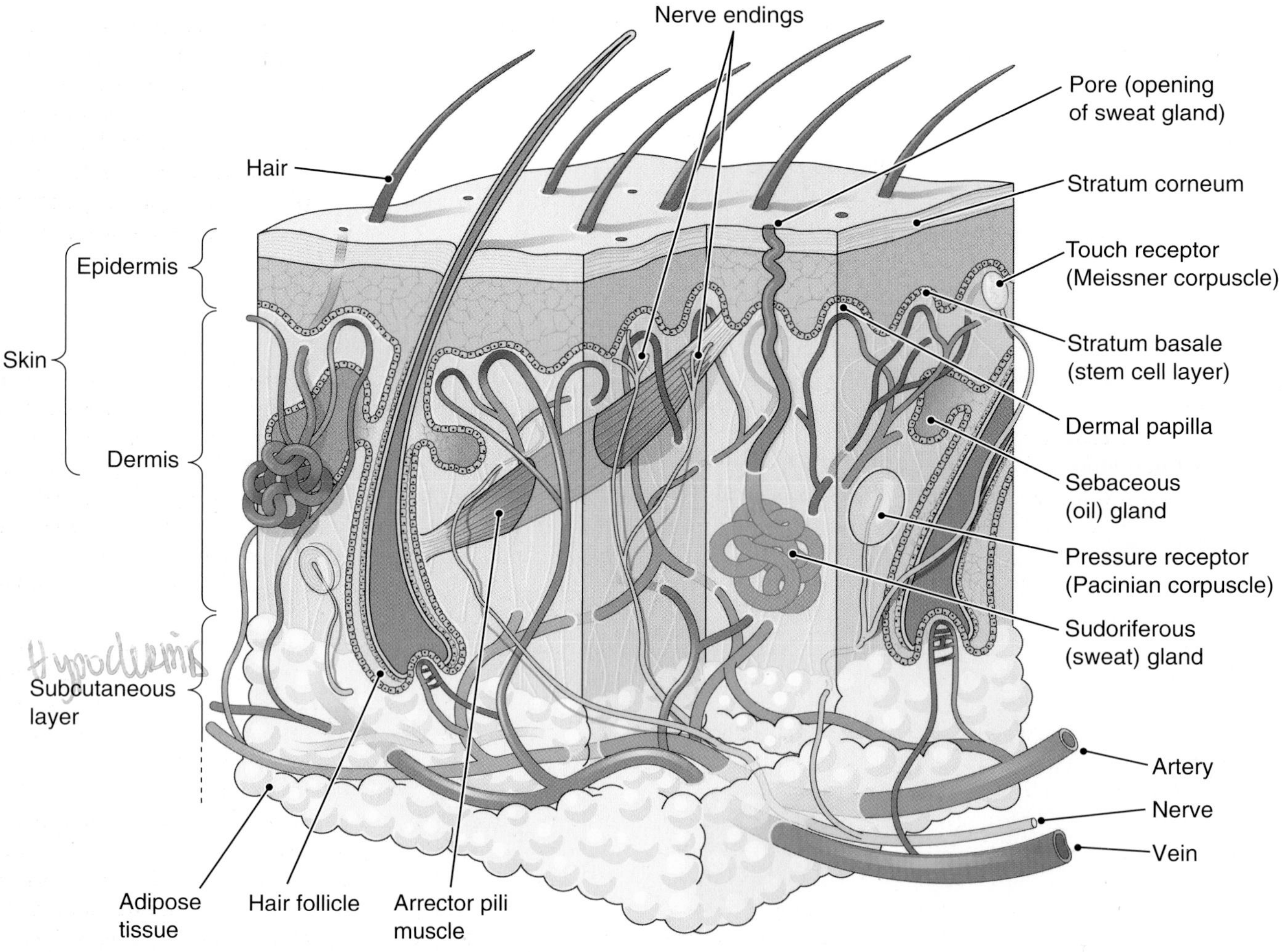

Figure 5-1 Cross section of the skin. KEY POINT The dermis and epidermis make up the skin. The skin and its associated structures make up the integumentary system. ZOOMING IN How is the epidermis supplied with oxygen and nutrients? What tissue is located beneath the skin?

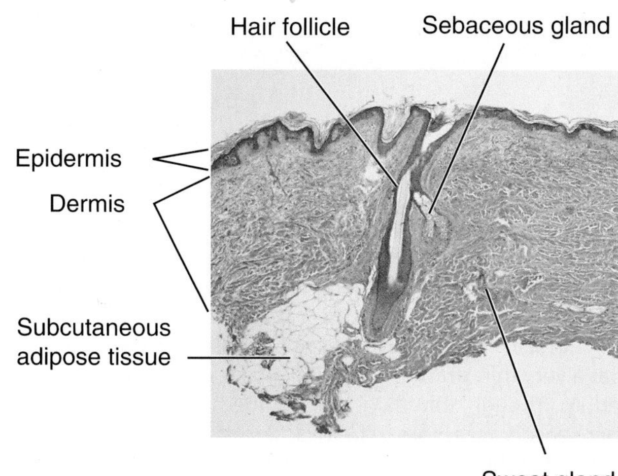

Figure 5-2 Microscopic view of thin skin. Tissue layers and some accessory structures are labeled. (Reprinted with permission from Cormack DH. *Essential Histology*, 2nd ed. Philadelphia, PA: Lippincott Williams & Wilkins, 2001.)

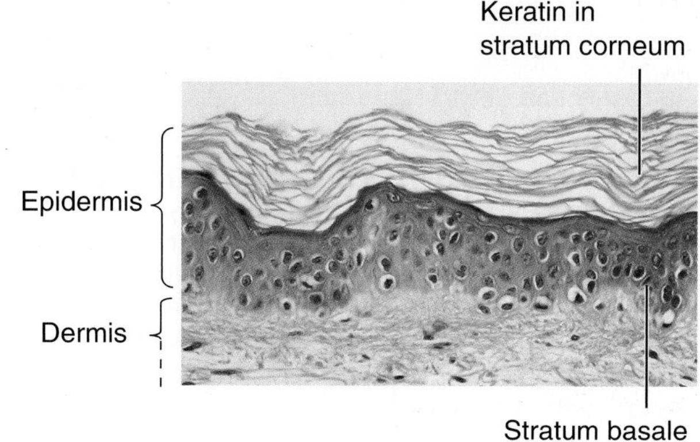

Figure 5-3 Upper portion of the skin. KEY POINT Layers of keratin in the stratum corneum are visible at the surface. Below are layers of stratified squamous epithelium making up the remainder of the epidermis. (Reprinted with permission from Cormack DH. *Essential Histology*, 2nd ed. Philadelphia, PA: Lippincott Williams & Wilkins, 2001.)

- The **dermis**, which has a framework of connective tissue and contains many blood vessels, nerve endings, and glands.

Figure 5-2 is a photograph of the skin as seen through a microscope showing the layers and some accessory structures.

EPIDERMIS

The epidermis is the skin's surface portion, the outermost cells of which are constantly lost through wear and tear. Because there are no blood vessels in the epidermis, the cells must be nourished by capillaries in the underlying dermis. New epidermal cells are produced from stem cells in the deepest layer, which is closest to the dermis. The cells in this layer, the **stratum basale** (bas-A-le), or *stratum germinativum* (jer-min-a-TI-vum), are constantly dividing and producing new cells, which are then pushed upward toward the skin surface. As the epidermal cells die from the gradual loss of nourishment, they undergo changes. Mainly, their cytoplasm is replaced by large amounts of a protein called **keratin** (KER-ah-tin), which thickens and protects the skin (Fig. 5-3).

By the time epidermal cells approach the surface, they have become flat and keratinized, or cornified, forming the uppermost layer of the epidermis, the **stratum corneum** (KOR-ne-um). The stratum corneum is a protective layer and is more prominent in thick skin than in thin skin. Cells at the surface are constantly being lost and replaced from below, especially in areas of the skin that are subject to wear and tear, as on the face, soles of the feet, and palms of the hands. Although this process of **exfoliation** (eks-fo-le-A-shun) occurs naturally at all times, many cosmetics companies sell products to promote exfoliation, presumably to "enliven" and "refresh" the skin.

Between the stratum basale and the stratum corneum are additional layers of stratified epithelium that vary in number and quantity depending on the skin's thickness.

Some cells in the deepest layer of the epidermis produce **melanin** (MEL-ah-nin), a dark pigment that colors the skin and protects it from sunlight's harmful rays. The cells that produce this pigment are the **melanocytes** (MEL-ah-no-sites). Irregular patches of melanin are called freckles.

DERMIS

The **dermis** has a framework of elastic connective tissue and is well supplied with blood vessels and nerves. It is called the "true skin" because it carries out the skin's vital functions. Because of dermal elasticity the skin can stretch, even dramatically as in pregnancy, with little damage. Most of the skin's accessory structures, including the sweat glands, the oil glands, and the hair, are located in the dermis and may extend into the subcutaneous layer under the skin.

Like the epidermis, the dermis varies in thickness in different areas. Some places, such as the soles of the feet and the palms of the hands, are covered with very thick layers of skin, whereas others, such as the eyelids, are covered with very thin and delicate layers (see Box 5-1).

Portions of the dermis extend upward into the epidermis, allowing blood vessels to get closer to the superficial cells (see Fig. 5-1). These extensions, or **dermal papillae**, can be seen on the surface of thick skin, such as at the tips of the fingers and toes. Here they form a distinct pattern of ridges that help to prevent slipping, as when grasping an object. The unchanging patterns of the ridges are determined by heredity. Because they are unique to each person, fingerprints and footprints can be used for identification.

Box 5-1 A Closer Look

Thick and Thin Skin: Getting a Grip on Their Differences

The skin is the largest organ in the body, weighing about 4 kg. Though it appears uniform in structure and function, its thickness in fact varies. Many of the functional differences between skin regions reflect the thickness of the epidermis and not the skin's overall thickness. Based on epidermal thickness, skin can be categorized as **thick** (about 1 mm deep) or **thin** (about 0.1 mm deep).

Areas of the body exposed to significant friction (the palms, fingertips, and bottoms of the feet and toes) are covered with thick skin. It is composed of a thick stratum corneum and an extra layer not found in thin skin, the stratum lucidum, both of which make thick skin resistant to abrasion. Thick skin is also characterized by epidermal ridges (e.g., fingerprints) and numerous sweat glands, but lacks hair and sebaceous (oil) glands. These adaptations make the thick skin covering the hands and feet effective for grasping or gripping. The dermis of thick skin also contains many sensory receptors, giving the hands and feet a superior sense of touch.

Thin skin covers body areas not exposed to much friction. It has a very thin stratum corneum and lacks a distinct stratum lucidum. Though thin skin lacks epidermal ridges and has fewer sensory receptors than thick skin, it has several specializations that thick skin does not. Most thin skin is covered with hair, which may help prevent heat loss from the body. In fact, hair is most densely distributed in skin that covers regions of great heat loss—the head, axillae (armpits), and groin. Thin skin also contains numerous sebaceous glands, making it supple and free of cracks that might let infectious organisms enter.

SUBCUTANEOUS LAYER

The dermis rests on the **subcutaneous** (sub-ku-TA-ne-us) **layer**, sometimes referred to as the hypodermis or the superficial fascia (see Fig. 5-1). This layer connects the skin to the underlying muscles. It consists of loose connective tissue and large amounts of adipose (fat) tissue. The fat serves as insulation and as a reserve energy supply. Continuous bundles of elastic fibers connect the subcutaneous tissue with the dermis, so there is no clear boundary between the two.

The blood vessels that supply the skin with nutrients and oxygen and help to regulate body temperature run through the subcutaneous layer. This tissue is also rich in nerves and nerve endings, including those that supply nerve impulses to and from the dermis and epidermis. The thickness of the subcutaneous layer varies in different parts of the body; it is thinnest on the eyelids and thickest on the abdomen.

CHECKPOINTS 

5-1 What is the name of the system that comprises the skin and all its associated structures?

5-2 Moving from the superficial to the deeper layer, what are the names of the two layers of the skin?

5-3 What is the composition of the subcutaneous layer?

Accessory Structures of the Skin

The integumentary system includes some structures associated with the skin—glands, hair, and nails—that not only protect the skin itself but have some more generalized functions as well.

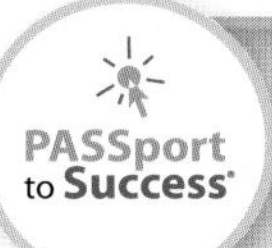

See the student resources on *thePoint* for a chart summarizing the skin's accessory structures.

SEBACEOUS (OIL) GLANDS

The **sebaceous** (se-BA-shus) **glands** are saclike in structure, and their oily secretion, **sebum** (SE-bum), lubricates the skin and hair and prevents drying. The ducts of the sebaceous glands open into the hair follicles (Fig. 5-4A).

Babies are born with a covering produced by these glands that resembles cream cheese; this secretion is called the **vernix caseosa** (VER-niks ka-se-O-sah), which literally means "cheesy varnish." Modified sebaceous glands, **meibomian** (mi-BO-me-an) **glands**, are associated with the eyelashes and produce a secretion that lubricates the eyes.

SUDORIFEROUS (SWEAT) GLANDS

The **sudoriferous** (su-do-RIF-er-us) **glands**, or sweat glands, are coiled, tubelike structures located in the dermis and the subcutaneous tissue (see Fig. 5-4B). Most of the sudoriferous glands function to cool the body. They release sweat, or perspiration, that draws heat from the skin as the moisture evaporates at the surface. These **eccrine** (EK-rin)-type sweat glands are distributed throughout the skin. Each gland has a secretory portion and an excretory tube that extends directly to the surface and opens at a pore (see also Fig. 5-1). Because sweat contains small amounts of dissolved salts and other wastes in addition to water, these glands also serve a minor excretory function.

Present in smaller number, the **apocrine** (AP-o-krin) sweat glands are located mainly in the armpits (axillae)

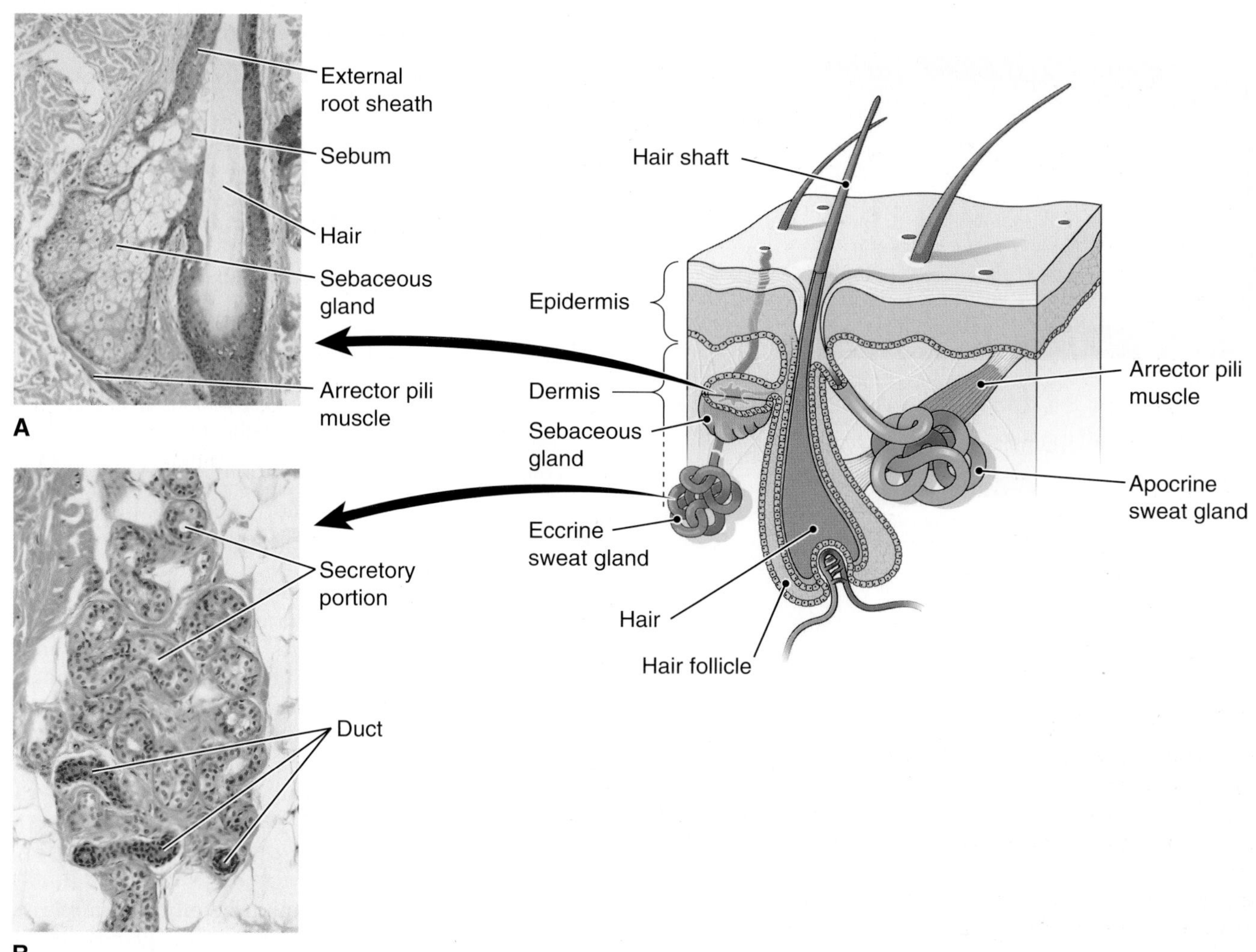

Figure 5-4 Portion of skin showing associated glands and hair. KEY POINT **A.** A sebaceous (oil) gland and its associated hair follicle. **B.** An eccrine (temperature-regulating) sweat gland. (A and B, Reprinted with permission from Cormack DH. *Essential Histology*, 2nd ed. Philadelphia, PA: Lippincott Williams & Wilkins, 2001.) ZOOMING IN How do the sebaceous glands and apocrine sweat glands secrete to the outside? What kind of epithelium makes up the sweat glands?

and groin area. These glands become active at puberty and release their secretions through the hair follicles in response to emotional stress and sexual stimulation. The apocrine glands release some cellular material in their secretions. Body odor develops from the action of bacteria in breaking down these organic cellular materials.

Several types of glands associated with the skin are modified sweat glands. These are the **ceruminous** (seh-RU-min-us) **glands** in the ear canal that produce ear wax, or **cerumen**; the **ciliary** (SIL-e-er-e) **glands** at the edges of the eyelids; and the **mammary glands** in the breasts.

HAIR

Almost all of the body is covered with hair, which in most areas is soft and fine. Hairless regions are the palms of the hands, soles of the feet, lips, nipples, and parts of the external genitalia. Hair is composed mainly of keratin and is not living. Each hair develops, however, from stem cells located in a bulb at the base of the **hair follicle**, a sheath of epithelial and connective tissue that encloses the hair **(see Fig. 5-4)**. Melanocytes in this growth region add pigment to the developing hair. Different shades of melanin produce the various hair colors we see in the population. The part of the hair that projects above the skin is the **shaft**; the portion below the skin is the hair's **root**.

Attached to most hair follicles is a thin band of involuntary muscle **(see Fig. 5-1)**. When a person is frightened or cold, this muscle contracts, raising the hair and forming "goose bumps" on the skin. The name of this muscle is **arrector pili** (ah-REK-tor PI-li), which literally means "hair raiser." This response is not important in humans, but is a warning sign in animals and helps animals with furry coats to conserve heat. As the arrector pili contracts, it presses on the sebaceous gland associated with the hair follicle, causing the release of sebum to lubricate the skin.

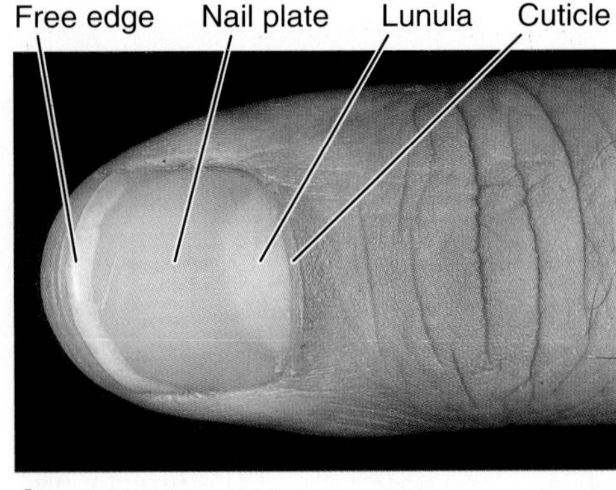

A

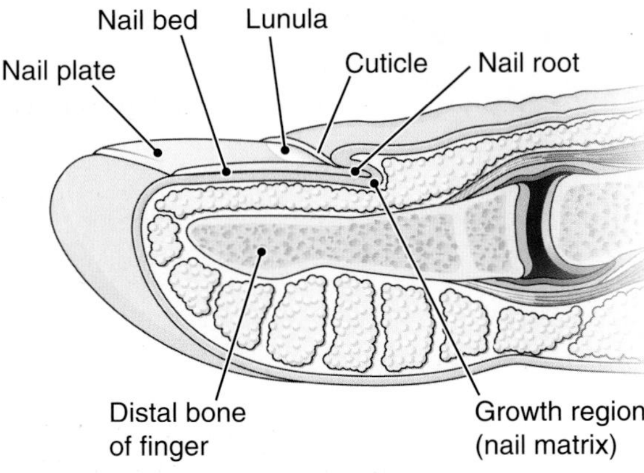

B

Figure 5-5 Nail structure. KEY POINT Nails protect the fingertips and toes. They form from epidermal cells at the nail root. **A.** Photograph of a nail, superior view. **B.** Midsagittal section of a fingertip. (A, Reprinted with permission from Bickley LS. *Bates' Guide to Physical Examination and History Taking*, 8th ed. Philadelphia, PA: Lippincott Williams & Wilkins, 2003.)

NAILS

Nails protect the fingers and toes and also help in grasping small objects with the hands. They are made of hardened keratin formed by the epidermis (Fig. 5-5). New cells develop continuously in a growth region (nail matrix) located under the nail's proximal end, a portion called the **nail root**. The remainder of the **nail plate** rests on a **nail bed** of epithelial tissue. The color of the dermis below the nail bed can be seen through the clear nail. The pale **lunula** (LU-nu-lah), literally "little moon," at the nail's proximal end appears lighter because it lies over the nail's thicker growing region. The **cuticle**, an extension of the stratum corneum, seals the space between the nail plate and the skin above the root.

CHECKPOINTS 

5-4 What is the name of the skin glands that produce an oily secretion?

5-5 What is the scientific name for the sweat glands?

5-6 What is the name of the sheath in which a hair develops?

5-7 Where are the active cells that produce a nail located?

Functions of the Integumentary System

Among the main functions of the integumentary system are the following:

- protection against infection
- protection against dehydration (drying)
- regulation of body temperature
- collection of sensory information

PROTECTION AGAINST INFECTION

Intact skin forms a primary barrier against invasion of pathogens. The cells of the stratum corneum form a tight interlocking pattern that resists penetration. The surface cells are constantly shed, thus mechanically removing pathogens. Rupture of this barrier, as in cases of wounds or burns, invites infection of deeper tissues. The skin also protects against bacterial toxins (poisons) and some harmful chemicals in the environment.

PROTECTION AGAINST DEHYDRATION

Both keratin in the epidermis and the oily sebum released to the skin's surface from the sebaceous glands help to waterproof the skin and keep it moist and supple, even in dry environments. These substances also prevent excessive water loss by evaporation. The skin itself forms a boundary that encloses body fluids, limiting water loss. When the skin is burned, fluid losses are significant, and burn patients commonly complain of intense thirst.

REGULATION OF BODY TEMPERATURE

Both the loss of excess heat and protection from cold are important functions of the integumentary system. Indeed, most of the blood flow to the skin is concerned with temperature regulation. In cold conditions, vessels in the skin constrict (become narrower) to reduce blood flow to the surface and diminish heat loss. The skin may become visibly pale under these conditions. In the skin of the ears, nose, and other exposed locations, special vessels that directly connect arteries and veins provide the volume of blood flow needed to prevent these structures from freezing.

To cool the body, the skin forms a large surface area for radiating body heat to the surrounding air. When the blood vessels dilate (widen), more blood is brought to the surface so that heat can dissipate. The other mechanism for cooling the body involves the sweat glands, as noted above. The evaporation of perspiration draws heat from the skin. A person feels uncomfortable on a hot and humid day because water does not evaporate as readily from the skin into the surrounding air. A dehumidifier makes one more comfortable even when the temperature remains high.

As is the case with so many body functions, temperature regulation is complex and involves other areas, including certain centers in the brain.

COLLECTION OF SENSORY INFORMATION

Because of its many nerve endings and other special receptors, the integumentary system may be regarded as one of the body's chief sensory organs. Free nerve endings detect pain and moderate changes in temperature. Other types of sensory receptors in the skin respond to light touch and deep pressure. **Figure 5-1** shows some free nerve endings, a touch receptor (Meissner corpuscle), and a deep pressure receptor (Pacinian corpuscle) in a section of skin.

Many of the reflexes that make it possible for humans to adjust themselves to the environment begin as sensory impulses from the skin. As elsewhere in the body, the skin receptors work with the brain and the spinal cord to accomplish these important functions.

OTHER ACTIVITIES OF THE INTEGUMENTARY SYSTEM

Substances can be absorbed through the skin in limited amounts. Some drugs—for example, estrogens, other steroids, anesthetics, and medications to control motion sickness—can be absorbed from patches placed on the skin (see Box 5-2). Most medicated ointments used on the skin, however, are for the treatment of local conditions only. Even medication injected into the subcutaneous tissues is absorbed very slowly.

There is also a minimal amount of excretion through the skin. Water and electrolytes are excreted in sweat (perspiration). Some nitrogen-containing wastes are eliminated through the skin, but even in disease, the amount of waste products excreted by the skin is small.

Vitamin D needed for the development and maintenance of bone tissue is manufactured in the skin under the effects of ultraviolet (UV) radiation in sunlight.

Note that the human skin does not "breathe." The pores of the epidermis serve only as outlets for perspiration from the sweat glands and sebum (oil) from the sebaceous glands. They are not used for exchange of gases.

CHECKPOINTS 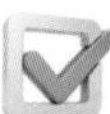

☐ 5-8 What two substances produced in the skin help to prevent dehydration?

☐ 5-9 What two mechanisms involving the skin are used to regulate temperature?

Color of the Skin

Skin color is determined by pigments present in the skin itself and in blood circulating through the skin. The three main pigments that impart color to the skin are:

- Melanin, the skin's main pigment. In addition to its presence in the skin, it is found in the hair, the middle coat of the eyeball, the iris of the eye, and certain

Box 5-2 *Clinical Perspectives*

Medication Patches: No Bitter Pill to Swallow

For most people, pills are a convenient way to take medication, but for others, they have drawbacks. Pills must be taken at regular intervals to ensure consistent dosing, and they must be digested and absorbed into the bloodstream before they can begin to work. For those who have difficulty swallowing or digesting pills, **transdermal (TD) patches** offer an effective alternative to some oral medications.

TD patches deliver a consistent dose of medication that diffuses at a constant rate through the skin into the bloodstream. There is no daily schedule to follow, nothing to swallow, and no stomach upset. TD patches can also deliver medication to unconscious patients, who would otherwise require intravenous drug delivery. TD patches are used in hormone replacement therapy, to treat heart disease, to manage pain, and to suppress motion sickness. Nicotine patches are also used as part of programs to quit smoking.

TD patches must be used carefully. Drug diffusion through the skin takes time, so it is important to know how long the patch must be in place before it is effective. It is also important to know how long the medication's effects will persist after the patch is removed. Because the body continues to absorb what has already diffused into the skin, removing the patch does not entirely remove the medicine. Also, increased heat may elevate drug absorption to dangerous levels.

A recent advance in TD drug delivery is **iontophoresis**. Based on the principle that like charges repel each other, this method uses a mild electric current to move ionic drugs through the skin. A small electrical device attached to the patch uses positive current to "push" positively charged drug molecules through the skin, and a negative current to push negatively charged ones. Even though very low levels of electricity are used, people with pacemakers should not use iontophoretic patches. Another disadvantage is that they can move only ionic drugs through the skin.

tumors. It is common to all races, but darker people have a much larger quantity in their tissues. The melanin in the skin helps to protect against sunlight's damaging UV radiation. Thus, skin that is exposed to the sun shows a normal increase in this pigment, a response we call tanning.

- Hemoglobin (he-mo-GLO-bin), the pigment that carries oxygen in red blood cells (further described in Chapters 12 and 16). It gives blood its color and is visible in the skin through vessels in the dermis.
- Carotene, a skin pigment derived from carrots and other orange and yellow vegetables. It is related to vitamin A and is stored in fatty tissue.

CHECKPOINTS 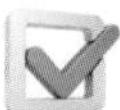

☐ **5-10** What are some pigments that impart color to the skin?

Repair of the Integument

Repair of the integument after injury can occur only in areas that have actively dividing stem cells or cells that can be triggered to divide by injury. These cells are found in the skin's epithelial tissues, and to a lesser extent, connective tissues. Mainly they are located in the stratum basale of the epidermis and in the hair follicles of the dermis. If both layers of the skin are destroyed along with their stem cells, healing may require skin grafts.

Repair of a skin wound or lesion begins after blood has clotted and an inflammatory response occurs. Blood brought to the damaged area brings growth factors that promote the activity of restorative cells and agents that break down tissue debris and fight infection. New vessels branch from damaged capillaries and grow into the injured tissue. Fibroblasts (fiber-producing cells) manufacture collagen to close the gap made by the wound. If the wound is large, underlying tissue may contract to bring the edges of the wound closer together.

A large injury requires extensive growth of new connective tissue, which develops from within the wound. This new tissue sometimes forms a **scar**, also called a **cicatrix** (SIK-ah-triks), which may continue to show at the surface as a white line.

FACTORS THAT AFFECT HEALING

Wound healing is a complex process involving multiple body systems. It is affected by

- Nutrition—A complete and balanced diet will provide the nutrients needed for cell regeneration. All required vitamins and minerals are important, especially vitamins A and C, which are needed for collagen production.
- Blood supply—The blood brings oxygen and nutrients to the tissues and also carries away waste materials and toxins (poisons) that might form during the healing process. White blood cells attack invading bacteria at the site of the injury. Tissues that have an abundant blood supply tend to heal faster than tissues that do not.
- Infection—Contamination prolongs inflammation and interferes with the formation of materials needed for wound repair.
- Age—Healing is generally slower among the elderly reflecting their slower rate of cell replacement. The elderly also may have a lowered immune response to infection.

CHECKPOINT 

☐ **5-11** What two categories of tissues repair themselves most easily?

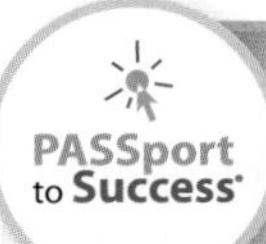

See the student resources on *thePoint* to view an animation on wound healing.

Effects of Aging on the Integumentary System

As people age, wrinkles, or crow's feet, develop around the eyes and mouth owing to the loss of fat, elastic fibers, and collagen in the underlying tissues. The dermis becomes thinner, and the skin may become transparent and lose its elasticity, an effect sometimes called "parchment skin." Pigment formation decreases with age. However, there may be localized areas of extra pigmentation in the skin with the formation of brown spots ("liver spots"), especially on areas exposed to the sun (e.g., the back of the hands). Circulation to the dermis decreases, so white skin looks paler.

The hair does not replace itself as rapidly as before and thus becomes thinner on the scalp and elsewhere on the body. Decreased melanin production leads to gray or white hair. Hair texture changes as the hair shaft becomes less dense, and hair, like the skin, becomes drier as sebum production decreases.

The sweat glands decrease in number, so there is less output of perspiration and lowered ability to withstand heat. The elderly are also more sensitive to cold because of having less fat in the skin and poor circulation. The fingernails may flake, become brittle, or develop ridges, and toenails may become discolored or abnormally thickened.

Care of the Skin

The most important factors in caring for the skin are those that ensure good general health. Proper nutrition and adequate circulation are vital to skin maintenance. Regular cleansing removes dirt and dead skin debris and sustains the slightly acid environment that inhibits bacterial growth. Careful handwashing with soap and water, with attention to the under-nail areas, is a simple measure that reduces the spread of disease.

The skin needs protection from excessive exposure to the UV radiation in sunlight. The radiation causes genetic mutations in skin cells that interfere with repair mechanisms and may lead to cancer. Note that radiation exposure in tanning booths is no safer than sun tanning. Excessive UV radiation also causes premature skin aging, including wrinkling, discoloration ("age spots" or "liver spots"), and a "leathery" texture. Appropriate applications of sunscreens before and during time spent in the sun, especially after swimming, can prevent UV-related skin damage. Limiting sun exposure during midday and covering up with protective clothing are also important. These are all lessons Paul learned in the course of his case study.

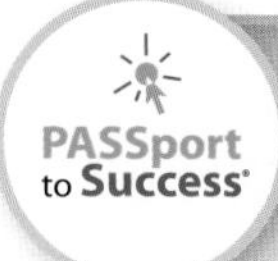

Observation and care of the skin are important in nursing as well as other healthcare professions. The student resources on *thePoint* have information on nursing careers.

A&P in Action Revisited

Squamous Cell Carcinoma

Paul was edgy during the 3 days before he telephoned the dermatologist's office. *What if I have skin cancer? Even if it's treatable, I may have a scar—and right smack in the center of my face!* Finally, he made the call, and learned from Dr. Nielsen that he did indeed have a small squamous cell carcinoma.

"I recommend that you consult Dr. Morris, a local surgeon who specializes in a procedure that guarantees the removal of all abnormal cells," the dermatologist advised. "Mohs surgery is done in stages, with the surgeon first removing just the visible lesion and then checking microscopically to be sure that the margins of the excised tissue are free of cancerous cells. If not, additional tissue is removed by degrees until the margins are clean."

Fortunately, Dr. Morris had to repeat the procedure only once after the first pathology examination to be sure of success. Paul left reassured after several hours. Dr. Morris was confident that Paul was safe from the cancer and that scarring would be minimal. "Let's make an appointment for a follow-up visit when I'll remove the stitches and you can see for yourself," he said.

That evening Paul described his day to his wife and told of his additional instructions. "I need to see my regular dermatologist every 6 months now, as I may be prone to these types of carcinomas." Paul can't undo earlier damage, but he can prevent further insult to his skin by wearing sunscreen outdoors and reapplying it often. The doctor also advised him to cover up in the sun and avoid times of high sun intensity. "Come to think of it," Paul said to his wife, "that's good advice for you too!"

In this case, we saw the carcinogenic effect of sun damage on the integumentary system. Unfortunately for Paul, the effects of years of sun damage are not limited to his skin. In Chapter 10, *The Sensory System*, we learn how sun exposure can affect other systems as well.

Chapter Wrap-Up

Summary Overview

A detailed chapter outline with space for note taking is on *thePoint*. The figure below illustrates the main topics covered in this chapter.

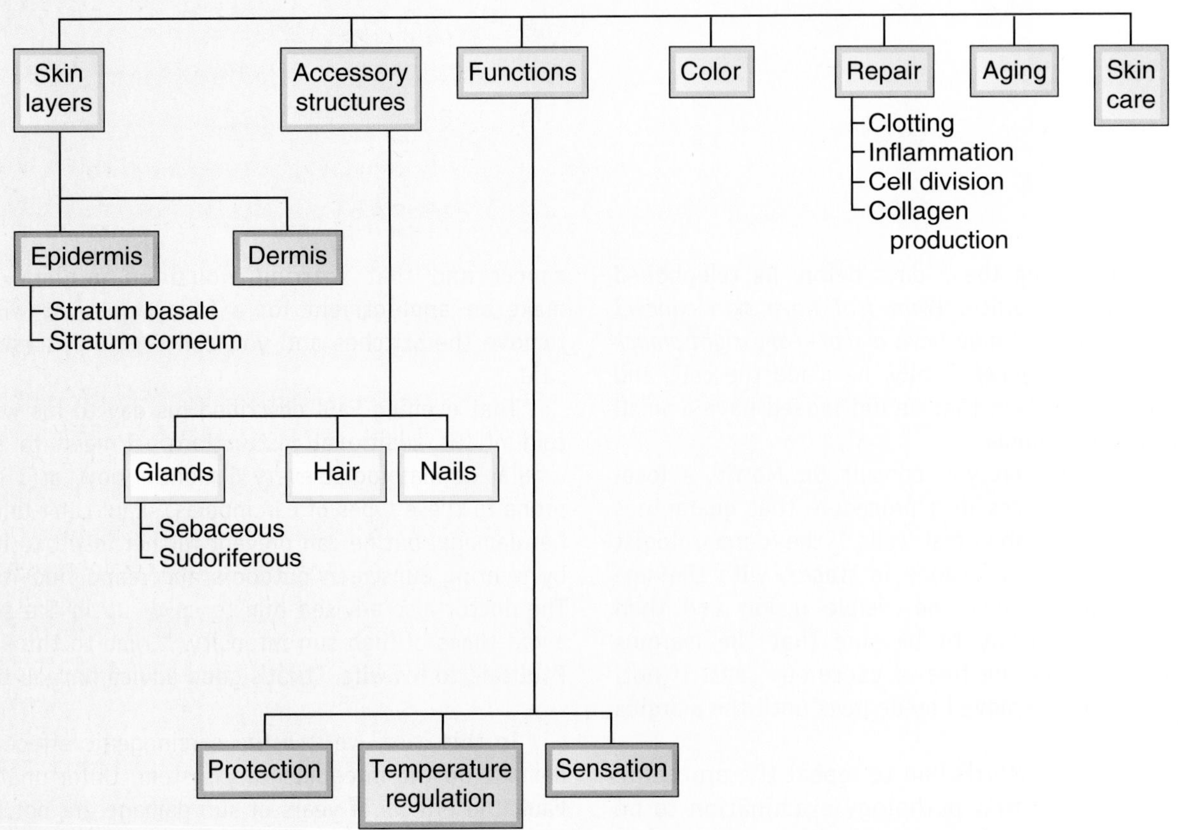

Key Terms

The terms listed below are emphasized in this chapter. Knowing them will help you organize and prioritize your learning. These and other boldface terms are defined in the Glossary with phonetic pronunciations.

apocrine
arrector pili
cerumen
cuticle
dermis
eccrine
epidermis
exfoliation
follicle
integument
keratin
lunula
melanin
melanocyte
papilla
scar
sebaceous
sebum
stratum
subcutaneous
sudoriferous

Word Anatomy

Medical terms are built from standardized word parts (prefixes, roots, and suffixes). Learning the meanings of these parts can help you remember words and interpret unfamiliar terms.

WORD PART	MEANING	EXAMPLE
Structure of the Skin		
derm/o	skin	The *epidermis* is the outermost layer of the skin.
corne/o	cornified, keratinized	The stratum *corneum* is the outermost thickened, keratinized layer of the skin.
melan/o	dark, black	A *melanocyte* is a cell that produces the dark pigment melanin.
sub-	under, below	The *subcutaneous* layer is under the skin.
Accessory Structures of the Skin		
ap/o-	separation from, derivation from	The *apocrine* sweat glands release some cellular material in their secretions
pil/o	hair	The *arrector pili* muscle raises the hair to produce "goose bumps."

Questions for Study and Review

BUILDING UNDERSTANDING

Fill in the blanks

1. The skin and its associated structures form the _____ system.
2. Cells of the stratum corneum contain large amounts of a protein called _____.
3. Sweat glands located in the axillae and groin are called _____ sweat glands.
4. The name of the muscle that raises the hair is _____.
5. A dark-colored pigment that protects the skin from ultraviolet light is called _____.

Matching > Match each numbered item with the most closely related lettered item.

___ **6.** Skin sensitivity characterized by intense itching and inflammation

___ **7.** The lowermost dividing epithelial layer of skin

___ **8.** Accessory structure of skin that senses deep touch

___ **9.** A modified sweat gland that produces ear wax

___ **10.** Accessory structure of skin that lubricates the eye

a. pressure receptor

b. stratum basale

c. ceruminous gland

d. stratum corneum

e. meibomian gland

Multiple Choice

____ **11.** The epidermis is _____ to the dermis.

a. superficial
b. deep
c. lateral
d. medial

____ **12.** The layer of skin that has its own blood supply is the

a. epidermis
b. dermis
c. hypodermis
d. subcutaneous layer

____ **13.** Fingerprints and footprints are formed by

a. melanocytes
b. Meissner corpuscles
c. Pacinian corpuscles
d. dermal papillae

____ **14.** The _____ glands are responsible for temperature regulation.

a. papillary
b. sudoriferous
c. ciliary
d. ceruminous

____ **15.** Nails grow from the

a. lunula
b. cuticle
c. nail bed
d. nail root

UNDERSTANDING CONCEPTS

16. Compare and contrast the epidermis, dermis, and hypodermis. How are the outermost cells of the epidermis replaced?

17. Describe the location and function of the two types of skin glands.

18. What are the four most important functions of the skin?

19. Describe the events associated with skin wound healing.

20. What changes may occur in the skin with age?

CONCEPTUAL THINKING

21. Skin is the largest organ in your body. Why is it considered to be an organ?

22. In Paul's case, sun damage caused skin cancer. Which layer of skin was damaged? Why is this layer most likely to become cancerous?

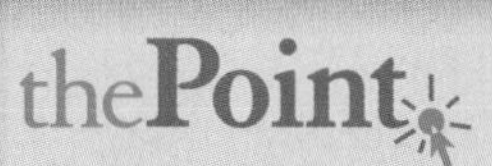

For more questions, see the learning activities on *thePoint*.

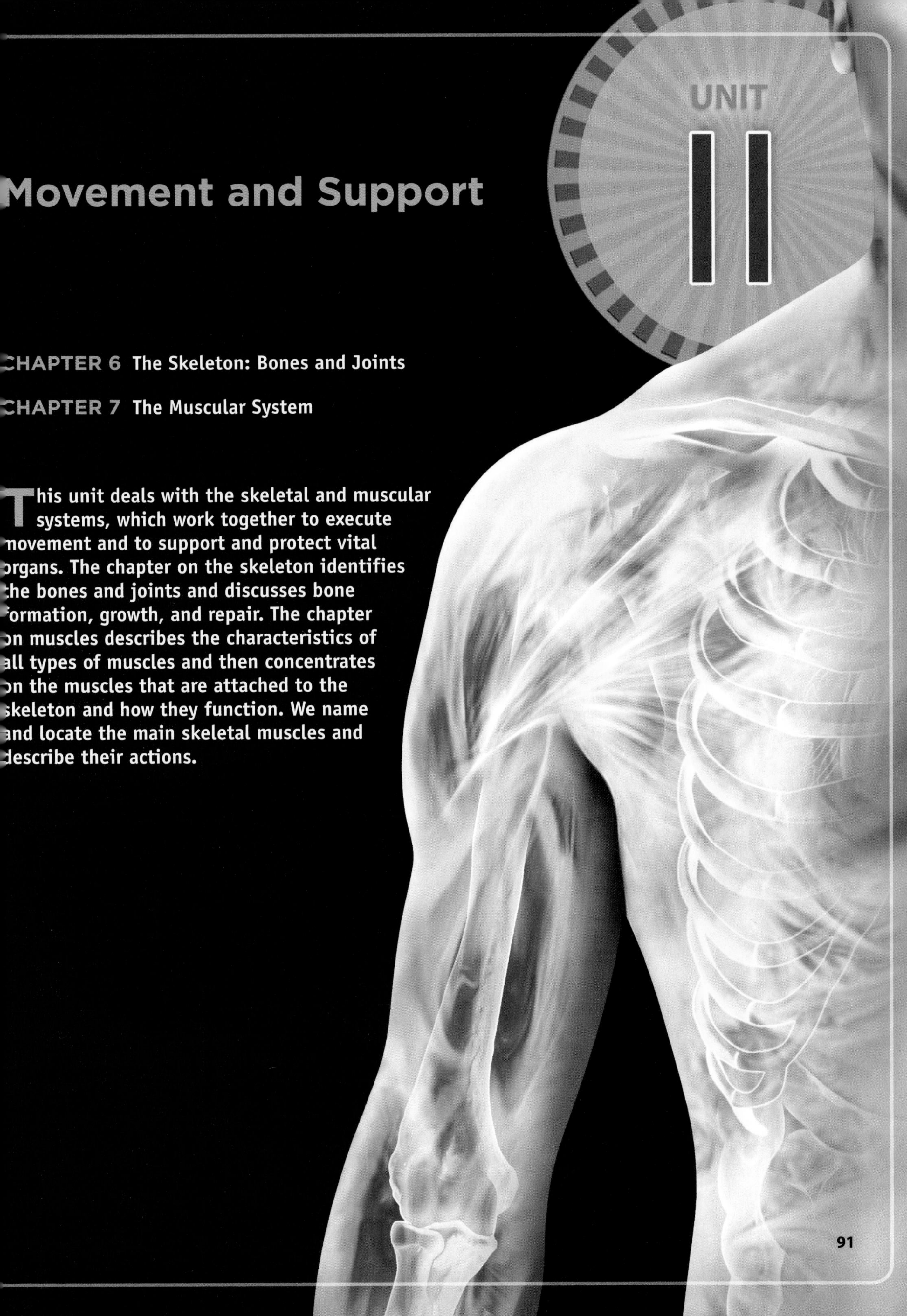

UNIT II

Movement and Support

This unit deals with the skeletal and muscular systems, which work together to execute movement and to support and protect vital organs. The chapter on the skeleton identifies the bones and joints and discusses bone formation, growth, and repair. The chapter on muscles describes the characteristics of all types of muscles and then concentrates on the muscles that are attached to the skeleton and how they function. We name and locate the main skeletal muscles and describe their actions.

CHAPTER

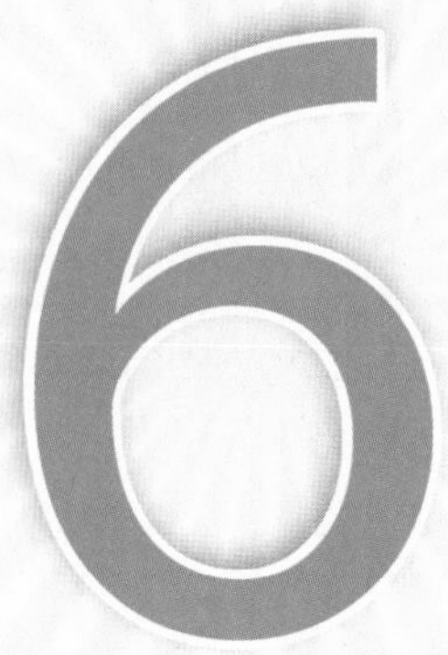

The Skeleton: Bones and Joints

A&P in Action

Reggie's Case: A Footballer's Fractured Femur

"Donnelly throws deep for a touchdown. Wilson makes a beautiful catch! Ooh, a nasty hit from number 26." The crowd roared their approval for the wide receiver. On the ground, Reggie Wilson knew that something was wrong with his hip. In fact, he thought he had actually heard the bone break! It didn't take long for the coaches and medical staff to realize that Reggie needed help. And it didn't take long for the ambulance to get him to the trauma center closest to the stadium.

At the hospital, the emergency team examined Reggie. His injured leg appeared shorter than the other and was adducted and laterally rotated—all signs of a hip fracture. An x-ray confirmed the team's suspicions: Reggie had sustained an intertrochanteric fracture of his right femur. He would need surgery, but luckily for Reggie, the fracture line extended from the greater trochanter to the lesser trochanter and didn't involve the femoral neck. This meant that the blood supply to the femoral head was not in danger, so the surgery would be more straightforward.

In the operating room, the surgical team applied traction to Reggie's right leg, pulling on it to reposition the broken ends of his proximal femur back into anatomic position (verified with another x-ray). Then, the orthopedic surgeon made an incision beginning at the tip of the greater trochanter and continuing distally along the lateral thigh through the skin, subcutaneous fat, and vastus lateralis muscle. After exposing the proximal femur, the surgeon drilled a hole and installed a titanium screw through the greater trochanter, neck, and into the femoral head. He then positioned a titanium plate over the screw and fastened it to the femoral shaft with four more screws. Confident that the broken ends of the femur were firmly held together, the surgeon closed the wound with sutures and skin staples. Reggie was then wheeled into the recovery room.

The surgical team successfully realigned the fractured ends of Reggie's femur. Now Reggie's body will begin the healing process. In this chapter, we learn more about bones and joints. Later in the chapter, we see how Reggie's skeletal system is repairing itself.

PASSport to Success®

Ancillaries At-A-Glance

Visit *thePoint* to access the PASSport to Success and the following resources. For guidance in using these resources most effectively, see pp. ix–xviii.

Learning TOOLS

- Learning Style Self Assessment
- Live Advise Online Student Tutoring
- Tips for Effective Studying

Learning RESOURCES

- E-book: Chapter 6
- Web Figure: Bone markings and formations
- Web Figure: Skeletal features of the anterior and lateral head and neck
- Web Figure: Skeletal features of the posterior head and neck
- Web Figure: Skeletal features of the scapula, shoulder, and torso
- Web Figure: Skeletal features of the arm
- Web Figure: Skeletal features of the thigh
- Web Figure: Skeletal features of the leg and foot
- Web Chart: Bones of the skull
- Animation: Bone Growth
- Health Professions: Radiologic Technologist
- Detailed Chapter Outline
- Answers to Questions for Study and Review
- Audio Pronunciation Glossary

Learning ACTIVITIES

- Pre-Quiz
- Visual Activities
- Kinesthetic Activities
- Auditory Activities

Learning Outcomes

After careful study of this chapter, you should be able to:

1. List the functions of bones, ***p. 94***
2. Describe the structure of a long bone, ***p. 94***
3. Differentiate between compact bone and spongy bone with respect to structure and location, ***p. 95***
4. Name the three different types of cells in bone and describe the functions of each, ***p. 95***
5. Explain how a long bone grows, ***p. 95***
6. Name and describe various markings found on bones, ***p. 97***
7. Name, locate, and describe the bones in the axial skeleton, ***p. 98***
8. Describe the normal curves of the spine and explain their purpose, ***p. 102***
9. Name, locate, and describe the bones in the appendicular skeleton, ***p. 103***
10. Describe three types of joints and give examples of each, ***p. 109***
11. Demonstrate six types of movement that occur at synovial joints, ***p. 111***
12. Describe how the skeletal system changes with age, ***p. 113***
13. Using the case study, discuss the process of bone repair, ***pp. 92, 114***
14. Show how word parts are used to build words related to the skeleton (see Word Anatomy at the end of the chapter), ***p. 116***

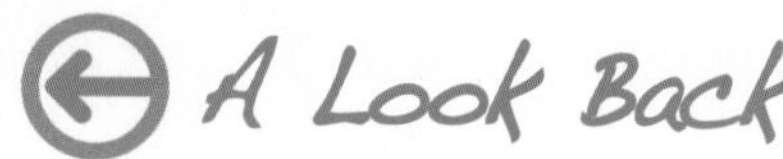

Bone tissue is the most dense form of the connective tissues introduced in Chapter 4. We now describe its characteristics in greater detail and show how it is built into the skeletal system.

The skeleton is the strong framework on which the body is constructed. Much like the frame of a building, the skeleton must be strong enough to support and protect all the body structures. Bones work with muscles to produce movement at the joints. The bones and joints, together with supporting connective tissue, form the skeletal system.

Bones

Bones have a number of functions, several of which are not evident in looking at the skeleton. They:

- form a sturdy framework for the entire body
- protect delicate structures, such as the brain and the spinal cord
- work as levers with attached muscles to produce movement
- store calcium salts, which may be resorbed into the blood if calcium is needed
- produce blood cells (in the red marrow)

BONE STRUCTURE

The complete bony framework of the body, known as the **skeleton** (Fig. 6-1), consists of 206 bones. It is divided into a central portion, the axial skeleton, and the extremities, which make up the appendicular skeleton. The individual bones in these two divisions are described in detail later in this chapter. The bones of the skeleton can be of several different shapes. They may be flat (ribs, cranium), short (carpals of wrist, tarsals of ankle), or irregular (vertebrae, facial bones). The most familiar shape, however, is the **long bone**, the type of bone that makes up almost all of the skeleton of the arms and legs. The long narrow shaft of this type of bone is called the **diaphysis** (di-AF-ih-sis). At the center of the diaphysis is a **medullary** (MED-u-lar-e) **cavity**, which contains bone marrow. The long bone also has two irregular ends, a proximal and a distal **epiphysis** (eh-PIF-ih-sis) (Fig. 6-2).

Bone Marrow Bones contain two kinds of marrow. **Red marrow** is found in the spongy bone at the ends of the long bones and at the center of other bones (see Fig. 6-2). Red bone marrow manufactures blood cells. **Yellow marrow** is found chiefly in the central cavities of the long bones. Yellow marrow is composed largely of fat.

Bone Membranes Bones are covered on the outside (except at the joint region) by a membrane called the **periosteum** (per-e-OS-te-um) (see Fig. 6-2). This membrane's inner layer contains cells (osteoblasts) that are essential in bone formation, not only during growth but also in the repair of injuries. Blood vessels in the periosteum play an important role in the nourishment of bone tissue. Nerve fibers in the periosteum make their presence known when a person suffers a fracture or receives a blow, such as on the shinbone. A thinner membrane, the **endosteum** (en-DOS-te-um), lines the bone's marrow cavity; it too contains cells that aid in the growth and repair of bone tissue.

Bone Tissue Bones are not lifeless. Even though the spaces between the cells of bone tissue—called **osseous** (OS-e-us) **tissue**—are permeated with hard mineral deposits of calcium salts, the cells themselves are very much alive. Bones are organs, with their own systems of blood vessels, lymphatic vessels, and nerves.

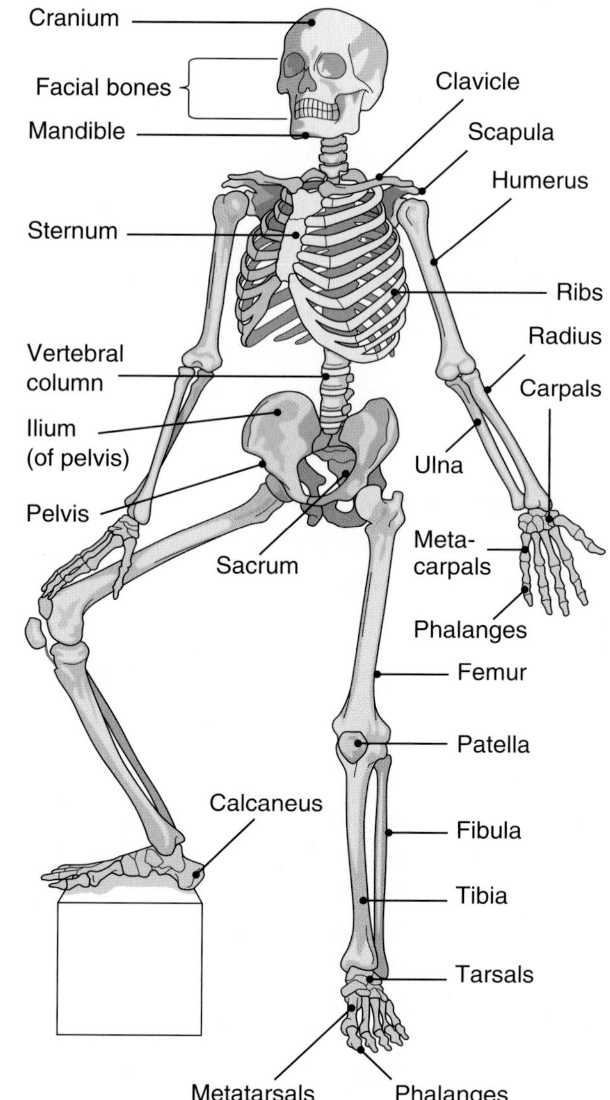

Figure 6-1 The skeleton. KEY POINT: The skeleton is divided into two portions. The axial skeleton is shown here in *yellow*; the appendicular, in *blue*.

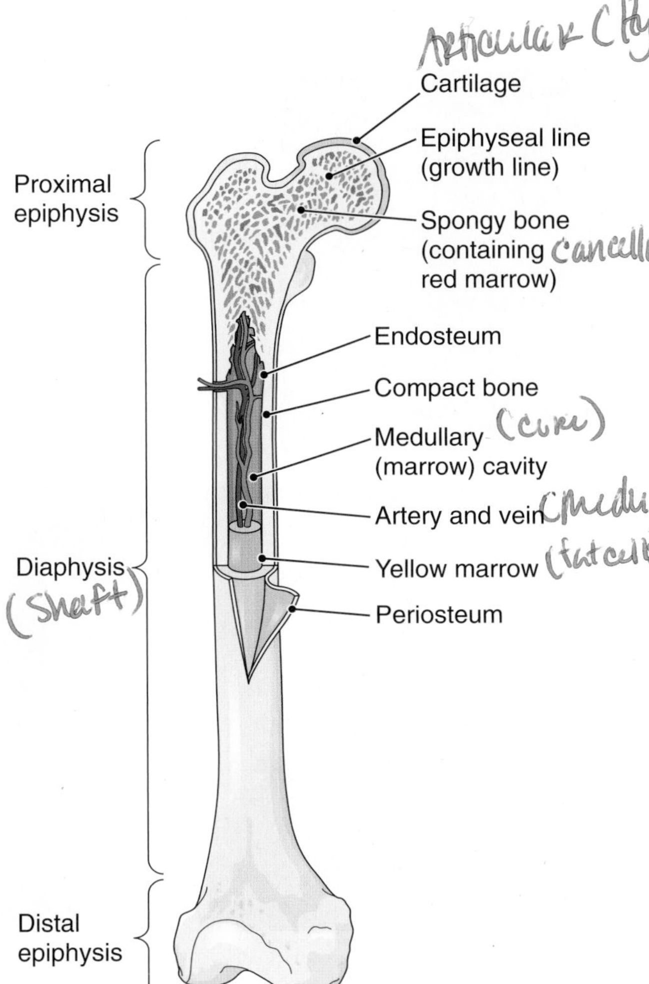

Figure 6-2 The structure of a long bone. KEY POINT A long bone has a long, narrow shaft, the diaphysis, and two irregular ends, the epiphyses. The medullary cavity has yellow marrow. Red marrow is located in spongy bone. ZOOMING IN What are the membranes on the outside and the inside of a long bone called?

There are two types of osseous tissue: compact and spongy. **Compact bone** is hard and dense **(Fig. 6-3)**. This tissue makes up the main shaft of a long bone and the outer layer of other bones. The cells in this type of bone are located in rings of bone tissue around a **central canal**, also called a *haversian* (ha-VER-shan) *canal* containing nerves and blood vessels. The bone cells live in spaces (lacunae) between the rings and extend out into many small radiating channels so that they can be in contact with nearby cells. Each ringlike unit with its central canal makes up an **osteon** (OS-te-on) or haversian system **(see Fig. 6-3B)**. Forming channels across the bone, from one side of the shaft to the other, are many **perforating** (Volkmann) **canals**, which also house blood vessels and nerves.

The second type of bone tissue, called **spongy bone**, or cancellous bone, has more spaces than compact bone. It is made of a meshwork of small, bony plates filled with red marrow. Spongy bone is found at the epiphyses (ends) of the long bones and at the center of other bones. It also lines the medullary cavity of long bones. **Figure 6-3C** shows a photograph of both compact and spongy bone tissue.

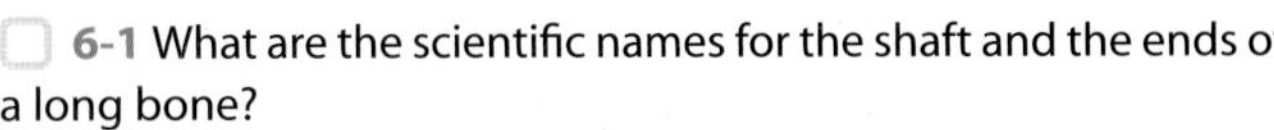

CHECKPOINTS

- 6-1 What are the scientific names for the shaft and the ends of a long bone?
- 6-2 What are the two types of osseous (bone) tissue and where is each type found?

BONE GROWTH, MAINTENANCE, AND REPAIR

The process of bone formation begins in the earliest weeks of embryonic life and continues until young adulthood. Even after skeletal growth is complete, bone cells actively maintain and repair bone tissue.

Fetal Ossification During early development, the embryonic skeleton is at first composed almost entirely of cartilage. (Portions of the skull and a few other bones develop from fibrous connective tissue.) The conversion of cartilage to bone, a process known as **ossification**, begins during the second and third months of embryonic life. At this time, bone-building cells, called **osteoblasts** (OS-te-o-blasts), become active. First, they begin to manufacture the **matrix**, which is the material located between the cells. This intercellular substance contains large quantities of **collagen** (KOL-ah-jen), a fibrous protein that gives the tissue strength and resilience. Then, with the help of enzymes, calcium compounds are deposited within the matrix.

Once this intercellular material has hardened, the cells remain enclosed within the lacunae (small spaces) in the matrix. These cells, now known as **osteocytes** (OS-te-o-sites), are still living and continue to maintain the existing bone matrix, but they do not produce new bone tissue. When bone has to be remodeled or repaired later in life, new osteoblasts develop from stem cells in the endosteum and periosteum. You will see the importance of these cells in Reggie's case study.

Formation of a Long Bone In a long bone, the transformation of cartilage into bone begins at the center of the shaft during fetal development. Around the time of birth, secondary bone-forming centers, or **epiphyseal** (ep-ih-FIZ-e-al) **plates**, develop across the ends of the bones. The long bones continue to grow in length at these centers by calcification of new cartilage through childhood and into the late teens. Finally, by the late teens or early 20s, the bones stop growing in length. Each epiphyseal plate hardens and can be seen in x-ray films as a thin line, the epiphyseal line, across the end of the bone **(see Figs. 6-2 and 6-3C)**. Physicians can judge a bone's future growth by the appearance of these lines on x-ray films.

As a bone grows in length, the shaft is remodeled as well, becoming wider as the central marrow cavity increases in size.

Bone Resorption One other cell type found in bone develops from a type of white blood cell (monocyte). These large, multinucleated **osteoclasts** (OS-te-o-klasts)

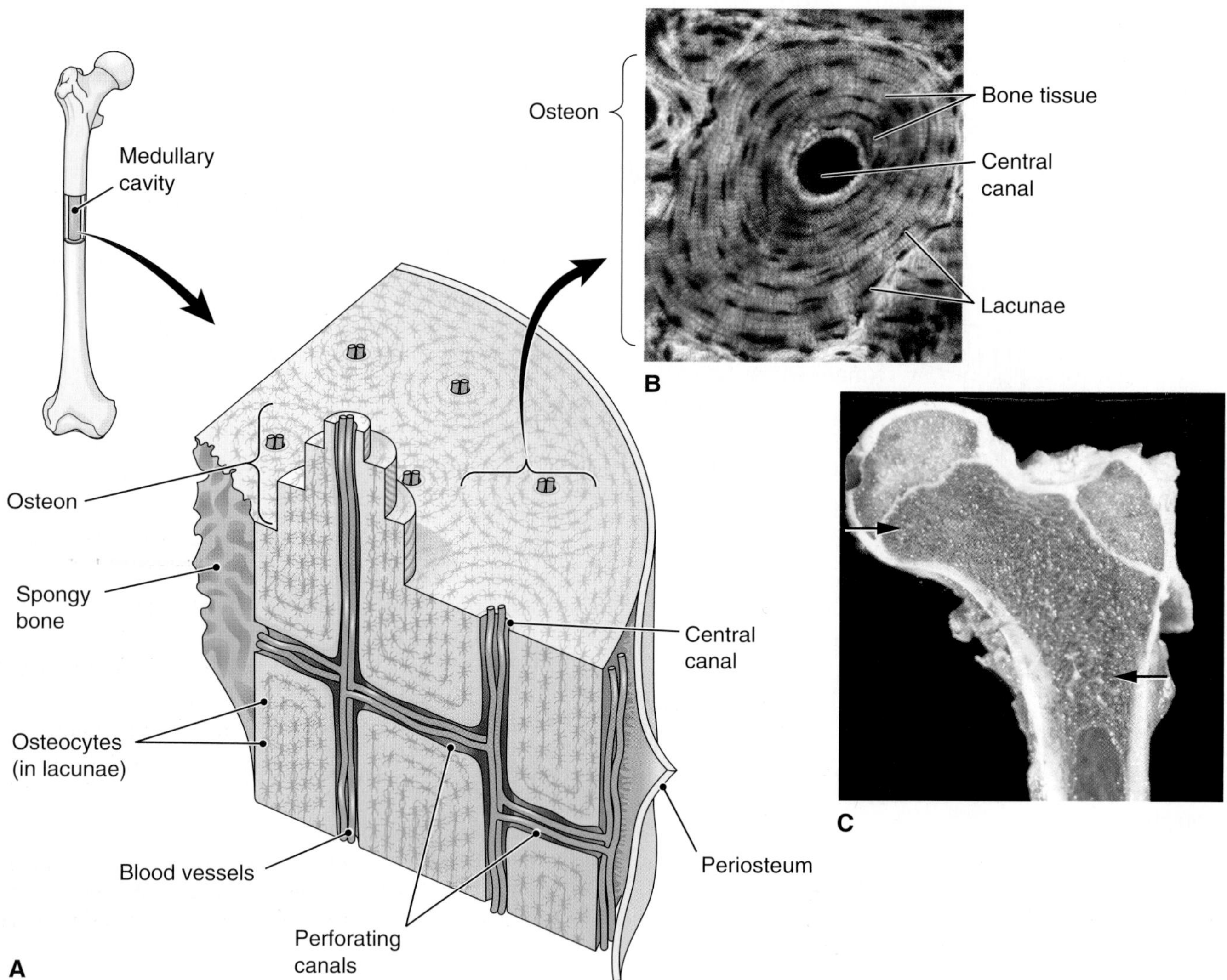

Figure 6-3 **Bone tissue.** KEY POINT There are two types of bone tissue—compact and spongy. **A.** This section shows osteocytes (bone cells) within osteons (haversian systems) in compact bone. It also shows the canals that penetrate the tissue. **B.** Microscopic view of compact bone in cross section (×300) showing a complete osteon. In living tissue, osteocytes (bone cells) reside in spaces (lacunae) and extend out into channels that radiate from these spaces. (Reprinted with permission from Gartner LP, Hiatt JL. *Color Atlas of Histology*, 4th ed. Baltimore, MD: Lippincott Williams & Wilkins, 2005). **C.** Longitudinal section of a long bone showing both types of bone tissue. There is an outer layer of compact bone; the remainder of the tissue is spongy bone, shown by the arrows. Transverse growth lines are also visible. (Reprinted with permission from Rubin R, Strayer DS. *Rubin's Pathology: Clinicopathologic Foundations of Medicine,* 5th ed. Baltimore, MD: Lippincott Williams & Wilkins, 2007). ZOOMING IN What cells are located in the spaces of compact bone?

are responsible for the process of **resorption**, which is the breakdown of bone tissue. Resorption is necessary for bone remodeling: as bone is added to some areas, it is resorbed from others, as seen in formation of a long bone. Resorption is also necessary for repair of bone injury. In addition, bone tissue is resorbed when the body needs its stored minerals.

Both the formation and resorption of bone tissue are regulated by hormones. Vitamin D promotes calcium absorption from the intestine. Another hormone involved in these processes is produced by glands in the neck. Parathyroid hormone from the parathyroid glands, located at the posterior of the thyroid, causes bone resorption and release of calcium into the blood. The sex hormones, estrogen and testosterone, also contribute to bone growth and maintenance. Hormones are discussed more fully in Chapter 11.

The processes of bone resorption and bone formation continue throughout life, more actively in some places than in others, as bones are subjected to wear and tear or injuries. The bones of small children are relatively pliable because they contain a larger proportion of cartilage and are undergoing active bone formation. Bones increase in density until the early 20s in females and the late 20s in males, at which point bones are at peak density and strength. Most people maintain peak bone density until about age 40. As people age, there is a slowing of bone tissue renewal. As a result, the bones become weaker and damage heals more slowly.

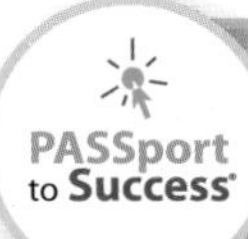

See the student resources on *thePoint* to view the animation *Bone Growth*, showing the growth process in a long bone.

BONE MARKINGS

In addition to their general shape, bones have other distinguishing features, or **bone markings**. These markings include raised areas and depressions, which help to form joints or serve as points for muscle attachments, and various holes, which allow the passage of nerves and blood vessels. Some of these identifying features are described next.

Projections

- **Head**—a rounded, knoblike end separated from the rest of the bone by a slender region, the neck
- **Process**—a large projection of a bone, such as the superior process of the ulna in the forearm that creates the elbow
- **Condyle** (KON-dile)—a rounded projection; a small projection above a condyle is an epicondyle
- **Crest**—a distinct border or ridge, often rough, such as over the top of the hip bone
- **Spine**—a sharp projection from the surface of a bone, such as the spine of the scapula (shoulder blade)

Depressions or Holes

- **Foramen** (fo-RA-men)—a hole that allows a vessel or a nerve to pass through or between bones. The plural is foramina (fo-RAM-ih-nah).

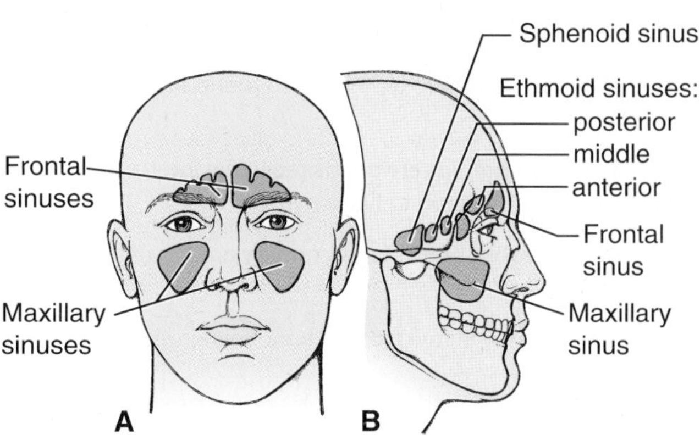

Figure 6-4 **Sinuses** KEY POINT A sinus is a cavity or hollow space, such as the air-filled chambers in certain skull bones. **A.** Anterior view of the skull showing sinuses. **B.** Lateral view.

- **Sinus** (SI-nus)—A cavity or hollow space. Most commonly, an air-filled chamber found in some skull bones. (Fig. 6-4) These sinuses are named for the bones in which they are located, as described below.
- **Fossa** (FOS-sah)—a depression on a bone surface. The plural is fossae (FOS-se).
- **Meatus** (me-A-tus)—a short channel or passageway, usually the external opening of a canal. An example is the channel in the skull's temporal bone that leads to the inner ear.

Examples of these and other markings can be seen on the bones illustrated in this chapter. To find out how these markings can be used in healthcare, see Box 6-1, Landmarking: Seeing with Your Fingers.

Box 6-1 *Clinical Perspectives*

Landmarking: Seeing with Your Fingers

Most body structures lie beneath the skin, hidden from direct view except in dissection. A technique called **landmarking** allows healthcare providers to locate hidden structures simply and easily. Bony prominences, or landmarks, can be palpated (felt) beneath the skin to serve as reference points for locating other internal structures. Landmarking is used during physical examinations and surgeries, when giving injections, and for many other clinical procedures. The lower tip of the sternum, the xiphoid process, is a reference point in the administration of CPR.

Practice landmarking by feeling for some of the other bony prominences. You can feel the joint between the mandible and the temporal bone of the skull (the temporomandibular joint, or TMJ) anterior to the ear canal as you move your lower jaw up and down. Feel for the notch in the sternum (breast bone) between the clavicles (collar bones). Approximately 4 cm below this notch you will feel a bump called the sternal angle. This prominence is an important landmark because its location marks where the trachea splits to deliver air to both lungs. Move your fingers lateral to the sternal angle to palpate the second ribs, important landmarks for locating the heart and lungs. Feel for the most lateral bony prominence of the shoulder, the acromion process of the scapula (shoulder blade). Two to three fingerbreadths down from this point is the correct injection site into the deltoid muscle of the shoulder. Place your hands on your hips and palpate the iliac crest of the hip bone. Move your hands forward until you reach the anterior end of the crest, the anterior superior iliac spine (ASIS). Feel for the part of the bony pelvis that you sit on. This is the ischial tuberosity. This and the ASIS are important landmarks for locating safe injection sites in the gluteal region.

CHECKPOINTS 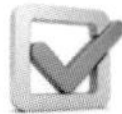

☐ 6-3 What are the three types of cells found in bone and what is the role of each?

☐ 6-4 What compounds are deposited in the intercellular matrix of the embryonic skeleton to harden it?

☐ 6-5 What are the centers for secondary growth of a long bone called?

☐ 6-6 What are some functions of bone markings?

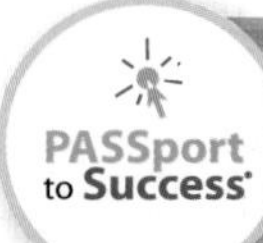

See the student resources on *thePoint* to view bone markings on an illustration of a whole skeleton.

Bones of the Axial Skeleton

As noted earlier, the skeleton may be divided into two main groups of bones (see Fig. 6-1):

- The **axial** (AK-se-al) **skeleton** consists of 80 bones and includes the bony framework of the head and the trunk. Think of the axial skeleton as the body's "axis."
- The **appendicular** (ap-en-DIK-u-lar) **skeleton** consists of 126 bones and forms the framework for the **extremities** (limbs) and for the shoulders and hips. Think of the appendicular skeleton as the body's "appendages."

We describe the axial skeleton first and then proceed to the appendicular skeleton. A table at the end of this section summarizes all of the bones described. Also see Appendix 3: Dissection Atlas, Figures A3-1 and A3-2, for pictures of a complete human skeleton, both anterior and posterior views. You can refer to these pictures as you study this chapter.

FRAMEWORK OF THE SKULL

The bony framework of the head, called the **skull,** is subdivided into two parts: the cranium and the facial portion. Refer to Figures 6-5 and 6-6, which show different views of the skull, as you study the following descriptions. The individual bones are color coded to help you identify them as you study the skull in different views.

Note the many features of the skull bones as you examine these illustrations. For example, openings in the base of the skull provide spaces for the entrance and exit of many blood vessels, nerves, and other structures. Bone projections and depressions (fossae) provide for muscle attachment. Some portions protect delicate structures, for example, the eye orbit (socket) and the part of the temporal bone at the lateral skull that encloses the inner ear. The sinuses provide lightness and serve as resonating chambers for the voice (which is why your voice sounds better to you as you are speaking than it sounds when you hear it played back as a recording).

Cranium This rounded chamber that encloses the brain is composed of eight distinct cranial bones.

- The **frontal bone** forms the forehead, the anterior of the skull's roof, and the roof of the eye orbit. The **frontal sinuses** communicate with the nasal cavities (see Fig. 6-6). These sinuses and others near the nose are described as **paranasal sinuses.**
- The two **parietal** (pah-RI-eh-tal) bones form most of the top and the sidewalls of the cranium.
- The two **temporal bones** form part of the sides and some of the base of the skull. Each contains the ear canal, the eardrum, and the ear's entire middle and inner portions. The **mastoid process** of the temporal bone projects downward immediately behind the outer ear. It is a place for muscle attachments and contains air cells that make up the **mastoid sinus** (see Fig. 6-5 B,C).
- The **ethmoid** (ETH-moyd) **bone** is a light, fragile bone located between the eyes (see Fig. 6-5 A,D). It forms a part of the medial wall of the eye orbit, a small portion of the cranial floor, and most of the nasal cavity roof. It also forms the superior and middle nasal conchae (KON-ke), bony plates that extend into the nasal cavity (the name *concha* means "shell") (see Fig. 6-6). The mucous membranes covering the conchae help to filter, warm, and moisten air as it passes through the nose. The ethmoid houses several air cells (spaces), comprising some of the paranasal sinuses. A thin, platelike, downward extension of this bone (the perpendicular plate) forms much of the nasal septum, a midline partition in the nose (see Fig. 6-5A).
- The **sphenoid** (SFE-noyd) **bone,** when seen from a superior view, resembles a bat with its wings extended. It lies at the base of the skull anterior to the temporal bones and forms part of the eye orbit. It contains the sphenoid sinuses. It also contains a depression called the **sella turcica** (SEL-ah TUR-sih-ka), literally "Turkish saddle," that holds and protects the pituitary gland like a saddle (see Fig. 6-5D).
- The **occipital** (ok-SIP-ih-tal) **bone** forms the skull's posterior portion and a part of its base. The **foramen magnum**, located at the base of the occipital bone, is a large opening through which the spinal cord communicates with the brain (see Figs. 6-5C,D).

Uniting the skull bones is a type of flat, immovable joint known as a **suture** (SU-chur) (see Fig. 6-5B). Some of the most prominent cranial sutures are as follows:

- The coronal (ko-RO-nal) suture joins the frontal bone with the two parietal bones along the coronal plane.
- The squamous (SKWA-mus) suture joins the temporal bone to the parietal bone on the cranium's lateral surface (named because it is in a flat portion of the skull).
- The lambdoid (LAM-doyd) suture joins the occipital bone with the parietal bones in the posterior cranium (named because it resembles the Greek letter lambda).

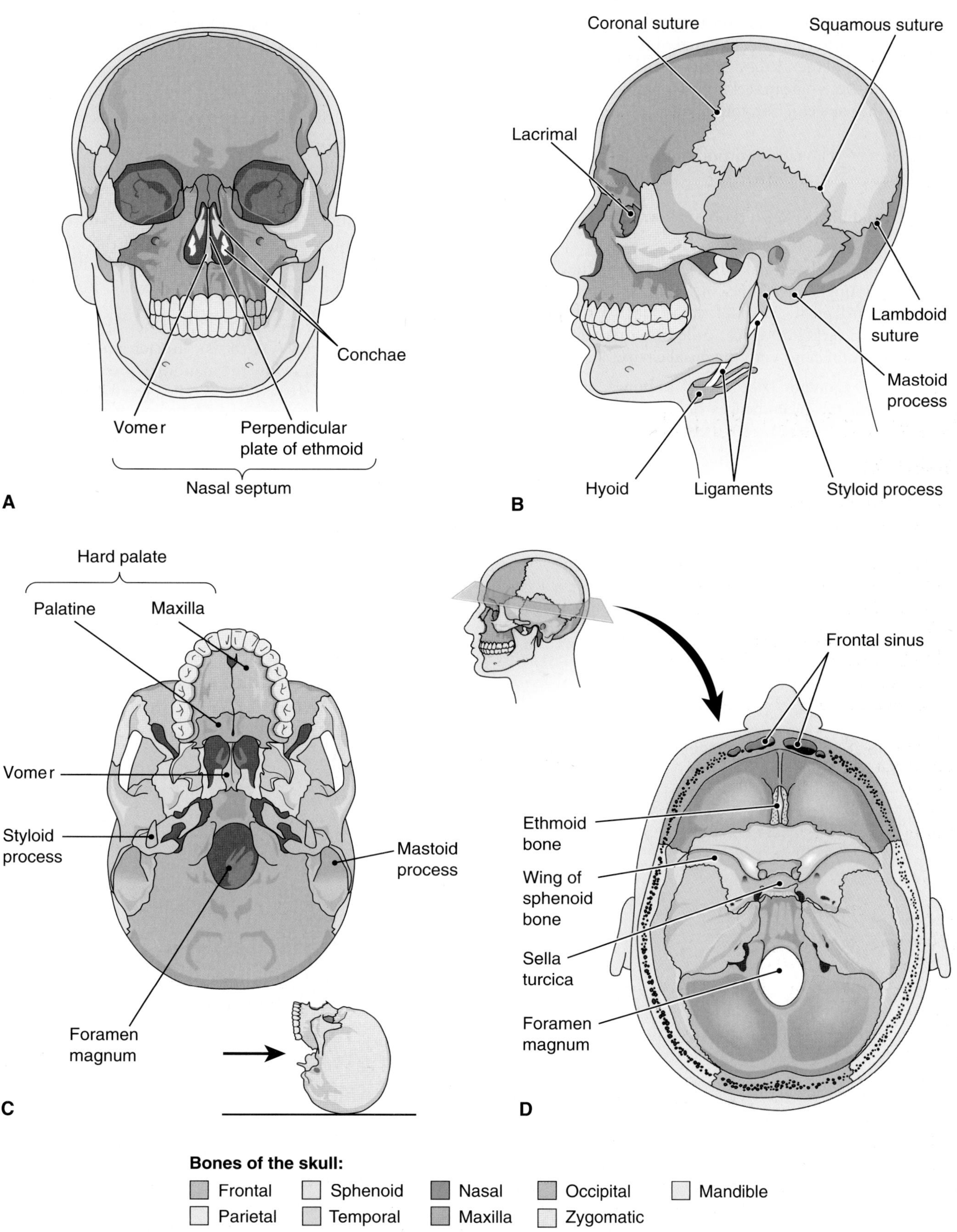

6

Figure 6-5 **The skull. A.** Anterior view. **B.** Left lateral view. **C.** Inferior view. The mandible (lower jaw) has been removed. **D.** Floor of cranium, superior view. The internal surfaces of some of the cranial bones are visible. ZOOMING IN What type of joint is between the bones of the skull? What two bones make up each side of the hard palate? What is a foramen?

- The sagittal (SAJ-ih-tal) suture joins the two parietal bones along the superior midline of the cranium, along the sagittal plane. Although this suture is not visible in **Figure 6-5B**, you can feel it if you press your fingertips along the top center of your skull.

Facial Bones The facial portion of the skull is composed of 14 bones **(see Fig. 6-5A)**:

- The **mandible** (MAN-dih-bl), or lower jaw bone, is the skull's only movable bone.
- The two **maxillae** (mak-SIL-e) fuse in the midline to form the upper jaw bone, including the anterior part of the hard palate (roof of the mouth). Each maxilla contains a large air space, called the **maxillary sinus,** that communicates with the nasal cavity.
- The two **zygomatic** (zi-go-MAT-ik) **bones**, one on each side, form the prominences of the cheeks. The zygomatic forms an arch over the cheek with a process of the temporal bone **(see Fig. 6-5B)**.
- Two slender **nasal bones** lie side by side, forming the bridge of the nose.
- The two **lacrimal** (LAK-rih-mal) **bones**, each about the size of a fingernail, form the anterior medial wall of each orbital cavity.
- The **vomer** (VO-mer), shaped like the blade of a plow, forms the inferior part of the nasal septum **(see Figs. 6-5A,C)**.
- The paired **palatine** (PAL-ah-tine) **bones** form the posterior part of the hard palate **(see Figs. 6-5C and 6-6)**.
- The two **inferior nasal conchae** (KON-ke) extend horizontally along the lateral wall (side) of the nasal cavities. (As noted, the paired superior and middle conchae are part of the ethmoid bone, as shown in **Fig. 6-6**).

In addition to the cranial and facial bones, there are three tiny bones, or **ossicles** (OS-sik-ls), in each middle ear (see Chapter 11) and, just below the mandible (lower jaw), a single horseshoe, or U-shaped, bone called the **hyoid** (HI-oyd) **bone**, to which the tongue and other muscles are attached **(see Fig. 6-5B)**.

Infant Skull The infant's skull has areas in which the bone formation is incomplete, leaving membranous "soft spots," properly called **fontanels** (fon-tah-NELS) **(Fig. 6-7)**. These

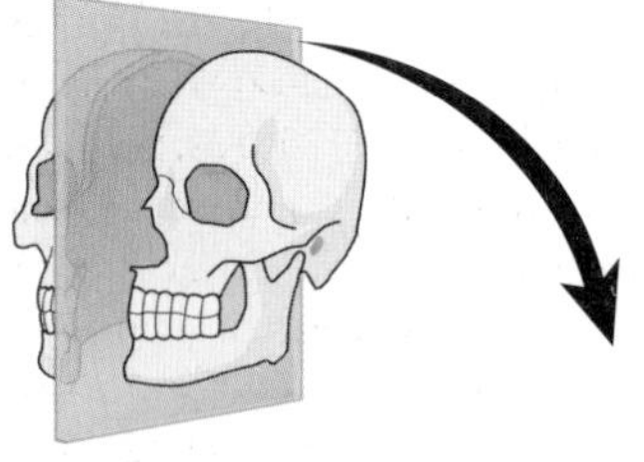

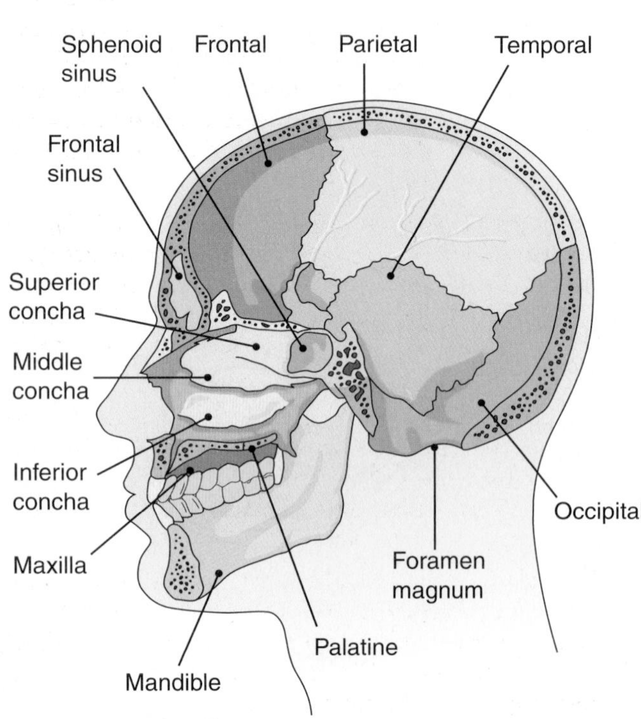

Figure 6-6 The skull, sagittal section. ZOOMING IN What bone makes up the superior and middle conchae?

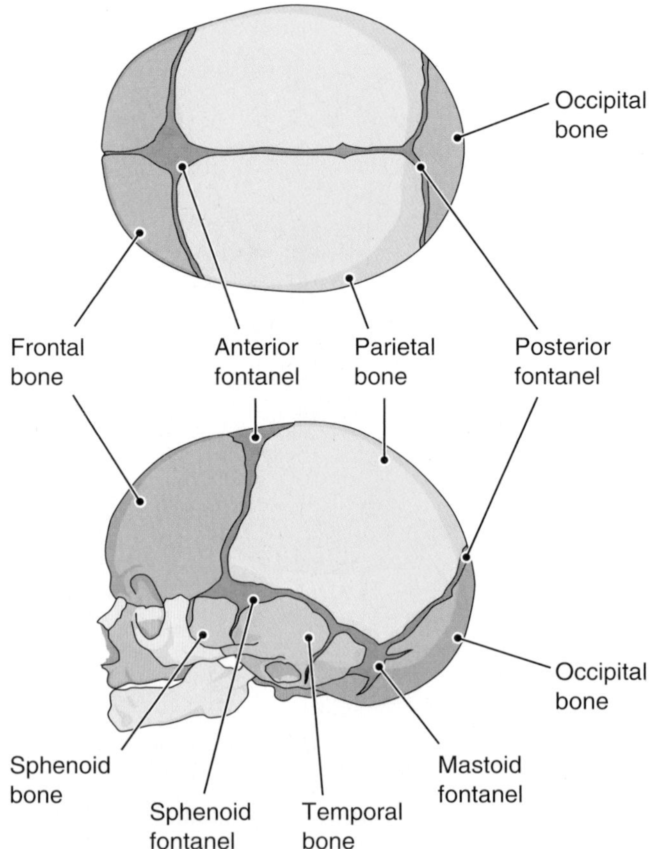

Figure 6-7 Infant skull, showing fontanels. KEY POINT Fibrous membranes between the skull bones allow the skull to compress during childbirth. Sutures later form in these areas. ZOOMING IN Which is the largest fontanel?

flexible regions allow the skull to compress and change shape during the birth process. They also allow for rapid brain growth during infancy. Although there are a number of fontanels, named for their location or the bones they border, the largest and most recognizable is near the front of the skull at the junction of the two parietal bones and the frontal bone. This anterior fontanel usually does not close until the child is about 18 months old.

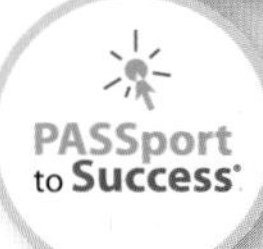

See the student resources on *thePoint* for a summary table of the cranial and facial bones and supplementary pictures of the anterior and posterior head and neck.

FRAMEWORK OF THE TRUNK

The bones of the trunk include the spine, or **vertebral** (VER-teh-bral), **column**, and the bones of the chest, or **thorax** (THO-raks).

Vertebral Column This bony sheath for the spinal cord is made of a series of irregularly shaped bones. These number 33 or 34 in the child, but because of fusions that occur later in the lower part of the spine, there usually are just 26 separate bones in the adult spinal column. **Figure 6-8** shows a lateral view of the vertebral column.

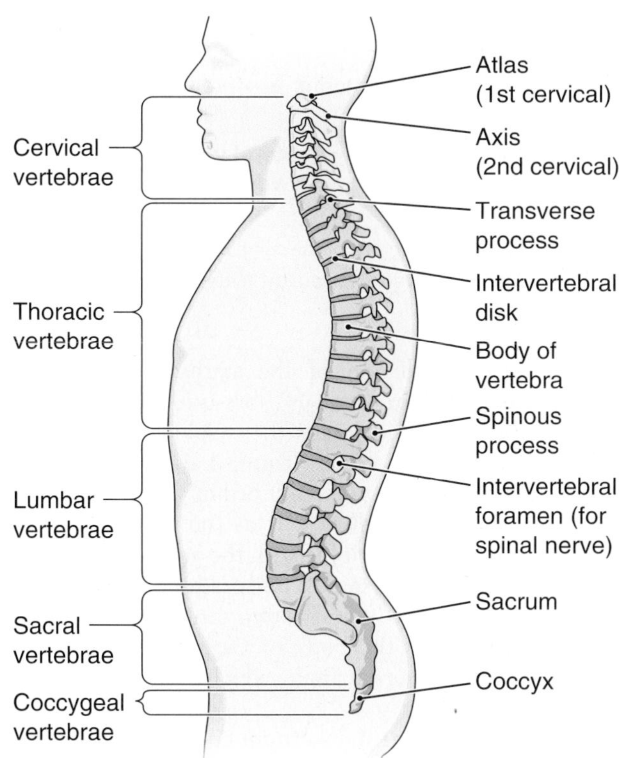

Figure 6-8 Vertebral column, left lateral view.
KEY POINT The adult spine has five regions and four curves. ZOOMING IN From an anterior view, which group(s) of vertebrae form a convex curve? Which group(s) form a concave curve?

Each **vertebra** (VER-teh-brah) (aside from the first two) has a drum-shaped **body** located anteriorly (toward the front) that serves as the weight-bearing part; disks of cartilage between the vertebral bodies absorb shock and provide flexibility **(Fig. 6-9)**. In the center of each vertebra is a large hole, or foramen. When all the vertebrae are linked in series by strong connective tissue bands (ligaments), these spaces form the spinal canal, a bony cylinder that protects the spinal cord. Projecting posteriorly (toward the back) from the bony arch that encircles the spinal cord is the **spinous process**, which usually can be felt just under the skin of the back. Projecting laterally is a **transverse process** on each side. These processes are attachment points for muscles. Other processes form joints with adjacent vertebrae. A lateral view of the vertebral column shows a series of **intervertebral foramina**, formed between the vertebrae as they join together. Spinal nerves emerge from the spinal cord through these openings **(see Fig. 6-8)**.

The bones of the vertebral column are named and numbered from superior to inferior and according to location. There are five groups:

- The **cervical** (SER-vih-kal) **vertebrae,** seven in number (C1 to C7), are located in the neck. The first vertebra, called the **atlas,** supports the head **(Fig. 6-10)**. (This vertebra is named for the mythologic character who was able to support the world in his hands.) When you nod your head, the skull rocks on the atlas at the occipital bone. The second cervical vertebra, the **axis (see Fig. 6-10)**, serves as a pivot when you turn your head from side to side. It has an upright tooth-like part, the dens, that projects into the atlas as a pivot point. The absence of a body in these vertebrae allows for the extra movement. Only the cervical vertebrae have a hole in the transverse process on each side **(see Fig. 6-9)**. These **transverse foramina** accommodate blood vessels and nerves that supply the neck and head.
- The **thoracic vertebrae,** 12 in number (T1 to T12), are located in the chest. They are larger and stronger than the cervical vertebrae and have a longer spinous process that points downward **(see Fig. 6-9)**. The posterior ends of the 12 pairs of ribs are attached to these vertebrae.
- The **lumbar vertebrae,** five in number (L1 to L5), are located in the small of the back. They are larger and heavier than the vertebrae superior to them and can support more weight **(see Fig. 6-9)**. All of their processes are shorter and thicker.
- The **sacral** (SA-kral) **vertebrae** are five separate bones in the child. They eventually fuse to form a single bone, called the **sacrum** (SA-krum), in the adult. Wedged between the two hip bones, the sacrum completes the posterior part of the bony pelvis.
- The **coccygeal** (kok-SIJ-e-al) **vertebrae** consist of four or five tiny bones in the child. These later fuse to form a single bone, the **coccyx** (KOK-siks), or tail bone, in the adult.

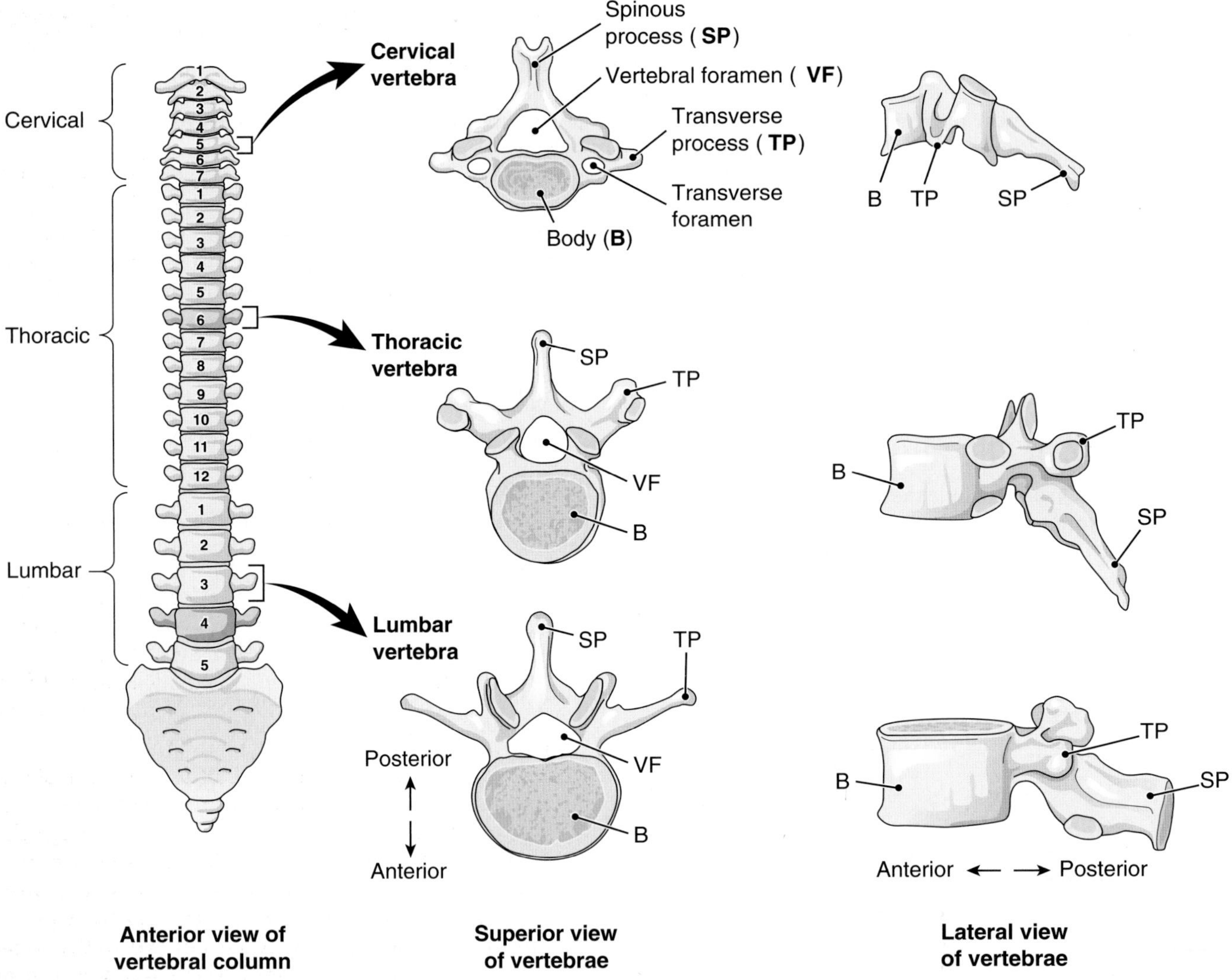

Figure 6-9 The vertebral column and vertebrae. KEY POINT The vertebrae in different regions of the spine have distinctive features. The blue areas on the vertebrae show points of contact with other bones. ZOOMING IN Which vertebrae are the largest and heaviest? Why?

Curves of the Spine When viewed from the side, the adult vertebral column shows four curves, corresponding to the four vertebral groups **(see Fig. 6-8)**. In the fetus, the entire column is concave forward (like a letter "C" and your spine when you assume a "fetal position"). This is the primary curve.

When an infant begins to assume an erect posture, secondary curves develop. The cervical curve is convex and appears as the baby holds its head up at about 3 months of age. The lumbar curve is also convex and appears when the child begins to walk. The thoracic and sacral curves remain the two primary concave curves. These curves of the vertebral column provide some of the resilience and spring so essential in balance and movement.

Thorax The bones of the thorax form a cone-shaped cage **(Fig. 6-11)**. Twelve pairs of **ribs** form the bars of this cage, completed anteriorly by the **sternum** (STER-num), or breastbone. These bones enclose and protect the heart, lungs, and other organs contained in the thorax.

The superior portion of the sternum is a roughly triangular **manubrium** (mah-NU-bre-um) that joins laterally on the right and left with a clavicle (collarbone). (The name manubrium comes from a Latin word meaning "handle.") The point on the manubrium where the clavicle joins can be seen on **Figure 6-11** as the clavicular notch. Laterally, the manubrium joins with the anterior ends of the first pair of ribs. The sternum's **body** is long and bladelike. It joins along each side with ribs two through seven. Where the manubrium joins the body of the sternum, there is a slight elevation, the **sternal angle**, which easily can be felt as a surface landmark.

The inferior end of the sternum consists of a small tip that is made of cartilage in youth but becomes bone in the adult. This is the **xiphoid** (ZIF-oyd) **process.** It is used as a landmark for cardiopulmonary resuscitation (CPR) to locate the region for chest compression.

All 12 ribs on each side are attached to the vertebral column posteriorly. However, variations in the anterior

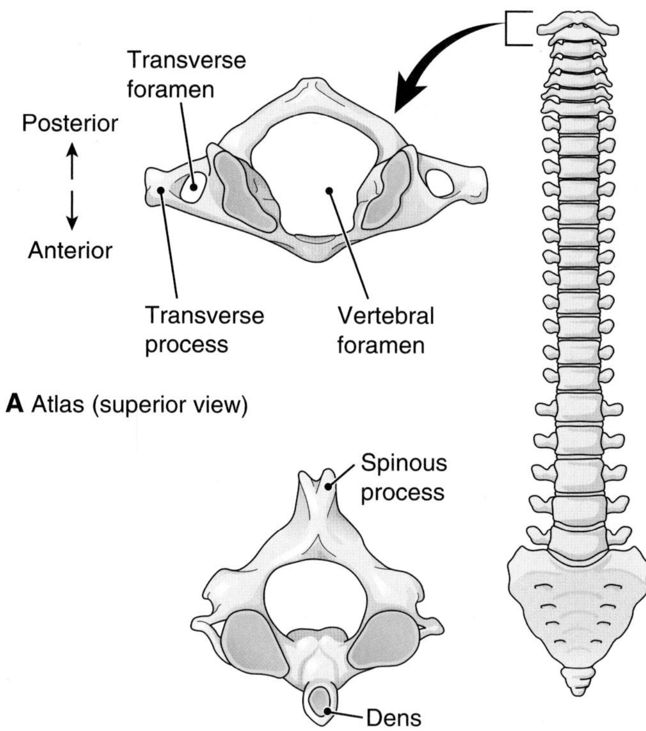

Figure 6-10 The first two cervical vertebrae. KEY POINT The first two cervical vertebrae are adapted to support the skull and allow for movements of the head in different directions. **A.** The atlas (first cervical vertebra), superior view. **B.** The axis (second cervical vertebra), superior view. ZOOMING IN What is missing in these two vertebrae that is present in all other vertebrae?

attachment of these slender, curved bones have led to the following classification:

- **True ribs,** the first seven pairs, are those that attach directly to the sternum by means of individual extensions called *costal* (KOS-tal) *cartilages.*
- **False ribs** are the remaining 5 pairs. Of these, the 8th, 9th, and 10th pairs attach to the cartilage of the rib above. The last 2 pairs have no anterior attachment at all and are known as **floating ribs.**

The spaces between the ribs, called *intercostal spaces*, contain muscles, blood vessels, and nerves.

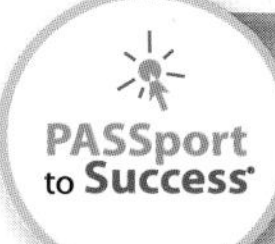

See the student resources on *thePoint* for additional pictures of the skeleton of the torso.

CHECKPOINTS

- 6-7 What bones make up the skeleton of the trunk?
- 6-8 What are the five regions of the vertebral column?

Bones of the Appendicular Skeleton

The appendicular skeleton may be considered in two divisions: upper and lower. The upper division on each side includes the shoulder, the arm (between the shoulder and the elbow), the forearm (between the elbow and the wrist), the wrist, the hand, and the fingers. The lower division includes the hip (part of the pelvic girdle), the thigh (between the hip and the knee), the leg (between the knee and the ankle), the ankle, the foot, and the toes.

THE UPPER DIVISION OF THE APPENDICULAR SKELETON

The bones of the upper division may be divided into two groups, the shoulder girdle and the upper extremity.

The Shoulder Girdle The shoulder girdle consists of two bones (Fig. 6-12).

- The **clavicle** (KLAV-ih-kl), or collarbone, is a slender bone with two shallow curves. It joins the sternum anteriorly and the scapula laterally and helps to support the shoulder. Because it often receives the full force of falls on outstretched arms or of blows to the shoulder, it is the most frequently broken bone.
- The **scapula** (SKAP-u-lah), or shoulder blade, is shown from anterior and posterior views in Figure 6-12. The **spine** of the scapula is the posterior raised ridge that can be felt behind the shoulder in the upper portion of the back. Muscles that move the arm attach to fossae (depressions), known as the **supraspinous fossa** and the **infraspinous fossa,** superior and inferior to the scapular spine. The **acromion** (ah-KRO-me-on) is the process that joins the clavicle. You can feel this as the highest point of your shoulder. Below the acromion there is a shallow socket, the **glenoid cavity,** that forms a ball-and-socket joint with the arm bone (humerus). Medial to the glenoid cavity is the **coracoid** (KOR-ah-koyd) **process,** to which muscles attach.

The Upper Extremity The upper extremity is also referred to as the upper limb, or simply the arm, although technically, the arm is only the region between the shoulder and the elbow. The region between the elbow and wrist is the forearm. The upper extremity consists of the following bones:

- The proximal bone is the **humerus** (HU-mer-us), or arm bone (Fig. 6-13). The head of the humerus articulates (forms a joint) with the glenoid cavity of the scapula. The distal end has a projection on each side, the medial and lateral **epicondyles** (ep-ih-KON-diles), to which tendons attach, and a midportion, the **trochlea** (TROK-le-ah), that forms a joint with the ulna of the forearm. (The name comes from a word that means "pulley wheel" because of its shape.)
- The forearm bones are the **ulna** (UL-nah) and the **radius** (RA-de-us). In the anatomic position, the ulna lies on

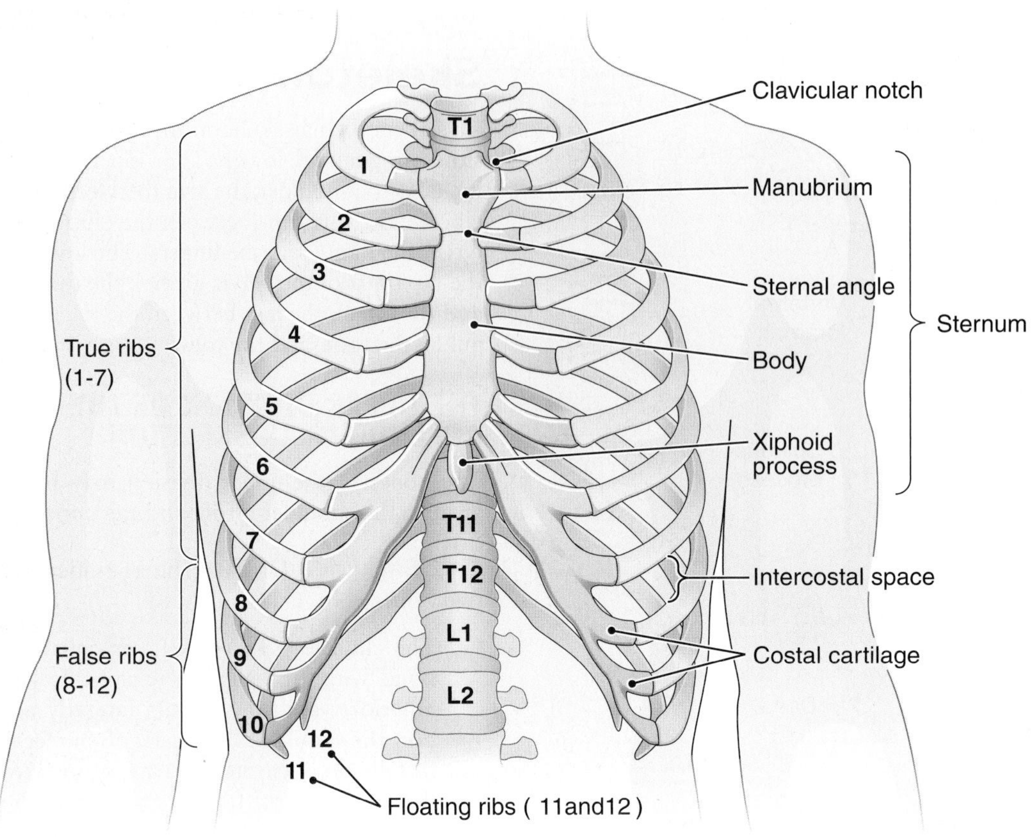

Figure 6-11 Bones of the thorax, anterior view. KEY POINT The first 7 pairs of ribs are the true ribs; pairs 8 through 12 are the false ribs, of which the last 2 pairs are also called floating ribs. ZOOMING IN To what bones do the costal cartilages attach?

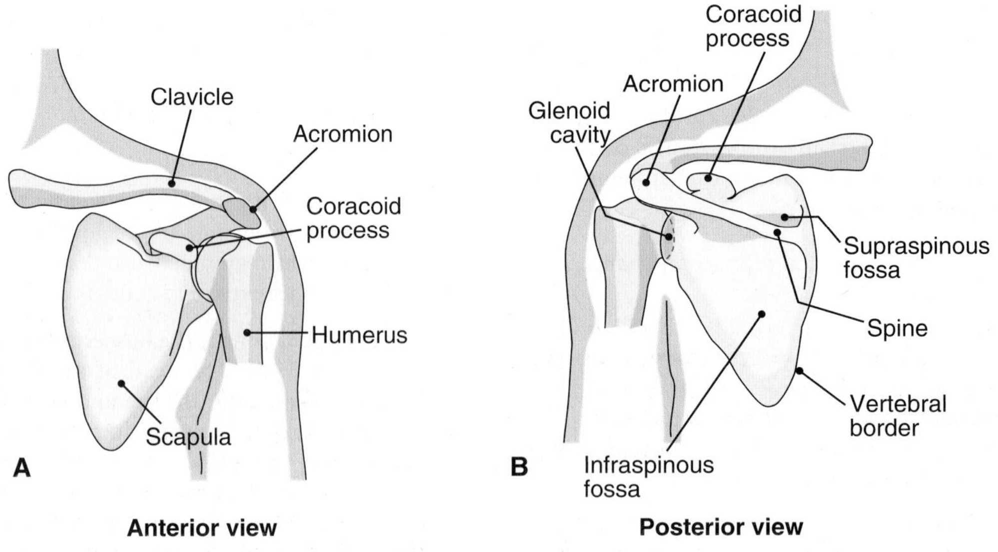

Figure 6-12 The shoulder girdle. KEY POINT The shoulder girdle consists of the clavicle and scapula. **A.** Bones of the left shoulder girdle, anterior view. **B.** Bones of the left shoulder girdle, posterior view. ZOOMING IN What does the prefix *supra* mean? What does the prefix *infra* mean?

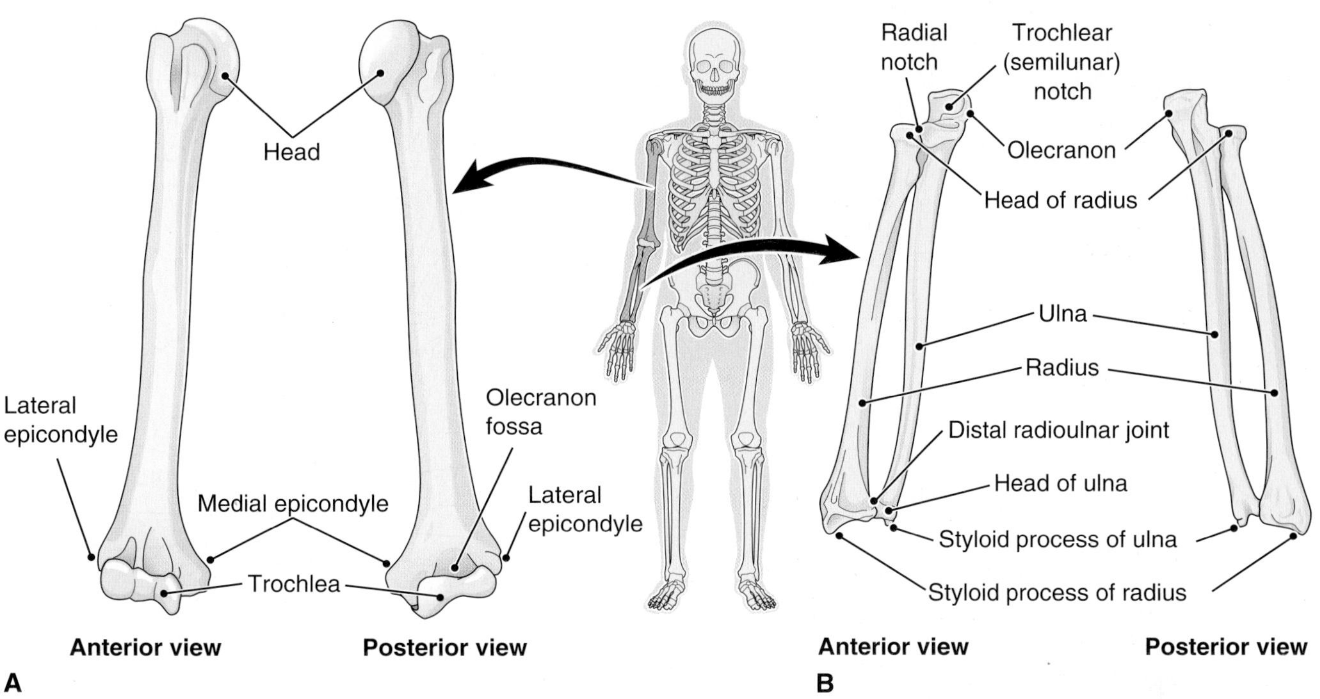

Figure 6-13 Bones of the upper extremity. KEY POINT The upper extremity consists of the arm and forearm. **A.** The humerus of the right arm in anterior and posterior view. **B.** The radius and ulna of the right forearm in anterior and posterior view. ZOOMING IN What is the medial bone of the forearm?

the medial side of the forearm in line with the little finger, and the radius lies laterally, above the thumb **(see Fig. 6-13)**. When the forearm is supine, with the palm up or forward, the two bones are parallel; when the forearm is prone, with the palm down or back, the distal end of the radius rotates around the ulna so that the shafts of the two bones are crossed **(Fig. 6-14)**. In this position, a distal projection (styloid process) of the ulna shows at the outside of the wrist.

The proximal end of the ulna has the large **olecranon** (o-LEK-rah-non), a process that forms the point of the elbow **(Fig. 6-15)**. At the posterior elbow joint, the olecranon fits into a depression of the distal humerus, the **olecranon fossa.** The trochlea of the distal humerus fits into the ulna's deep **trochlear notch**, allowing a hinge action at the elbow joint. This ulnar depression, because of its deep half-moon shape, is also known as the semilunar notch **(see Fig. 6-15)**.

- The wrist contains eight small **carpal** (KAR-pal) **bones** arranged in two rows of four each. The names of these eight different bones are given in **Figure 6-16**. Note that the anatomic wrist, comprised of the carpal bones, is actually the heel of the hand. We wear a "wristwatch" over the distal ends of the radius and ulna.
- Five **metacarpal bones** are the framework for the palm of each hand. Their rounded distal ends form the knuckles.
- There are 14 **phalanges** (fah-LAN-jeze), or finger bones, in each hand, two for the thumb and three for each finger. Each of these bones is called a **phalanx** (FA-lanx). They are identified as the proximal, which is attached to a metacarpal; the middle; and the distal. Note that the thumb has only two phalanges, a proximal and a distal **(see Fig. 6-16)**.

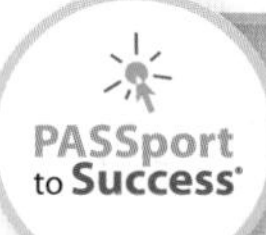

See the student resources on *thePoint* for additional pictures of the upper extremity's skeleton.

THE LOWER DIVISION OF THE APPENDICULAR SKELETON

The bones of the lower division also fall into two groups, the pelvis and the lower extremity.

The Pelvic Bones The hip bone, or **os coxae**, begins its development as three separate bones that later fuse **(Fig. 6-17)**. These individual bones are the following:

- The **ilium** (IL-e-um) forms the upper, flared portion. The **iliac** (IL-e-ak) **crest** is the curved rim along the ilium's superior border. It can be felt just below the waist. At either end of the crest are two bony projections. The most prominent of these is the **anterior superior iliac spine**, which is often used as a surface landmark in diagnosis and treatment.
- The **ischium** (IS-ke-um) is the lowest and strongest part. The **ischial** (IS-ke-al) **spine** at the posterior of the pelvic

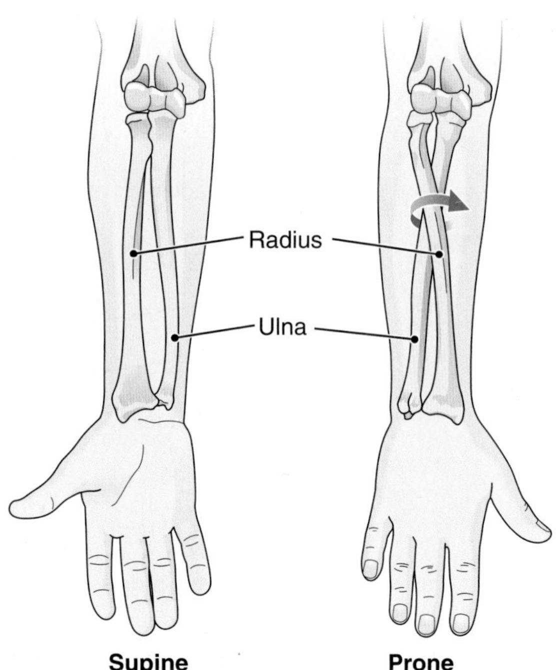

Figure 6-14 **Movements of the forearm.** KEY POINT When the palm is supine (facing up or forward), the radius and ulna are parallel. When the palm is prone (facing down or to the rear), the radius crosses over the ulna.

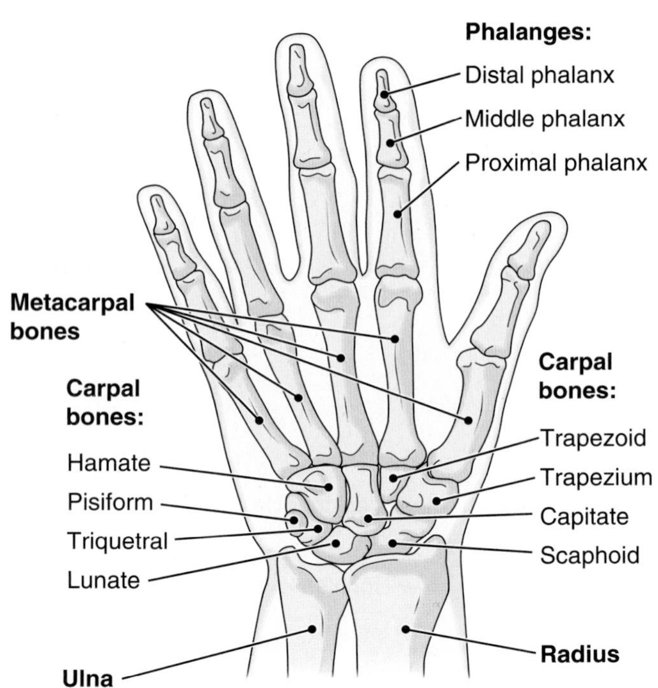

Figure 6-16 **Bones of the right hand, anterior view.** ZOOMING IN How many phalanges are there on each hand?

outlet is used as a reference point during childbirth to indicate the progress of the presenting part (usually the baby's head) down the birth canal. Just inferior to this spine is the large **ischial tuberosity**, which helps support the trunk's weight when a person sits down. You may sometimes be aware of this ischial projection when sitting on a hard surface for a while.

- The **pubis** (PU-bis) forms the anterior part of the os coxae. The joint formed by the union of the two hip bones anteriorly is called the **pubic symphysis** (SIM-fih-sis). This joint becomes more flexible late in pregnancy to allow for passage of the baby's head during childbirth.

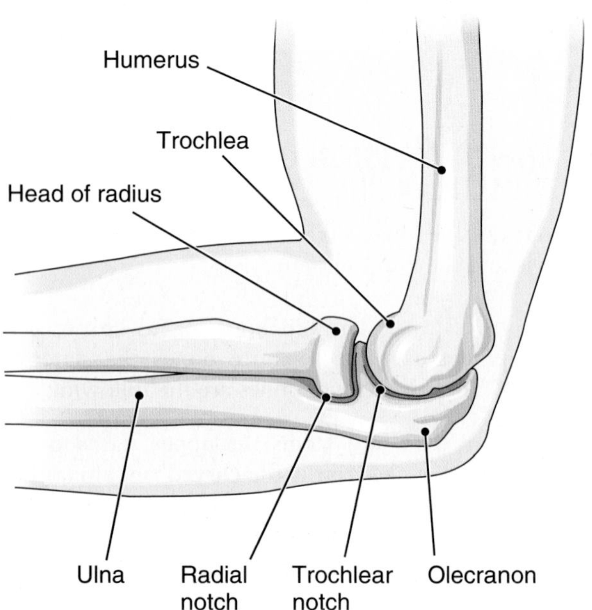

Figure 6-15 **Left elbow, lateral view.** ZOOMING IN What part of what bone forms the bony prominence of the elbow?

Portions of all three pelvic bones contribute to the formation of the **acetabulum** (as-eh-TAB-u-lum), the deep socket that holds the head of the femur (thigh bone) to form the hip joint **(see Fig. 6-17)**.

The largest foramina in the entire body are found near the anterior of each hip bone on either side of the pubic symphysis. This opening is named the **obturator** (OB-tu-ra-tor) **foramen** **(see Fig. 6-17)**, referring to the fact that it is partially closed by a membrane and has only a small opening for passage of blood vessels and a nerve.

The two ossa coxae join in forming the pelvis, a strong bony girdle completed posteriorly by the sacrum and coccyx of the spine. The pelvis supports the trunk and the organs in the lower abdomen, or pelvic cavity, including the urinary bladder, the internal reproductive organs, and parts of the intestine.

The female pelvis is adapted for pregnancy and childbirth **(Fig. 6-18)**. Some ways in which the female pelvis differs from that of the male are

- It is lighter in weight.
- The ilia are wider and more flared.
- The pubic arch, the anterior angle between the pubic bones, is wider.

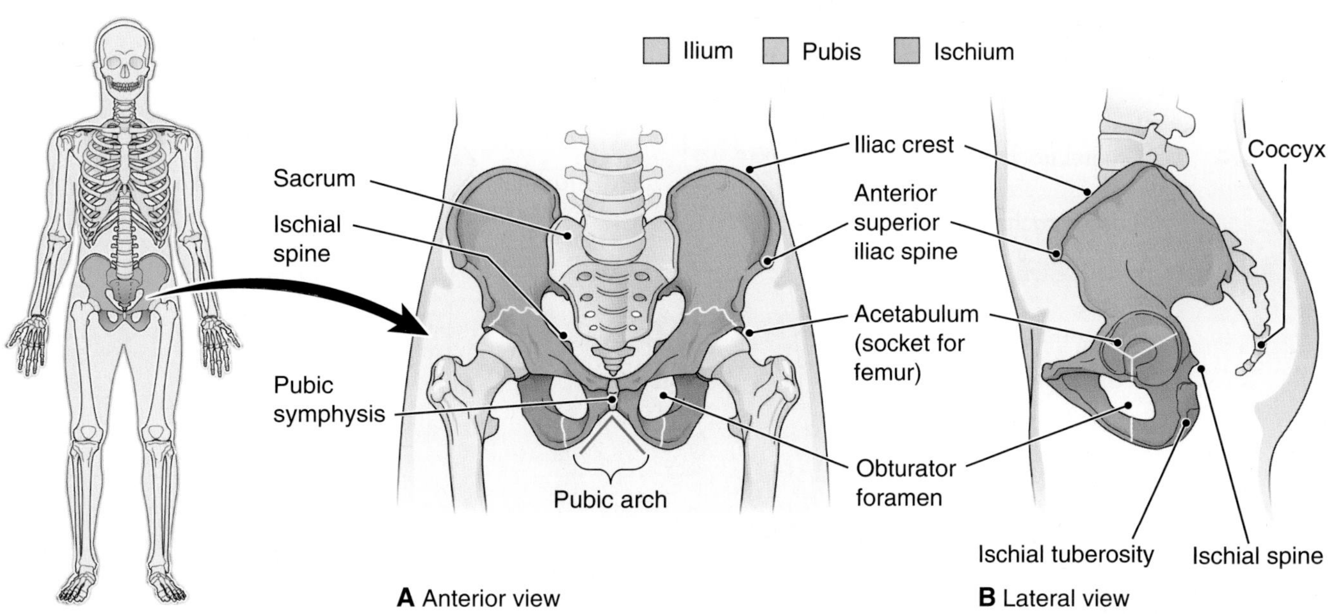

Figure 6-17 The pelvic bones. KEY POINT The hip bone, or os coxae, is formed of three fused bones. **A.** Anterior view. **B.** Lateral view showing the joining of the three pelvic bones to form the acetabulum. ZOOMING IN What bone is nicknamed the "sit bone"?

- The pelvic inlet, the upper opening, bordered by the pubic joint and sacrum, is wider and more rounded.
- The pelvic outlet, the lower opening, bordered by the pubic joint and coccyx, is larger.
- The sacrum and coccyx are shorter and less curved.

The Lower Extremity The lower extremity is also referred to as the lower limb, or simply the leg, although technically the leg is only the region between the knee and the ankle. The portion of the extremity between the hip and the knee is the thigh. The lower extremity consists of the following bones:

- The **femur** (FE-mer), the thigh bone, is the longest and strongest bone in the body. Proximally, it has a large ball-shaped head that joins the os coxae (Fig. 6-19). The large lateral projection near the head of the femur is the **greater trochanter** (tro-KAN-ter), used as a surface landmark. The **lesser trochanter,** a smaller elevation, is located on the medial side. On the posterior surface, there is a long central ridge, the **linea aspera** (literally "rough line"), which is a point for attachment of hip muscles. The distal anterior **patellar surface** articulates with the knee cap. The femur is the bone involved in Reggie's case study.

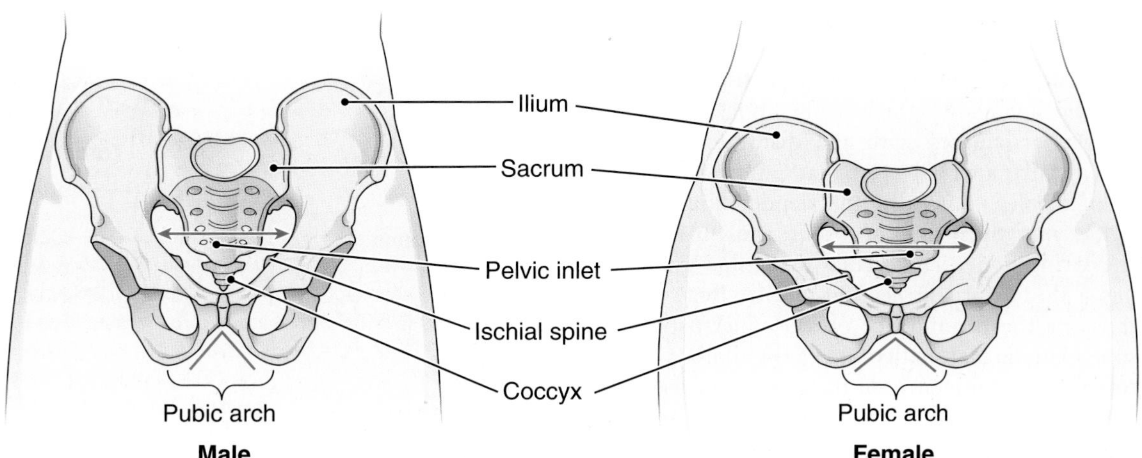

Figure 6-18 Comparison of male and female pelvis, anterior view. KEY POINT The female pelvis is adapted for pregnancy and childbirth. Note the broader angle of the pubic arch and the wider pelvic outlet in the female. Also, the ilia are wider and more flared; the sacrum and coccyx are shorter and less curved.

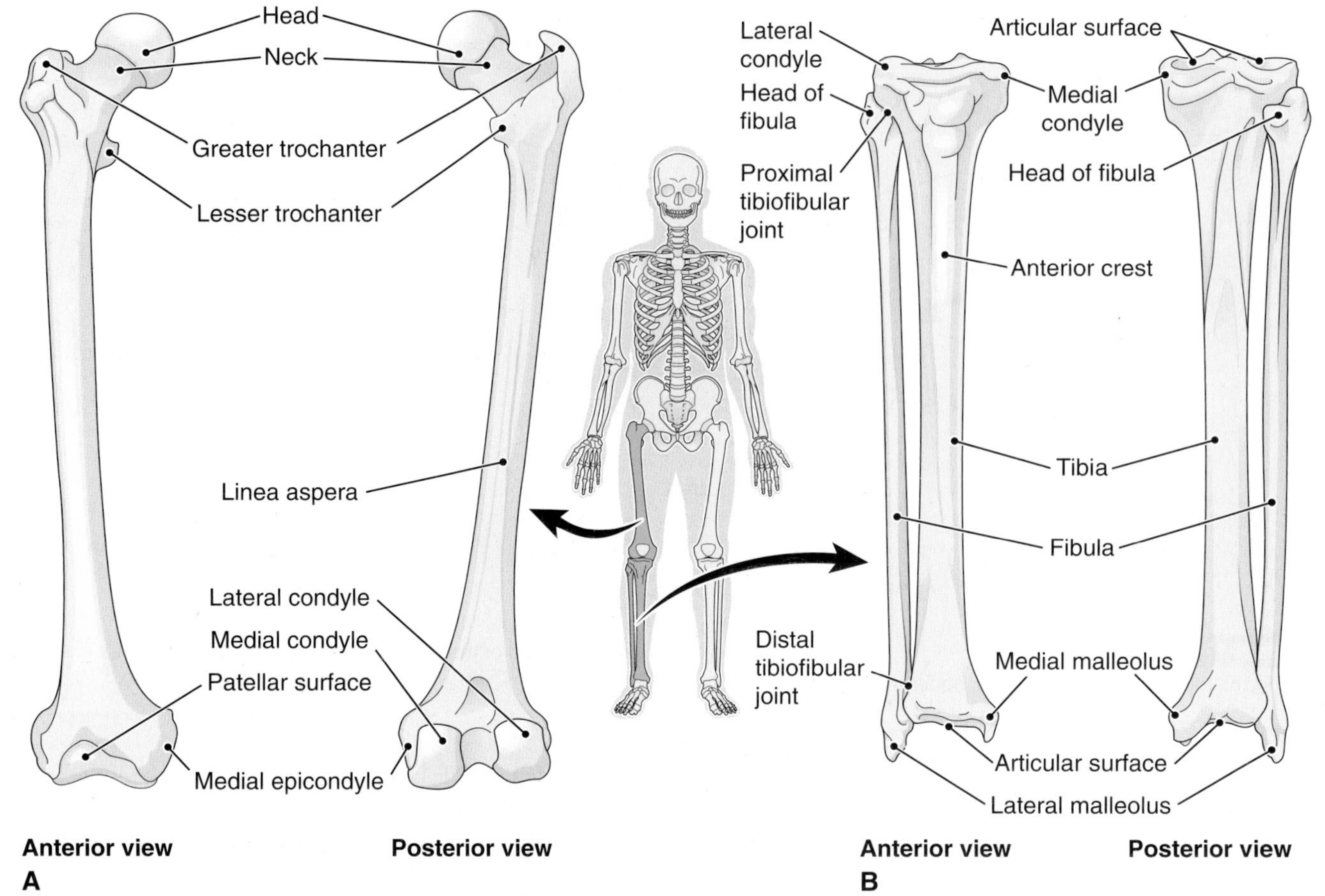

Figure 6-19 Bones of the lower extremity. KEY POINT The lower extremity consists of the thigh and leg. **A.** The femur of the right thigh. **B.** The tibia and fibula of the right leg. ZOOMING IN What is the lateral bone of the leg? Which bone of the leg is weight bearing?

- The **patella** (pah-TEL-lah), or kneecap **(see Fig. 6-1)**, is embedded in the tendon of the large anterior thigh muscle, the quadriceps femoris, where it crosses the knee joint. It is an example of a **sesamoid** (SES-ah-moyd) **bone,** a type of bone that develops within a tendon or a joint capsule.
- There are two bones in the leg **(see Fig. 6-19)**. Medially (on the great toe side), the **tibia,** or shin bone, is the longer, weight-bearing bone. Its proximal surface articulates with the distal femur. The tibia has a sharp anterior crest that can be felt at the surface of the leg. Laterally, the slender **fibula** (FIB-u-lah) does not reach the knee joint; thus, it is not a weight-bearing bone. The **medial malleolus** (mal-LE-o-lus) is a downward projection at the tibia's distal end; it forms the prominence on the inner aspect of the ankle. The **lateral malleolus**, at the fibula's distal end, forms the prominence on the outer aspect of the ankle. Most people think of these projections as their "ankle bones," whereas, in truth, they are features of the tibia and fibula.
- The structure of the foot is similar to that of the hand. However, the foot supports the body's weight, so it is stronger and less mobile than the hand. There are seven **tarsal bones** associated with the ankle and foot. These are named and illustrated in **Figure 6-20**. The largest of these is the **calcaneus** (kal-KA-ne-us), or heel bone. The **talus** above it forms the ankle joint with the tibia.

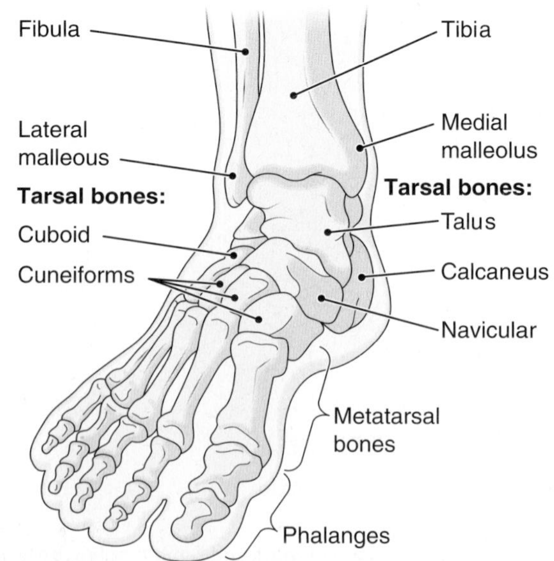

Figure 6-20 Bones of the right foot. ZOOMING IN Which tarsal bone is the heel bone? Which tarsal bone forms a joint with the tibia?

6

Table 6-1 Bones of the Skeleton

Region	Bones	Description
Axial Skeleton		
Skull		
Cranium	Cranial bones (8)	Chamber enclosing the brain; houses the ear and forms part of the eye socket
Facial portion	Facial bones (14)	Form the face and chambers for sensory organs
Hyoid		U-shaped bone under lower jaw; used for muscle attachments
Ossicles	Ear bones (3)	Transmit sound waves through middle ear
Trunk		
Vertebral column	Vertebrae (26)	Enclose the spinal cord
Thorax	Sternum	Anterior bone of the thorax
	Ribs (12 pair)	Enclose the organs of the thorax
Appendicular Skeleton		
Upper division		
Shoulder girdle	Clavicle	Anterior; between sternum and scapula
	Scapula	Posterior; anchors muscles that move arm
Upper extremity	Humerus	Arm bone
	Ulna	Medial bone of forearm
	Radius	Lateral bone of forearm
	Carpals (8)	Wrist bones
	Metacarpals (5)	Bones of palm
	Phalanges (14)	Bones of fingers
Lower division		
Pelvis	Os coxae (2)	Join sacrum and coccyx of vertebral column to form the bony pelvis
Lower extremity	Femur	Thigh bone
	Patella	Kneecap
	Tibia	Medial bone of leg
	Fibula	Lateral bone of leg
	Tarsal bones (7)	Ankle bones
	Metatarsals (5)	Bones of instep
	Phalanges (14)	Bones of toes

- Five **metatarsal bones** form the framework of the instep, and the heads of these bones form the ball of the foot (see Fig. 6-20).
- The **phalanges** of the toes are counterparts of those in the fingers. There are three of these in each toe except for the great toe, which has only two.

See Table 6-1 for a summary outline of all the bones of the skeleton.

CHECKPOINT 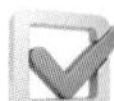

6-9 What division of the skeleton consists of the bones of the shoulder girdle, hip, and extremities?

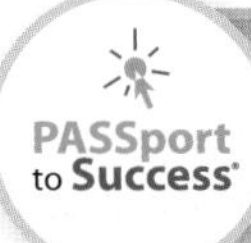

See the student resources on *thePoint* for additional pictures of the skeleton of the pelvis and lower extremity.

The Joints

An **articulation**, or **joint**, is an area of junction or union between two or more bones. Joints are classified into three main types on the basis of the material between the adjoining bones. They may also be classified according to the degree of movement permitted (Table 6-2):

- **Fibrous joint.** The bones in this type of joint are held together by fibrous connective tissue. An example is a **suture** (SU-chur) between bones of the skull. This type of joint is immovable and is termed a **synarthrosis** (sin-ar-THRO-sis).
- **Cartilaginous joint.** The bones in this type of joint are connected by cartilage. Examples are the joint between the pubic bones of the pelvis—the pubic symphysis—and the joints between the bodies of the vertebrae. This type of joint is slightly movable and is termed an **amphiarthrosis** (am-fe-ar-THRO-sis).
- **Synovial** (sin-O-ve-al) **joint.** The bones in this type of joint have a potential space between them called the

Table 6-2 Joints

Type	Movement	Material between the Bones	Examples
Fibrous	Immovable (synarthrosis)	No joint cavity; fibrous connective tissue between bones	Sutures between skull bones
Cartilaginous	Slightly movable (amphiarthrosis)	No joint cavity; cartilage between bones	Pubic symphysis; joints between vertebral bodies
Synovial	Freely movable (diarthrosis)	Joint cavity containing synovial fluid	Gliding, hinge, pivot, condyloid, saddle, ball-and-socket joints

joint cavity, which contains a small amount of thick, colorless fluid. This lubricant, **synovial fluid,** resembles uncooked egg white (*ov* is the root, meaning "egg") and is secreted by the membrane that lines the joint cavity. The synovial joint is freely movable and is termed a **diarthrosis** (di-ar-THRO-sis). Most of the body's joints are synovial joints; they are described in more detail next.

MORE ABOUT SYNOVIAL JOINTS

The bones in freely movable joints are held together by **ligaments,** bands of fibrous connective tissue. Additional ligaments reinforce and help stabilize the joints at various points (Fig. 6-21). Also, for strength and protection, there is a **joint capsule** of connective tissue that encloses each joint

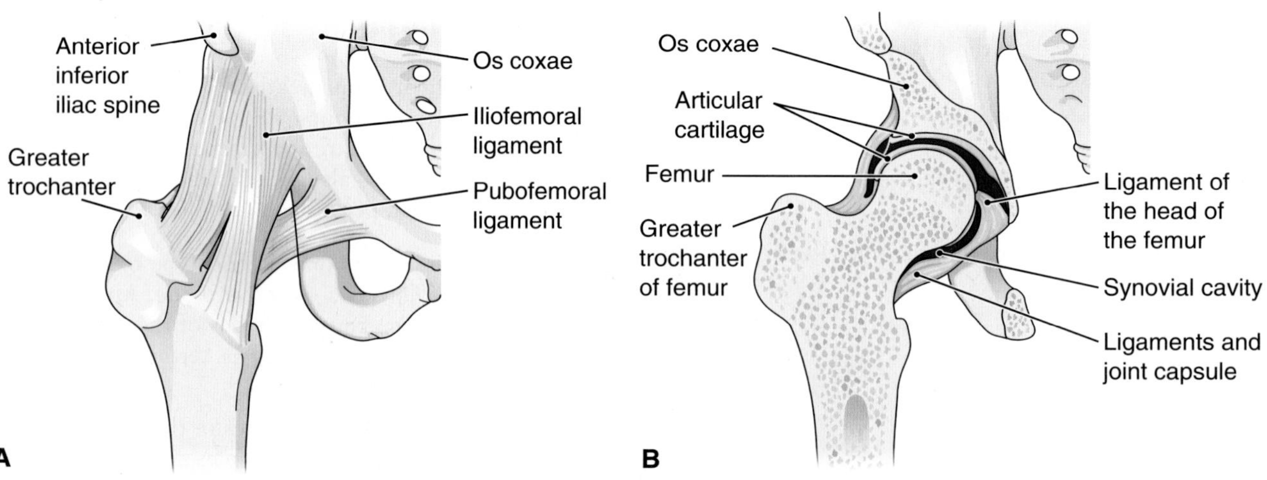

Figure 6-21 Structure of a synovial joint. KEY POINT Connective tissue structures stabilize and protect synovial joints. **A.** Anterior view of the hip joint showing ligaments that reinforce and stabilize the joint. **B.** Frontal section through right hip joint showing protective structures. ZOOMING IN What is the purpose of the greater trochanter of the femur? What type of tissue covers and protects the ends of the bones?

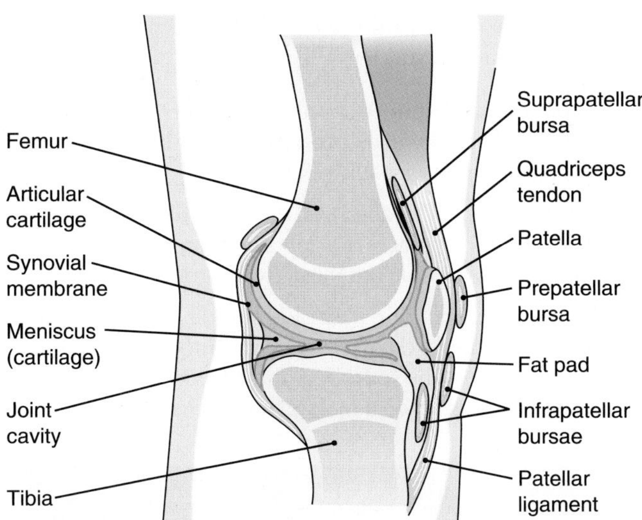

Figure 6-22 The knee joint, sagittal section. Protective structures are also shown.

and is continuous with the periosteum of the bones (see Fig. 6-21B). The bone surfaces in freely movable joints are protected by a smooth layer of hyaline cartilage called the **articular** (ar-TIK-u-lar) **cartilage**. Some complex joints may have additional cushioning cartilage between the bones, such as the crescent-shaped medial meniscus (meh-NIS-kus) and lateral meniscus in the knee joint (Fig. 6-22). Fat may also appear as padding around a joint.

Near some joints are small sacs called **bursae** (BER-se), which are filled with synovial fluid (see Fig. 6-22). These lie in areas subject to stress and help ease movement over and around the joints. Inflammation of a bursa, as a result of injury or irritation, is called **bursitis.**

Movement at Synovial Joints The chief function of the freely movable joints is to allow for changes of position and so provide for motion. These movements are named to describe changes in the positions of body parts (Fig. 6-23) from the anatomic position. Experiment with moving your body in these different directions as you read these descriptions and examine the illustrations. There are four kinds of angular movement, or movement that changes the angle between bones:

- **Flexion** (FLEK-shun) is a bending motion that decreases the angle between bones, as in bending the fingers to close the hand.
- **Extension** is a straightening motion that increases the angle between bones, as in straightening the fingers to open the hand. In **hyperextension**, a part is extended beyond its anatomic position, as in opening the hand to its maximum by hyperextending the fingers or hyperextending the thigh at the hip in preparation for kicking a ball from a standing position.
- **Abduction** (ab-DUK-shun) is movement away from the midline of the body, as in moving the arm straight out to the side.

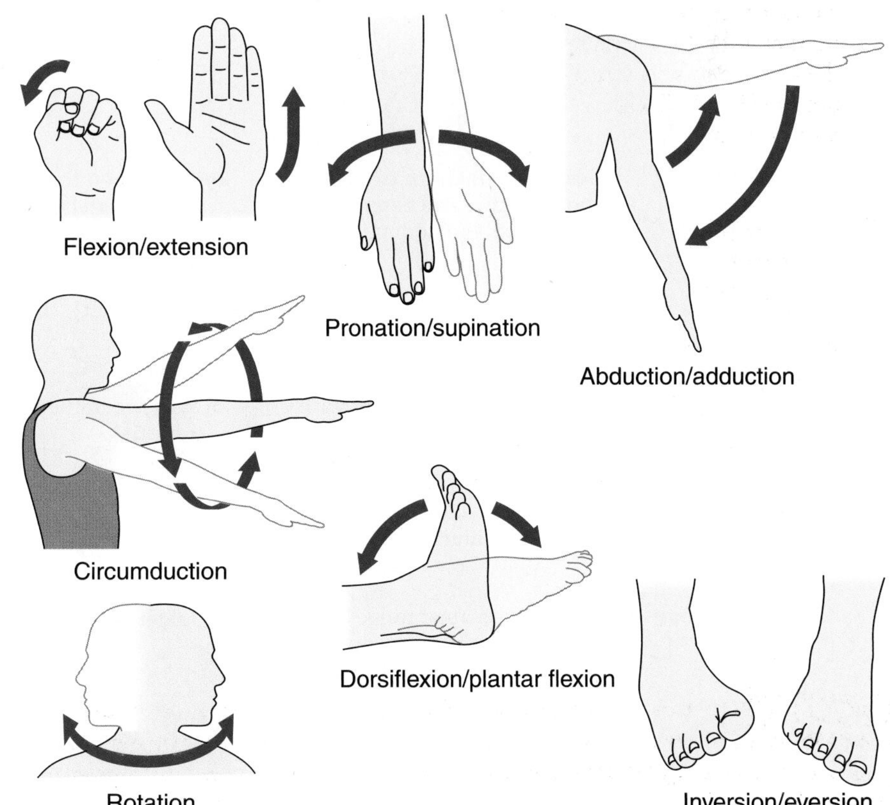

Figure 6-23 Movements at synovial joints. KEY POINT Synovial joints allow the greatest range of motion. All movements are in reference to the anatomic position.

- **Adduction** is movement toward the midline of the body, as in bringing the arm back to its original position beside the body.

A combination of these angular movements enables one to execute a movement referred to as **circumduction** (ser-kum-DUK-shun). To perform this movement, stand with your arm outstretched and draw a large imaginary circle in the air. Note the smooth combination of flexion, abduction, extension, and adduction that makes circumduction possible.

Rotation refers to a twisting or turning of a bone on its own axis, as in turning the head from side to side to say "no," or rotating the forearm to turn the palm up and down.

There are special movements that are characteristic of the forearm and the ankle:

- **Supination** (su-pin-A-shun) is the act of turning the palm up or forward; **pronation** (pro-NA-shun) turns the palm down or backward.
- **Inversion** (in-VER-zhun) is the act of turning the sole inward, so that it faces the opposite foot; **eversion** (e-VER-zhun) turns the sole outward, away from the body.
- In **dorsiflexion** (dor-sih-FLEK-shun), the foot is bent upward at the ankle, narrowing the angle between the leg and the top of the foot; in **plantar flexion,** the toes point downward, as in toe dancing, flexing the arch of the foot.

Table 6-3 Synovial Joints

Type of Joint	Type of Movement	Examples
Gliding joint	Flat bone surfaces slide over one another with little change in the joint angle	Joints in the wrist and ankles **(Figs. 6-16 and 6-20)**
Hinge joint	Allows movement in one direction, changing the angle of the bones at the joint, as in flexion and extension	Elbow joint; joints between phalanges of fingers and toes **(Figs. 6-15, 6-16 and 6-20)**
Pivot joint	Allows rotation around the length of the bone	Joint between the first and second cervical vertebrae; joint at proximal ends of the radius and ulna **(Figs. 6-8 and 6-14)**
Condyloid joint	Allows movement in two directions flexion and extension, abduction and adduction	Joint between the metacarpal and the first phalanx of the finger (knuckle) **(Fig. 6-16)**; joint between the occipital bone of the skull and the first cervical vertebra (atlas) **(Fig. 6-8)**
Saddle joint	Like a condyloid joint, but with deeper articulating surfaces and movement in three directions, rotation in addition to flexion and extension, abduction and adduction	Joint between the wrist and the metacarpal bone of the thumb **(Fig. 6-16)**
Ball-and-socket joint	Allows the greatest range of motion. Permits movement in three directions around a central point, as in circumduction.	Shoulder joint and hip joint **(Figs. 6-12 and 6-24)**

Types of Synovial Joints Synovial joints are classified according to the types of movement they allow, as described and illustrated in **Table 6-3**. Locate these types of joints on your body and demonstrate the different movements they allow. Listed in order of increasing range of motion, they are

- Gliding joint—two relatively flat bone surfaces slide over each other with little change in the joint angle. Examples are the joints between the tarsal and carpal bones.
- Hinge joint—a convex surface of one bone fits into the concave surface of another bone, allowing movement in one direction. Hinge joints allow flexion and extension only. Examples are the elbow joint and the joints between the phalanges.
- Pivot joint—a rounded or pointed portion of one bone fits into a ring in another bone. This joint allows rotation only, as in the joint between the atlas and axis of the cervical spine or the proximal joint between the radius and ulna that allows rotation of the forearm.
- Condyloid joint—an oval-shaped projection of one bone fits into an oval-shaped depression on another bone. This joint allows movement in two directions: flexion and extension and abduction and adduction. Examples are the joints between the metacarpal bones and the proximal phalanges of the fingers.
- Saddle joint—similar to the condyloid joint, but deeper and allowing greater range of motion. One bone fits into a saddle-like depression on another bone. It allows movement in three directions: flexion and extension, abduction and adduction, and rotation. An example is the joint between the wrist and the metacarpal of the thumb.
- Ball-and-socket joint—a ball-like surface of one bone fits into a deep cuplike depression in another bone. It allows the greatest range of motion in three directions, as in circumduction. Examples are the shoulder and hip joints.

CHECKPOINTS 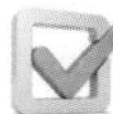

- [ ] **6-10** What are the three types of joints classified according to the type of material between the adjoining bones?
- [ ] **6-11** What is the most freely movable type of joint?

6

Effects of Aging on the Skeletal System

The aging process includes significant changes in all connective tissues, including bone. There is a loss of calcium salts and a decreased ability to form the protein framework on which calcium salts are deposited. Cellular metabolism slows, so bones are weaker, less dense, and more fragile; fractures and other bone injuries heal more slowly. Muscle tissue is also lost throughout adult life. Loss of balance and diminished reflexes may lead to falls. Thus, there is a tendency to decrease the exercise that is so important to the maintenance of bone tissue. To learn about ways to slow bone degeneration, see **Box 6-2**. Three Steps Toward a Strong and Healthy Skeleton.

Changes in the vertebral column with age lead to a loss in height. Approximately 1.2 cm (about 0.5 in.) are lost each 20 years beginning at 40 years of age, owing primarily to a thinning of the intervertebral disks (between the bodies

Box 6-2 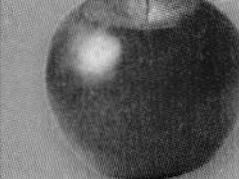 *Health Maintenance*

Three Steps toward a Strong and Healthy Skeleton

The skeleton is the body's framework. It supports and protects internal organs, helps to produce movement, and manufactures blood cells. Bone also stores nearly all of the body's calcium, releasing it into the blood when needed for processes such as nerve transmission, muscle contraction, and blood clotting. Proper nutrition, exercise, and a healthy lifestyle can help the skeleton perform all these essential roles.

A well-balanced diet supplies the nutrients and energy needed for strong, healthy bones. Calcium, phosphorus, and magnesium make up the mineral crystals of bone and confer strength and rigidity. Foods rich in both calcium and phosphorus include dairy products, fish, beans, and leafy green vegetables. When body fluids become too acidic, bone releases calcium and phosphate and is weakened. Both magnesium and potassium help regulate the pH of body fluids, with magnesium also helping bone absorb calcium. Foods rich in magnesium and potassium include beans, potatoes, and leafy green vegetables. Bananas and dairy products are high in potassium.

Protein supplies the amino acids needed to make collagen, which gives bone tissue flexibility. Meat, poultry, fish, eggs, dairy, soy, and nuts are excellent sources of protein.

Vitamin C helps stimulate collagen synthesis, and vitamin D helps the digestive system absorb calcium into the bloodstream, making it available for bone. Most fruits and vegetables are rich in vitamin C. Few foods supply vitamin D. Reliable sources include fatty fish and fortified milk. Liver, butter, and eggs also contain very small amounts.

Like muscle, bone becomes weakened with disuse. Consistent exercise promotes a stronger, denser skeleton by stimulating bone to absorb more calcium and phosphate from the blood, reducing the risk of osteoporosis. A healthy lifestyle also includes avoiding smoking and excessive alcohol consumption, both of which decrease bone calcium and inhibit bone growth. High levels of caffeine in the diet may also rob the skeleton of calcium.

of the vertebrae). Even the vertebral bodies themselves may lose height in later years. The costal (rib) cartilages become calcified and less flexible, and the chest may decrease in diameter by 2 to 3 cm (about 1 in.), mostly in the lower part. Many of these structures can be observed by x-ray studies.

At the joints, reduction of collagen in bone, tendons, and ligaments contributes to the diminished flexibility so often experienced by older people. Thinning of articular cartilage and loss of synovial fluid may contribute to joint damage. By the process of calcification, minerals may be deposited in and around the joints, especially at the shoulder, causing pain and limiting mobility.

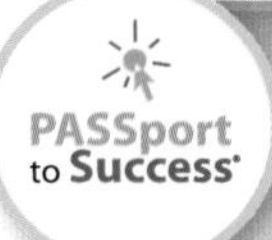
PASSport
to Success

See the student resources on *thePoint* for information on careers in radiology.

A&P in Action

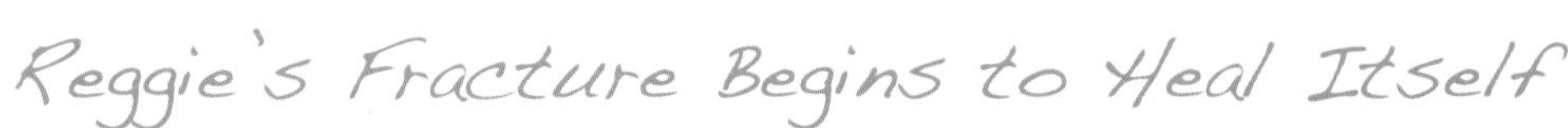
Reggie's Fracture Begins to Heal Itself

"So, Doc, what's the chance my leg's going to heal up enough to play football again?" asked Reggie. "Well," replied the doctor, "It's going to take some time before you're catching footballs again, but once your hip heals, it will be better than new."

The surgeon knew that even before the surgery to realign its broken ends, Reggie's femur had already begun to heal itself. Immediately after the injury occurred on the football field, a blood clot formed around the fracture. A day or two later, chemical messengers within the clot would stimulate blood vessels from the periosteum and endosteum to invade the clot, bringing connective tissue cells with them. Over the next several weeks, fibroblasts and chondroblasts in the clot would secrete collagen and cartilage, converting it into a soft callus. Meanwhile, macrophages would remove the remains of the blood clot and osteoclasts would digest dead bone tissue. Soon after, osteoblasts in the callus would convert it into spongy bone called a hard callus. Months after the injury, osteoclasts and osteoblasts would work together to remodel the outer layers of the hard callus into compact bone, resulting in a repair even stronger than the original bone tissue in Reggie's femur.

During this case, we saw how fractured bones are repaired using screws and plates. We also saw that the body has its own "orthopedic surgeons"—cells like osteoblasts and osteoclasts, which can engineer a bone repair that is even stronger than the original. Although Reggie's skeletal system is beginning to repair itself, he is not out of danger yet. In Chapter 14, a blood clot puts Reggie's life in jeopardy.

Chapter Wrap-Up

Summary Overview

A detailed chapter outline with space for note-taking is on *thePoint*. The figure below illustrates the main topics covered in this chapter.

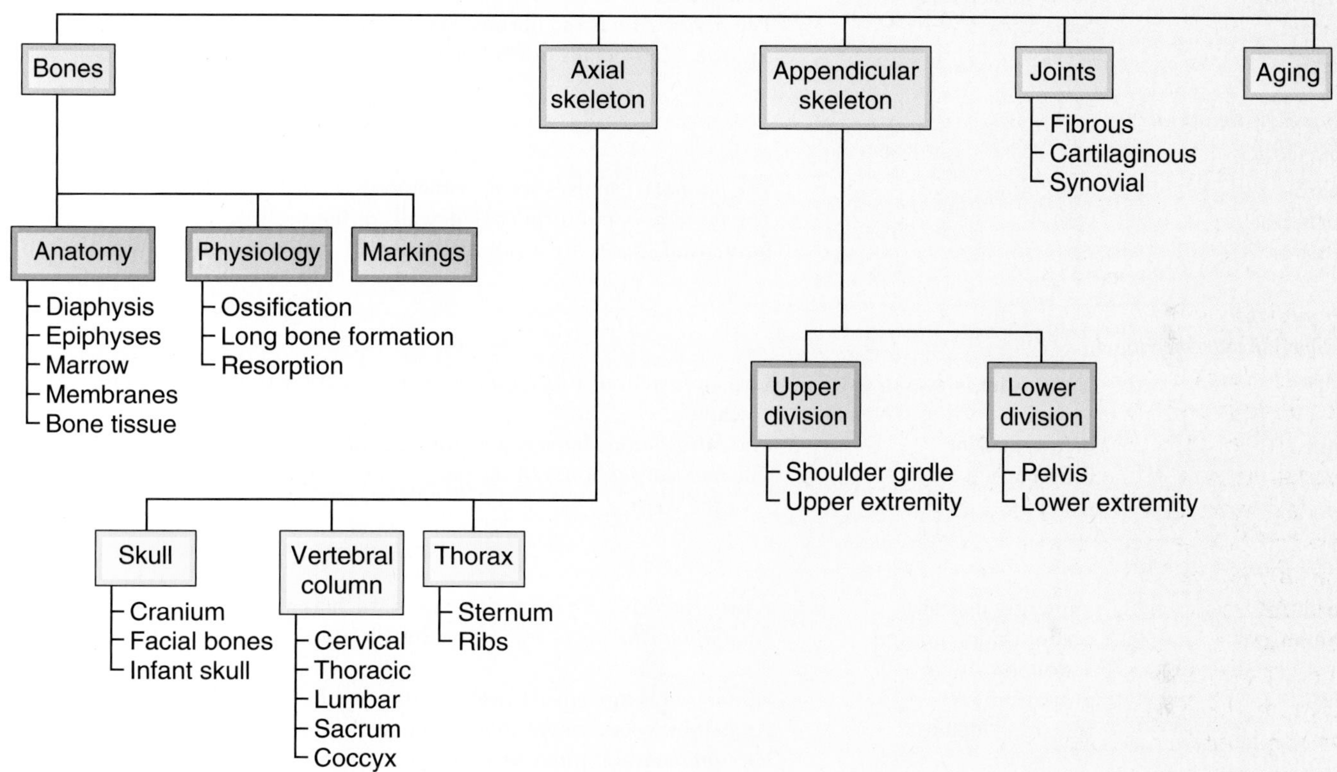

Key Terms

The terms listed below are emphasized in this chapter. Knowing them will help you organize and prioritize your learning. These and other boldface terms are defined in the Glossary with phonetic pronunciations.

amphiarthrosis
articulation
bursa
circumduction
diaphysis
diarthrosis
endosteum
epiphysis
extremity
fontanel
joint
marrow
osteoblast
osteoclast
osteocyte
osteon
periosteum
resorption
skeleton
synarthrosis
synovial

Word Anatomy

Scientific terms are built from standardized word parts (prefixes, roots, and suffixes). Learning the meanings of these parts can help you remember words and interpret unfamiliar terms.

WORD PART	MEANING	EXAMPLE
Bones		
dia-	through, between	The *diaphysis*, or shaft, of a long bone is between the two ends, or epiphyses.
oss, osse/o	bone, bone tissue	*Osseous* tissue is another name for bone tissue.
oste/o	bone, bone tissue	The *periosteum* is the fibrous membrane around a bone.
-clast	break	An *osteoclast* breaks down bone in the process of resorption.
Bones of the Axial Skeleton		
para-	near	The *paranasal* sinuses are near the nose.
pariet/o	wall	The *parietal* bones form the sidewalls of the skull.
cost/o	rib	*Intercostal* spaces are located between the ribs.
Bones of the Appendicular Skeleton		
supra-	above, superior	The *supraspinous* fossa is a depression superior to the spine of the scapula.
infra-	below, inferior	The *infraspinous* fossa is a depression inferior to the spine of the scapula.
meta-	near, beyond	The *metacarpal* bones of the palm are near and distal to the carpal bones of the wrist.
The Joints		
arthr/o	joint, articulation	A *synarthrosis* is an immovable joint, such as a suture.
amphi-	on both sides, around, double	An *amphiarthrosis* is a slightly movable joint.
ab-	away from	*Abduction* is movement away from the midline of the body.
ad-	toward, added to	*Adduction* is movement toward the midline of the body.
circum-	around	*Circumduction* is movement around a joint in a circle.

Questions for Study and Review

BUILDING UNDERSTANDING

Fill in the blanks

1. The shaft of a long bone is called the _____.

2. The structural unit of compact bone is the _____.

3. Red bone marrow manufactures _____.

4. Bones are covered by a connective tissue membrane called _____.

5. Bone matrix is produced by _____.

Matching > Match each numbered item with the most closely related lettered item.

___ **6.** A rounded bony projection

___ **7.** A sharp bony prominence

___ **8.** A hole through bone

___ **9.** A bony depression

___ **10.** An air-filled bony cavity

a. condyle

b. foramen

c. fossa

d. sinus

e. spine

Multiple Choice

___ **11.** Which cells resorb bone?

a. osteoblasts
b. osteoclasts
c. osteocytes
d. osteons

___ **12.** Which bone contains the mastoid process?

a. occipital bone
b. femur
c. temporal bone
d. humerus

___ **13.** Which bone contains the greater trochanter?

a. humerus
b. ulna
c. femur
d. tibia

___ **14.** Which joint is freely movable?

a. arthrotic
b. amphiarthrotic
c. diarthrotic
d. synarthrotic

___ **15.** What kind of synovial joint is the hip?

a. gliding
b. hinge
c. pivot
d. ball and socket

UNDERSTANDING CONCEPTS

16. List five functions of bone and describe how a long bone's structure enables it to carry out each of these functions.

17. Explain the differences between the terms in each of the following pairs:

a. osteoblast and osteocyte
b. periosteum and endosteum
c. compact bone and spongy bone
d. epiphysis and diaphysis
e. axial skeleton and appendicular skeleton

18. Discuss the process of long bone formation during fetal development and childhood. What role does resorption play in bone formation?

19. Name the bones of the

a. cranium and face
b. thoracic cavity, vertebral column, and pelvis
c. upper and lower limbs

20. List the structural differences between the male and female pelvis.

21. Name three effects of aging on the skeletal system.

22. Differentiate between the terms in each of the following pairs:

a. flexion and extension
b. abduction and adduction
c. supination and pronation
d. inversion and eversion
e. circumduction and rotation
f. dorsiflexion and plantar flexion

CONCEPTUAL THINKING

23. The vertebral bodies are much larger in the lower back than the neck. What is the functional significance of this structural difference?

24. Six-year-old Emily is admitted to the emergency room with a fracture of the right radius. Radiography reveals that the fracture crosses the distal epiphyseal plate. What concerns should Emily's healthcare team have about the location of her injury?

25. In the case story, Reggie presented with three typical signs of hip fracture—shortening, adduction, and lateral rotation of the affected limb. What causes these signs? (HINT—the skeleton is part of the musculoskeletal system.)

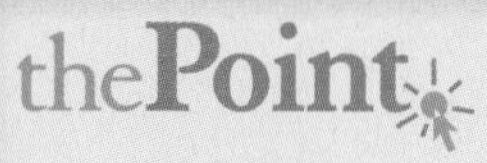

For more questions, see the learning activities on *thePoint.*

CHAPTER

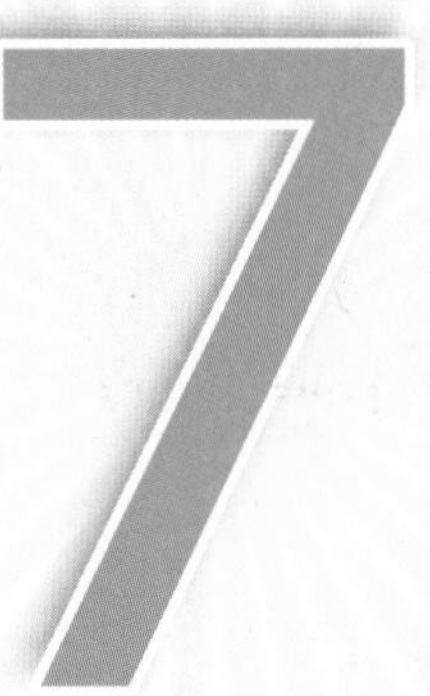

The Muscular System

A&P in Action

Sue's Case: A Muscle Mystery

Dr. Mathews glanced at his patient's chart as he stepped into the consulting room to see her. Sue Pritchard was 26 years old, white, and, according to her medical history, relatively healthy. "Hi Sue. It's been a while since your last visit. What can I do for you today?" asked the doctor.

"I'm probably making a mountain out of a molehill," Sue replied. "But, I've been having some odd symptoms that are starting to worry me. For the last couple of weeks I've noticed that my right hand is getting weak. Just the other day, I had barely enough strength to hold my coffee cup! On top of that, I've had trouble walking. I haven't fallen down or anything, but I feel like I'm off balance."

Based on Sue's description of her symptoms, Dr. Mathews initially suspected a problem with her muscular system. He checked her hand strength and verified that her right hand was weaker than her left—unusual since she was right-handed. He had Sue bend and straighten her arm at the elbows, and stand on her tip toes. Again, he noticed right-sided weakness. He compared both of Sue's arms and observed slight atrophy of the flexor muscles in her right upper limb. He tested several of her reflexes and noted that the responses in her biceps brachii and quadriceps femoris muscles were exaggerated in her right limbs. He had Sue do a few simple coordination tests like touching her nose and standing on one foot. As in the previous tests, Sue seemed to have more difficulty with right-sided tasks than left. "Have you had any pain or tingling in your arms or legs lately?" the doctor asked.

"Yes!" answered Sue. "In fact, last night I had a cramp in my right leg that was so painful I had to get out of bed and walk it off. And, my fingertips have been tingling on and off for the last few days too."

Dr. Mathews quickly recognized that Sue's problem was not just limited to her muscular system. It also appeared that her nervous system was involved.

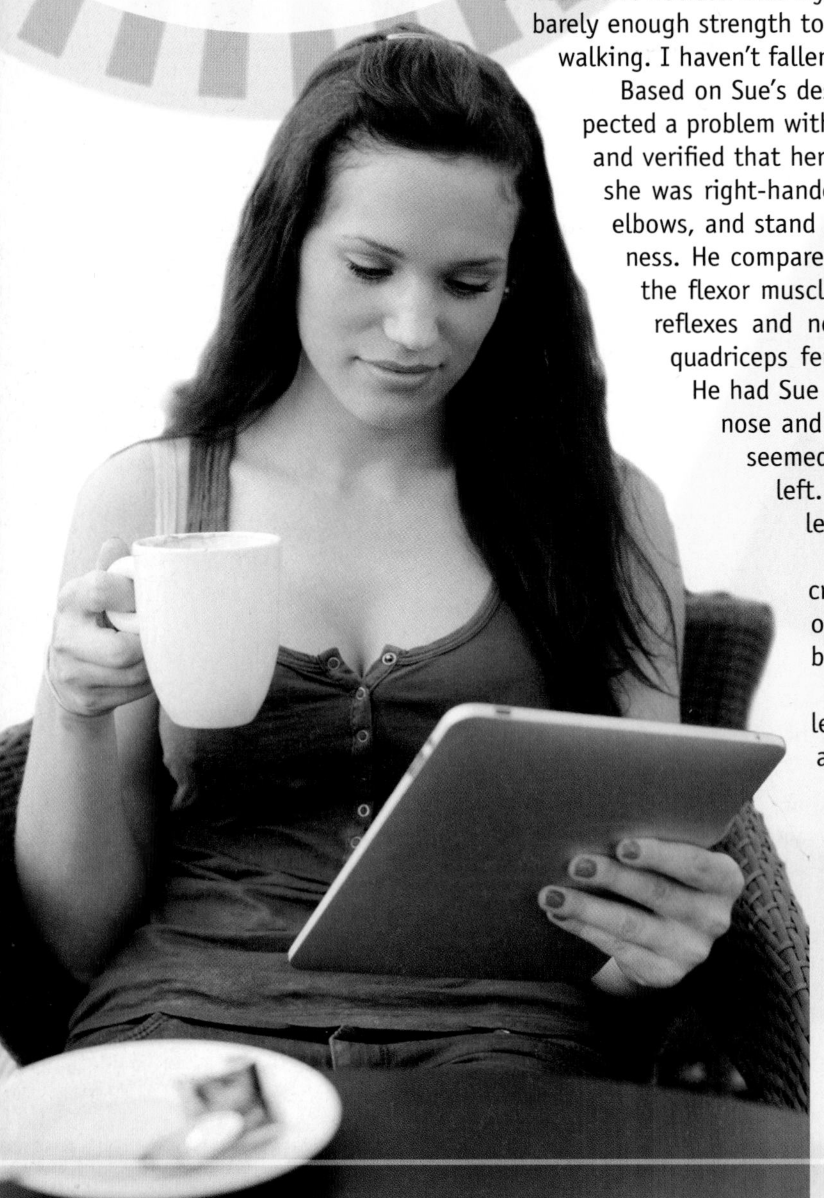

Dr. Mathews' knowledge of the structure and function of the muscular system helps him to diagnose medical conditions. In this chapter, you learn about muscle tissue and the connection it has with nervous tissue. Later in the chapter, we find out more about Sue's condition.

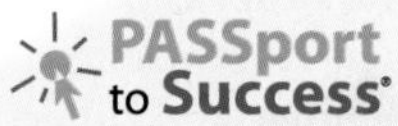

Ancillaries At-A-Glance

Visit *thePoint* to access the PASSport to Success and the following resources. For guidance in using these resources most effectively, see pp. ix–xviii.

Learning TOOLS

- Learning Style Self Assessment
- Live Advise Online Student Tutoring
- Tips for Effective Studying

Learning RESOURCES

- E-book: Chapter 7
- Web Figure: Muscles of the lateral head and neck
- Web Figure: Muscles of the anterior head and neck
- Web Figure: Muscles of the chest and shoulder
- Web Figure: Muscles of the shoulder and upper back
- Web Figure: Anatomy of the rotator cuff
- Web Figure: Muscles of the anterior forearm and arm
- Web Figure: Muscles of the posterior arm
- Web Figure: Muscles of the posterior forearm
- Web Figure: Muscles of the thigh, anterior view
- Web Figure: Muscles of the leg, anterior view
- Web Figure: Muscles of the leg, posterior view
- Animation: The Neuromuscular Junction
- Health Professions: Physical Therapist
- Detailed Chapter Outline
- Answers to Questions for Study and Review
- Audio Pronunciation Glossary

Learning Outcomes

After careful study of this chapter, you should be able to:

1. Compare the three types of muscle tissue, ***p. 120***
2. Describe three functions of skeletal muscle, ***p. 121***
3. Explain how skeletal muscles contract, ***p. 123***
4. List compounds stored in muscle cells that are used to generate energy, ***p. 125***
5. Explain what happens in muscle cells contracting anaerobically, ***p. 125***
6. Cite the effects of exercise on muscles, ***p. 126***
7. Compare isotonic and isometric contractions, ***p. 127***
8. Explain how muscles work together to produce movement, ***p. 128***
9. Compare the workings of muscles and bones to lever systems, ***p. 128***
10. Explain how muscles are named, ***p. 130***
11. Name some of the major muscles in each muscle group and describe the location and function of each, ***p. 131***
12. Describe how muscles change with age, ***p. 139***
13. Identify and locate the muscles involved in the tests carried out in the case study, ***pp. 118, 140***
14. Show how word parts are used to build words related to the muscular system (see Word Anatomy at the end of the chapter), ***p. 142***

Learning ACTIVITIES

- Pre-Quiz
- Visual Activities
- Kinesthetic Activities
- Auditory Activities

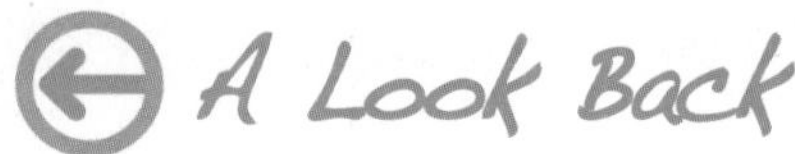

The voluntary muscles discussed in this chapter attach to the skeleton to create the movements described in Chapter 6. We also see in this chapter how membrane receptors and the membrane potential introduced in Chapter 3 function in muscle contraction.

Types of Muscle

There are three kinds of muscle tissue: smooth, cardiac, and skeletal muscle, as introduced in Chapter 4. After a brief description of all three types (Table 7-1), this chapter concentrates on skeletal muscle.

SMOOTH MUSCLE

Smooth muscle makes up the walls of the hollow body organs as well as those of the blood vessels and respiratory passageways. It contracts involuntarily and produces the wavelike motions of peristalsis that move substances through a system. Smooth muscle can also regulate the diameter of an opening, such as the central opening of blood vessels, or produce contractions of hollow organs, such as the uterus.

Smooth muscle fibers (cells) are tapered at each end and have a single, central nucleus. The cells appear smooth under the microscope because they do not contain the visible bands, or **striations**, that are seen in the other types of muscle cells. Smooth muscle may contract in response to a nerve impulse, hormonal stimulation, stretching, and other stimuli. The muscle contracts and relaxes slowly and can remain contracted for a long time.

CARDIAC MUSCLE

Cardiac muscle, also involuntary, makes up the heart's wall and creates the pulsing action of that organ. The cells of cardiac muscle are striated, like those of skeletal muscle. They differ in having one nucleus per cell and branching interconnections. The membranes between the cells are specialized to allow electric impulses to travel rapidly through them, so that contractions can be better coordinated. These membranes appear as dark lines between the cells (see Table 7-1) and are called intercalated (in-TER-kah-la-ted) disks, because they are "inserted between" the cells. The electric impulses that produce cardiac muscle contractions are generated within the muscle itself but can be modified by nervous stimuli and hormones.

SKELETAL MUSCLE

When viewed under the microscope, skeletal muscle cells appear heavily striated. The arrangement of protein threads within the cell that produces these striations is described later. The cells are very long and cylindrical, and because

Table 7-1 Comparison of the Different Types of Muscle

	Smooth	Cardiac	Skeletal
Location	Wall of hollow organs, vessels, respiratory, passageways	Wall of heart	Attached to bones
Cell characteristics	Tapered at each end, branching networks, nonstriated	Branching networks; special membranes (intercalated disks) between cells; single nucleus; lightly striated	Long and cylindrical; multinucleated; heavily striated
Control	Involuntary	Involuntary	Voluntary
Action	Produces peristalsis; contracts and relaxes slowly; may sustain contraction	Pumps blood out of heart; self-excitatory but influenced by nervous system and hormones	Produces movement at joints; stimulated by nervous system; contracts and relaxes rapidly

of their great length compared to other cells, they are often described as muscle *fibers*. They have multiple nuclei per cell because, during development, groups of precursor cells (myoblasts) fuse to form large multinucleated cells. Each mature muscle fiber contracts as a single unit when stimulated.

A division of the nervous system, the voluntary, or somatic, nervous system, stimulates skeletal muscle to contract, and the tissue usually contracts and relaxes rapidly. Because it is under conscious control, skeletal muscle is described as voluntary.

Skeletal muscle is so named because most of these muscles are attached to bones and produce movement at the joints. There are a few exceptions. The muscles of the abdominal wall, for example, are partly attached to other muscles, and the muscles of facial expression are attached to the skin. Skeletal muscles constitute the largest amount of the body's muscle tissue, making up about 40% of the total body weight. This muscular system is composed of more than 600 individual skeletal muscles. Although each one is a distinct structure, muscles usually act in groups to execute body movements.

CHECKPOINTS 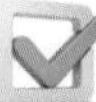

☐ 7-1 What are the three types of muscle?

The Muscular System

The three primary functions of skeletal muscles are

- Movement of the skeleton. Muscles are attached to bones and contract to change the position of the bones at a joint.
- Maintenance of posture. A steady partial contraction of muscle, known as **muscle tone**, keeps the body in position. Some of the muscles involved in maintaining posture are the large muscles of the thighs, back, neck, and shoulders as well as the abdominal muscles.
- Generation of heat. Muscles generate most of the heat needed to keep the body at 37°C (98.6°F). Heat is a natural by-product of muscle cell metabolism. When we are cold, muscles can boost their heat output by the rapid small contractions we know of as shivering.

7

MUSCLE STRUCTURE

In forming whole muscles, individual muscle fibers (cells) are arranged in bundles, or **fascicles** (FAS-ih-kls), held together by fibrous connective tissue **(Fig. 7-1)**. These layers are as follows:

- The **endomysium** (en-do-MIS-e-um) is the deepest layer of this connective tissue and surrounds the individual fibers in the fascicles.

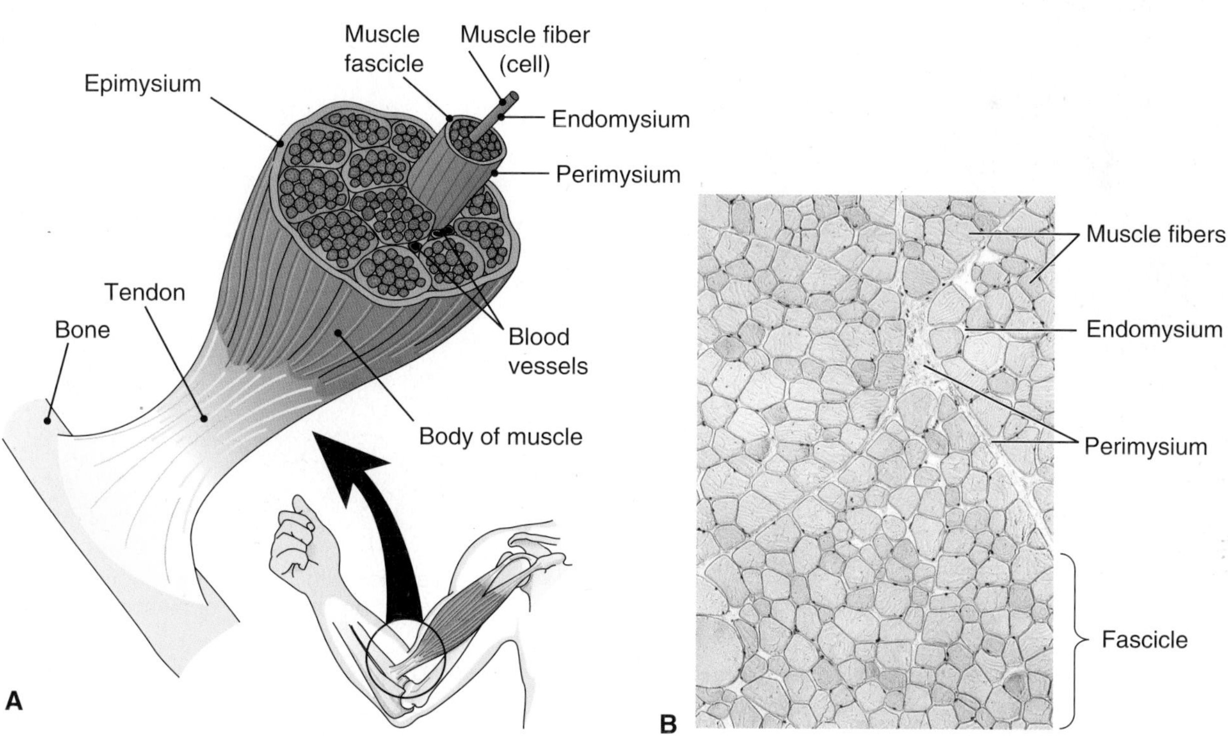

Figure 7-1 **Structure of a skeletal muscle.** KEY POINT Muscles are held together by layers of connective tissue. These layers merge to form the tendon that attaches the muscle to a bone. **A.** Muscle structure. **B.** Muscle tissue seen under a microscope. Portions of several fascicles are shown with connective tissue coverings. (B, Reprinted with permission from Gartner LP, Hiatt JL. *Color Atlas of Histology*, 3rd ed. Philadelphia, PA: Lippincott Williams & Wilkins, 2000.) ZOOMING IN What is the innermost layer of connective tissue in a muscle? What layer of connective tissue surrounds a fascicle of muscle fibers?

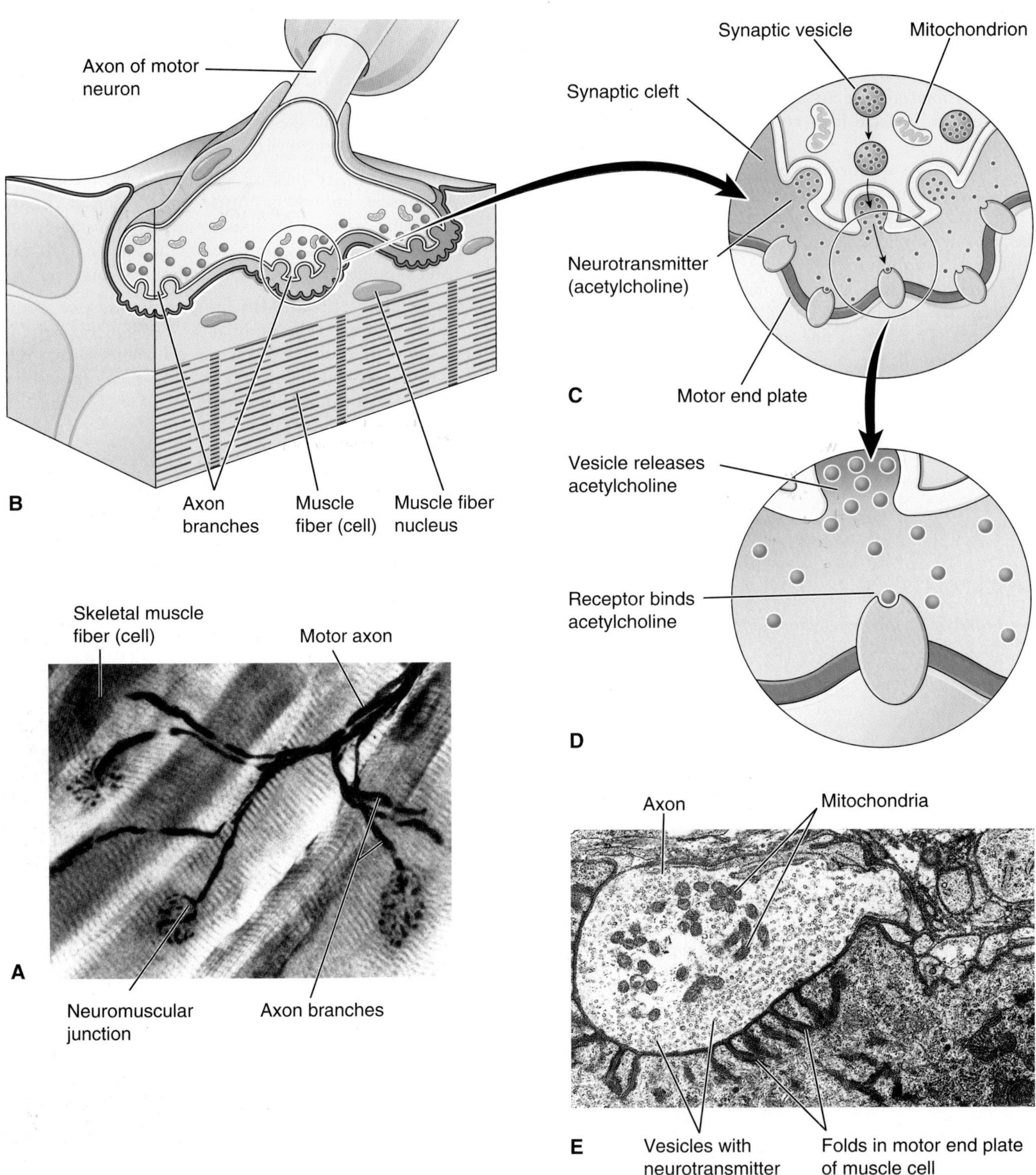

Figure 7-2 **Nerve supply to a skeletal muscle and the neuromuscular junction (NMJ).** KEY POINT Motor neurons stimulate skeletal muscle cells at the NMJ. **A.** A motor axon branches to stimulate multiple muscle fibers (cells). **B.** An axon branch makes contact with the membrane of a muscle fiber (cell) at the NMJ. **C.** Enlarged view of the NMJ showing release of neurotransmitter (acetylcholine) into the synaptic cleft. **D.** Acetylcholine attaches to receptors in the motor end plate, whose folds increase surface area. **E.** Electron microscope photograph of the NMJ. (A, Reprinted with permission from Cormack DH. *Essential Histology*, 2nd ed. Philadelphia, PA: Lippincott Williams & Wilkins, 2001. E, Courtesy of A. Sima.)

- The **perimysium** (per-ih-MIS-e-um) is a connective tissue layer around each fascicle.
- The **epimysium** (ep-ih-MIS-e-um) is a connective tissue sheath that encases the entire muscle. The epimysium forms the innermost layer of the **deep fascia**, the tough, fibrous sheath that encloses and defines a muscle.

Note that all these layers are named with prefixes that describe their position: *endo* meaning "within," *peri* meaning "around," *epi* meaning "above." (These prefixes are added to the root *my/o*, meaning "muscle.") All of these supporting tissues merge to form the **tendon**, a band of connective tissue that attaches a muscle to a bone (see Fig. 7-1).

MUSCLE CELLS IN ACTION

Nerve impulses coming from the brain and the spinal cord stimulate skeletal muscle fibers (see Chapter 8). Because these impulses are traveling away from the central nervous system (CNS), they are described as *motor impulses* (as contrasted to sensory impulses traveling toward the CNS), and the neurons (nerve cells) that carry these impulses are described as motor neurons. As the neuron contacts the muscle, its axon (fiber) branches to supply from a few to hundreds of individual muscle cells, or in some cases more than 1,000 (Fig. 7-2A).

A single neuron and all the muscle fibers it stimulates comprise a **motor unit**. Small motor units are used in fine coordination, as in movements of the eye. Larger motor units are used for maintaining posture or for broad movements, such as walking or swinging a tennis racquet.

The Neuromuscular Junction The point at which a nerve fiber contacts a muscle cell is called the **neuromuscular junction** (NMJ) (see Fig. 7-2). It is here that a chemical classified as a **neurotransmitter** is released from the neuron to stimulate the muscle fiber. The specific neurotransmitter released here is **acetylcholine** (as-e-til-KO-lene), abbreviated ACh, which is found elsewhere in the body as well. A great deal is known about the events that occur at this junction, and this information is important in understanding muscle action.

The NMJ is an example of a **synapse** (SIN-aps), a point of communication between a neuron and another cell (the term comes from a Greek word meaning "to clasp"). At every synapse, there is a tiny space, the **synaptic cleft,** across which the neurotransmitter must travel. Until its release, the neurotransmitter is stored in tiny membranous sacs, called vesicles, in the nerve fiber's endings. Once released, the neurotransmitter crosses the synaptic cleft and attaches to receptors, which are proteins embedded in the muscle cell membrane. The membrane forms multiple folds at this point, and these serve to increase surface area and hold a maximum number of receptors. The muscle cell's receiving membrane is known as the **motor end plate.**

In Chapter 3, we discussed the electrical potential of plasma membranes, that is, the voltage difference on the two sides of the membrane. Muscle fibers and nerve cells, moreover, show the property of **excitability**. Based on alternate opening and closing of ion channels in the membrane, they are able to transmit a change in the membrane potential, like an electric current, along the membrane. When a muscle is stimulated at the NMJ, an electric impulse is generated that spreads rapidly along the muscle cell membrane. This spreading wave of electric current is called the **action potential** because it calls the muscle cell into action. Chapter 8 provides more information on synapses and the action potential and more information that applies to Sue's problems in the case study.

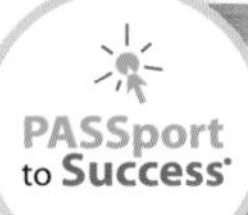

See the student resources on *thePoint* to view the animation *The Neuromuscular Junction*.

Contraction Another important property of muscle tissue is **contractility**. This is a muscle fiber's capacity to undergo shortening, becoming thicker. Studies of muscle chemistry and observation of cells under the powerful electron microscope have increased our understanding of how muscle cells work.

These studies reveal that each skeletal muscle fiber contains many threads, or filaments, made of two kinds of proteins, called **actin** (AK-tin) and **myosin** (MI-o-sin). Filaments made of actin are thin and light; those made of myosin are thick and dark. The filaments are present in alternating bundles within the muscle cell (Fig. 7-3). It is

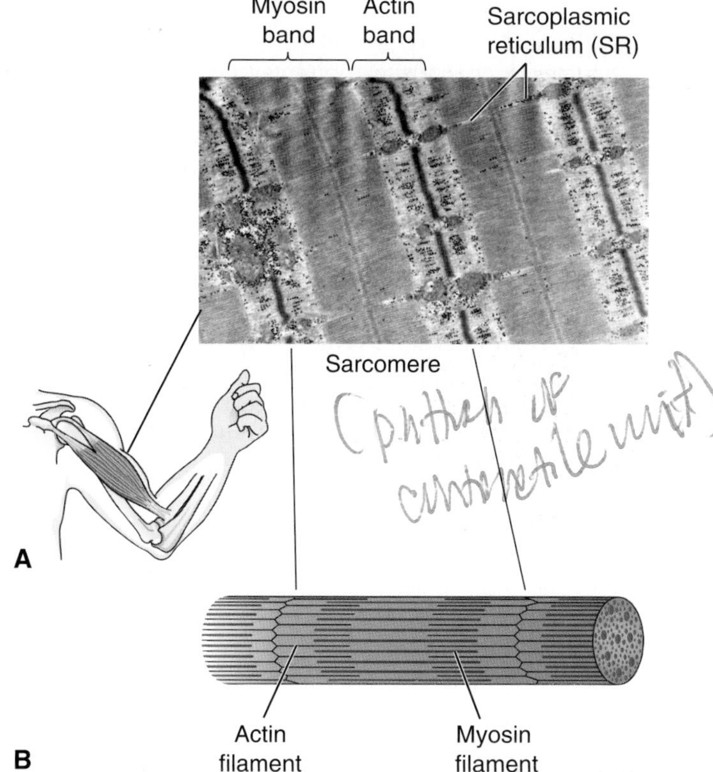

Figure 7-3 Detailed structure of a skeletal muscle cell. KEY POINT **A.** Photomicrograph of skeletal muscle cell (×6,500). Actin makes up the light band and myosin makes up the dark band. The dark line in the actin band marks points where actin filaments are held together. A sarcomere is a contracting subunit of skeletal muscle. The sarcoplasmic reticulum is the ER of muscle cells. **B.** Diagram of the photographic image. (A, Reprinted with permission from Mills SE. *Histology for Pathologists*, 3rd ed. Philadelphia, PA: Lippincott Williams & Wilkins, 2006.)

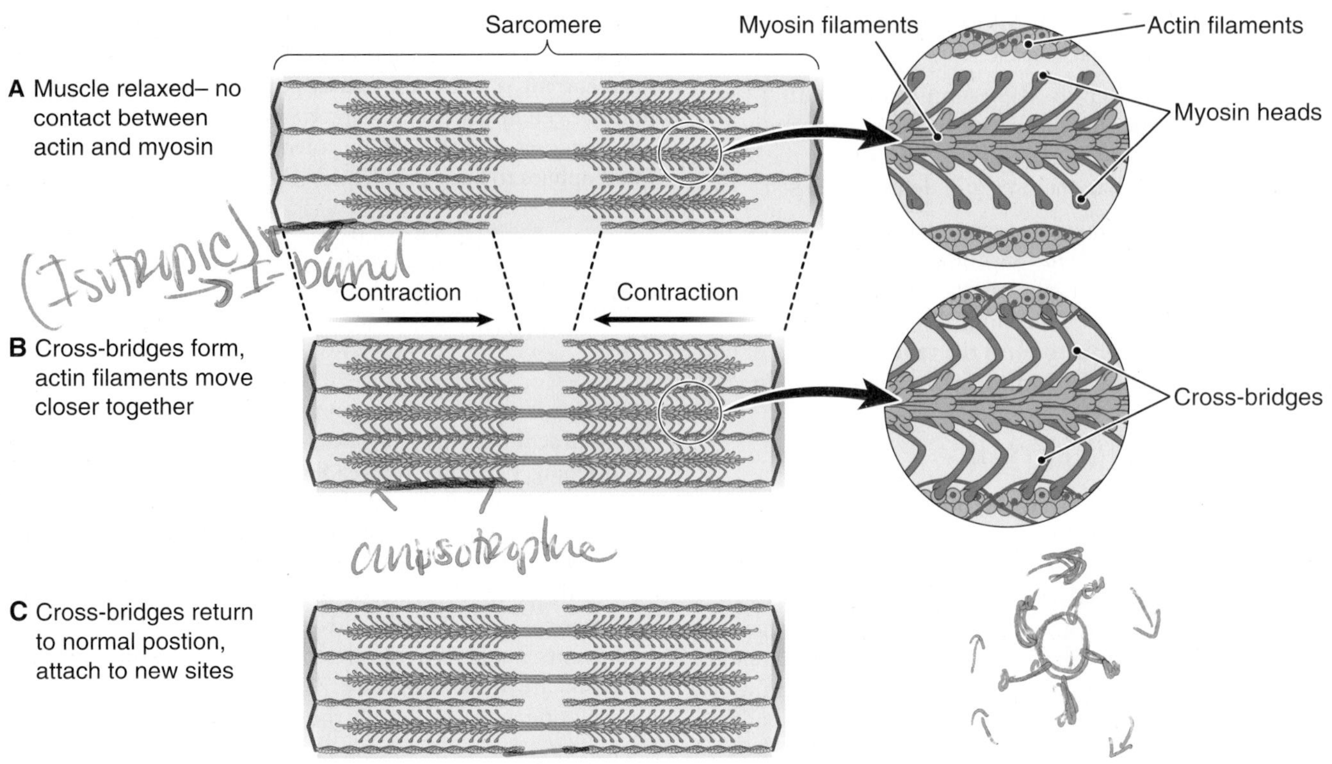

Figure 7-4 **Sliding filament mechanism of skeletal muscle contraction.** KEY POINT Muscle contraction depends on the interaction of actin and myosin filaments within the cell. **A.** Muscle is relaxed and there is no contact between the actin and myosin filaments. **B.** Cross-bridges form and the actin filaments are moved closer together as the muscle fiber contracts. **C.** The cross-bridges return to their original position and attach to new sites to prepare for another pull on the actin filaments and further contraction. ZOOMING IN Do the actin or myosin filaments change in length as contraction proceeds?

the alternating bands of light actin and heavy myosin filaments that give skeletal muscle its striated appearance. They also give a view of what occurs when muscles contract.

Note that the actin and myosin filaments overlap where they meet, just as your fingers overlap when you fold your hands together. A contracting subunit of skeletal muscle is called a **sarcomere** (SAR-ko-mere). It consists of a band of myosin filaments and the actin filaments on each side of them (see Fig. 7-3) The myosin molecules are shaped like two golf clubs twisted together with their paddle-like heads projecting away from the sarcomere's center. The actin molecules are twisted together like two strands of beads, each bead having a myosin binding site (Fig. 7-4).

Figure 7-4 shows a section of muscle as it contracts. In movement, the myosin heads "latch on" to the actin filaments in their overlapping region, forming attachments between the filaments that are described as *cross-bridges*. Using the energy of stored ATP, the myosin heads, like the oars of a boat moving water, pull all the actin strands closer together within each sarcomere. New ATP molecules trigger the release of the myosin heads and move them back to position for another "power stroke." With repeated movements, the overlapping filaments slide together, and the muscle fiber contracts, becoming shorter and thicker. This action is aptly named the *sliding filament mechanism* of muscle contraction. Note that the filaments overlap increasingly as the cell contracts. (In reality, not all the myosin heads are moving at the same time. About one-half are forward at any time, and the rest are preparing for another swing.) During contraction, each sarcomere becomes shorter, but the individual filaments do not change in length. As in shuffling a deck of cards, as you push the cards together, the deck becomes smaller, but the cards do not change in length.

The Role of Calcium In addition to actin, myosin, and ATP, calcium is needed for muscle contraction. It enables cross-bridges to form between actin and myosin so the sliding filament action can begin. When muscles are at rest, two additional proteins called **troponin** (tro-PO-nin) and **tropomyosin** (tro-po-MI-o-sin) block the sites on actin filaments where cross-bridges can form (Fig. 7-5). When calcium attaches to the troponin, these proteins move aside, uncovering the binding sites. In resting muscles, the calcium is not available because it is stored within the cell's endoplasmic reticulum, which, in muscle cells, is called the **sarcoplasmic reticulum** (SR). Calcium is released into the cytoplasm only when the cell is stimulated by a nerve fiber. Muscles relax when nervous stimulation stops, and the calcium is then pumped back into the SR, ready for the next contraction.

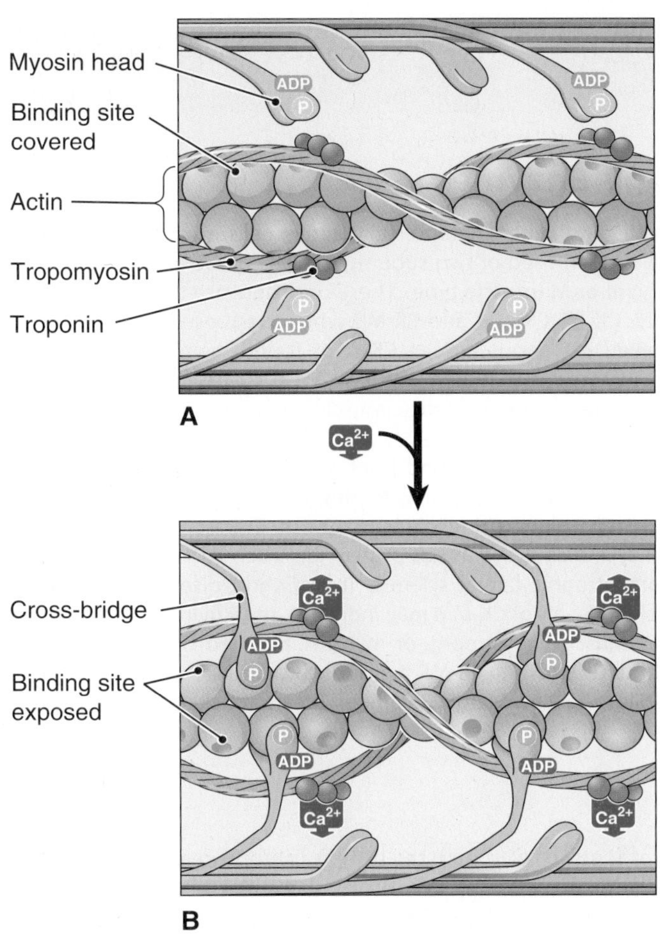

Figure 7-5 Role of calcium in muscle contraction.
KEY POINT Calcium unblocks sites where cross-bridges can form between actin and myosin filaments to begin muscle contraction. **A.** Troponin and tropomyosin cover the binding sites where cross-bridges can form between actin and myosin. **B.** Calcium shifts troponin and tropomyosin away from binding sites so cross-bridges can form.

A summary of the events in a muscle contraction is as follows:

1. ACh is released from a neuron ending into the synaptic cleft at the NMJ.
2. ACh binds to the muscle's motor end plate and produces an action potential.
3. The action potential travels to the SR.
4. The SR releases calcium into the cytoplasm.
5. Calcium shifts troponin and tropomyosin so that binding sites on actin are exposed.
6. Myosin heads bind to actin, forming cross-bridges.
7. Using stored energy, myosin heads pull actin filaments together within the sarcomeres and the cell shortens.
8. New ATP is used to detach myosin heads and move them back to position for another "power stroke."
9. Muscle relaxes when stimulation ends and the calcium is pumped back into the SR.

The phenomenon of rigor mortis, a state of rigidity that occurs after death, illustrates ATP's crucial role in muscle contraction. Shortly after death, muscle cells begin to degrade. Calcium escapes into the cytoplasm, and the muscle filaments slide together. Metabolism has ceased, however, and there is no ATP to disengage the filaments, so they remain locked in a contracted state. Rigor mortis lasts about 24 hours, gradually fading as enzymes break down the muscle filaments.

CHECKPOINTS 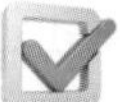

- 7-2 What are the three main functions of skeletal muscle?
- 7-3 What is the name of the special synapse where a nerve cell makes contact with a muscle cell?
- 7-4 What neurotransmitter is involved in the stimulation of skeletal muscle cells?
- 7-5 What are the two properties of muscle cells that are needed for response to a stimulus?
- 7-6 What filaments interact to produce muscle contraction?
- 7-7 What mineral is needed for interaction of the contractile filaments?

7

ENERGY SOURCES

As noted earlier, all muscle contraction requires energy in the form of ATP. Most of this energy is produced by the oxidation (commonly called "burning") of nutrients within the cell's mitochondria, especially the oxidation of glucose and fatty acids. Metabolism that requires oxygen is described as *aerobic* (the root *aer/o* means "air" or "gas," but in this case refers to oxygen).

Storage Compounds The circulating blood constantly brings nutrients and oxygen to the cells, but muscle cells also store a small supply of each for rapid ATP generation, such as during vigorous exercise. For example

- **Myoglobin** (mi-o-GLO-bin) stores additional oxygen. This compound is similar to the hemoglobin in blood, but is located specifically in muscle cells, as indicated by the root *my/o* in its name.
- **Glycogen** (GLI-ko-jen) is the storage form of glucose. It is a polysaccharide made of multiple glucose molecules and it can be broken down into glucose when needed by the muscle cells.
- Fatty acids are stored as triglycerides formed into fat droplets. These droplets can be broken down into fatty acids when needed by the muscle cells.

Anaerobic Metabolism Oxidation is very efficient and yields a large amount of ATP, but it is relatively slow, so it cannot supply enough energy for the first few seconds of muscle contraction. Also, it requires an abundant oxygen supply. During strenuous activity, oxygen delivery to the tissues cannot keep up with the demands of hard-working

Box 7-1 *A Closer Look*

Creatine Kinase: Muscle's Backup Energy Enzyme

At rest, muscle cells store some of the ATP they produce in the sarcoplasm. But the amount stored is sufficient for only a few seconds of contraction, and it takes several more seconds before anaerobic glycolyis and oxidation can replenish it. So, how do muscle fibers power their contractions in the meantime? They have a backup energy source called creatine phosphate to tide them over.

When muscle cells are resting, they manufacture creatine phosphate by transferring energy from ATP to creatine, a substance produced by the liver, pancreas, and kidneys. When muscle cells are exercising actively, they transfer that energy to ADP to create ATP. There is enough creatine phosphate in the sarcoplasm to produce 4 or 5 times the original amount of stored ATP—enough to power the cell until the other ATP-producing reactions take over.

Creatine kinase (CK) catalyzes the transfer of energy from creatine phosphate to ADP. CK is found in all muscle cells and other metabolically active cells, such as neurons. It is composed of two subunits, which can be either *B* (brain type) or *M* (muscle type). Therefore, there are three forms of CK: CK-BB, CK-MM, and CK-MB, which are present at different levels in various tissues. CK-BB is found mainly in nervous and smooth muscle tissue. CK-MM is found predominantly in skeletal muscle. Cardiac muscle contains both CK-MM and CK-MB.

Normally, the blood level of creatine kinase is low, but damage to CK-containing tissues increases it. Thus, clinicians can use blood CK levels in diagnosis. Elevated blood CK-BB may indicate a nervous system disorder, such as stroke or amyotrophic lateral sclerosis (Lou Gehrig disease). Elevated blood levels of CK-MM may indicate a muscular disorder, such as muscular dystrophy or myositis. Elevated blood levels of both CK-MM and CK-MB may indicate cardiac muscle damage following a myocardial infarction (heart attack).

muscles. Under these conditions, the cells use faster mechanisms of ATP production that do not require oxygen. These processes are described as *anaerobic* (*an-* means "not" or "without"), and are as follows:

1. Breakdown of **creatine** (KRE-ah-tin) **phosphate**. Creatine phosphate is a compound similar to ATP, in that it has a high energy bond that breaks down to release energy. This energy is used to make ATP for muscle contraction. It generates ATP very rapidly, but its supply is limited (see Box 7-1).
2. **Anaerobic glycolysis**. This process breaks glucose down incompletely without using oxygen (*glyc/o* means "glucose" and *-lysis* means "separation"). A few ATPs are generated in these reactions, as is a by-product called lactic acid, which is later oxidized for energy when oxygen is available.

Changing conditions limit the continuation of anaerobic metabolism. When a person stops exercising, enough ATP must be generated to reestablish a resting state by oxidizing any accumulated lactic acid and replenishing stored materials. The person must take in extra oxygen by continued rapid breathing, known as *excess postexercise oxygen consumption*. Chapter 18 has more details on metabolism.

Muscle Fatigue It is commonly thought that muscles tire because they are out of ATP or because lactic acid accumulates. In fact, fatigue in nonathletes frequently originates in the nervous system, not the muscles. People unaccustomed to strenuous exercise find the sensations it generates unpleasant and, consciously or unconsciously, reduce the nervous impulses to skeletal muscles. It is difficult to overcome the brain's inhibition and truly fatigue a muscle, that is, take it to the point that it no longer responds to stimuli. True muscle fatigue has many causes, and may depend on individual factors, fitness and genetic makeup for example, and the type of exercise involved. These causes include depletion of glycogen reserves, inadequate oxygen supply, or the accumulation of phosphates from ATP breakdown.

EFFECTS OF EXERCISE

Regular exercise results in a number of changes in muscle tissue, as the muscle cells adapt to the increased workload. The changes depend on the type of exercise. Resistance training, such as weight lifting, causes muscle cells to increase in size, a condition known as hypertrophy (hi-PER-tro-fe). Larger muscle cells contain more myofibrils and can form more cross-bridges, so they can generate more force. Resistance training also increases muscle stores of creatine phosphate and glycogen, so that muscle cells can use anaerobic metabolism to generate a large amount of ATP in a short time. Muscle hypertrophy is stimulated by hormones, especially the male sex steroids. Box 7-2 has information on how some athletes abuse these steroids to increase muscle size and strength, but at the expense of their health.

Aerobic exercise, that is, exercise that increases oxygen consumption, such as running, biking, or swimming, leads to improved muscular endurance. Endurance training increases the muscle cells' blood supply and number of mitochondria, improving their ability to generate ATP aerobically and to get rid of waste products. Endurance-trained

Box 7-2 Hot Topics

Anabolic Steroids: Winning at All Costs?

Anabolic steroids mimic the effects of the male sex hormone testosterone by promoting metabolism and stimulating growth. These drugs are legally prescribed to promote muscle regeneration and prevent atrophy from disuse after surgery. However, some athletes also purchase them illegally, using them to increase muscle size and strength and improve endurance.

When steroids are used illegally to enhance athletic performance, the doses needed are large enough to cause serious side effects. They increase blood cholesterol levels, which may lead to atherosclerosis, heart disease, kidney failure, and stroke. They damage the liver, making it more susceptible to cancer and other diseases, and suppress the immune system, increasing the risk of infection and cancer. In men, steroids cause impotence, testicular atrophy, low sperm count, infertility, and the development of female sex characteristics, such as breasts (gynecomastia). In women, steroids disrupt ovulation and menstruation and produce male sex characteristics, such as breast atrophy, enlargement of the clitoris, increased body hair, and deepening of the voice. In both sexes, steroids increase the risk for baldness and, especially in men, cause mood swings, depression, and violence.

7

muscles can contract more frequently and for longer periods without fatiguing.

Cardiovascular changes are perhaps the most important physical benefits of endurance exercise. You can think of endurance exercise as "strength training for the heart." That organ has to pump up to five times as much blood during endurance exercise as it does at rest. The heart muscle (especially the left ventricle) adapts to its increased workload by growing larger and stronger. Its increased pumping efficiency means that the heart doesn't have to work very hard at rest, so the resting heart rate declines. Endurance exercise also benefits the vascular system by decreasing the amount of less healthy (LDL) cholesterol in the blood and reducing blood pressure. These vascular changes may derive in part from the reduced body fat and improved psychological well-being that result from regular physical activity. Whatever the cause of the improved cardiovascular function, it's well established that, aside from not smoking, exercise is the most important thing you can do to improve your health.

The benefits of one form of exercise do not significantly carry over to the other—endurance exercise does not significantly increase muscle strength, and resistance training does not significantly increase muscle endurance. An exercise program thus should include both methods, with periods of warm-up and cool-down before and after working out. Stretching generally improves the range of motion at the joints and improves balance. However, studies show that static stretching that is, holding an extended position for 30 seconds to 2 minutes, just before a strenuous workout, actually decreases muscle strength and increases the risk of injury.

TYPES OF MUSCLE CONTRACTIONS

Muscle tone refers to a muscle's partially contracted state that is normal even when the muscle is not in use. The maintenance of this tone, or **tonus** (TO-nus), is due to the action of the nervous system in keeping the muscles in a constant state of readiness for action. Muscles that are little used soon become flabby, weak, and lacking in tone.

In addition to the partial contractions that are responsible for muscle tone, there are two other types of contractions on which the body depends:

- In **isotonic** (i-so-TON-ik) **contractions**, the tone or tension within the muscle remains the same, but muscle length changes and the muscle bulges as it accomplishes work (*iso-* means "same" or "equal" and *ton* means "tension"). Within this category, there are two forms of contraction:
    - **Concentric contractions.** These contractions are more familiar, as they produce more obvious changes in position. In concentric contractions, a muscle as a whole shortens to produce movement. Try flexing your arm at the elbow to pick up a dumbbell or heavy can. The anterior arm flexors, the biceps brachii and brachialis, move the forearm at the elbow, lifting the weight, and you can see that the muscles change shape and bulge outward.
    - **Eccentric contractions.** In these contractions, the muscle lengthens as it exerts force. Think of gradually lowering that dumbbell or heavy can. The arm flexors tense as they lengthen. These contractions strengthen muscles considerably, but are more likely to cause soreness later, perhaps because of microscopic tears in the muscle fibers.
- In **isometric** (i-so-MET-rik) **contractions,** there is no change in muscle length but there is a great increase in muscle tension (*metr/o* means "measure"). Pushing against an immovable force produces an isometric contraction, as in trying to lift a weight that is too heavy to move. Try pushing the palms of your hands hard

against each other. There is no movement, but you can feel the increased tension in your arm muscles.

Most body movements involve a combination of both isotonic and isometric contractions. When walking, for example, some muscles contract isotonically to propel the body forward, but at the same time, other muscles are contracting isometrically to keep your body in position.

CHECKPOINTS 

- 7-8 What compound is formed in oxidation of nutrients that supplies the energy for contraction?
- 7-9 What acid accumulates during anaerobic metabolism?
- 7-10 What are the two main types of muscle contraction?

The Mechanics of Muscle Movement

Most muscles have two or more points of attachment to the skeleton. The muscle is attached to a bone at each end by means of a cordlike extension called a **tendon** (Fig. 7-6). All of the connective tissue within and around the muscle merges to form the tendon, which then attaches directly to the bone's periosteum (see Fig. 7-1). In some instances, a broad sheet called an **aponeurosis** (ap-o-nu-RO-sis) may attach muscles to bones or to other muscles.

In moving the bones, one end of a muscle is attached to a more freely movable part of the skeleton, and the other end is attached to a relatively stable part. The less movable (more fixed) attachment is called the **origin;** the attachment to the body part that the muscle puts into action is called the **insertion.** When a muscle contracts, it pulls on both attachment points, bringing the more movable insertion closer to the origin and thereby causing movement of the body part. Figure 7-6 shows the action of the biceps brachii (in the upper arm) in flexing the arm at the elbow. The insertion on the radius of the forearm is brought toward the origin at the scapula of the shoulder girdle.

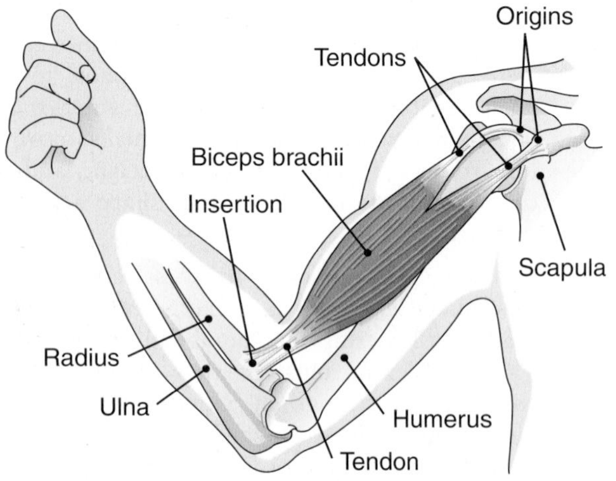

Figure 7-6 **Muscle attachments to bones.** KEY POINT Tendons attach muscles to bones. The stable point is the origin; the movable point is the insertion. In this diagram, three attachments are shown—two origins and one insertion. ZOOMING IN Does contraction of the biceps brachii produce flexion or extension at the elbow?

MUSCLES WORK TOGETHER

Many of the skeletal muscles function in pairs. An **agonist** (AG-on-ist) is any muscle that performs a given movement. The muscle that produces a movement opposite to that of the agonist is termed the **antagonist** (an-TAG-on-ist) (the prefix *anti-* means "against.") Clearly, for any given movement, the antagonist must relax when the agonist contracts. For example, when the brachialis at the anterior arm contracts to flex the arm, the triceps brachii at the back must relax; when the triceps brachii contracts to extend the arm, the brachialis must relax. In addition to agonists and antagonists, there are also muscles that steady body parts or assist agonists. These "helping" muscles are called **synergists** (SIN-er-jists), because they work with the agonist to accomplish a movement (*syn-* means "together" and *erg/o* means "work.") For example, the biceps brachii is a synergist to the brachialis in flexing the arm.

As the muscles work together, actions are coordinated to accomplish many complex movements. Note that during development, the nervous system must gradually begin to coordinate our movements. A child learning to walk or to write, for example, may use muscles unnecessarily at first or fail to use appropriate muscles when needed.

LEVERS AND BODY MECHANICS

Proper body mechanics help conserve energy and ensure freedom from strain and fatigue; conversely, such ailments as lower back pain—a common complaint—can be traced to poor body mechanics. Body mechanics have special significance to healthcare workers, who frequently must move patients and handle cumbersome equipment. Maintaining the body segments in correct alignment also affects the vital organs that are supported by the skeleton.

If you have had a course in physics, recall your study of levers. A lever is simply a rigid bar that moves about a fixed pivot point, the fulcrum. There are three classes of levers, which differ only in the location of the fulcrum (F), the effort (E), or force, and the resistance (R), the weight or load:

- In a first-class lever, the fulcrum is located between the resistance and the effort; a seesaw or a scissors is an example of this class (Fig. 7-7A).
- The second-class lever has the resistance located between the fulcrum and the effort; a wheelbarrow or a mattress lifted at one end is an illustration of this class (see Fig. 7-7B).

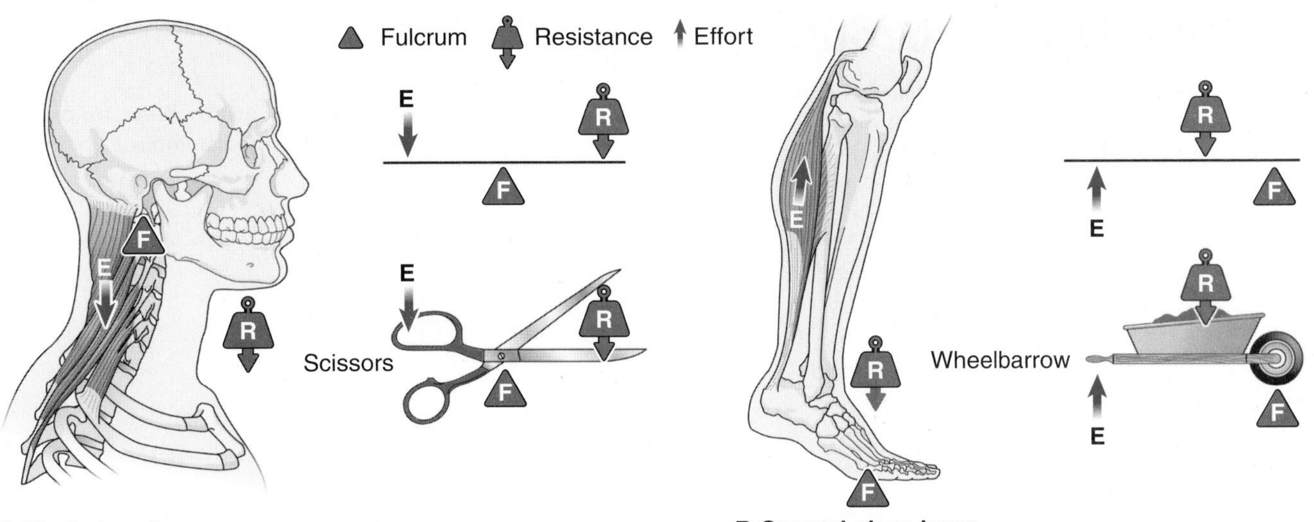

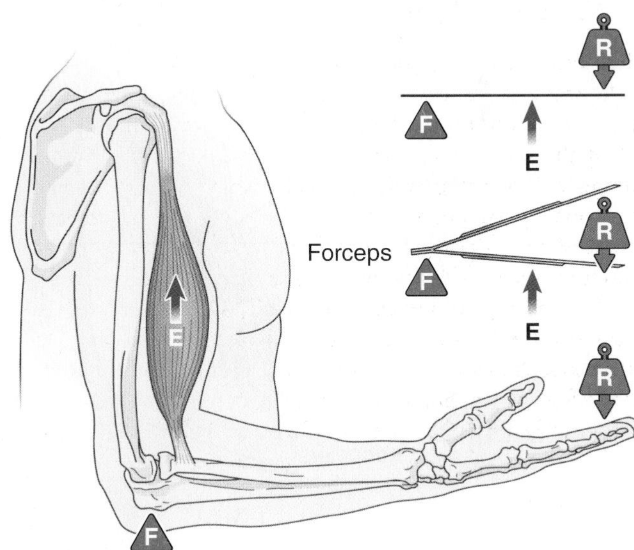

Figure 7-7 **Levers.** KEY POINT Muscles work with bones as lever systems to produce movement. Three classes of levers are shown along with tools and anatomic examples that illustrate each type. R, resistance (weight); E, effort (force); F, fulcrum (pivot point). ZOOMING IN In a third-class lever system, where is the fulcrum with regard to the effort and the resistance?

- In the third-class lever, the effort is between the resistance and the fulcrum. A forceps or a tweezers is an example of this type of lever. The effort is applied in the tool's center, between the fulcrum, where the pieces join, and the resistance at the tip (see Fig. 7-7C).

The musculoskeletal system can be considered a system of levers, in which the bone is the lever, the joint is the fulcrum, and the force is applied by a muscle. An example of a first-class lever in the body is using the muscles at the back of the neck to lift the head at the joint between the skull's occipital bone and the first cervical vertebra (atlas) (see Fig. 7-7). A second-class lever is exemplified by raising your weight to the ball of your foot (the fulcrum) using the calf muscles.

However, there are very few examples of first- and second-class levers in the body. Most lever systems in the body are of the third-class type. A muscle usually inserts past a joint and exerts force between the fulcrum and the resistance. That is, the fulcrum is behind both the point of effort and the weight. As shown in Figure 7-7C, when the biceps brachii flexes the forearm at the elbow, the muscle exerts its force at its insertion on the radius. The weight of the hand and forearm creates the resistance, and the fulcrum is the elbow joint, which is behind the point of effort.

By understanding and applying knowledge of levers to body mechanics, healthcare workers can reduce their risk of musculoskeletal injury while carrying out their numerous clinical tasks.

CHECKPOINTS

- ☐ 7-11 What are the names of the two attachment points of a muscle and how do they function?
- ☐ 7-12 What is the name of the muscle that produces a movement as compared with the muscle that produces an opposite movement?
- ☐ 7-13 Of the three classes of levers, which one represents the action of most muscles?

Skeletal Muscle Groups

The study of muscles is made simpler by grouping them according to body regions. Knowing how muscles are named can also help in remembering them. A number of different characteristics are used in naming muscles, including the following:

- location, using the name of a nearby bone, for example, or a position, such as lateral, medial, internal, or external

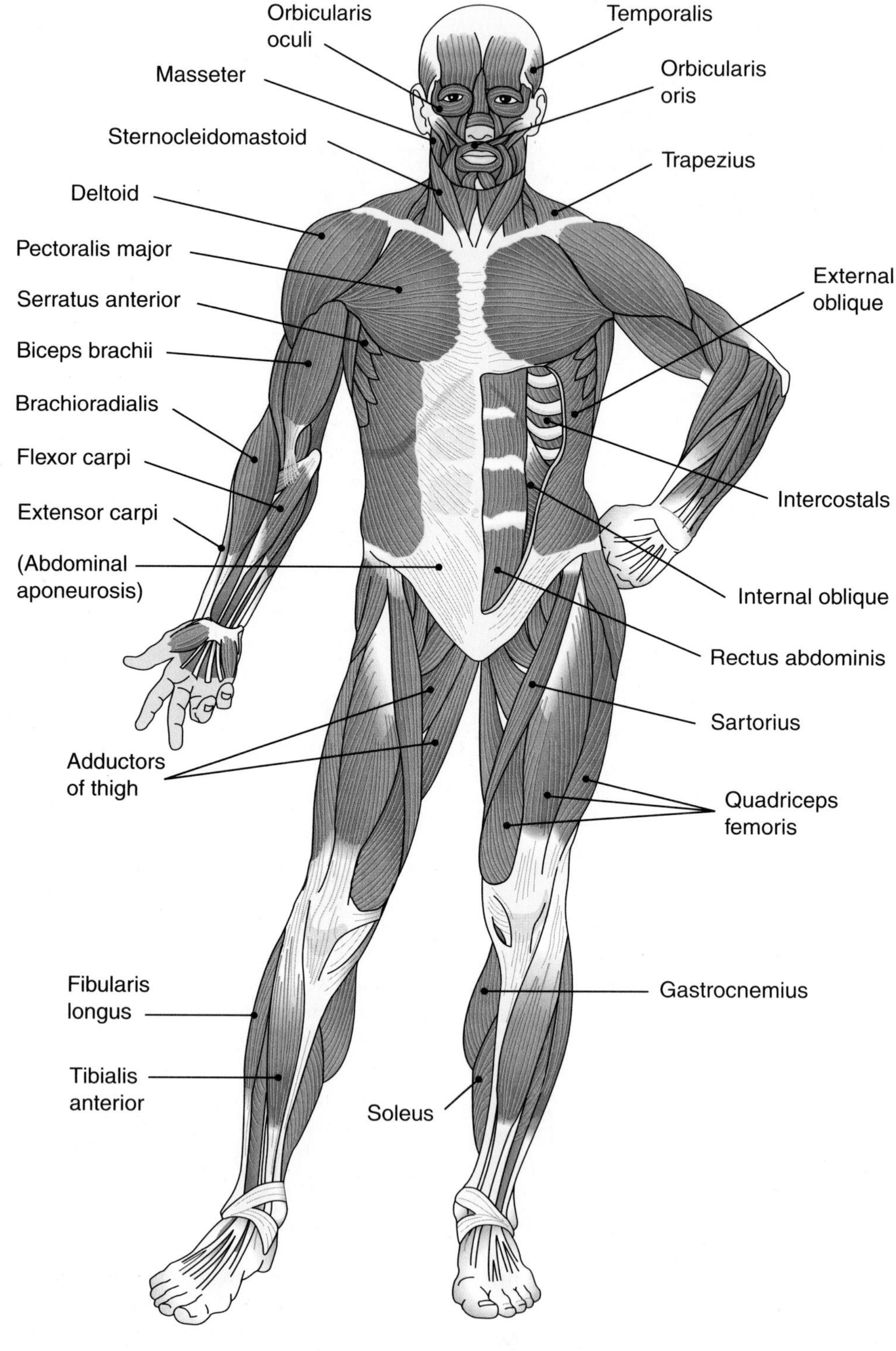

Figure 7-8 **Superficial muscles, anterior view.** An associated structure is labeled in parentheses. An aponeurosis is a broad, sheetlike tendon.

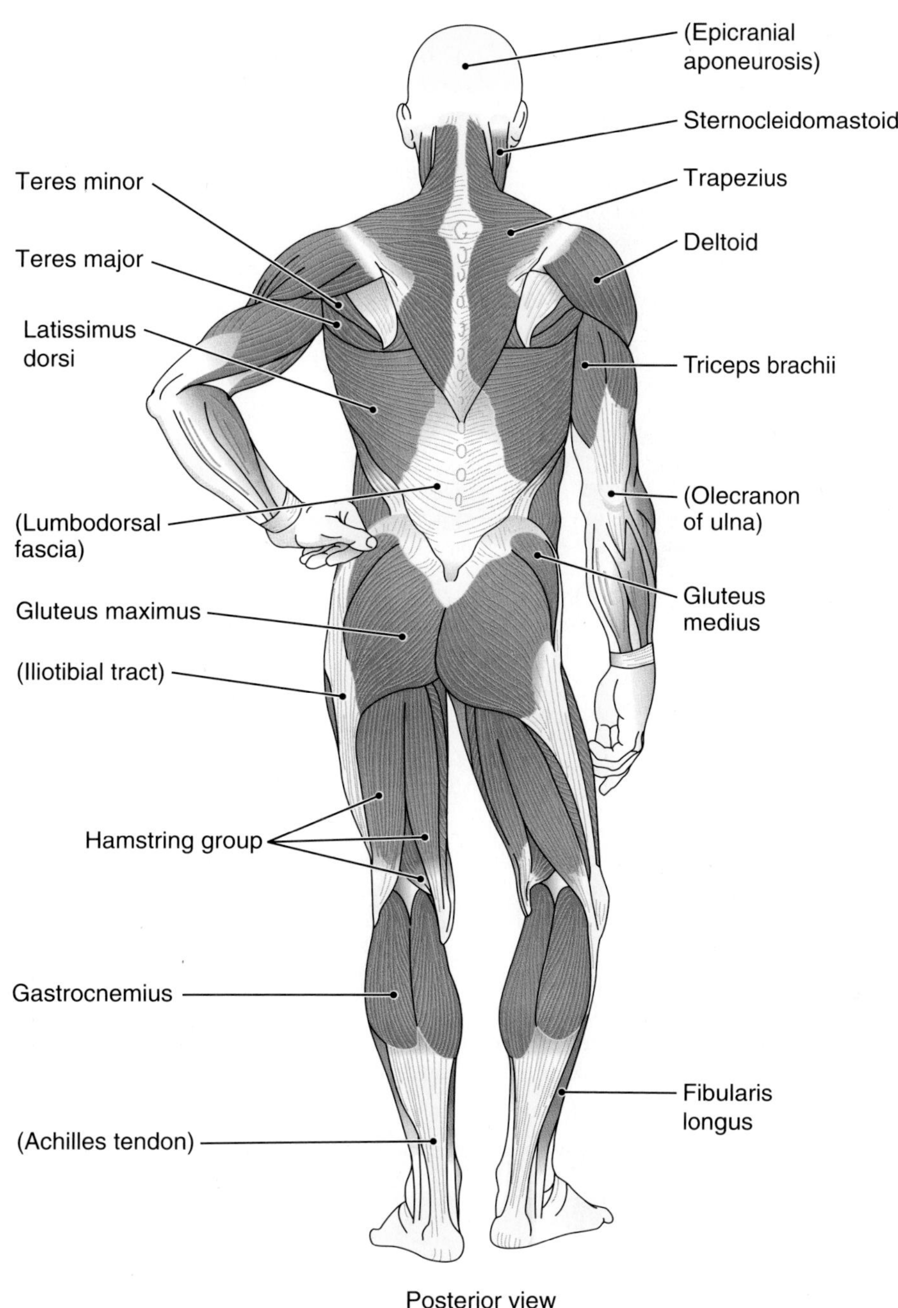

Figure 7-9 **Superficial muscles, posterior view.** Associated structures are labeled in parentheses.

- size, using terms such as maximus, major, minor, longus, or brevis
- shape, such as circular (orbicularis), triangular (deltoid), or trapezoid (trapezius)
- direction of fibers, including straight (rectus) or angled (oblique)
- number of heads (attachment points), as indicated by the suffix *-ceps*, as in biceps, triceps, and quadriceps
- action, as in flexor, extensor, adductor, abductor, or levator

Often, more than one feature is used in naming. Refer to Figures 7-8 and 7-9 as you study the locations and functions of the superficial skeletal muscles, and try to figure out the basis for each name. Although they are described in the singular, most of the muscles are present on both sides of the body.

MUSCLES OF THE HEAD

The principal muscles of the head are those of facial expression and of mastication (chewing) (Fig. 7-10, Table 7-2).

The muscles of facial expression include ring-shaped ones around the eyes and the lips, called the **orbicularis** (or-bik-u-LAH-ris) **muscles** because of their shape (think of "orbit"). The muscle surrounding the eye is called the **orbicularis oculi** (OK-u-li), whereas the lip muscle is the

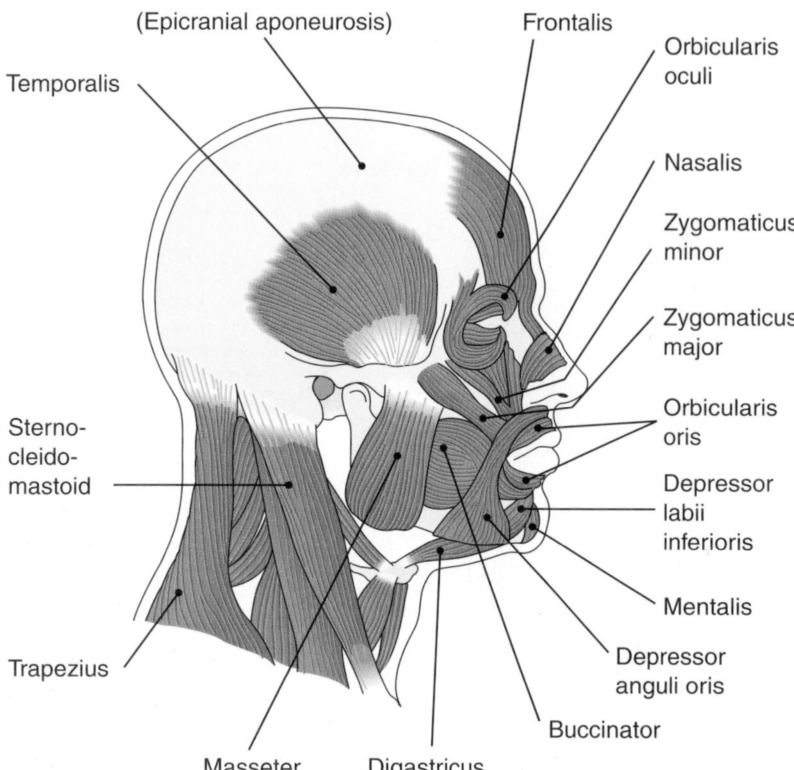

Figure 7-10 **Muscles of the head.** An associated structure is labeled in parentheses. ZOOMING IN Which of the muscles in this illustration are named for a nearby bone?

orbicularis oris. These muscles all have antagonists. For example, the **levator palpebrae** (PAL-pe-bre) **superioris**, or lifter of the upper eyelid, is the antagonist for the orbicularis oculi.

One of the largest muscles of expression forms the fleshy part of the cheek and is called the **buccinator** (BUK-se-na-tor). Used in whistling or blowing, it is sometimes referred to as the trumpeter's muscle. You can readily think of other muscles of facial expression: for instance, the antagonists of the orbicularis oris can produce a smile, a sneer, or a grimace. There are a number of scalp muscles that lift the eyebrows or draw them together into a frown.

There are four pairs of mastication (chewing) muscles, all of which insert on and move the mandible. The largest are the **temporalis** (TEM-po-ral-is), which is superior to the ear, and the **masseter** (mas-SE-ter) at the angle of the jaw.

Table 7-2 Muscles of the Head and Neck[a]

Name	Location	Function
Orbicularis oculi	Encircles eyelid	Closes eye
Levator palpebrae superioris (deep muscle; not shown)	Posterior orbit to upper eyelid	Opens eye
Orbicularis oris	Encircles mouth	Closes lips
Buccinator	Fleshy part of cheek	Flattens cheek; helps in eating, whistling, and blowing wind instruments
Temporalis	Above and near ear	Closes jaw
Masseter	At angle of jaw	Closes jaw
Sternocleidomastoid	Along lateral neck, to mastoid process	Flexes head; rotates head toward opposite side from muscle

[a]*These and other muscles of the face are shown in Figure 7-10.*

The tongue has two muscle groups. The first group, called the *intrinsic muscles,* is located entirely within the tongue. The second group, the *extrinsic muscles*, originates outside the tongue. It is because of these many muscles that the tongue has such remarkable flexibility and can perform so many different functions. Consider the intricate tongue motions involved in speaking, chewing, and swallowing. **Figure 7-10** shows some additional muscles of the face.

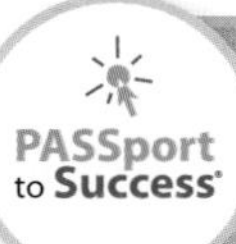

See the student resources on *thePoint* to view additional pictures of head and neck musculature.

MUSCLES OF THE NECK

The neck muscles tend to be ribbon-like and extend vertically or obliquely in several layers and in a complex manner **(see Fig. 7-10, Table 7-2)**. The one you will hear of most frequently is the **sternocleidomastoid** (ster-no-kli-do-MAS-toyd), sometimes referred to simply as the sternomastoid. This strong muscle extends superiorly from the sternum across the lateral neck to the mastoid process of the temporal bone. When the left and right muscles work together, they bring the head forward on the chest (flexion). Working alone, each muscle tilts and rotates the head so as to orient the face toward the side opposite that muscle.

A portion of the trapezius muscle (described later) is located at the posterior neck, where it helps hold the head up (extension). Other large deep muscles are the chief extensors of the head and neck.

MUSCLES OF THE UPPER EXTREMITIES

Muscles of the upper extremities include the muscles that determine the position of the shoulder, the anterior and posterior muscles that move the arm, and the muscles that move the forearm and hand.

7

Muscles that Move the Shoulder and Arm The position of the shoulder depends to a large extent on the degree of contraction of the **trapezius** (trah-PE-ze-us), a triangular muscle that covers the posterior neck and extends across the posterior shoulder to insert on the clavicle and scapula **(see Figs. 7-8 and 7-9, Table 7-3)**. The trapezius muscles enable one to raise the shoulders and pull them back. The superior portion of each trapezius can also extend the head and turn it from side to side.

The **latissimus** (lah-TIS-ih-mus) **dorsi** is the wide muscle of the back and lateral trunk **(see Fig. 7-9)**. It originates from the vertebral spine in the middle and lower back and covers the inferior half of the thoracic region, forming the posterior portion of the axilla (armpit). The fibers of each muscle converge to a tendon that inserts on the humerus. The latissimus dorsi powerfully extends the arm, bringing it down forcibly as, for example, in swimming.

Table 7-3 Muscles of the Upper Extremities[a]

Name	Location	Function
Trapezius	Posterior neck and upper back to clavicle and scapula	Raises shoulder and pulls it back; superior portion extends and turns head
Latissimus dorsi	Middle and lower back, to humerus	Extends and adducts arm behind back
Pectoralis major	Superior, anterior chest, to humerus	Flexes and adducts arm across chest; pulls shoulder forward and downward
Serratus anterior	Inferior to axilla on lateral chest, to scapula	Moves shoulder forward; aids in raising arm, punching, or reaching forward
Deltoid	Covers shoulder joint, to lateral humerus	Abducts arm; flexes and extends arm at shoulder
Biceps brachii	Anterior arm along humerus, to radius	Flexes forearm at elbow and supinates the forearm and hand
Brachialis	Deep to biceps brachii; inserts at anterior elbow joint	Forceful flexor of forearm
Brachioradialis	Lateral forearm from distal end of humerus to distal end of radius	Flexes forearm at elbow
Triceps brachii	Posterior arm, to ulna	Extends forearm to straighten upper extremity
Flexor carpi group	Anterior forearm, to hand	Flexes hand
Extensor carpi group	Posterior forearm, to hand	Extends hand
Flexor digitorum group	Anterior forearm, to fingers	Flexes fingers
Extensor digitorum group	Posterior forearm, to fingers	Extends fingers

[a]*These and other muscles of the upper extremities are shown in Figures 7-8, 7-9, and 7-11.*

A large **pectoralis** (pek-to-RAL-is) **major** is located on either side of the superior chest (see Fig. 7-8). This muscle arises from the sternum, the upper ribs, and the clavicle and forms the anterior "wall" of the axilla; it inserts on the superior humerus. The pectoralis major flexes and adducts the arm, pulling it across the chest.

The **serratus** (ser-RA-tus) **anterior** is below the axilla, on the lateral chest (see Fig. 7-8). It originates on the upper eight or nine ribs on the lateral and anterior thorax and inserts in the scapula on the side toward the vertebrae. The serratus anterior moves the scapula forward when, for example, one is pushing something. It also aids in raising the arm above the horizontal level.

The **deltoid** covers the shoulder joint and is responsible for the roundness of the upper arm just inferior to the shoulder (see Figs. 7-8 and 7-9). This muscle is named for its triangular shape, which resembles the Greek letter delta. Arising from the shoulder girdle (clavicle and scapula), the deltoid fibers converge to insert on the lateral surface of the humerus. Contraction of this muscle abducts the arm, raising it laterally to the horizontal position. The anterior portion flexes and rotates the shoulder, whereas the posterior portion extends and rotates the shoulder.

The shoulder joint allows for a very wide range of movements. This freedom of movement is possible because the humerus fits into a shallow scapular socket, the glenoid cavity. This joint requires the support of four deep muscles and their tendons, which compose the **rotator cuff.** The four muscles are the supraspinatus, infraspinatus, teres minor, and subscapularis, known together as SITS, based on the first letters of their names.

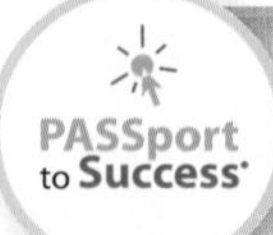

See the student resources on *thePoint* to view additional pictures of muscles that move the shoulder and arm and also the muscles of the rotator cuff.

Muscles that Move the Forearm and Hand The **biceps brachii** (BRA-ke-i), located at the anterior arm along the humerus, is the muscle you usually display when you want to "flex your muscles" to show your strength (Fig. 7-11). The root *brachi* means "arm," and is found in the names of several arm muscles. The biceps brachii inserts on the radius. It flexes the forearm and supinates the hand. The **brachialis** (bra-ke-AL-is) lies deep to the biceps brachii

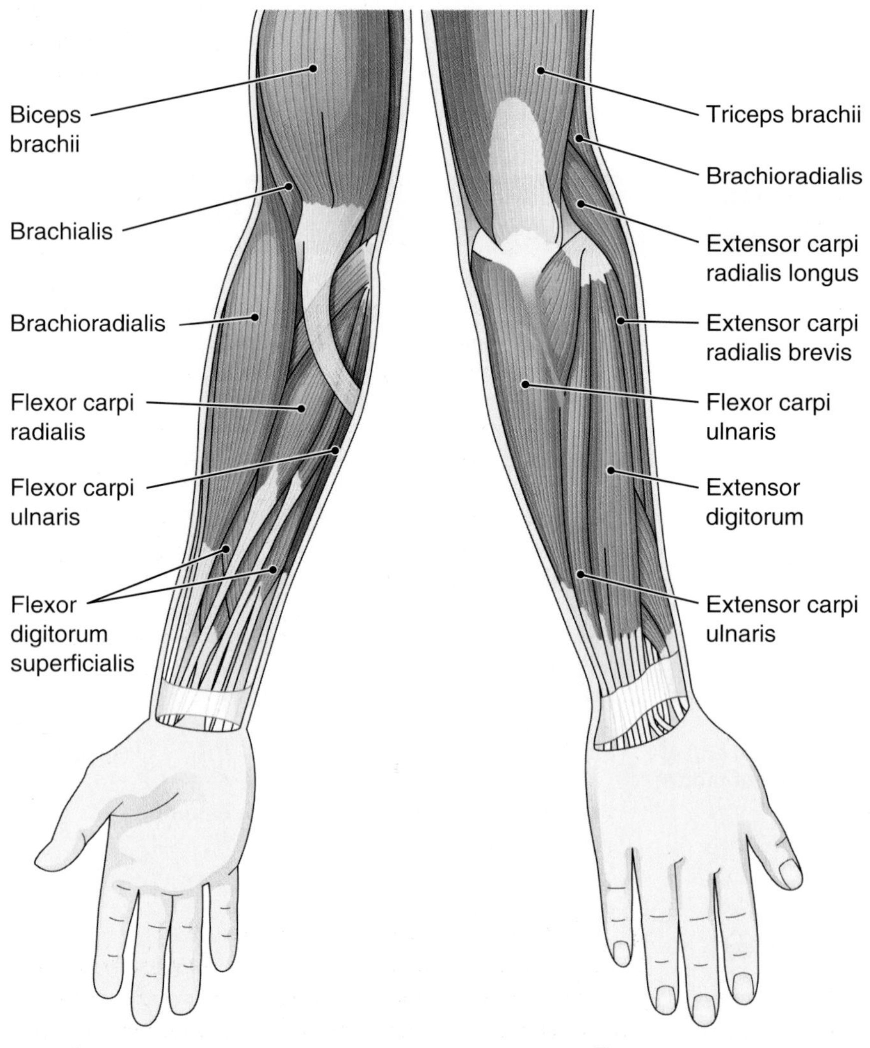

Figure 7-11 Muscles that move the forearm and hand. ZOOMING IN What does carpi refer to in the names of muscles? Digitorum?

and inserts distally over the anterior elbow joint. It flexes the forearm forcefully in all positions, sustains flexion, and steadies the forearm's slow extension.

Another forearm flexor at the elbow is the **brachioradialis** (bra-ke-o-ra-de-A-lis), a prominent forearm muscle that originates at the distal humerus and inserts on the distal radius (see Fig. 7-11).

The **triceps brachii**, located on the posterior arm, inserts on the olecranon of the ulna (see Fig. 7-11B). It is used to straighten the arm, as in lowering a weight from an arm curl. It is also important in pushing because it converts the arm and forearm into a sturdy rod.

Most of the muscles that move the hand and fingers originate from the radius and the ulna (see Fig. 7-11). Some of them insert on the carpal bones of the wrist, whereas others have long tendons that cross the wrist and insert on bones of the hand and the fingers.

The **flexor carpi** and the **extensor carpi muscles** are responsible for many hand movements (see Fig. 7-11). Muscles that produce finger movements are the several **flexor digitorum** (dij-e-TO-rum) and the **extensor digitorum muscles.** The names of these muscles may include bones they are near, their action, or their length, for example, *longus* for long and *brevis* for short.

Special muscle groups in the fleshy parts of the hand execute the intricate movements that can be performed with the thumb and the fingers. The thumb's freedom of movement has been one of humankind's most useful capacities.

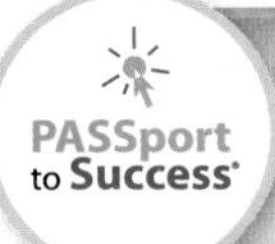

See the student resources on *thePoint* for additional pictures of the muscles that move the forearm and hand.

MUSCLES OF THE TRUNK

The trunk muscles include the muscles involved in breathing, the thin muscle layers of the abdomen, and the muscles of the pelvic floor. The following discussion also includes the deep muscles of the back that support and move the vertebral column.

Muscles of Respiration The most important muscle involved in the act of breathing is the **diaphragm.** This dome-shaped muscle forms the partition between the thoracic cavity above and the abdominal cavity below (Fig. 7-12). When the diaphragm contracts, the central dome-shaped portion is pulled downward, thus enlarging the thoracic cavity from top to bottom.

The **intercostal muscles** are attached to and fill the spaces between the ribs. The external and internal intercostals run at angles in opposite directions. Contraction of the intercostal muscles elevates the ribs, thus enlarging the thoracic cavity from side to side and from anterior to posterior. Additional muscles of the neck, chest, and abdomen are employed in forceful breathing. The mechanics of breathing are described in Chapter 16.

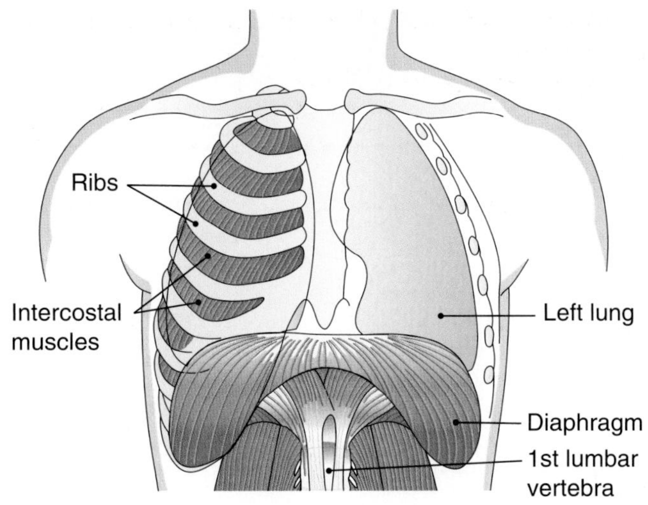

Figure 7-12 **Muscles of respiration.** KEY POINT The diaphragm is the main muscle of respiration. The left lung and ribs are also shown.

Muscles of the Abdomen and Pelvis The abdominal wall has three muscle layers that extend from the back (dorsally) and around the sides (laterally) to the front (ventrally) (Fig. 7-13, Table 7-4). They are the **external oblique** on the exterior, the **internal oblique** in the middle, and the **transversus abdominis**, the innermost. The connective tissue from

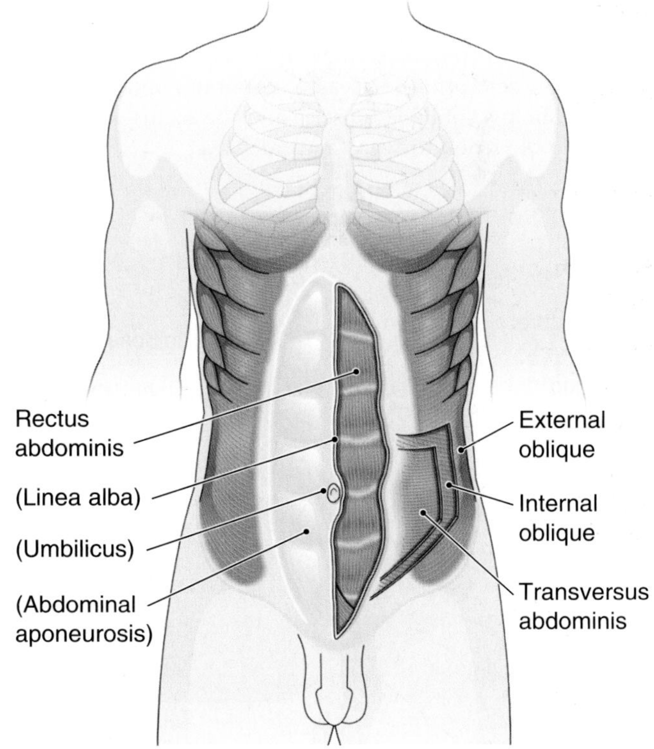

Figure 7-13 **Muscles of the abdominal wall.** KEY POINT Thin layers of muscle tissue with fibers running in different directions give strength to the abdominal wall. Surface tissue is removed here on the right side to show deeper muscles. Associated structures are labeled in parentheses. ZOOMING IN What does rectus mean? Oblique?

Table 7-4 Muscles of the Trunk[a]

Name	Location	Function
Diaphragm	Dome-shaped partition between thoracic and abdominal cavities	Dome descends to enlarge thoracic cavity from top to bottom
Intercostals	Between ribs	Elevate ribs and enlarge thoracic cavity
Muscles of abdominal wall: External oblique Internal oblique Transversus abdominis Rectus abdominis	Anterolateral abdominal wall	Compress abdominal cavity and expel substances from body; flex spinal column
Levator ani	Pelvic floor	Aids defecation
Erector spinae (deep; not shown)	Group of deep vertical muscles between the sacrum and skull	Extends vertebral column to produce erect posture

[a]*These and other muscles of the trunk are shown in Figures 7-12, 7-13, and 7-14.*

these muscles extends anteriorly and encloses the vertical **rectus abdominis** of the anterior abdominal wall. The fibers of these muscles, as well as their connective tissue extensions (aponeuroses), run in different directions, resembling the layers in plywood and resulting in a strong abdominal wall. The midline meeting of the aponeuroses forms a whitish area called the **linea alba** (LIN-e-ah AL-ba), which is an important abdominal landmark. It extends from the tip of the sternum to the pubic joint (see Fig. 7-13).

These four pairs of abdominal muscles act together to protect the internal organs and compress the abdominal cavity, as in coughing, emptying the bladder (urination) and bowel (defecation), sneezing, vomiting, and childbirth (labor). The two oblique muscles and the rectus abdominis help bend the trunk forward and sideways.

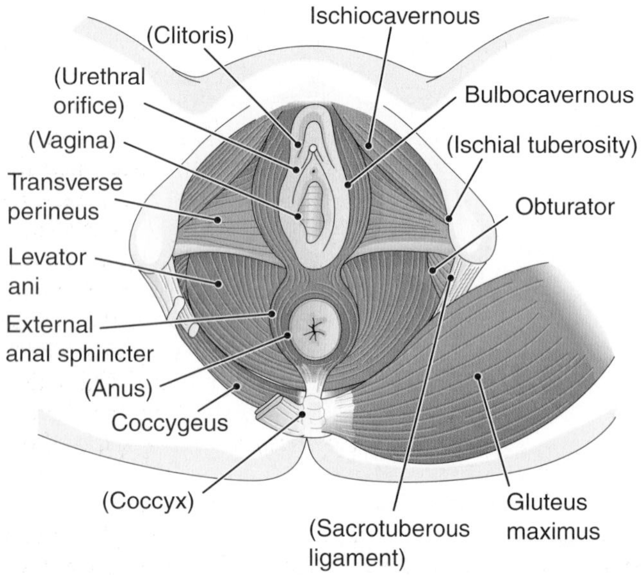

Figure 7-14 Muscles of the female perineum (pelvic floor). Associated structures are labeled in parentheses.

The pelvic floor, or **perineum** (per-ih-NE-um), has its own form of diaphragm, shaped somewhat like a shallow dish. One of the principal muscles of this pelvic diaphragm is the **levator ani** (le-VA-tor A-ni), which acts on the rectum and thus aids in defecation. The superficial and deep muscles of the female perineum are shown in Figure 7-14 along with some associated structures.

Deep Muscles of the Back The deep muscles of the back, which act on the vertebral column itself, are thick vertical masses that lie under the trapezius and latissimus dorsi and thus are not illustrated. The **erector spinae** muscles make up a large group located between the sacrum and the skull. These muscles extend the spine and maintain the vertebral column in an erect posture. Even deeper muscles lie beneath the lumbodorsal fascia. These small muscles extend the vertebral column in the lumbar region.

MUSCLES OF THE LOWER EXTREMITIES

The muscles in the lower extremities, among the longest and strongest muscles in the body, are specialized for locomotion and balance. They include the muscles that move the thigh and leg and those that control movement of the foot.

Muscles that Move the Thigh and Leg The **gluteus maximus** (GLU-te-us MAK-sim-us), which forms much of the buttock's fleshy part, is relatively large in humans because of its support function when a person is standing erect (see Fig. 7-9, Table 7-5).This muscle extends the thigh and is important in walking and running. The **gluteus medius**, which is partially covered by the gluteus maximus, abducts the thigh. It is one of the sites used for intramuscular injections.

The **iliopsoas** (il-e-o-SO-as) arises from the ilium and the bodies of the lumbar vertebrae; it crosses the anterior hip joint to insert on the femur (Fig. 7-15A). It is a powerful

Table 7-5 Muscles of the Lower Extremities[a]

Name	Location	Function
Gluteus maximus	Superficial buttock, to femur	Extends thigh
Gluteus medius	Deep buttock, to femur	Abducts thigh
Iliopsoas	Crosses anterior hip joint, to femur	Flexes thigh
Adductor group (e.g., Adductor longus, adductor magnus)	Medial thigh, to femur	Adducts thigh
Sartorius	Crosses anterior thigh; from ilium to medial tibia	Flexes thigh and leg (to sit cross-legged)
Gracilis	Pubic bone to medial surface of tibia	Adducts thigh at hip; flexes leg at knee
Quadriceps femoris:	Anterior thigh, to tibia	Extends leg
Rectus femoris		
Vastus medialis		
Vastus lateralis		
Vastus intermedius (deep; not shown)		
Hamstring group:	Posterior thigh; ischium and femur to tibia and fibula	Flexes leg at knee; extends and rotates thigh at hip
Biceps femori		
Semimembranosus		
Semitendinosus		
Gastrocnemius	Posterior leg, to calcaneus, inserting by the Achilles tendon	Plantar flexes foot (as in tiptoeing)
Soleus	Posterior leg deep to gastrocnemius	Plantar flexes foot
Tibialis anterior	Anterior and lateral leg, to foot	Dorsiflexes foot at ankle (as in walking on heels); inverts foot (sole inward)
Fibularis (peroneus) longus	Lateral leg, to foot	Everts foot (sole outward)
Flexor digitorum group	Posterior leg and foot to inferior surface of phalanges	Flexes toes
Extensor digitorum group	Anterior surface of leg bones to superior surface of phalanges	Extends toes

[a]*These and other muscles of the lower extremities are shown in Figures 7-15 and 7-16.*

thigh flexor and helps keep the trunk from falling backward when one is standing erect.

The **adductor muscles** are located on the medial thigh (see Fig. 7-15). They arise from the pubis and ischium and insert on the femur. These strong muscles press the thighs together, as in grasping a saddle between the knees when riding a horse. They include the **adductor longus** and **adductor magnus.**

The **sartorius** (sar-TO-re-us) is a long, narrow muscle that begins at the iliac spine, winds downward and medially across the anterior thigh, and ends on the tibia's superior medial surface (see Fig. 7-15). It is called the tailor's muscle because it is used in crossing the legs in the manner of tailors, who in days gone by sat cross-legged on the floor. The **gracilis** (grah-SIL-is) extends from the pubic bone to the medial tibia. It adducts the thigh at the hip and flexes the leg at the knee.

The anterior and lateral femur are covered by the **quadriceps femoris** (KWOD-re-seps FEM-or-is), a large muscle that has four heads of origin (see Fig. 7-15A). The individual parts are as follows: in the center, covering the anterior thigh, the **rectus femoris;** on either side, the **vastus medialis** and **vastus lateralis;** deeper in the center, the **vastus intermedius.** One of these muscles (rectus femoris) originates from the ilium, and the other three are from the femur, but all four have a common tendon of insertion on the tibia. You may remember that this is the tendon that encloses the patella (kneecap). This muscle extends the leg, as in kicking a ball.

The iliotibial tract is a thickened band of fascia that covers the lateral thigh muscles. It extends from the ilium of the hip to the superior tibia and reinforces the fascia of the thigh (fascia lata) (see Fig. 7-15).

The **hamstring muscles** are located in the posterior thigh (see Fig. 7-15B). They originate on the ischium and femur and you can feel their tendons behind the knee as they descend to insert on the tibia and fibula. The hamstrings flex the leg at the knee as in kneeling. They also extend and rotate the thigh at the hip. Individually, moving from lateral

Figure 7-15 **Muscles of the thigh.** Associated structures are labeled in parentheses. ZOOMING IN How many muscles make up the quadriceps femoris?

to medial position, they are the **biceps femoris**, the **semimembranosus**, and the **semitendinosus**. The name of this muscle group refers to the tendons at the posterior of the knee by which these muscles insert on the leg.

Muscles that Move the Foot The **gastrocnemius** (gas-trok-NE-me-us) is the chief muscle of the calf of the leg (its name means "belly of the leg") (Fig. 7-16). It has been called the toe dancer's muscle because it is used in standing on tiptoe. It ends near the heel in a prominent cord called the **Achilles tendon** (see Fig. 7-16B), which attaches to the calcaneus (heel bone). The Achilles tendon is the largest tendon in the body. According to Greek mythology, the region above the heel was the only place on his body where the hero Achilles was vulnerable, and if the Achilles tendon is cut, it is impossible to walk. The **soleus** (SO-le-us) is a flat muscle deep to the gastrocnemius. It also inserts by means of the Achilles tendon and, like the gastrocnemius, flexes the foot at the ankle.

Another leg muscle that acts on the foot is the **tibialis** (tib-e-A-lis) **anterior**, located on the anterior region of the leg (see Fig. 7-16A). This muscle performs the opposite function of the gastrocnemius. Walking on the heels uses the tibialis anterior to raise the rest of the foot off the ground (dorsiflexion). This muscle is also responsible for inversion of the foot. The muscle for the foot's eversion is the **fibularis** (fib-u-LA-ris) **longus**, also called the peroneus (per-o-NE-us) longus, located on the lateral leg. This muscle's long tendon crosses under the foot, forming a sling that supports the transverse (metatarsal) arch.

The toes, like the fingers, are provided with flexor and extensor muscles. The tendons of the extensor muscles are located in the superior part of the foot and insert on the superior surface of the phalanges (toe bones). The flexor digitorum tendons cross the sole of the foot and insert on the undersurface of the phalanges (see Fig. 7-16).

CHECKPOINTS  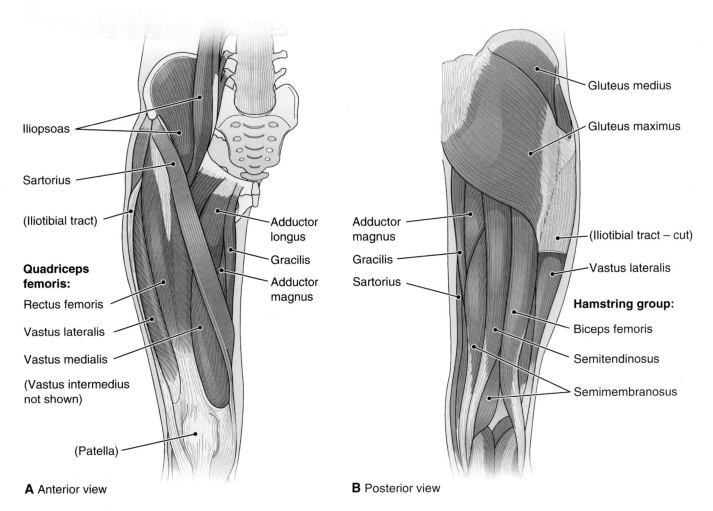

- 7-14 What muscle is most important in breathing?
- 7-15 What structural feature gives strength to the muscles of the abdominal wall?

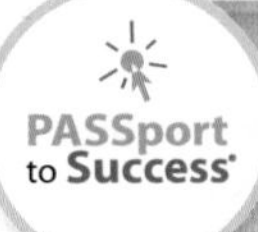

See the student resources on *thePoint* for additional pictures of the muscles that move the lower extremity.

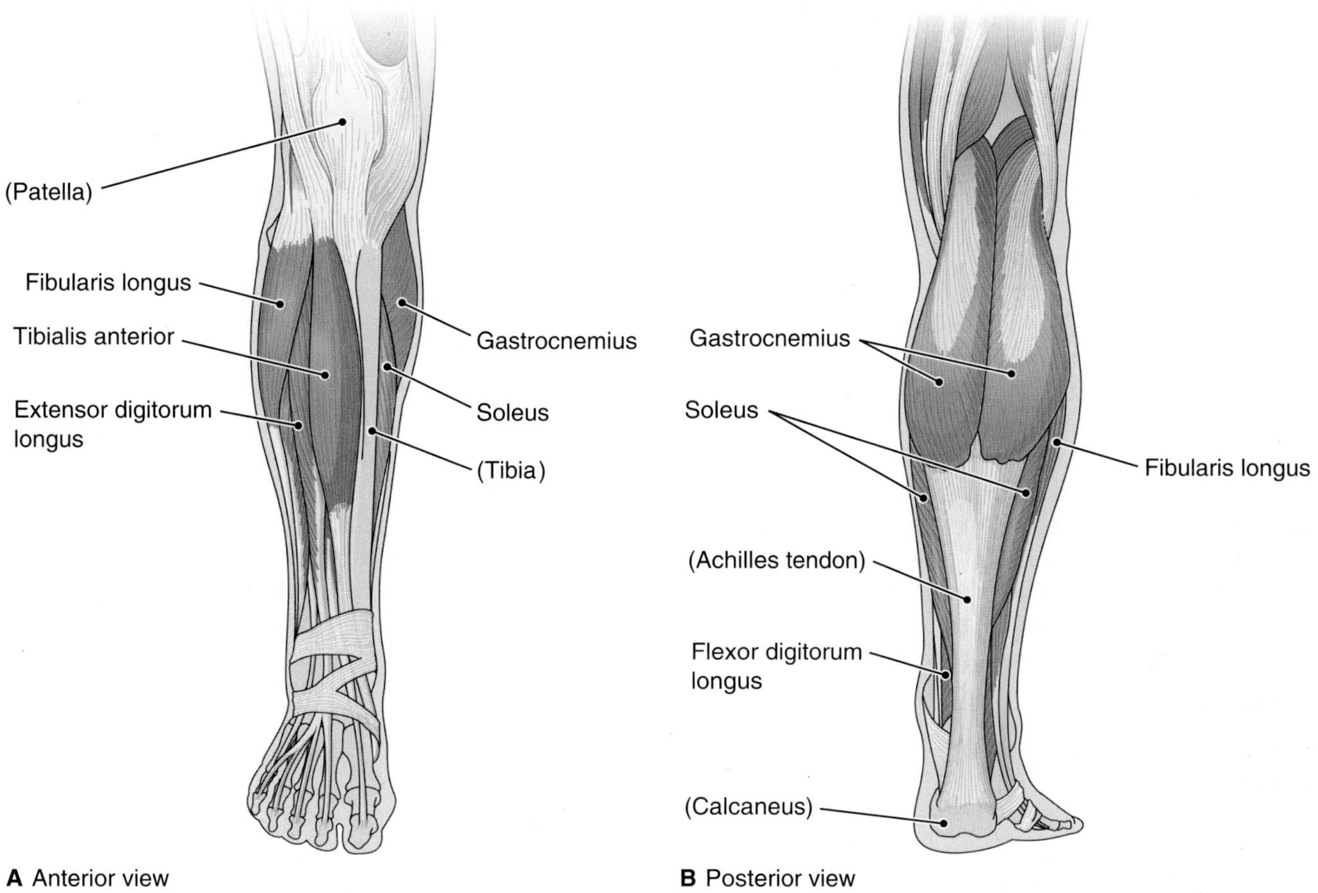

(Patella)
Fibularis longus
Tibialis anterior
Extensor digitorum longus
Gastrocnemius
Soleus
(Tibia)

A Anterior view

Gastrocnemius
Soleus
Fibularis longus
(Achilles tendon)
Flexor digitorum longus
(Calcaneus)

B Posterior view

Figure 7-16 **Muscles that move the foot.** KEY POINT Associated structures are labeled in parentheses. ZOOMING IN On what bone does the Achilles tendon insert?

Effects of Aging on Muscles

Beginning at about 40 years of age, there is a gradual loss of muscle cells with a resulting decrease in the size of each individual muscle. There is also a loss of power, notably in the extensor muscles, such as the large sacrospinalis near the vertebral column. This causes the "bent-over" appearance of a hunchback (kyphosis). Sometimes, there is a tendency to bend (flex) the hips and knees. In addition to the previously noted changes in the vertebral column (see Chapter 6), these effects on the extensor muscles result in a further decrease in the elderly person's height. Activity and exercise throughout life delay and decrease these undesirable effects of aging. Even among the elderly, resistance exercise, such as weight lifting, increases muscle strength and function.

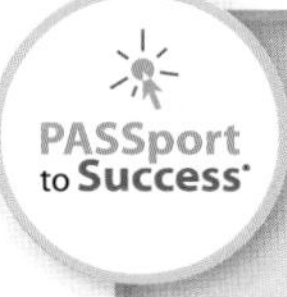

See the student resources on *thePoint* for information on careers in physical therapy and how physical therapists help delay the effects of aging on muscles.

A&P in Action Revisited

Sue's Multiple Sclerosis

Having finished the physical examination of his patient, Dr. Mathews thought carefully about what he had discovered. Sue, a 26-year-old white female, presented with muscle weakness, atrophy, and abnormal reflexes localized to the right side of her body. At first, it seemed likely that Sue was suffering from a muscular system disorder. Muscular dystrophy is characterized by muscle deterioration and weakness, but the doctor knew that the disease is genetic and its effects appear during childhood. Myasthenia gravis, a disorder of the NMJ, is also characterized by muscle weakness and appears during adulthood. But, it usually begins affecting muscles of the head, not the limbs. Fibromyalgia syndrome affects adults and is associated with widespread muscle aches. This didn't seem to fit either because Sue's disorder was localized to her right side.

It was Sue's report of pain and tingling in her right limbs that provided the last clue Dr. Mathews needed to make his diagnosis. Sue probably had a disorder of the nervous system called multiple sclerosis. The disease is characterized by both muscular and nervous symptoms, which first appear in adults and are sometimes localized to one side of the body. After explaining his findings to Sue, Dr. Mathews ordered an MRI of her brain and spinal cord and referred her to a neurologist for further treatment.

During this case, Dr. Mathews examined Sue's muscular system. He quickly realized that Sue's symptoms suggested that she had a nervous system disorder. The case study in Chapter 8, The Nervous System: The Spinal Cord and Spinal Nerves, will follow Sue as she learns more about her disorder.

Chapter Wrap-Up

Summary Overview

A detailed chapter outline with space for note-taking is on *thePoint*. The figure below illustrates the main topics covered in this chapter.

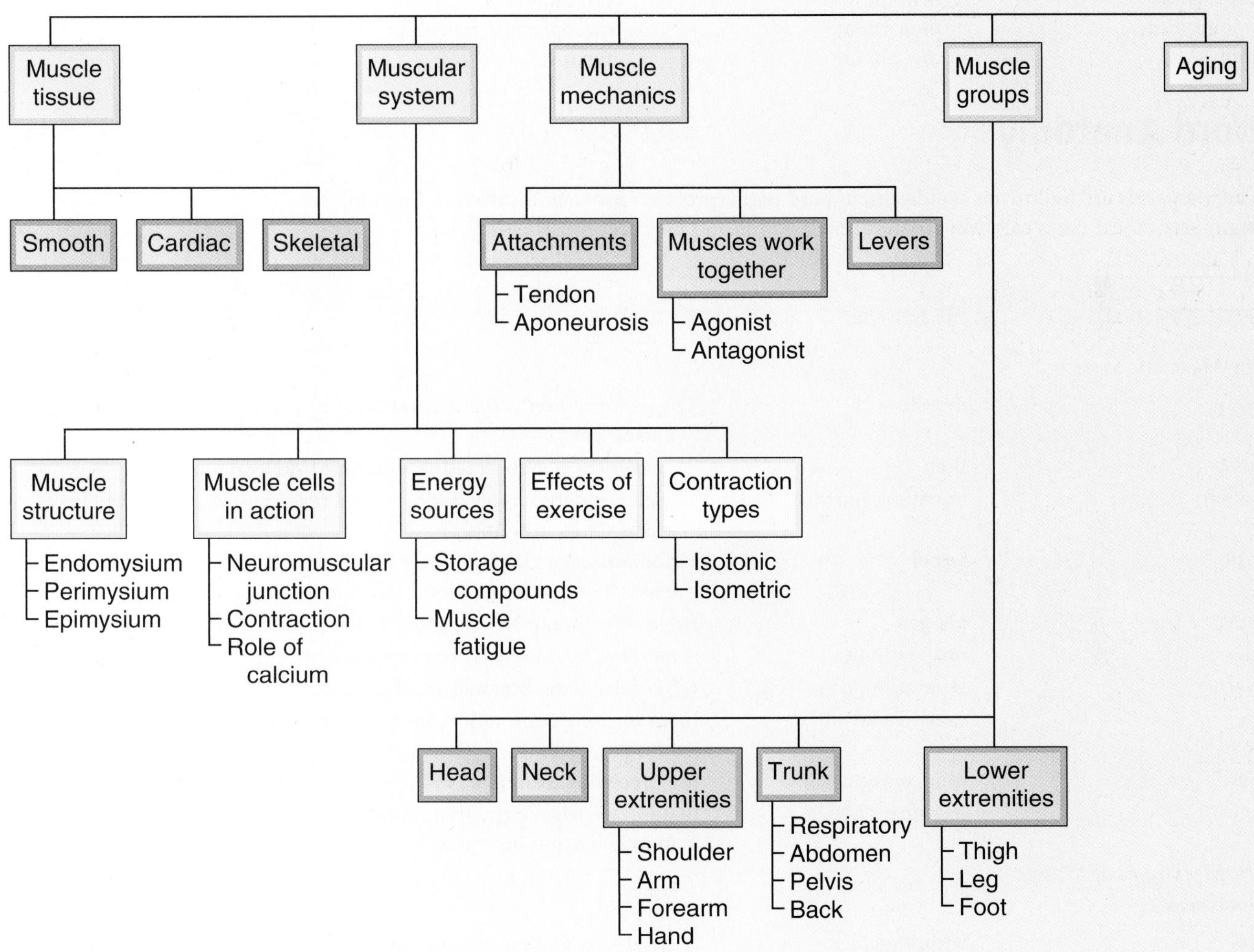

Key Terms

The terms listed below are emphasized in this chapter. Knowing them will help you organize and prioritize your learning. These and other boldface terms are defined in the Glossary with phonetic pronunciations.

acetylcholine
actin
agonist
antagonist
aponeurosis
contractility
endomysium
epimysium
excitability
fascicle
glycogen
insertion
isometric
isotonic
motor unit
myoglobin
myosin
neuromuscular junction
neurotransmitter
origin
perimysium
sarcomere
sarcoplasmic reticulum
synapse
synergist
tendon
tonus
tropomyosin
troponin

Word Anatomy

Scientific terms are built from standardized word parts (prefixes, roots, and suffixes). Learning the meanings of these parts can help you remember words and interpret unfamiliar terms.

WORD PART	MEANING	EXAMPLE
The Muscular System		
my/o	muscle	The *endomysium* is the deepest layer of connective tissue around muscle cells.
sarc/o	flesh	A *sarcomere* is a contracting subunit of skeletal muscle.
troph/o	nutrition, nurture	Muscles undergo *hypertrophy*, an increase in size, under the effects of resistance training.
vas/o	vessel	*Vasodilation* (widening) of the blood vessels in muscle tissue during exercise brings more blood into the tissue.
aer/o	air, gas	An *aerobic* organism can grow in the presence of air (oxygen).
an-	not, without	*Anaerobic* metabolism does not require oxygen.
-lysis	separation, dissolving	*Glycolysis* is the breakdown of glucose
iso-	same, equal	In an *isotonic* contraction, muscle tone remains the same, but the muscle shortens.
ton/o	tone, tension	See preceding example.
metr/o	measure	In an *isometric* contraction, muscle length remains the same, but muscle tension increases.
The Mechanics of Muscle Movement		
syn-	with, together	A *synapse* is a point of communication between a neuron and another cell
erg/o	work	*Synergists* are muscles that work together.
Skeletal Muscle Groups		
brachi/o	arm	The biceps *brachii* and triceps brachii are in the arm.
quadr/i	four	The *quadriceps* muscle group consists of four muscles.

Questions for Study and Review

BUILDING UNDERSTANDING

Fill in the blanks

1. Individual muscle fibers are arranged in bundles called _____.
2. The point at which a nerve fiber contacts a muscle cell is called the _____.
3. A contraction in which there is no change in muscle length but there is a great increase in muscle tension is _____.
4. A contracting subunit of skeletal muscle is called a(n) _____.
5. A skeletal muscle's partially contracted state that is normal even when the muscle is not in use is called _____.

Matching > Match each numbered item with the most closely related lettered item.

___ **6.** Extends vertebral column to produce erect posture
___ **7.** Elevate ribs and enlarge thoracic cavity
___ **8.** Flattens cheeks
___ **9.** Aids in defecation
___ **10.** Closes eye

a. levator ani
b. buccinator
c. orbicularis oris
d. erector spinae
e. intercostal muscles

Multiple Choice

___ **11.** From superficial to deep, what is the correct order of muscle structure?
a. deep fascia, epimysium, perimysium, and endomysium
b. epimysium, perimysium, endomysium, and deep fascia
c. deep fascia, endomysium, perimysium, and epimysium
d. endomysium, perimysium, epimysium, and deep fascia

___ **12.** What is the function of calcium ions in skeletal muscle contraction?
a. bind to receptors on the motor end plate to stimulate muscle contraction
b. cause a pH change in the cytoplasm to trigger muscle contraction
c. bind to the myosin-binding sites on actin so that myosin will have something to attach to
d. bind to regulatory proteins so that the myosin-binding sites on the actin can be exposed

___ **13.** Which structure is a broad flat extension that attaches muscle to bone?
a. tendon
b. fascicle
c. aponeurosis
d. motor end plate

___ **14.** Which lever is responsible for forearm flexion?
a. first-class
b. second-class
c. third-class
d. fourth-class

___ **15.** Which muscle is most involved in the act of breathing?
a. sternocleidomastoid
b. pectoralis major
c. intercostal
d. diaphragm

UNDERSTANDING CONCEPTS

16. Compare smooth, cardiac, and skeletal muscle with respect to location, structure, and function. Briefly explain how each type of muscle is specialized for its function.
17. Describe four substances stored in skeletal muscle cells that are used to manufacture a constant supply of ATP.
18. Name and describe muscle(s) that
    - **a.** open and close the eye
    - **b.** close the jaw
    - **c.** flex and extend the head
    - **d.** flex and extend the forearm
    - **e.** flex and extend the hand and fingers
    - **f.** flex and extend the leg
    - **g.** flex and extend the foot and toes

19. During a Cesarean section, a transverse incision is made through the abdominal wall. Name the muscles incised and state their functions.

20. What effect does aging have on muscles? What can be done to resist these effects?

CONCEPTUAL THINKING

21. Margo recently began "working out" and jogs three times a week. After her jog, she is breathless and her muscles ache. From your understanding of muscle physiology, describe what has happened inside of Margo's skeletal muscle cells. How do Margo's muscles recover from this? If Margo continues to exercise, what changes would you expect to occur in her muscles?

22. Alfred suffered a mild stroke, leaving him partially paralyzed on his left side. Physical therapy was ordered to prevent left-sided atrophy. Prescribe some exercises for Alfred's shoulder and thigh.

23. In Sue's case, her disorder prevents motor impulses from arriving at neuromuscular junctions. With this in mind, explain why one of her symptoms is muscle wasting (called atrophy).

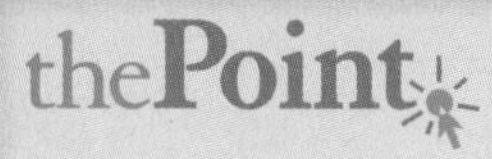

For more questions, see the learning activities on *thePoint.*

UNIT III

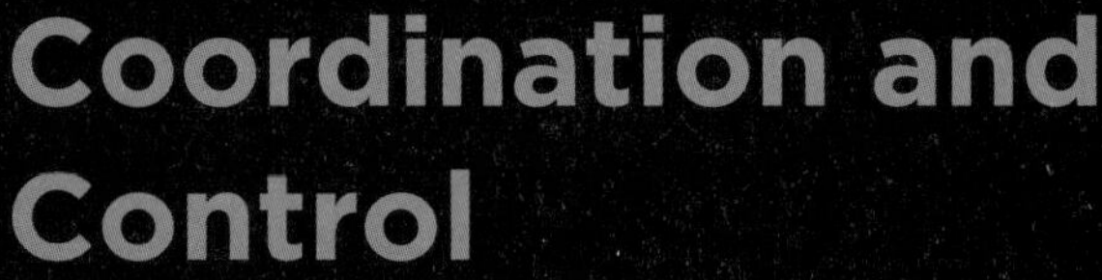

Three chapters in this unit describe the nervous system and some of its many parts and complex functions, including those of the sensory system. The last chapter in this unit discusses hormones and the organs that produce them. Working with the nervous system, these hormones play an important role in coordination and control.

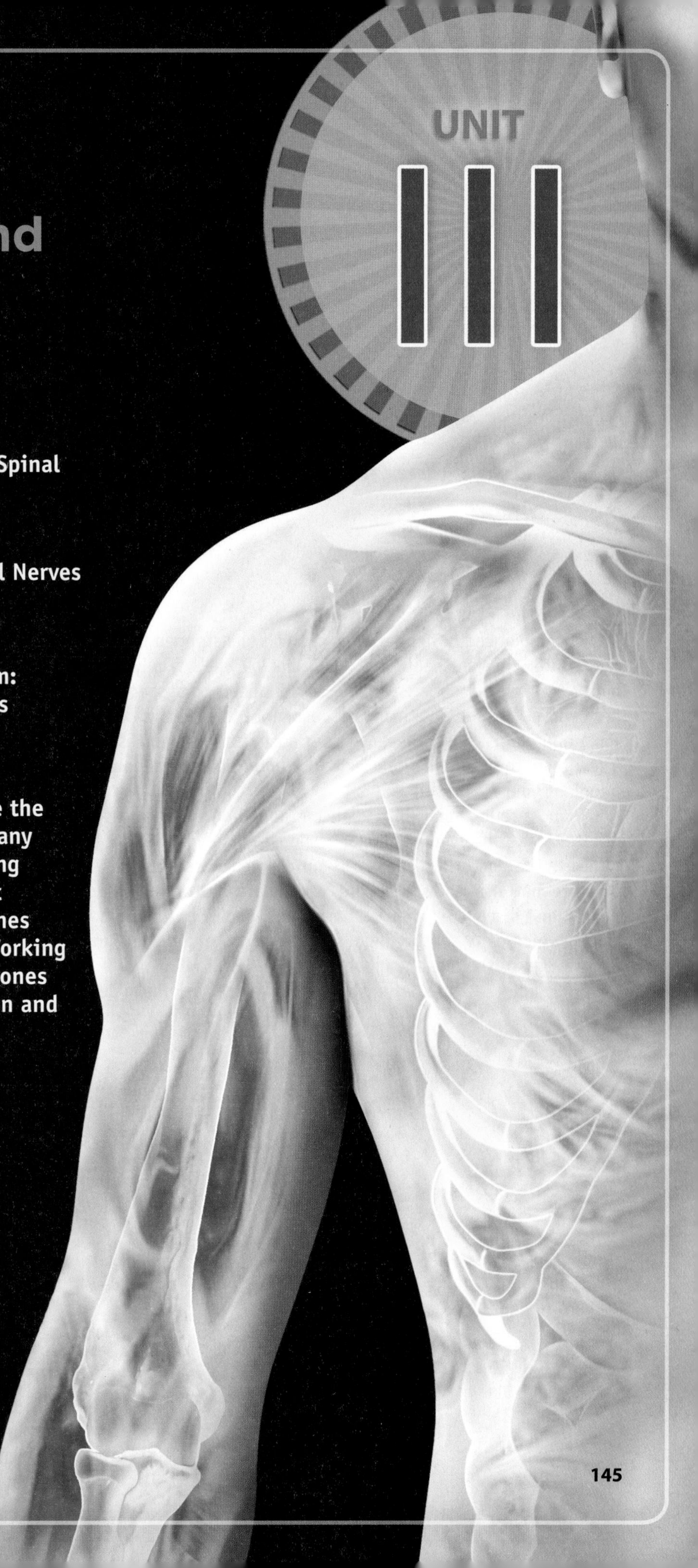

CHAPTER 8

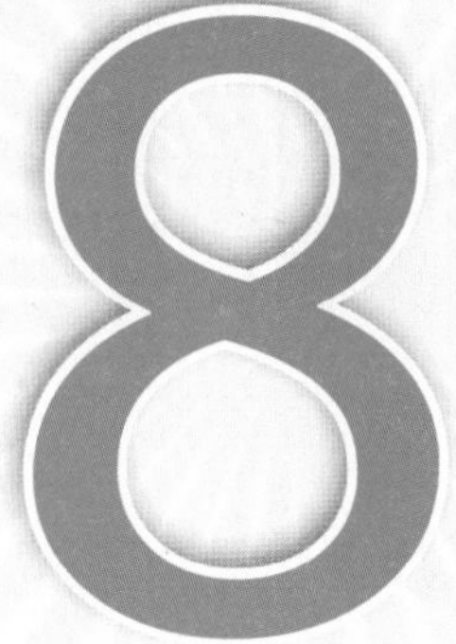

The Nervous System: The Spinal Cord and Spinal Nerves

A&P in Action

Sue's Second Case: The Importance of Myelin

Dr. Jensen glanced at her patient's chart as she stepped into the consulting room to see her. Sue Pritchard was 26 years old, white, and had been referred to her by Sue's family physician. According to her chart, Sue had presented with motor and sensory deficits, which led her doctor to suspect she had multiple sclerosis (MS). In addition to the referral, her doctor had ordered a magnetic resonance image (MRI) of her brain and spinal cord. "Hi Sue. My name is Dr. Jensen. I'm a neurologist, which means I specialize in the diagnosis and treatment of nervous system disorders. Let's start with a few tests to determine how well your brain and spinal cord communicate with the rest of your body. Then, we'll take a look at your MRI results."

Using a reflex hammer, Dr. Jensen tapped on the tendons of several muscles in Sue's arms and legs to elicit stretch reflexes. She observed abnormal responses—a typical sign of damage to the parts of the spinal cord that control reflexes. The doctor also detected muscle weakness in Sue's limbs—an indication of damage to the descending tracts of white matter in the spinal cord, which carry motor nerve impulses from the brain to skeletal muscle. In addition, the neurologist discovered that Sue's sense of touch was impaired—an indication of damage to the spinal cord's ascending tracts, which carry sensory impulses from receptors in the skin to the brain. Dr. Jensen had discovered that Sue exhibited several of the most common clinical signs of MS.

After the physical examination, Dr. Jensen showed Sue the results of the MRI scan done earlier. "Here's the MRI of your spinal cord. You can see that it is surrounded by bones called vertebrae, which protect it from injury. The nervous tissue making up the spinal cord is organized into two regions—this inner region called gray matter, and this outer one called white matter. If you look closely at the white matter, you can see several damaged areas, which we call lesions. They are causing many of your symptoms because they prevent your spinal cord from transmitting impulses between your brain and the rest of your body. These lesions, or scleroses, are what give multiple sclerosis its name."

The clinical and diagnostic evidence shows that Sue has MS—a disease of neurons in the central nervous system (CNS). In this chapter, we learn more about neurons and the spinal cord, one part of the CNS.

PASSport to Success

Ancillaries At-A-Glance

Visit *thePoint* to access the PASSport to Success and the following resources. For guidance in using these resources most effectively, see pp. ix–xviii.

Learning TOOLS

- Learning Style Self-Assessment
- Live Advise Online Student Tutoring
- Tips for Effective Studying

Learning RESOURCES

- E-book: Chapter 8
- Web Figure: The cauda equina
- Web Chart: Neuroglia
- Animation: The Synapse and the Nerve Impulse
- Animation: The Action Potential
- Animation: The Myelin Sheath
- Animation: The Reflex Arc
- Health Professions: Occupational Therapist
- Detailed Chapter Outline
- Answers to Questions for Study and Review
- Audio Pronunciation Glossary
- Auditory Activities

Learning ACTIVITIES

- Pre-Quiz
- Visual Activities
- Kinesthetic Activities
- Auditory Activities

Learning Outcomes

After careful study of this chapter, you should be able to:

1. Outline the organization of the nervous system according to structure and function, ***p. 148***
2. Describe the structure of a neuron, ***p. 149***
3. Describe how neuron fibers are built into a nerve, ***p. 151***
4. Explain the purpose of neuroglia, ***p. 152***
5. Diagram and describe the steps in an action potential, ***p. 153***
6. Explain the role of myelin in nerve conduction, ***p. 153***
7. Explain the role of neurotransmitters in impulse transmission at a synapse, ***p. 154***
8. Describe the distribution of gray and white matter in the spinal cord, ***p. 156***
9. Describe and name the spinal nerves and three of their main plexuses, ***p. 156***
10. List the components of a reflex arc, ***p. 159***
11. Define a simple reflex and give several examples of reflexes, ***p. 160***
12. Compare the location and functions of the sympathetic and parasympathetic nervous systems, ***p. 162***
13. Explain the role of cellular receptors in the action of neurotransmitters in the autonomic nervous system, ***p. 162***
14. Using the case study, describe the importance of myelin on motor and sensory function, ***pp. 146, 164***
15. Show how word parts are used to build words related to the nervous system (see Word Anatomy at the end of the chapter), ***p. 166***

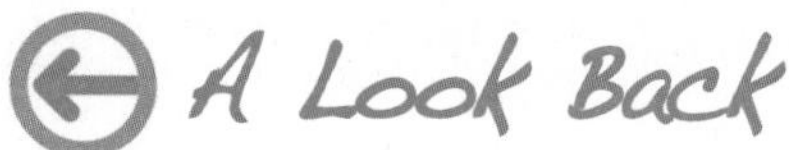

In Chapter 3, we learned about the electric charge, or potential, on the plasma membrane. In Chapter 7, we discussed synapses between cells, the importance of neurotransmitters, and generation of an action potential to activate muscle cells. Now, we put this information together in describing the nervous system's activities as it transmits information and coordinates responses to changes in the environment.

Overview of the Nervous System

No body system is capable of functioning alone. All are interdependent and work together as one unit to maintain normal conditions, or homeostasis. The nervous system serves as the chief coordinating agency for all systems. Conditions both within and outside the body are constantly changing. The nervous system must detect and respond to these changes (known as *stimuli*) so that the body can adapt itself to new conditions.

The nervous system can be compared with a large corporation, in which market researchers (sensory receptors) feed information into middle management (the spinal cord), who then transmit information to the chief executive officer or CEO (the brain). The CEO organizes and interprets the information and then sends instructions out to workers (effectors) who carry out appropriate actions for the good of the company. These instructions are communicated via e-mails, which, like the body's nerves, carry information throughout the system.

Although all parts of the nervous system work in coordination, portions may be grouped together on the basis of either structure or function.

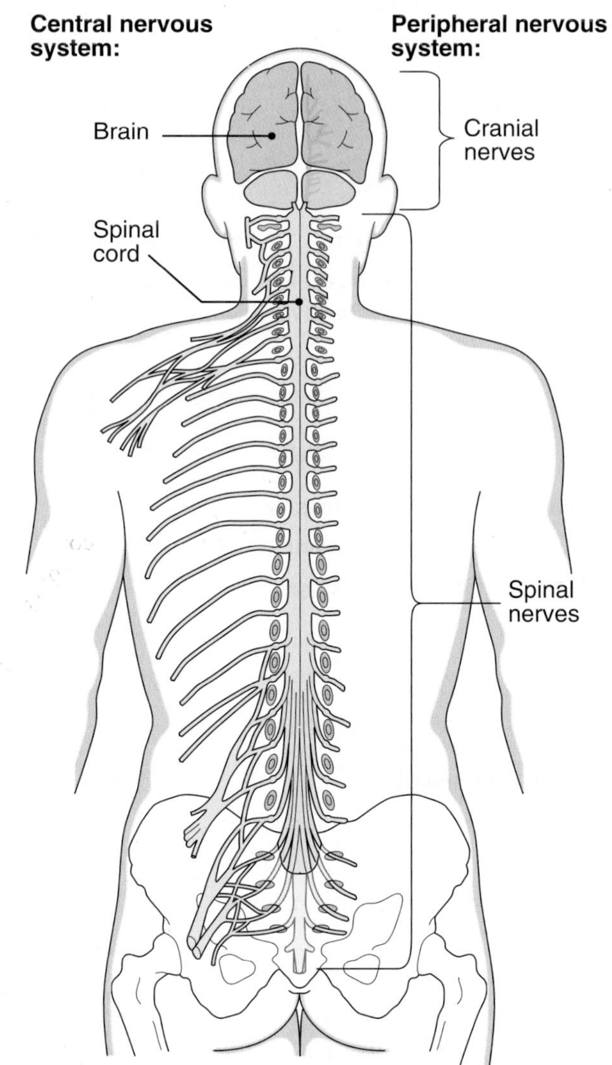

Figure 8-1 Anatomic divisions of the nervous system, posterior view. KEY POINT The nervous system is divided structurally into a central nervous system and a peripheral nervous system. ZOOMING IN What structures make up the central nervous system? The peripheral nervous system?

STRUCTURAL DIVISIONS

The anatomic, or structural, divisions of the nervous system are as follows **(Fig. 8-1)**:

- The **central nervous system** (CNS) includes the brain and spinal cord.
- The **peripheral** (per-IF-er-al) **nervous system** (PNS) is made up of all the nerves outside the CNS. It includes all the **cranial nerves** that carry impulses to and from the brain and all the **spinal nerves** that carry messages to and from the spinal cord.

The CNS and PNS together include all of the nervous tissue in the body.

FUNCTIONAL DIVISIONS OF THE PNS

Functionally, the PNS is divided according to whether control is voluntary or involuntary and according to what type of tissue is stimulated **(Table 8-1)**. Any tissue or organ that carries out a nervous system command is called an **effector,** all of which are muscles or glands.

The **somatic nervous system** is controlled voluntarily (by conscious will), and all its effectors are skeletal muscles (described in Chapter 7). The nervous system's involuntary division is called the **autonomic nervous system** (ANS), making reference to its automatic activity. It is also called the **visceral nervous system** because its effectors are smooth muscle, cardiac muscle, and glands, which are found in the soft body organs, the viscera. The ANS is described in more detail later in this chapter.

Although these divisions are helpful for study purposes, the lines that divide the nervous system according to function are not as distinct as those that classify the

Table 8-1 Functional Divisions of the Peripheral Nervous System

Division	Control	Effectors
Somatic nervous system	Voluntary	Skeletal muscle
Autonomic nervous system	Involuntary	Smooth muscle, cardiac muscle, and glands

system structurally. Although skeletal muscles *can* be controlled voluntarily, they may function commonly without conscious control. The diaphragm, for example, a skeletal muscle, typically functions in breathing without conscious thought. In addition, we have certain rapid reflex responses involving skeletal muscles—drawing the hand away from a hot stove, for example—that do not involve the brain. In contrast, people can be trained to consciously control involuntary functions, such as blood pressure and heart rate, by training techniques known as *biofeedback*.

CHECKPOINTS 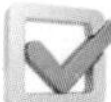

☐ 8-1 What are the two divisions of the nervous system based on structure?

☐ 8-2 What division of the PNS is voluntary and controls skeletal muscles? What division is involuntary and controls smooth muscle, cardiac muscle, and glands?

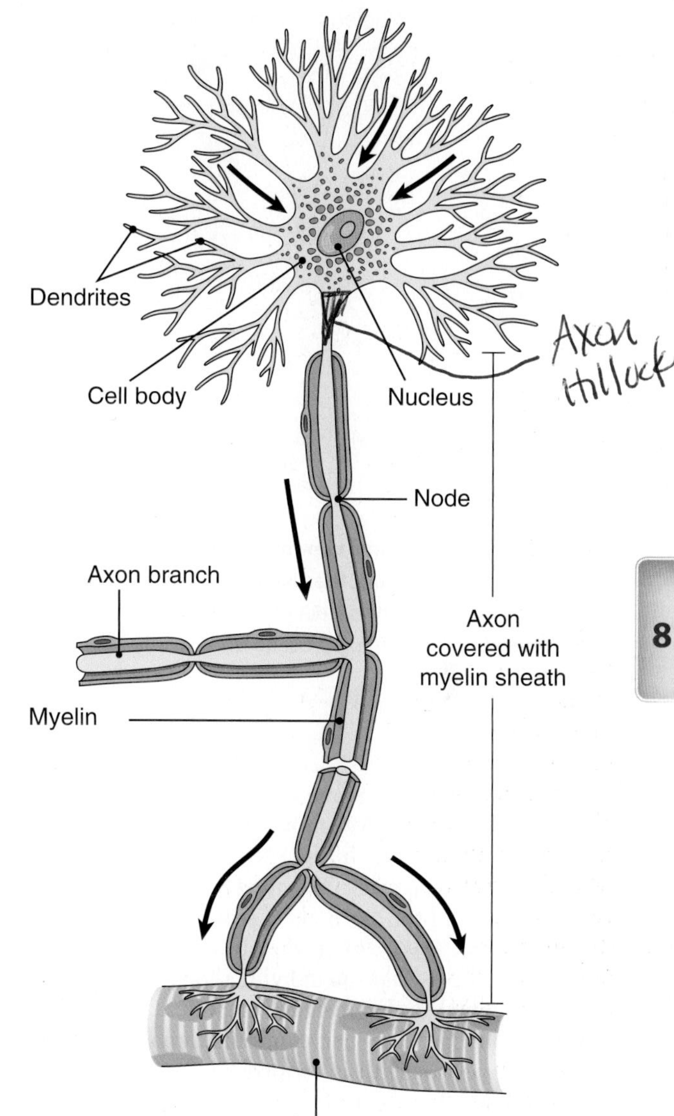

Figure 8-2 Diagram of a motor neuron. KEY POINT A neuron has fibers extending from the cell body. Dendrites carry impulses toward the cell body; axons carry impulses away from the cell body. The break in the axon denotes length. The arrows show the direction of the nerve impulse. ZOOMING IN Is the neuron shown here a sensory or a motor neuron? Is it part of the somatic or visceral nervous system? Explain.

Neurons and Their Functions

The functional cells of the nervous system are highly specialized cells called **neurons** (Fig. 8-2). These cells have a unique structure related to their function.

STRUCTURE OF A NEURON

The main portion of each neuron, the cell body, contains the nucleus and other organelles typically found in cells. A distinguishing feature of the neurons, however, is the long, threadlike fibers that extend out from the cell body and carry impulses across the cell (Fig. 8-3).

Dendrites and Axons Two kinds of fibers extend from the neuron cell body: dendrites and axons.

- **Dendrites** are neuron fibers that conduct impulses *to* the cell body. Most dendrites have a highly branched, treelike appearance (see Fig. 8-2). In fact, the name comes from a Greek word meaning "tree." Dendrites function as **receptors** in the nervous system. That is, they receive a stimulus that begins a neural pathway. In Chapter 10, we describe how the dendrites of the sensory system may be modified to respond to a specific type of stimulus, such as pressure or taste.
- **Axons** (AK-sons) are neuron fibers that conduct impulses *away from* the cell body (see Fig. 8-2). These impulses may be delivered to another neuron, to a muscle, or to a gland. An axon is a single fiber, which may be quite long, but it may give off branches and its ending is branched.

8

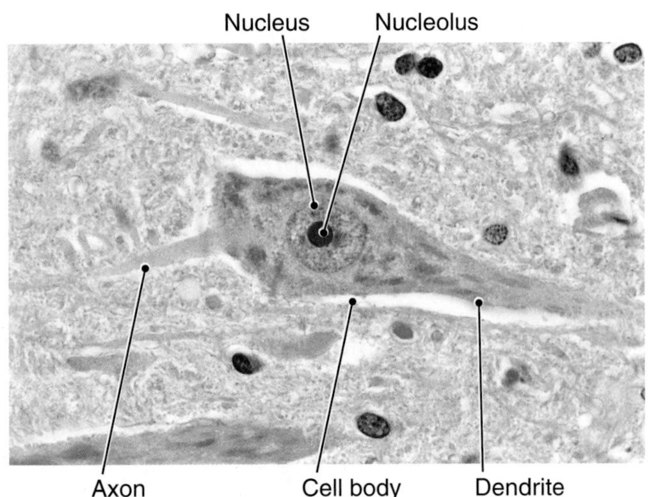

Figure 8-3 **Microscopic view of a neuron.** Based on staining properties and structure, the fiber on the left is identified as an axon; the fiber on the right is a dendrite. The clear space around the axon is caused by the staining procedure.

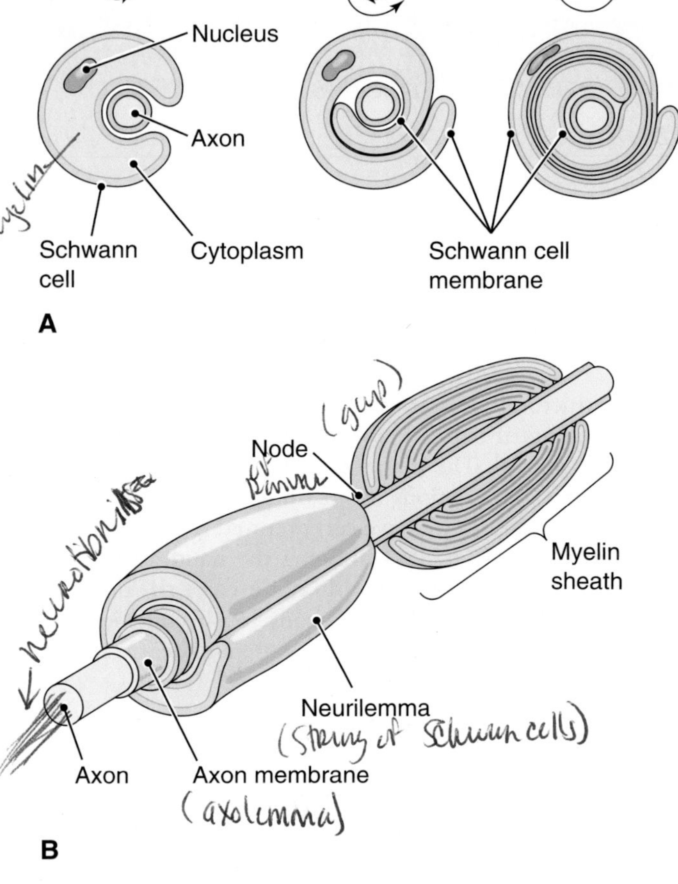

Figure 8-4 **Formation of a myelin sheath.** KEY POINT The myelin sheath is formed by Schwann cells in the peripheral nervous system. **A.** Schwann cells wrap around the axon, creating a myelin coating. **B.** The outermost layer of the Schwann cell forms the neurilemma. Spaces between the cells are the nodes (of Ranvier).

The Myelin Sheath Some axons are covered with a fatty material called **myelin** (MI-eh-lin) that insulates and protects the fiber (see Fig. 8-2). In the PNS, this covering is formed by specialized protective cells called **Schwann** (shvahn) **cells** that wrap around the axon like a jelly roll depositing layers of myelin (Fig. 8-4). When the sheath is complete, small spaces remain between the individual Schwann cells. These tiny gaps, called **nodes** (originally, nodes of Ranvier), are important in speeding nerve impulse conduction. In the CNS, the myelin sheath is formed by another type of cell, described later.

The Schwann cells' outermost membranes form a thin coating known as the **neurilemma** (nu-rih-LEM-mah). This covering is a part of the mechanism by which some peripheral nerves repair themselves when injured. Under some circumstances, damaged nerve cell fibers may regenerate by growing into the sleeve formed by the neurilemma. Because cells of the brain and the spinal cord are myelinated by cells other than Schwann cells, they have no neurilemma. If they are injured, the damage is almost always permanent. Even in the peripheral nerves, however, repair is a slow and uncertain process.

Myelinated axons, because of myelin's color, are called **white fibers** and are found in the **white matter** of the brain and spinal cord as well as most nerves throughout the body. The fibers and cell bodies of the **gray matter** are not covered with myelin.

TYPES OF NEURONS

The job of neurons is to relay information to or from the CNS or to different places within the CNS itself. There are three functional categories of neurons:

- **Sensory neurons,** also called *afferent neurons,* conduct impulses *to* the spinal cord and brain. For example, if you touch a sharp object with your finger, sensory neurons will carry impulses generated by the stimulus to the CNS for interpretation.
- **Motor neurons,** also called *efferent* neurons, carry impulses *from* the CNS to muscles and glands (effectors). For example, the CNS responds to the pain of touching a sharp object by directing skeletal muscles in your arm to flex and withdraw.
- **Interneurons,** also called *central* or *association neurons,* relay information from place to place within the CNS. Following our original example, in addition to immediate withdrawal from pain, impulses may travel to other parts of the CNS to help retain balance as you withdraw your hand or to help you learn how to avoid sharp objects!

NERVES AND TRACTS

Everywhere in the nervous system, neuron fibers are collected into bundles of varying size (Fig. 8-5). A fiber bundle located within the PNS is a **nerve**. A similar grouping, but located within the CNS, is a **tract**. Tracts are located both in the brain, where they conduct impulses between regions, and in the spinal cord, where they conduct impulses to and from the brain.

A nerve or tract can be compared to an electric cable made up of many wires. The "wires," the neuron fibers in a nerve or tract are bound together with connective tissue, just like muscle fibers in a muscle. As in muscles, the individual fibers are organized into groups called *fascicles*. The names of the connective tissue layers are similar to their names in muscles, but the root *neur/o*, meaning "nerve" is substituted for the muscle root *my/o*, as follows:

- Endoneurium is around an individual fiber.
- Perineurium is around a fascicle.
- Epineurium is around the whole nerve.

A nerve may contain all sensory fibers, all motor fibers, or a combination of both types of fibers. A few of the cranial nerves contain only sensory fibers conducting impulses toward the brain. These are described as **sensory** (afferent) **nerves**. A few of the cranial nerves contain only motor fibers conducting impulses away from the brain and these are classified as **motor** (efferent) **nerves**. However, most of the cranial nerves and *all* of the spinal nerves contain both sensory *and* motor fibers and are referred to as **mixed nerves**. Note that in a mixed nerve, impulses may be traveling in two directions (toward or away from the CNS), but each individual fiber in the nerve is carrying impulses in one direction only. Think of the nerve as a large highway. Traffic may be going north and south, for example, but each lane carries cars traveling in only one direction.

8

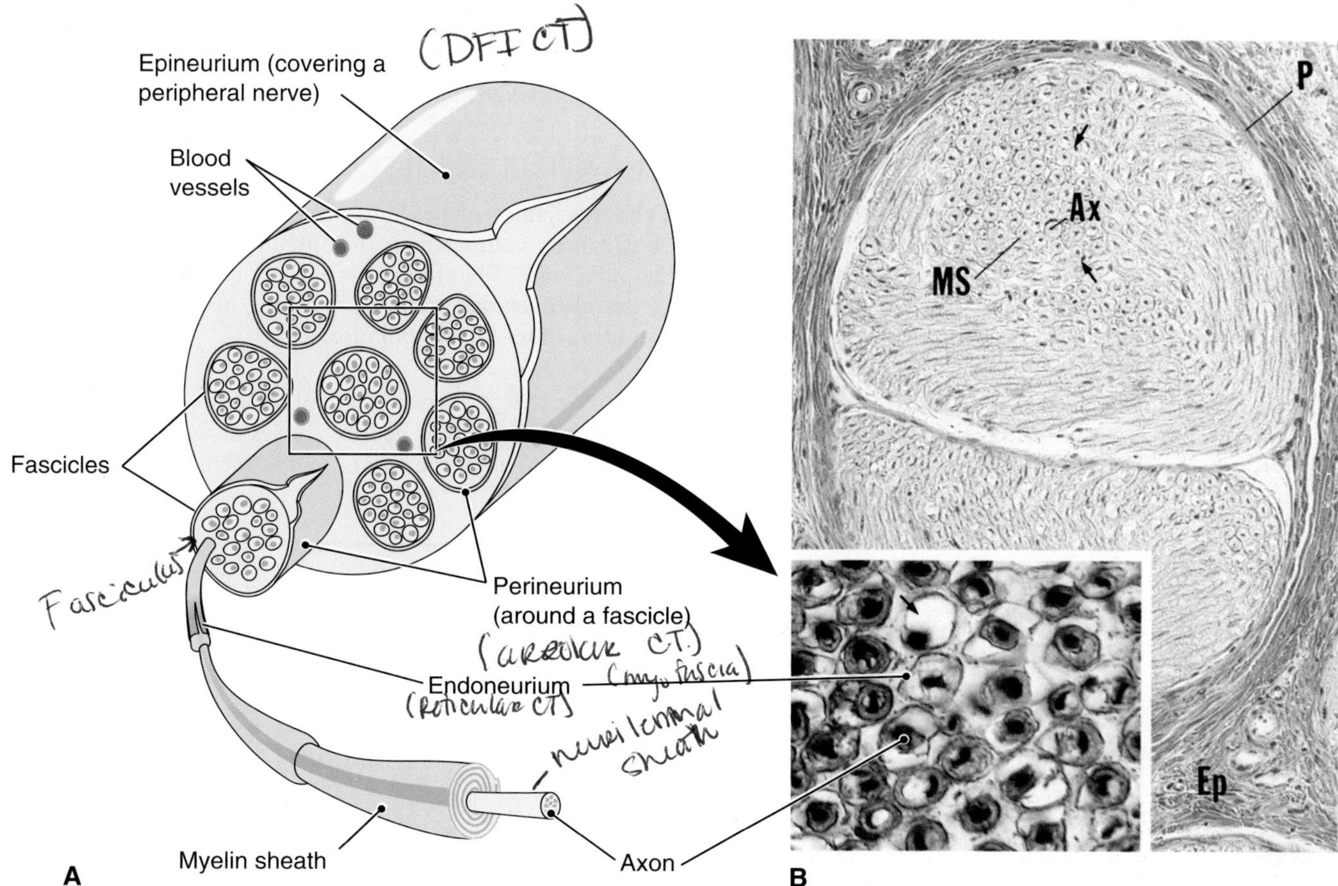

Figure 8-5 Structure of a nerve. KEY POINT Neuron fibers are collected in bundles called fascicles. Groups of fascicles make up a nerve. Connective tissue holds all components of the nerve together. **A.** Structure of a nerve showing neuron fibers and fascicles. **B.** Micrograph of a nerve (X132). Two fascicles are shown. Perineurium (P) surrounds each fascicle. Epineurium (Ep) is around the entire nerve. Individual axons (Ax) are covered with a myelin sheath (MS). Inset shows myelinated axons surrounded by endoneurium. (B, Reprinted with permission from Gartner LP, Hiatt JL. *Color Atlas of Histology*, 3rd ed. Philadelphia, PA: Lippincott Williams & Wilkins, 2000.) ZOOMING IN What is the deepest layer of connective tissue in a nerve? What is the outermost layer?

CHECKPOINTS 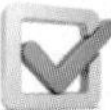

8-3 What is the name of the neuron fiber that carries impulses toward the cell body? What is the name of the fiber that carries impulses away from the cell body?

8-4 What color describes myelinated fibers? What color describes the nervous system's unmyelinated tissue?

8-5 What is a nerve? What is a tract?

8-6 What name is given to nerves that convey impulses toward the CNS? What name is given to nerves that transport away from the CNS?

Neuroglia

In addition to conducting tissue, the nervous system contains cells that support and protect the neurons. Collectively, these cells are called **neuroglia** (nu-ROG-le-ah) or **glial** (GLI-al) **cells**, from a Greek word meaning "glue." There are different types of neuroglia, each with specialized functions, some of which are the following:

- protect and nourish nervous tissue
- support nervous tissue and bind it to other structures
- aid in repair of cells
- act as phagocytes to remove pathogens and impurities
- regulate the composition of fluids around cells

Neuroglia appear throughout the CNS and PNS. The Schwann cells that form the myelin sheath in the PNS are one type of neuroglia. Cells that form the myelin sheath in the CNS are named *oligodendrocytes* (ol-ih-go-DEN-dro-sites) (literally meaning "cell with few dendrites"). Another example is shown in Figure 8-6. These cells are *astrocytes*, named for their starlike appearance. Astrocytes fulfill many of the functions listed above and also serve as stem cells in the regeneration of nervous tissue.

Unlike neurons, neuroglia continue to multiply throughout life. Because of their capacity to reproduce, most tumors of the nervous system are tumors of neuroglial tissue and not of nervous tissue itself.

CHECKPOINT 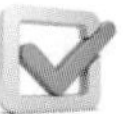

8-7 What is the name of the nervous system's nonconducting cells, which protect, nourish, and support the neurons?

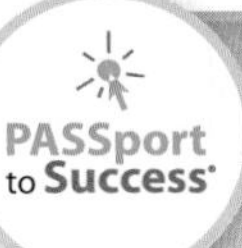

See the Student Resources on *thePoint* for a summary of the different neuroglial types.

The Nervous System at Work

The nervous system works by means of electric impulses sent along neuron fibers and transmitted from cell to cell at highly specialized junctions.

THE NERVE IMPULSE

The mechanics of nerve impulse conduction are complex but can be compared to the spread of an electric current along a wire. What follows is a brief description of the electrical changes that occur as a resting neuron is stimulated and transmits a nerve impulse.

The Resting State The plasma membrane of an unstimulated (resting) neuron carries an electric charge, or **potential**. At rest, the inside of the membrane is negative

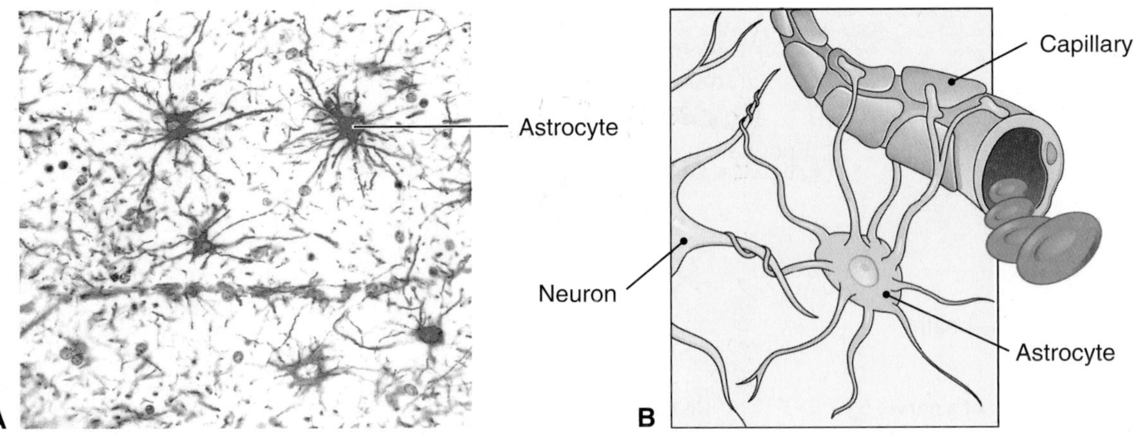

Figure 8-6 Astrocytes, a type of neuroglia. KEY POINT Astrocytes have several functions in the CNS, such as binding nervous tissue to other structures. **A.** Astrocytes in the white matter of the brain. **B.** An astrocyte binds a capillary to a neuron. (A, Reprinted with permission from Mills SE. *Histology for Pathologists*, 3rd ed. Philadelphia, PA: Lippincott Williams & Wilkins, 2006; B, Modified with permission from McConnell TH. *The Nature of Disease: Pathology for the Health Professions*. Baltimore, MA: Lippincott Williams & Wilkins, 2006.)

as compared with the outside. In this state, the membrane is said to be *polarized*. As in a battery, the separation of charges on either side of the membrane creates a possibility (potential) for generating energy. If there is a way for the charges to move toward each other, electricity (a nerve impulse) will be generated.

Also important for the generation of a nerve impulse are large concentration gradients for sodium and potassium ions across the plasma membrane. Sodium ions are more concentrated along the extracellular side of the plasma membrane than they are along the intracellular side of the membrane. Conversely, potassium ions are in higher concentration on the inside than on the outside of the membrane. The plasma membrane uses active transport to maintain these levels, as ions constantly are diffusing across the membrane in small amounts through channels known as *leak channels* and during nerve impulse transmission. (Remember that substances flow by diffusion from an area where they are in higher concentration to an area where they are in lower concentration.) This transport system requires energy from ATP and is described as the sodium–potassium pump or Na^+–K^+ pump.

The Action Potential A **nerve impulse** starts with a local reversal in the membrane potential caused by the movement of ions across the membrane. This sudden electrical change at the membrane is called an **action potential**, as mentioned in Chapter 7 in describing stimulation of skeletal muscles. A simple description of the events in an action potential is as follows (Fig. 8-7):

- Depolarization. A stimulus, such as an electrical, chemical, or mechanical signal of adequate force, causes specific channels in the membrane to open and allow Na^+ ions to flow into the cell. As these positive ions enter, they make the inside of the membrane less negative, thus reducing the membrane potential (electrical difference). This change is known as **depolarization** (see Fig. 8-7).
- Repolarization. In the next step of the action potential, K^+ channels open to allow K^+ to leave the cell. As the electric charge returns to its resting value, the membrane is undergoing **repolarization.** While the membrane is repolarizing, it does not respond to further stimulation. For this reason, the action potential spreads in one direction along the membrane from the point of excitation.

The action potential occurs rapidly—in less than one thousandth of a second, and is followed by a rapid return to the resting state. However, this local electrical change in the membrane stimulates an action potential at an adjacent point along the membrane (Fig. 8-8). In scientific terms, the channels in the membrane are "voltage dependent," that is, they respond to an electrical stimulus. And so, the action potential spreads along the membrane as a wave of electric current. The spreading action potential is the nerve impulse, and in fact, the term *action potential* is used to mean the nerve impulse. A stimulus is any force that can start an action potential by opening membrane channels and allowing Na^+ to enter the cell.

8

The Role of Myelin in Conduction As previously noted, some axons are coated with the fatty material myelin (see Fig. 8-4). If a fiber is not myelinated, the action potential spreads continuously along the cell's membrane (see Fig. 8-8). When myelin is present on an axon, however, it insulates the fiber against the spread of current. This would appear to slow or stop conduction along these fibers, but in fact, the myelin sheath speeds conduction. The reason is that the myelin causes the action potential to "jump" like a spark from node to node along the sheath (Fig. 8-9). This type of conduction, called **saltatory** (SAL-tah-to-re) **conduction** (from the Latin verb meaning "to leap"), is actually faster than continuous conduction, because fewer action potentials are needed for an impulse to travel a given distance. It is this type of conduction that is impaired in Sue's case of MS.

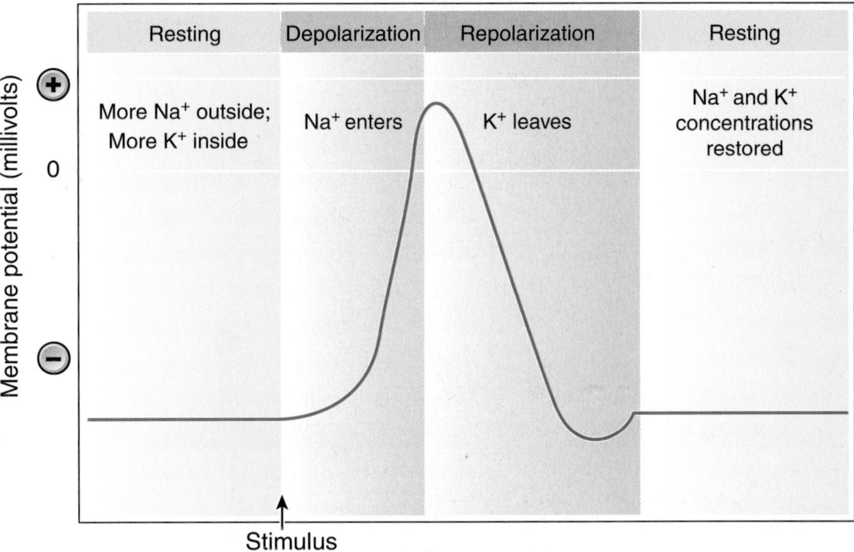

Figure 8-7 The action potential. KEY POINT In depolarization, Na^+ membrane-channels open and Na^+ enters the cell. In repolarization, K^+ membrane channels open and K^+ leaves the cell.

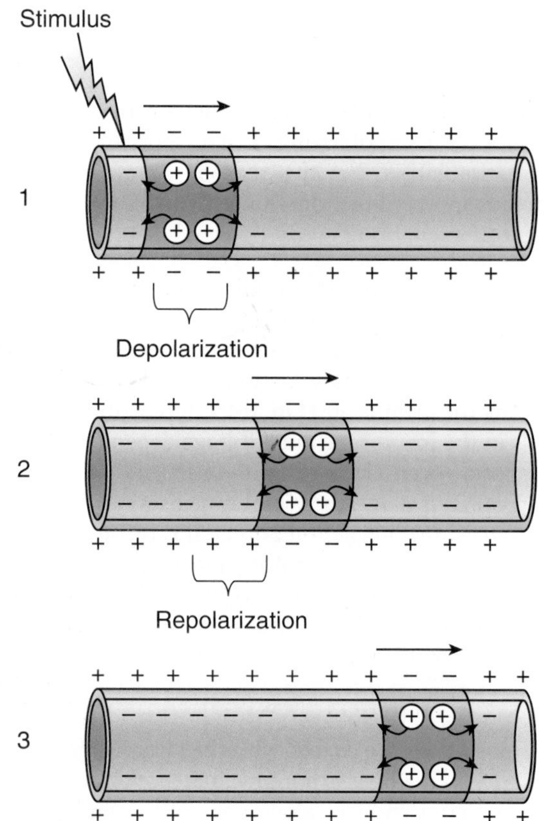

Figure 8-8 **A nerve impulse.** KEY POINT From a point of stimulation, a wave of depolarization followed by repolarization travels along the membrane of a neuron. This spreading action potential is a nerve impulse. ZOOMING IN What happens to the charge on the membrane at the point of an action potential?

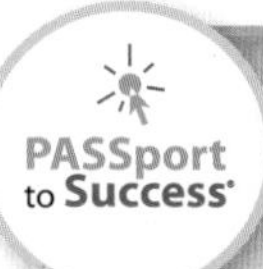

See the Student Resources on *thePoint* to view the animations *The Synapse and the Nerve Impulse, The Action Potential,* and *The Myelin Sheath.*

THE SYNAPSE

Neurons do not work alone; impulses must be transferred between neurons to convey information within the nervous system. The point of junction for transmitting the nerve impulse is the synapse **(Fig. 8-10)**. (There are also synapses between neurons and effector organs. We studied synapses between neurons and muscle cells in Chapter 7.) At a nerve-to-nerve synapse, transmission of an impulse usually occurs from the axon of one cell, the **presynaptic cell,** to the dendrite of another cell, the **postsynaptic cell.**

As described in Chapter 7, information must be passed from one cell to another at the synapse across a tiny gap between the cells, the synaptic cleft. Information usually crosses this gap by means of a neurotransmitter. While the cells at a synapse are at rest, the neurotransmitter is stored in many small vesicles (sacs) within the enlarged axon endings, usually called *end bulbs* or *terminal knobs,* but known by several other names as well.

When a nerve impulse traveling along a neuron membrane reaches the end of the presynaptic axon, some of these vesicles fuse with the membrane and release their neurotransmitter into the synaptic cleft (an example of exocytosis, as described in Chapter 3). The neurotransmitter then acts as a chemical signal to the postsynaptic cell.

On the postsynaptic receiving membrane, usually that of a dendrite, but sometimes another cell part, there are special sites, or **receptors,** ready to pick up and respond to specific neurotransmitters. Receptors in the postsynaptic cell's

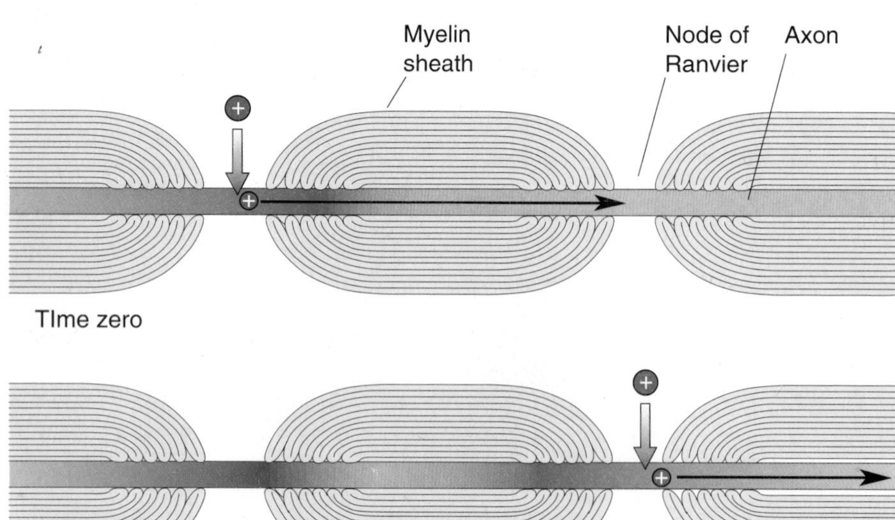

Figure 8-9 **Saltatory conduction.** KEY POINT The action potential along a myelinated axon jumps from node to node, speeding conduction. (Reprinted with permission from Bear MF et al. *Neuroscience, Exploring the Brain,* 3rd ed. Philadelphia, PA: Lippincott Williams & Wilkins, 2007.)

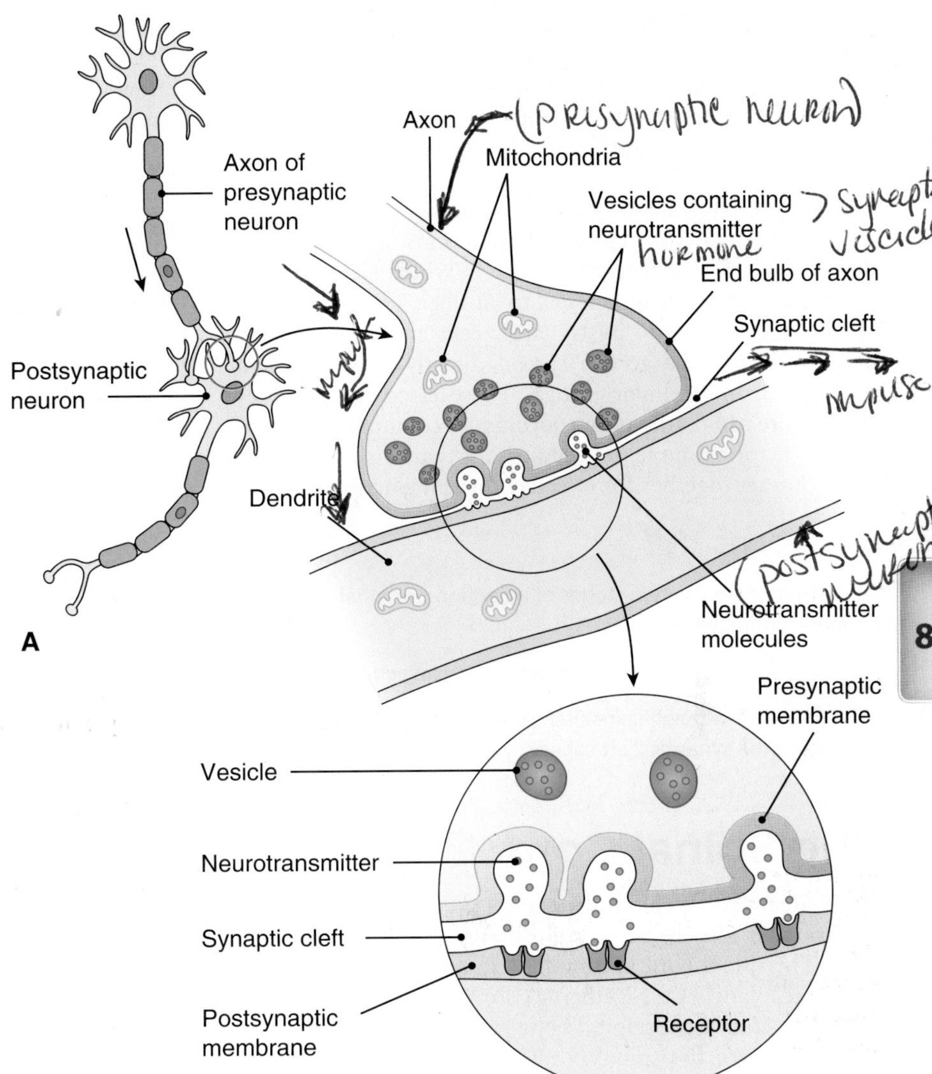

Figure 8-10 A synapse. KEY POINT Neurotransmitters carry impulses across a synaptic cleft. **A.** The end bulb of the presynaptic (transmitting) axon has vesicles containing neurotransmitter, which is released into the synaptic cleft to the membrane of the postsynaptic (receiving) cell. **B.** Close-up of a synapse showing receptors for neurotransmitter in the postsynaptic cell membrane.

membrane influence how or if that cell will respond to a given neurotransmitter.

Neurotransmitters Although there are many known neurotransmitters, some common ones are **norepinephrine** (nor-ep-ih-NEF-rin), **serotonin** (ser-o-TO-nin), **dopamine** (DO-pah-mene), and **acetylcholine** (as-e-til-KO-lene). Acetylcholine (ACh) is the neurotransmitter released at the neuromuscular junction.

It is common to think of neurotransmitters as stimulating the cells they reach; in fact, they have been described as such in this discussion. Note, however, that some of these chemicals inhibit the postsynaptic cell and keep it from reacting, as will be demonstrated later in discussions of the ANS.

The connections between neurons can be quite complex. One cell can branch to stimulate many receiving cells, or a single cell may be stimulated by a number of different axons. The cell's response is based on the total effects of all the neurotransmitters it receives at any one time.

After its release into the synaptic cleft, the neurotransmitter may be removed by several methods:

- It may slowly diffuse away from the synapse.
- It may be destroyed rapidly by enzymes in the synaptic cleft.
- It may be taken back into the presynaptic cell to be used again, a process known as *reuptake*.
- It may be taken up by neuroglial cells, specifically astrocytes.

The method of removal helps determine how long a neurotransmitter will act.

Many drugs that act on the mind, substances known as *psychoactive drugs*, function by affecting neurotransmitter activity in the brain. Prozac, for example, increases the level of the neurotransmitter serotonin by blocking its reuptake into presynaptic cells at synapses. This and other selective serotonin reuptake inhibitors prolong the neurotransmitter's activity and produce a mood-elevating effect. They are used to treat depression, anxiety, and obsessive–compulsive disorder. Similar psychoactive drugs prevent the reuptake of the neurotransmitters norepinephrine and dopamine. Another class of antidepressants prevents serotonin's enzymatic breakdown in the synaptic cleft, thus extending its action.

Electrical Synapses Not all synapses are chemically controlled. In smooth muscle, cardiac muscle, and also in the CNS, there is a type of synapse in which electrical signals travel directly from one cell to another. The membranes of the presynaptic and postsynaptic cells are close together and an electric charge can spread directly between them through an intercellular bridge. These electrical synapses allow more rapid and more coordinated communication. In the heart, for example, it is important that large groups of cells contract together for effective pumping action.

CHECKPOINTS 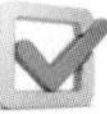

- 8-8 What are the two stages of an action potential and what happens during each?
- 8-9 What ions are involved in generating an action potential?
- 8-10 As a group, what are all the chemicals that carry information across the synaptic cleft called?

The Spinal Cord

The spinal cord is the link between the spinal nerves and the brain. It also helps to coordinate impulses within the CNS. The spinal cord is contained in and protected by the vertebrae, which fit together to form a continuous tube extending from the occipital bone to the coccyx (Fig. 8-11). In the embryo, the spinal cord occupies the entire spinal canal, extending down into the tail portion of the vertebral column. The bony column grows much more rapidly than the nervous tissue of the cord, however, and eventually, the end of the spinal cord no longer reaches the lower part of the spinal canal. This disparity in growth continues to increase, so that in adults, the spinal cord ends in the region just below the area to which the last rib attaches (between the first and second lumbar vertebrae).

STRUCTURE OF THE SPINAL CORD

The spinal cord has a small, irregularly shaped internal section of gray matter (unmyelinated tissue) surrounded by a larger area of white matter (myelinated axons) (see Fig. 8-11B,C). The internal gray matter is arranged so that a column of gray matter extends up and down dorsally, one on each side; another column is found in the ventral region on each side. These two pairs of columns, called the **dorsal horns** and **ventral horns**, give the gray matter a H-shaped appearance in cross section. The bridge of gray matter that connects the right and left horns is the **gray commissure** (KOM-ih-shure). In the center of the gray commissure is a small channel, the **central canal**, that contains cerebrospinal fluid (CSF), the liquid that circulates around the brain and spinal cord. A narrow groove, the **posterior median sulcus** (SUL-kus), divides the right and left portions of the posterior white matter. A deeper groove, the **anterior median fissure** (FISH-ure), separates the right and left portions of the anterior white matter.

ASCENDING AND DESCENDING TRACTS

The spinal cord is the pathway for sensory and motor impulses traveling to and from the brain. These impulses are carried in the thousands of myelinated axons in the spinal cord's white matter, which are subdivided into tracts (fiber bundles). Sensory impulses entering the spinal cord are transmitted toward the brain in **ascending tracts** of the white matter. Motor impulses traveling from the brain are carried in **descending tracts** toward the PNS. Damage to these tracts prevents transmission of impulses along the spinal cord. Box 8-1 contains information on treatment of these injuries.

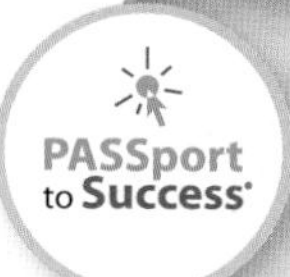

Occupational therapists often help to care for people with nervous system disorders. See the Student Resources on *thePoint* for more information about this career.

CHECKPOINTS 

- 8-11 How are the gray and white matter arranged in the spinal cord?
- 8-12 What is the purpose of the tracts in the spinal cord's white matter?

The Spinal Nerves

There are 31 pairs of spinal nerves, each pair numbered according to the level of the spinal cord from which it arises (see Fig. 8-11A). Note that the nerves that arise near the end of the cord travel in a group within the spinal canal until each exits from its appropriate intervertebral foramen. Together, the nerves resemble a horse's tail, and this region is aptly named the **cauda equina** (KAW-dah eh-KWI-nah).

Each nerve is attached to the spinal cord by two roots: the **dorsal root** and the **ventral root** (see Fig. 8-11B). On each dorsal root is a marked swelling of gray matter called the **dorsal root ganglion**, which contains the cell bodies of the sensory neurons. A **ganglion** (GANG-le-on) is any collection of nerve cell bodies located outside the CNS. Fibers from sensory receptors throughout the body lead to the dorsal roots and these dorsal root ganglia.

A spinal nerve's ventral root contains motor fibers that supply muscles and glands (effectors). The cell bodies of these neurons are located in the cord's ventral gray matter (ventral horns). Because the dorsal (sensory) and ventral (motor) roots combine to form the spinal nerve, all spinal nerves are mixed nerves.

Figure 8-11 **Spinal cord and spinal nerves. A.** Posterior view. Nerve plexuses (networks) are shown. Nerves from the distal cord form the cauda equina. **B.** Cross section of the spinal cord showing the organization of the gray and white matter. The roots of the spinal nerves are also shown. **C.** Microscopic view of the spinal cord in cross section (×5). (B, Reprinted with permission from Mills SE. *Histology for Pathologists*, 3rd ed. Philadelphia, PA: Lippincott Williams & Wilkins, 2006.) **ZOOMING IN** Is the spinal cord the same length as the spinal column? How does the number of cervical vertebrae compare to the number of cervical spinal nerves?

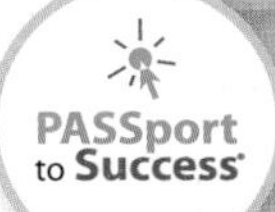

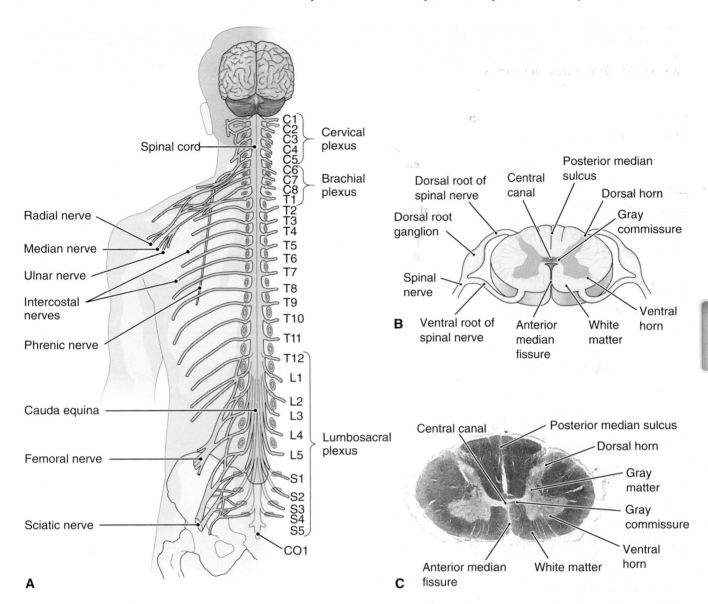

See the Student Resources on *thePoint* to view an illustration of the cauda equina.

BRANCHES OF THE SPINAL NERVES

Each spinal nerve continues only a short distance away from the spinal cord and then branches into small posterior divisions and larger anterior divisions. The posterior divisions distribute branches to the back. The anterior branches of the thoracic nerves 2 through 11 become the intercostal nerves supplying the regions between the ribs. The remaining anterior branches interlace to form networks called **plexuses** (PLEK-sus-eze), which then distribute branches to the body parts **(see Fig. 8-11)**. The three main plexuses are described as follows:

- The **cervical plexus** supplies motor impulses to the neck muscles and receives sensory impulses from the neck and the back of the head. The phrenic nerve, which activates the diaphragm, arises from this plexus.
- The **brachial** (BRA-ke-al) **plexus** sends numerous branches to the shoulder, arm, forearm, wrist, and

Box 8-1 *Hot Topics*

Spinal Cord Injury: Crossing the Divide

Approximately 13,000 new cases of traumatic spinal cord injury occur each year in the United States, the majority involving males ages 16 to 30. More than 80% of these injuries are due to motor vehicle accidents, acts of violence, and falls. Because neurons show little, if any, capacity to repair themselves, spinal cord injuries almost always result in a loss of sensory or motor function (or both), and therapy has focused on injury management rather than cure. However, scientists are investigating four improved treatment approaches:

- *Minimizing spinal cord trauma after injury.* Intravenous injection of the steroid methylprednisolone shortly after injury reduces swelling at the site of injury and improves recovery.
- *Using neurotrophins to induce repair in damaged nerve tissue.* Certain types of neuroglia produce chemicals called neurotrophins (e.g., nerve growth factor) that have promoted nerve regeneration in experiments.
- *Regulation of inhibitory factors that keep neurons from dividing.* "Turning off" these factors (produced by neuroglia) in the damaged nervous system may promote tissue repair. The factor called Nogo is an example.
- *Nervous tissue transplantation.* Successfully transplanted donor tissue may take over the damaged nervous system's functions.

hand. For example, the radial nerve emerges from the brachial plexus, as do the median and ulnar nerves.

- The **lumbosacral** (lum-bo-SA-kral) **plexus** supplies nerves to the pelvis and legs. The femoral nerve to the thigh is part of this plexus. The largest branch in this plexus is the **sciatic** (si-AT-ik) **nerve,** which leaves the dorsal part of the pelvis, passes beneath the gluteus maximus muscle, and extends down the posterior

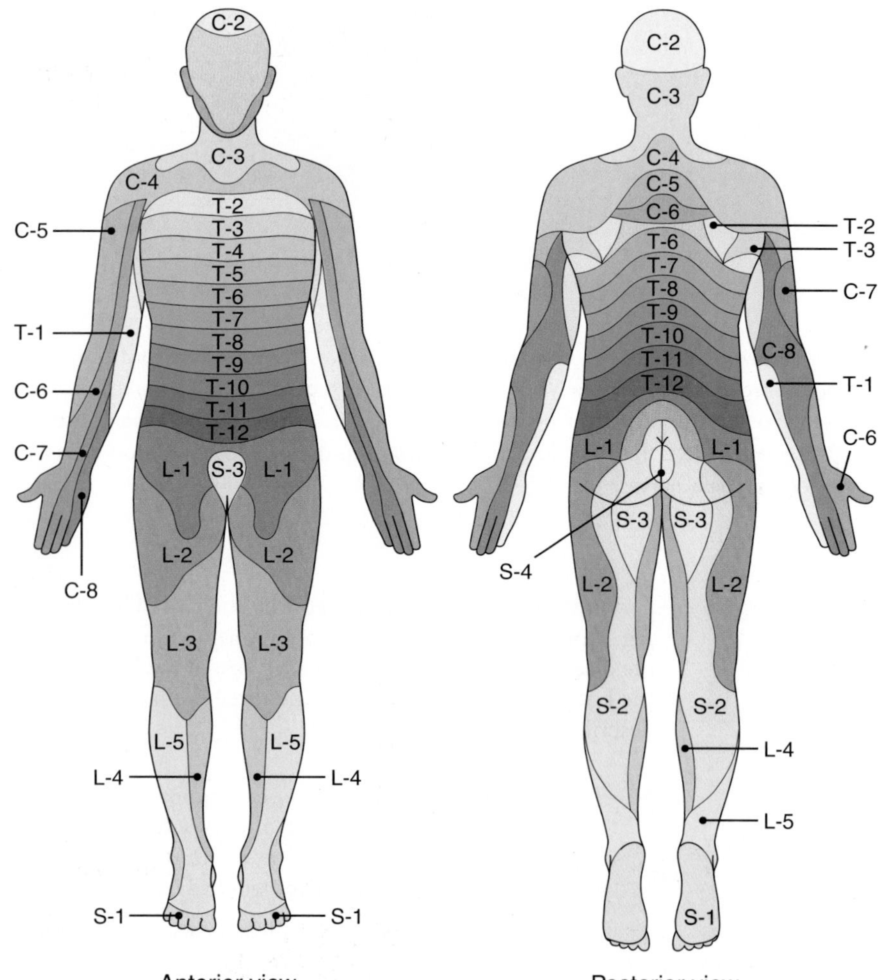

Figure 8-12 **Dermatomes.** KEY POINT A dermatome is a region of the skin supplied by a single spinal nerve. ZOOMING IN Which spinal nerves carry impulses from the skin of the toes? From the anterior hand and fingers?

thigh. At its beginning, it is nearly 1 in. thick, but it soon branches to the thigh muscles. Near the knee, it forms two subdivisions that supply the leg and the foot.

DERMATOMES

Sensory neurons from all over the skin, except for the skin of the face and scalp, feed information into the spinal cord through the spinal nerves. The skin surface can be mapped into distinct regions that are supplied by a single spinal nerve. Each of these regions is called a **dermatome** (DER-mah-tome) (Fig. 8-12).

Sensation from a given dermatome is carried over its corresponding spinal nerve. This information can be used to identify the spinal nerve or spinal segment that is involved in an injury, as sensation from its corresponding skin surface will be altered. In some areas, the dermatomes are not absolutely distinct. Some dermatomes may share a nerve supply with neighboring regions. For this reason, it is necessary to numb several adjacent dermatomes to achieve successful anesthesia.

CHECKPOINTS 

- 8-13 How many pairs of spinal nerves are there?
- 8-14 What types of fibers are in a spinal nerve's dorsal root? What types are in its ventral root?

Reflexes

As the nervous system develops, neural pathways are formed to coordinate responses. Most of these pathways are very complex, involving multiple neurons and interactions between different regions of the nervous system. Easier to study are simple pathways involving a minimal number of neurons. Responses controlled by some of these simpler pathways are useful in neurologic studies.

THE REFLEX ARC

A complete pathway through the nervous system from stimulus to response is termed a **reflex arc** (Fig. 8-13). This is the

8

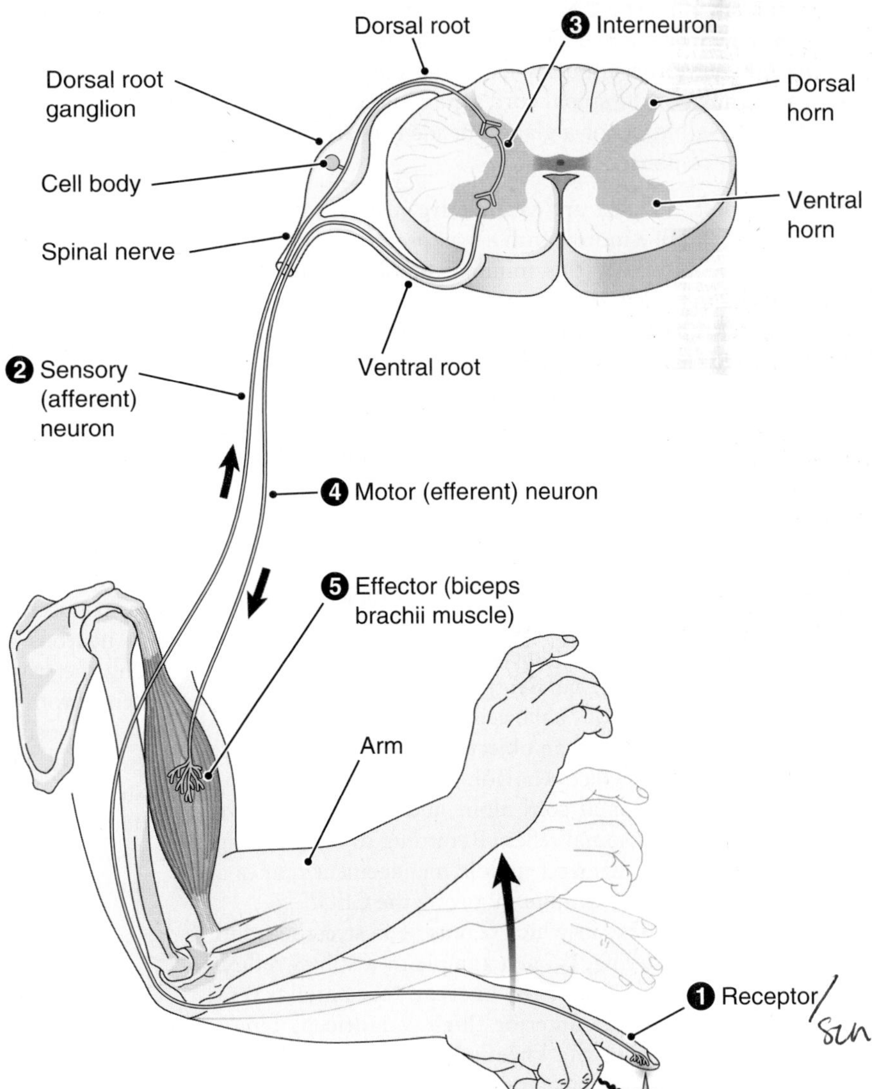

Figure 8-13 Typical reflex arc. KEY POINT Numbers show the sequence in the pathway of impulses through the spinal cord (*solid arrows*). Contraction of the biceps brachii results in flexion of the arm at the elbow. ZOOMING IN Is this a somatic or an autonomic reflex arc? What type of neuron is located between the sensory and motor neuron in the CNS?

Table 8-2 Components of a Reflex Arc

Component	Function
Receptor	End of a dendrite or specialized cell that responds to a stimulus
Sensory neuron	Transmits a nerve impulse toward the CNS
Central nervous	Coordinates sensory impulses and organizes a system response; usually requires interneurons
Motor neuron	Carries impulses away from the CNS toward the effector, a muscle or a gland
Effector	A muscle or gland outside the CNS that carries out a response

nervous system's basic functional pathway. The fundamental parts of a reflex arc are the following (Table 8-2):

1. **Receptor**—the end of a dendrite or some specialized receptor cell, as in a special sense organ, that detects a stimulus.
2. **Sensory neuron**—a cell that transmits impulses toward the CNS. Sensory impulses enter the dorsal horn of the spinal cord's gray matter.
3. **Central nervous system**—where impulses are coordinated and a response is organized. Interneurons transmit impulses within the CNS.
4. **Motor neuron**—a cell that carries impulses away from the CNS. Motor impulses leave the cord through the ventral horn of the spinal cord's gray matter.
5. **Effector**—a muscle or a gland outside the CNS that carries out a response.

At its simplest, a reflex arc can involve just two neurons, one sensory and one motor, with a synapse in the CNS. Few reflex arcs require only this minimal number of neurons. (The knee-jerk reflex described below is one of the few examples in humans.) Most reflex arcs involve many more, even hundreds, of connecting neurons within the CNS. The many intricate patterns that make the nervous system so responsive and adaptable also make it difficult to study, and investigation of the nervous system is one of the most active areas of research today.

REFLEX ACTIVITIES

Although reflex pathways may be quite complex, a **simple reflex** is a rapid, uncomplicated, and automatic response involving very few neurons. Reflexes are specific; a given stimulus always produces the same response. When you fling out an arm or leg to catch your balance, withdraw from a painful stimulus, or blink to avoid an object approaching your eyes, you are experiencing reflex behavior. A simple reflex arc that passes through the spinal cord alone and does not involve the brain is termed a **spinal reflex**. Returning to our opening corporation analogy, it's as if middle management makes a decision independently, without involving the CEO.

The **stretch reflex**, in which a muscle is stretched and responds by contracting, is one example of a spinal reflex. If you tap the tendon below the kneecap (the patellar tendon), the muscle of the anterior thigh (quadriceps femoris) contracts, eliciting the knee-jerk reflex. Such stretch reflexes may be evoked by appropriate tapping of most large muscles (such as the triceps brachii in the arm and the gastrocnemius in the calf of the leg). Because reflexes are simple and predictable, they are used in physical examinations to test the condition of the nervous system. In the case study, Dr. Jensen tested Sue's stretch reflexes to help in diagnosis.

CHECKPOINT 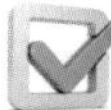

☐ 8-15 What is the name for a pathway through the nervous system from a stimulus to an effector?

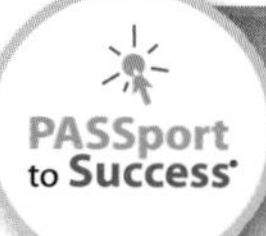

See the Student Resources on *thePoint* to view the animation *The Reflex Arc*.

The Autonomic Nervous System

The autonomic (visceral) nervous system regulates the action of the glands, the smooth muscles of hollow organs and vessels, and the heart muscle. These actions are carried out automatically; whenever a change occurs that calls for a regulatory adjustment, it is made without conscious awareness.

Most ANS studies concentrate on the motor portion of the system. All autonomic pathways contain two motor neurons connecting the spinal cord with the effector organ. The two neurons synapse in ganglia that serve as relay stations along the way. The first neuron, the preganglionic neuron, extends from the spinal cord to the ganglion. The second neuron, the postganglionic neuron, travels from the ganglion to the effector. This differs from the voluntary (somatic) nervous system, in which each motor nerve fiber extends all the way from the spinal cord to the skeletal muscle with no intervening synapse. Some of the autonomic fibers are within the spinal nerves; some are within the cranial nerves (see Chapter 9).

DIVISIONS OF THE AUTONOMIC NERVOUS SYSTEM

The ANS motor neurons are arranged in a distinct pattern, which has led to their separation for study purposes into **sympathetic** and **parasympathetic** divisions (Fig. 8-14), as described below and summarized in Table 8-3.

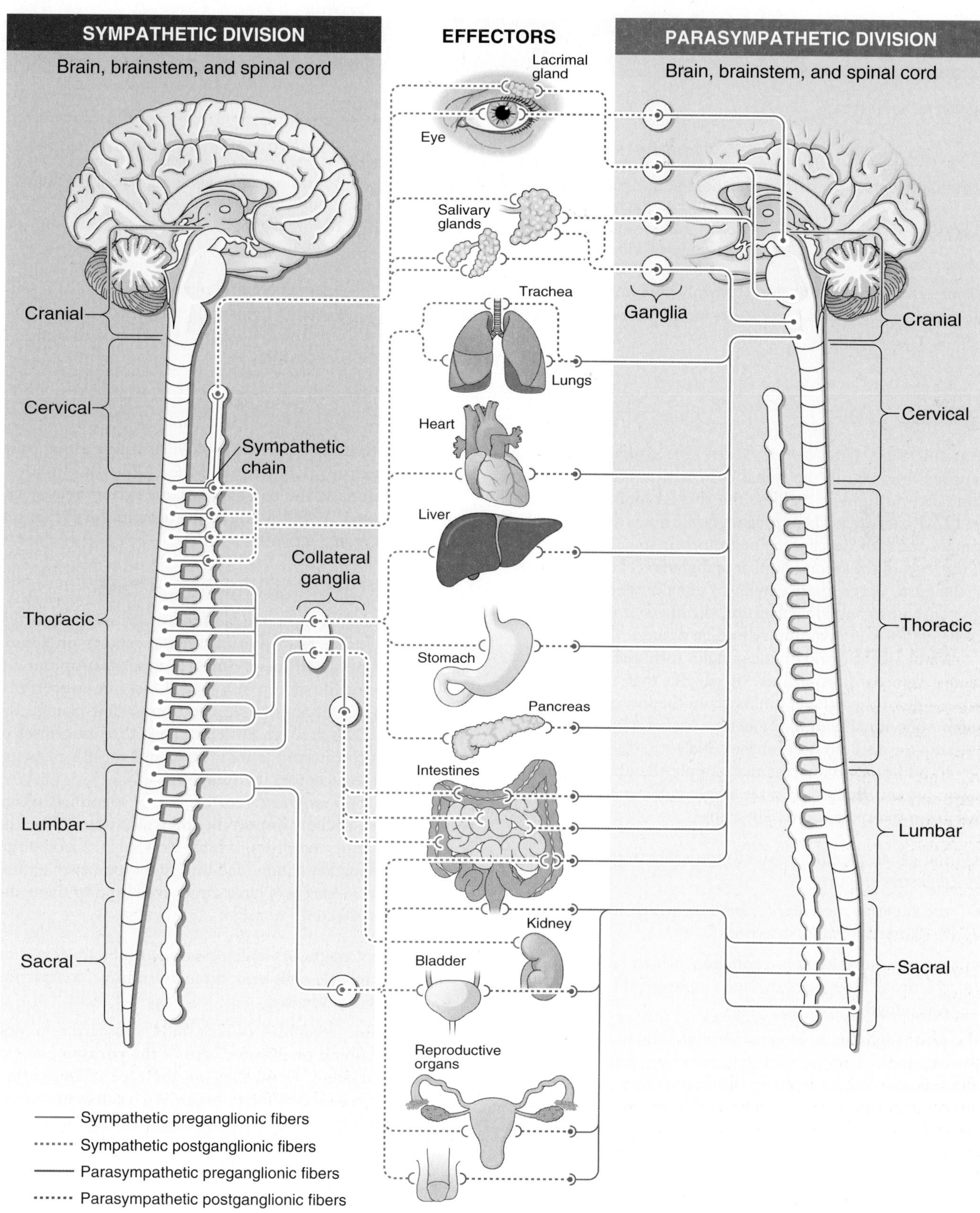

8

Figure 8-14 Autonomic nervous system. KEY POINT Most organs have both sympathetic and parasympathetic fibers. The diagram shows only one side of the body for each division. ZOOMING IN Which division of the autonomic nervous system has ganglia closer to the effector organ?

Table 8-3 Divisions of the Autonomic Nervous System

Characteristics	Divisions	
	Sympathetic nervous system	**Parasympathetic nervous system**
Origin of fibers	Thoracic and lumbar regions of the spinal cord; thoracolumbar	Brain stem and sacral regions of the spinal cord; craniosacral
Location of ganglia	Sympathetic chains and three single collateral ganglia (celiac, superior mesenteric, and inferior mesenteric)	Terminal ganglia in or near the effector organ
Neurotransmitter at effector	Mainly norepinephrine; adrenergic	Acetylcholine; cholinergic
Effects	Response to stress; fight-or-flight response	Reverses fight-or-flight (stress) (see Table 8-4) response; stimulates some activities

Sympathetic Nervous System The sympathetic motor neurons originate in the spinal cord with cell bodies in the thoracic and lumbar regions, the **thoracolumbar** (tho-rah-ko-LUM-bar) area. These preganglionic fibers arise from the spinal cord at the level of the first thoracic spinal nerve down to the level of the second lumbar spinal nerve. From this part of the cord, nerve fibers extend to ganglia where they synapse with postganglionic neurons, the fibers of which extend to the glands and involuntary muscle tissues.

Many of the sympathetic ganglia form the **sympathetic chains**, two cordlike strands of ganglia that extend along either side of the spinal column from the lower neck to the upper abdominal region. (Note that Figure 8-14 shows only one side for each division of the ANS.)

In addition, the nerves that supply the abdominal and pelvic organs synapse in three single **collateral ganglia** farther from the spinal cord. These are:

- the celiac ganglion, which sends fibers mainly to the digestive organs
- the superior mesenteric ganglion, which sends fibers to the large and small intestines
- the inferior mesenteric ganglion, which sends fibers to the distal large intestine and organs of the urinary and reproductive systems

The postganglionic neurons of the sympathetic system, with few exceptions, act on their effectors by releasing the neurotransmitter norepinephrine (noradrenaline), a compound similar in chemical composition and action to the hormone epinephrine (adrenalin). This system is therefore described as **adrenergic**, which means "activated by adrenaline."

Parasympathetic Nervous System The parasympathetic motor pathways begin in the **craniosacral** (kra-ne-o-SAK-ral) areas, with fibers arising from cell bodies in the brain stem (midbrain and medulla) and the lower (sacral) part of the spinal cord. From these centers, the first fibers extend to autonomic ganglia that are usually located near or within the walls of the effector organs and are called **terminal ganglia**. The pathways then continue along postganglionic neurons that stimulate the involuntary tissues.

The neurons of the parasympathetic system release the neurotransmitter ACh, leading to the description of this system as **cholinergic** (activated by ACh).

THE ROLE OF CELLULAR RECEPTORS

An important factor in the actions of neurotransmitters is their "docking sites," that is, their receptors on receiving (postsynaptic) cell membranes. A neurotransmitter fits into its receptor like a key in a lock. Once the neurotransmitter binds, the receptor initiates events that change the postsynaptic cell's activity. Different receptors' responses to the same neurotransmitter may vary, and a cell's response depends on the receptors it contains.

Among the many different classes of identified receptors, two are especially important and well studied. The first is the cholinergic receptors, which bind ACh. Cholinergic receptors are further subdivided into two types, each named for drugs that researchers have discovered bind to them and mimic ACh's effects:

- Nicotinic receptors (which bind nicotine) are found on skeletal muscle cells and stimulate muscle contraction when ACh is present.
- Muscarinic receptors (which bind muscarine, a poison) are found on effector cells of the parasympathetic nervous system. Depending on the type of muscarinic receptor in a given effector organ, ACh can either stimulate or inhibit a response. For example, ACh stimulates digestive organs but inhibits the heart.

The second class of receptors is the adrenergic receptors, which bind norepinephrine. They are found on effector cells of the sympathetic nervous system. They are further subdivided into alpha (α) and beta (β). Depending on the type of adrenergic receptor in a given effector organ, norepinephrine can either stimulate or inhibit a response. For example, norepinephrine stimulates the heart and inhibits the digestive organs.

Some drugs block specific receptors. For example, "beta-blockers" regulate the heart in cardiac disease by preventing β receptors from binding norepinephrine, the neurotransmitter that increases the rate and strength of heart contractions.

FUNCTIONS OF THE AUTONOMIC NERVOUS SYSTEM

Most organs are supplied by both sympathetic and parasympathetic fibers, and the two systems generally have opposite effects (Table 8-4). The sympathetic system tends to act as an accelerator for those organs needed to meet a stressful situation. It promotes what is called the **fight-or-flight response** because in the most primitive terms, the person must decide to stay and "fight it out" with the enemy or to run away from danger. The times when the sympathetic nervous system comes into play can be summarized by the four Es, that is, times of emergency, excitement, embarrassment, and exercise. If you think of what happens to a person who is in any of these situations, you can easily remember the effects of the sympathetic nervous system:

- Increase in the rate and force of heart contractions
- Increase in blood pressure due partly to the more effective heartbeat and partly to constriction of small arteries everywhere except the brain
- Dilation of blood vessels to skeletal muscles, bringing more blood to these tissues
- Dilation of the bronchial tubes to allow more oxygen to enter and more carbon dioxide to leave
- Stimulation of the central portion of the adrenal gland. This gland produces hormones that prepare the body to meet emergency situations in many ways (see Chapter 11). The sympathetic nerves and hormones from the adrenal gland reinforce each other
- Increase in basal metabolic rate
- Dilation of the eye's pupil and increase in distance focusing ability

The sympathetic system also acts as a brake on those systems not directly involved in the stress response, such as the urinary and digestive systems. If you try to eat while you are angry, you may note that your saliva is thick and so small in amount that you can swallow only with difficulty. Under these circumstances, when food does reach the stomach, it seems to stay there longer than usual.

The parasympathetic system normally acts as a balance for the sympathetic system once a crisis has passed. It is the "rest and digest" system. It causes constriction of the pupils, slowing of the heart rate, and constriction of the bronchial tubes. However, the parasympathetic nervous system also stimulates certain activities needed for maintenance of homeostasis. Among other actions, it promotes the formation and release of urine and activity of the digestive tract. Saliva, for example, flows more easily and profusely under its effects. These stimulatory actions are summarized by the acronym SLUDD: salivation, lacrimation (tear formation), urination, digestion, defecation.

8

CHECKPOINTS 

☐ 8-16 How many neurons are there in each motor pathway of the ANS?

☐ 8-17 Which division of the ANS stimulates a stress response? Which division reverses the stress response?

Table 8-4 Effects of the Sympathetic and Parasympathetic Systems on Selected Organs

Effector	Sympathetic system	Parasympathetic system
Pupils of eye	Dilation	Constriction
Lacrimal glands	None	Secretion of tears
Sweat glands	Stimulation	None
Digestive glands	Inhibition	Stimulation
Heart	Increased rate and strength of beat	Decreased rate of beat
Bronchi of lungs	Dilation	Constriction
Muscles of digestive system	Decreased contraction	Increased contraction
Kidneys	Decreased activity	None
Urinary bladder	Relaxation	Contraction and emptying
Liver	Increased release of glucose	None
Penis	Ejaculation	Erection
Adrenal medulla	Stimulation	None
Blood vessels	Constriction	Dilation, penis and clitoris only

A&P in Action Revisited

Sue Learns about Her MS

Sue, I can't really answer the question of why you developed multiple sclerosis," Dr. Jensen explained to her patient. "There is evidence that the disease has a genetic component but the environment, and perhaps even a virus, might be involved. We do know that MS affects women more frequently than men, and is more prevalent in areas like the northern United States and Canada. We also know that MS is an autoimmune disease. Normally, immune cells travel through the brain and spinal cord looking for pathogens. In MS, the immune cells make a mistake and cause inflammation in healthy nervous tissue. This inflammatory response damages neuroglial cells called oligodendrocytes. These cells form the myelin sheath that covers and insulates the axons of neurons much like the plastic covering on an electrical wire does. When the oligodendrocytes are damaged, they are unable to make this myelin sheath and the axons can't properly transmit nerve impulses. Right now, it appears that the largest areas of demyelination are in the white matter tracts of your spinal cord."

"Is there a medication I can take to stop the disease?" asked Sue.

"Unfortunately," replied the doctor, "there isn't a cure for MS yet. But, we can slow down the disease's progress using antiinflammatory drugs to decrease the inflammation and drugs called interferons that depress the immune response."

During this case, we saw that neurons carrying information to and from the CNS require myelin sheaths. Inflammation and subsequent damage of the myelin sheath in diseases like MS have profound effects on sensory and motor function. For more information about the inflammatory response and interferons, see Chapter 15.

Chapter Wrap-Up

Summary Overview

A detailed chapter outline with space for note-taking is on *thePoint*. The figure below illustrates the main topics covered in this chapter.

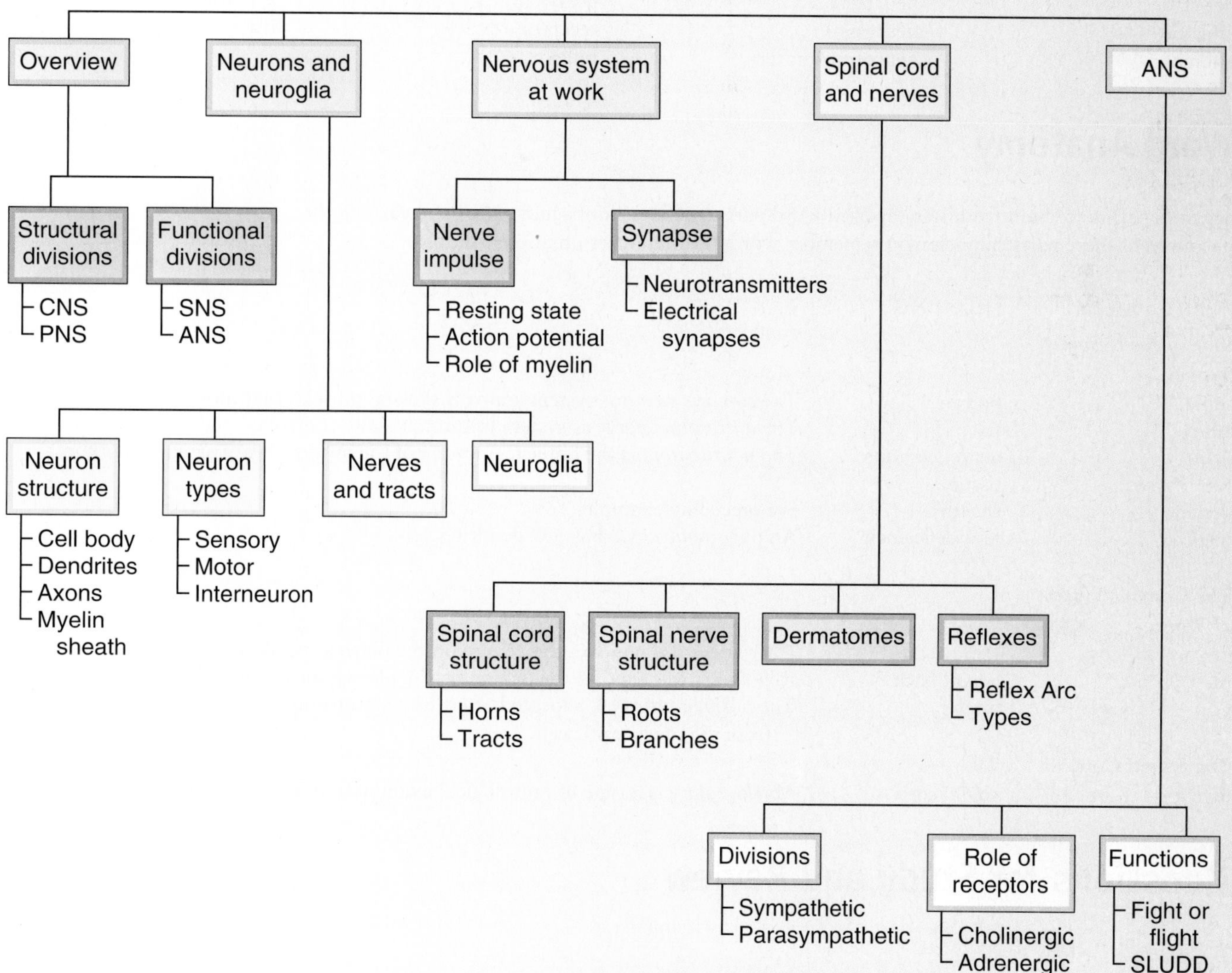

Key Terms

The terms listed below are emphasized in this chapter. Knowing them will help you organize and prioritize your learning. These and other boldface terms are defined in the Glossary with phonetic pronunciations.

acetylcholine
action potential
afferent
autonomic nervous system
axon
dendrite
effector
efferent
ganglion
interneuron
motor
nerve
nerve impulse
neuroglia
neuron
neurotransmitter
norepinephrine
parasympathetic nervous system
plexus
postsynaptic
presynaptic
receptor
reflex
repolarization
saltatory conduction
sensory
somatic nervous system
sympathetic nervous system
synapse
tract

Word Anatomy

Scientific terms are built from standardized word parts (prefixes, roots, and suffixes). Learning the meanings of these parts can help you remember words and interpret unfamiliar terms.

WORD PART	MEANING	EXAMPLE
Role of the Nervous System		
soma-	body	The *somatic* nervous system controls skeletal muscles that move the body.
aut/o	self	The *autonomic* nervous system is automatically controlled and is involuntary.
neur/i	nerve, nervous tissue	The *neurilemma* is the outer membrane of the myelin sheath around an axon.
-lemma	sheath	See preceding example.
olig/o-	few, deficiency	An *oligodendrocyte* has few dendrites.
The Nervous System at Work		
de-	remove	*Depolarization* removes the charge on the plasma membrane of a cell.
re-	again, back	*Repolarization* restores the charge on the plasma membrane of a cell.
post-	after	The *postsynaptic* cell is located after the synapse and receives neurotransmitter from the presynaptic cell.
The Spinal Cord		
myel/o	spinal cord	*Myelography* is a type of radiological examination of the spinal cord.

Questions for Study and Review

BUILDING UNDERSTANDING

Fill in the Blanks

1. The brain and spinal cord make up the _____ nervous system.
2. Action potentials are conducted away from the neuron cell body by the _____.
3. During an action potential, the flow of Na^+ into the cell causes _____.
4. In the spinal cord, sensory information travels in _____ tracts.
5. With few exceptions, the sympathetic nervous system uses the neurotransmitter _____ to act on effector organs.

Matching > Match each numbered item with the most closely related lettered item.

___ **6.** Cells that carry impulses from the CNS
___ **7.** Cells that carry impulses to the CNS
___ **8.** Cells that carry impulses within the CNS
___ **9.** Cells that detect a stimulus
___ **10.** Cells that carry out a response to a stimulus

a. receptors
b. effectors
c. sensory neurons
d. motor neurons
e. interneurons

Multiple Choice

___ **11.** Which system directly innervates skeletal muscles?
- **a.** central nervous system
- **b.** somatic nervous system
- **c.** parasympathetic nervous system
- **d.** sympathetic nervous system

___ **12.** Which neurotransmitter binds to muscarinic receptors?
- **a.** nicotine
- **b.** norepinephrine
- **c.** epinephrine
- **d.** acetylcholine

___ **13.** What is the correct order of synaptic transmission?
- **a.** postsynaptic neuron, synapse, and presynaptic neuron
- **b.** presynaptic neuron, synapse, and postsynaptic neuron
- **c.** presynaptic neuron, postsynaptic neuron, and synapse
- **d.** postsynaptic neuron, presynaptic neuron, and synapse

___ **14.** Where do afferent nerve fibers enter the spinal cord?
- **a.** dorsal horn
- **b.** ventral horn
- **c.** gray commissure
- **d.** central canal

___ **15.** What promotes the "fight-or-flight" response?
- **a.** sympathetic nervous system
- **b.** parasympathetic nervous system
- **c.** somatic nervous system
- **d.** reflex arc

UNDERSTANDING CONCEPTS

16. Differentiate between the terms in each of the following pairs:
- **a.** neurons and neuroglia
- **b.** vesicle and membrane receptor
- **c.** gray matter and white matter
- **d.** nerve and tract
- **e.** adrenergic and cholinergic

17. Describe an action potential. How does conduction along a myelinated fiber differ from conduction along an unmyelinated fiber?

18. Discuss the structure and function of the spinal cord.

19. Explain the reflex arc using stepping on a tack as an example.

20. Describe the anatomy of a spinal nerve. How many pairs of spinal nerves are there?

21. Define a *plexus*. Name the three main spinal nerve plexuses.

22. Differentiate between the functions of the sympathetic and parasympathetic divisions of the autonomic nervous system.

CONCEPTUAL THINKING

23. Clinical depression is associated with abnormal serotonin levels. Medications that block the removal of this neurotransmitter from the synapse can control the disorder. Based on this information is clinical depression associated with increased or decreased levels of serotonin? Explain your answer.

24. Mr. Hayward visits his dentist for a root canal and is given Novocaine, a local anesthetic, at the beginning of the procedure. Novocaine reduces membrane permeability to Na^+. What effect does this have on action potential?

25. In Sue's case, her symptoms were caused by demyelination in her central nervous system. Would her symptoms be the same or different if her spinal nerves were involved? Explain why.

thePoint **For more questions, see the learning activities on *thePoint.***

CHAPTER 9

The Nervous System: The Brain and Cranial Nerves

A&P in Action

Frank's Case: Blood Clot in the Brain

Ross loved his job as a physiotherapist. He especially enjoyed his current position at the hospital where he was a member of the brain injury team. His responsibility was to design and implement rehabilitation programs for patients recovering from brain injury.

When Ross arrived at work, there was a new medical chart waiting for him at his desk. He opened it and scanned its contents. Yesterday evening, Frank Carter, a 68-year-old African American, was transported by ambulance to the emergency room. According to Frank's wife, he had collapsed suddenly in their living room. Worried that he was having a heart attack, she called 911. At the hospital, Frank appeared confused and disoriented. His speech was slurred and he had difficulty forming words. He reported double vision, dizziness, and a severe headache. He had a history of high blood pressure and, according to his wife, had smoked a pack of cigarettes per day for most of his adult life. The emergency room physician examined Frank and noted muscle weakness and a diminished sense of touch on the right side of his face and arm. Based upon his neurological findings, the physician ordered an emergency CT scan of Frank's brain. The results of the scan indicated that there was a blood clot blocking Frank's left middle cerebral artery, preventing blood flow to his left cerebral hemisphere. Frank wasn't having a heart attack—he was having a stroke. The emergency physician administered tissue plasminogen activator to dissolve the clot and restore blood flow to his brain.

Frank's neurological symptoms are due to a lack of blood flow to a part of his brain called the cerebrum. In this chapter, we learn about the structure and function of the brain. We also revisit Frank and look at Ross' assessment of his stroke symptoms.

PASSport to Success

Ancillaries At-A-Glance

Visit *thePoint* to access the PASSport to Success and the following resources. For guidance in using these resources most effectively, see pp. ix–xviii.

Learning TOOLS

- Learning Style Self Assessment
- Live Advise Online Student Tutoring
- Tips for Effective Studying

Learning RESOURCES

- E-book: Chapter 9
- Health Professions: Speech Therapist
- Detailed Chapter Outline
- Answers to Questions for Study and Review
- Audio Pronunciation Glossary

Learning ACTIVITIES

- Pre-Quiz
- Visual Activities
- Kinesthetic Activities
- Auditory Activities

Learning Outcomes

After careful study of this chapter, you should be able to:

1. Give the location of the four main divisions of the brain, ***p. 170***
2. Name and describe the three meninges, ***p. 172***
3. Cite the function of cerebrospinal fluid and describe where and how this fluid is formed, ***p. 172***
4. Name and locate the lobes of the cerebral hemispheres, ***p. 173***
5. Cite one function of the cerebral cortex in each lobe of the cerebrum, ***p. 174***
6. Name two divisions of the diencephalon and cite the functions of each, ***p. 178***
7. Locate the three subdivisions of the brain stem and give the functions of each, ***p. 178***
8. Describe the cerebellum and identify its functions, ***p. 179***
9. Describe four techniques used to study the brain, ***p. 180***
10. List the names and functions of the 12 cranial nerves, ***p. 181***
11. Match some of the patient's signs and symptoms in the case study to the parts of his brain that were damaged by the stroke, ***pp. 168, 183***
12. Show how word parts are used to build words related to the nervous system (see Word Anatomy at the end of the chapter), ***p. 185***

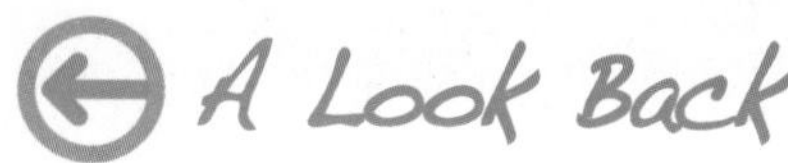

Having discussed the basics of nerve impulse conduction and the reflex arc, we now apply these fundamentals to a look at how the various brain regions coordinate information and orchestrate responses. As you might guess, this is a very complex topic, affecting activities from the cellular level to the highest abstract brain function.

Overview of the Brain

The brain is the control center of the nervous system, where sensory information is processed, responses are coordinated, and the higher functions of reasoning, learning, and memory occur. The brain occupies the cranial cavity and is surrounded by membranes, fluid, and the skull bones.

DIVISIONS OF THE BRAIN

For study purposes, the brain can be divided into four regions with specific activities. These divisions are in constant communication as they work together to regulate body functions (Fig. 9-1):

- The **cerebrum** (SER-e-brum) is the most superior and largest part of the brain. It is such a predominant portion of the brain that people often mean the cerebrum when they refer to "the brain."
- The **diencephalon** (di-en-SEF-ah-lon) is the area between the cerebral hemispheres and the brain stem. It includes the thalamus and the hypothalamus.
- The **brain stem** connects the cerebrum and diencephalon with the spinal cord. The superior portion of the brain stem is the **midbrain.** Inferior to the midbrain is the **pons** (ponz), followed by the **medulla oblongata** (meh-DUL-lah ob-long-GAH-tah). The pons connects the midbrain with the medulla, whereas the medulla connects the brain with the spinal cord through a large opening in the base of the skull (foramen magnum).
- The **cerebellum** (ser-eh-BEL-um) is located immediately below the posterior part of the cerebral hemispheres and is connected with the cerebrum, brain stem, and spinal cord by means of the pons. The word *cerebellum* means "little brain."

Each of these divisions is described in greater detail later in this chapter and summarized in Table 9-1 as a general chapter reference. See also Dissection Atlas A3-3.

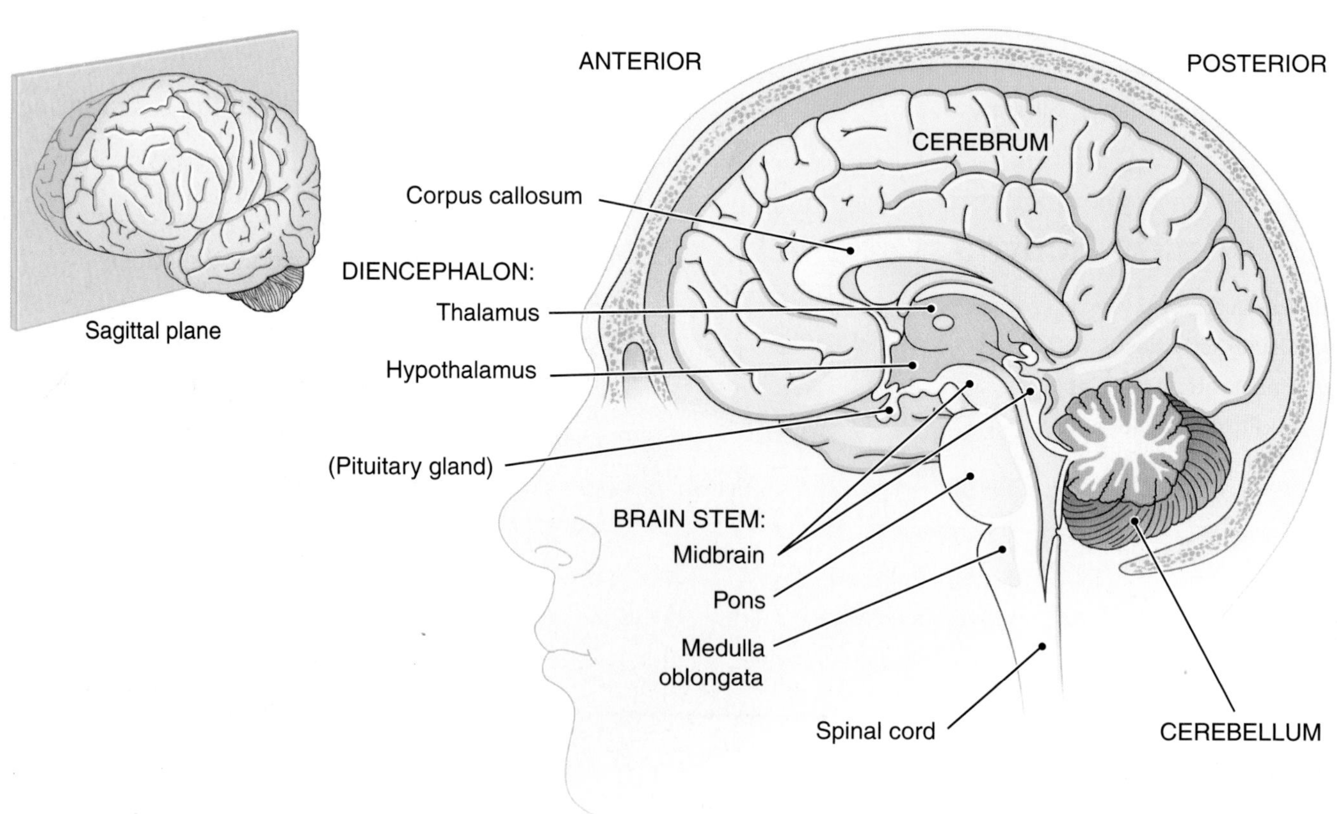

Figure 9-1 **Brain, sagittal section.** KEY POINT The four main divisions of the brain are the cerebrum, diencephalon, brain stem, and cerebellum. The pituitary gland is closely associated with the brain. ZOOMING IN What is the largest part of the brain? What part connects with the spinal cord?

Table 9-1 Organization of the Brain

Division	Description	Functions
CEREBRUM	Largest and most superior portion of the brain Divided into two hemispheres, each subdivided into lobes	Cortex (outer layer) is site for conscious thought, memory, reasoning, and abstract mental functions, all localized within specific lobes
DIENCEPHALON	Between the cerebrum and the brain stem Contains the thalamus and hypothalamus	Thalamus sorts and redirects sensory input. Hypothalamus maintains homeostasis, controls autonomic nervous system and pituitary gland
BRAIN STEM	Anterior region below the cerebrum	Connects cerebrum and diencephalon with spinal cord
Midbrain	Below the center of the cerebrum	Has reflex centers concerned with vision and hearing. Connects cerebrum with lower portions of the brain
Pons	Anterior to the cerebellum	Connects cerebellum with other portions of the brain. Helps to regulate respiration
Medulla oblongata	Between the pons and the spinal cord	Links the brain with the spinal cord. Has centers for control of vital functions, such as respiration and the heartbeat
CEREBELLUM	Below the posterior portion of the cerebrum Divided into two hemispheres	Coordinates voluntary muscles. Maintains balance and muscle tone

PROTECTIVE STRUCTURES OF THE BRAIN AND SPINAL CORD

The protective structures of the brain include the meninges, the cerebrospinal fluid (CSF), and the ventricles. Both the meninges and the CSF also protect the spinal cord.

Meninges The **meninges** (men-IN-jez) are three layers of connective tissue that surround both the brain and spinal cord to form a complete enclosure **(Fig. 9-2)**. The outermost of these membranes, the **dura mater** (DU-rah MA-ter), is the thickest and toughest of the meninges. (*Mater* is from the Latin meaning "mother," referring to the protective function of the meninges; *dura* means "hard.") Around the brain, the dura mater is in two layers, and the outer layer is fused to the cranial bones. In certain places, these two layers separate to provide venous channels, called **dural sinuses**, for the drainage of blood coming from the brain tissue. The dura is in a single layer around the spinal cord.

The middle layer of the meninges is the **arachnoid** (ah-RAK-noyd). This membrane is loosely attached to the deepest of the meninges by weblike fibers, allowing a space for the movement of CSF between these two membranes. (The arachnoid is named from the Latin word for spider because of its weblike appearance.)

The innermost layer around the brain, the **pia mater** (PI-ah MA-ter), is attached to the nervous tissue of the brain and spinal cord and follows all the contours of these structures **(see Fig. 9-2)**. The pia is made of a delicate connective tissue (*pia* meaning "tender" or "soft"). It holds blood vessels that supply nutrients and oxygen to the brain and spinal cord.

Cerebrospinal Fluid **Cerebrospinal** (ser-e-bro-SPI-nal) **fluid** (CSF) is a clear liquid that circulates in and around the brain and spinal cord **(Fig. 9-3)**. The function of the CSF is to support nervous tissue and to cushion shocks that would otherwise injure these delicate structures. This fluid also carries nutrients to the cells and transports waste products from the cells.

CSF flows freely through passageways in and around the brain and spinal cord and finally flows out into the subarachnoid space of the meninges. Much of the fluid then returns to the blood through projections called *arachnoid villi* in the dural sinuses **(see Figs. 9-2 and 9-3)**.

Ventricles CSF forms in four spaces within the brain called **ventricles** (VEN-trih-klz) **(Fig. 9-4)**. A vascular network in each ventricle, the **choroid** (KOR-oyd) **plexus**, forms CSF by filtration of the blood and by cellular secretion.

The four ventricles that produce CSF extend somewhat irregularly into the various parts of the brain. The first two, the largest, are the lateral ventricles in the two cerebral hemispheres. Their extensions into the lobes of the cerebrum are called **horns**. These paired ventricles communicate with a midline space, the third ventricle, by means of openings called **interventricular foramina** (fo-RAM-in-ah). The third ventricle is surrounded by the diencephalon. Continuing down from the third ventricle,

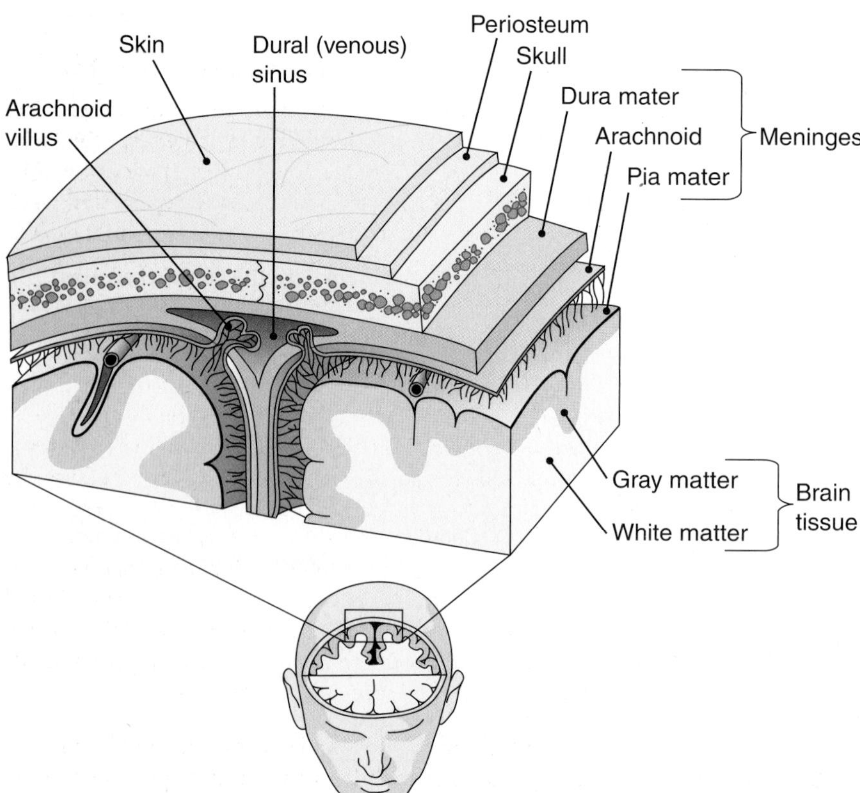

Figure 9-2 Frontal (coronal) section of the top of the head. The meninges and related parts are shown. KEY POINT The brain has many layers of protective substances. ZOOMING IN What are the channels formed where the dura mater divides into two layers? How many layers of meninges are there?

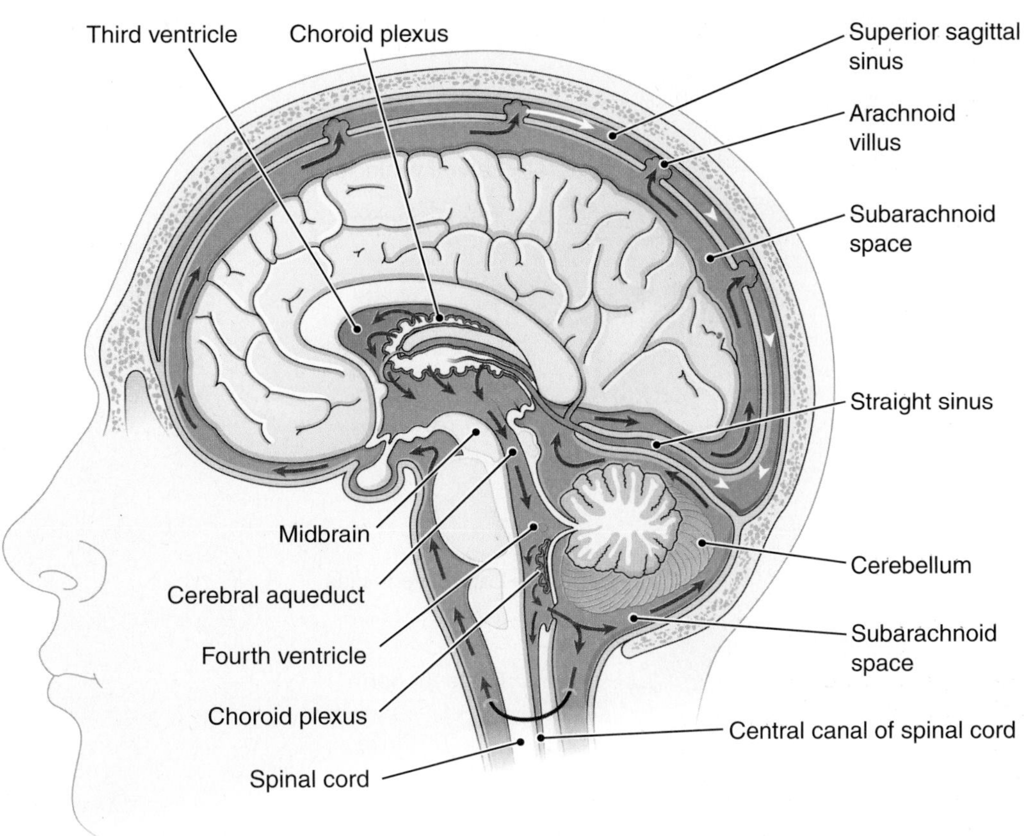

Figure 9-3 **Flow of cerebrospinal fluid (CSF).** KEY POINT Black arrows show the flow of CSF from the choroid plexuses and back to the blood in dural sinuses; white arrows show the flow of blood. (The actual passageways through which the CSF flows are narrower than those shown here, which have been enlarged for visibility.) ZOOMING IN Which ventricle is continuous with the central canal of the spinal cord?

a small canal, the **cerebral aqueduct**, extends through the midbrain into the fourth ventricle, which is located between the brain stem and the cerebellum. This ventricle is continuous with the central canal of the spinal cord. In the roof of the fourth ventricle are three openings that allow the escape of CSF to the area that surrounds the brain and spinal cord.

Boxes 9-1 and 9-2 present information on protecting the brain.

CHECKPOINTS 

- 9-1 What are the main divisions of the brain?
- 9-2 What are the names of the three layers of the meninges from the outermost to the innermost?
- 9-3 Where is CSF produced?

The Cerebrum

The cerebrum, the brain's largest portion, is divided into right and left cerebral (SER-e-bral) hemispheres by a deep groove called the longitudinal fissure **(Fig. 9-5)**. The two hemispheres have overlapping functions and are similarly subdivided.

DIVISIONS OF THE CEREBRAL HEMISPHERES

Each cerebral hemisphere is divided into four visible **lobes** named for the overlying cranial bones. These are the frontal, parietal, temporal, and occipital lobes **(see Fig. 9-5B)**. In addition, there is a small fifth lobe deep within each hemisphere that cannot be seen from the surface. Not much is known about this lobe, which is called the **insula** (IN-su-lah).

The outer nervous tissue of the cerebral hemispheres is gray matter that comprises the **cerebral cortex (see Fig. 9-2)**. This thin layer of gray matter (2 to 4 mm thick) is the most highly evolved portion of the brain and is responsible for conscious thought, reasoning, and abstract mental functions. Specific functions are localized in the cortex of the different lobes, as described in greater detail later.

The cortex is arranged in folds forming elevated portions known as **gyri** (JI-ri), singular *gyrus*. These raised areas are separated by shallow grooves called **sulci** (SUL-si), singular *sulcus*. Although there are many sulci, the following two are especially important landmarks:

- the **central sulcus**, which lies between the frontal and parietal lobes of each hemisphere at right angles to the longitudinal fissure **(see Fig. 9-5)**

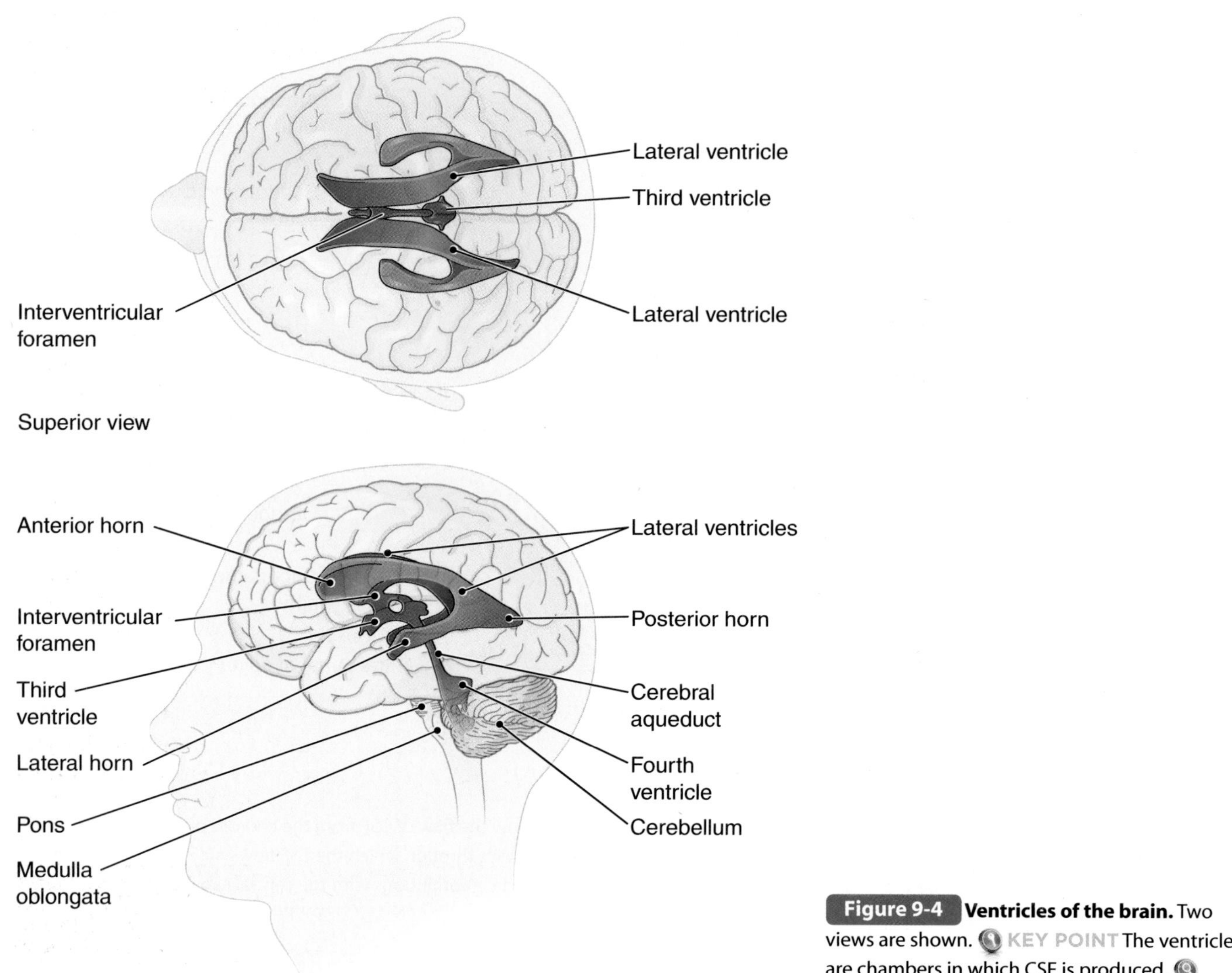

Figure 9-4 Ventricles of the brain. Two views are shown. KEY POINT The ventricles are chambers in which CSF is produced. ZOOMING IN Which are the largest ventricles?

- the **lateral sulcus,** which curves along the side of each hemisphere and separates the temporal lobe from the frontal and parietal lobes (see Fig. 9-5)

Internally, the cerebral hemispheres are made largely of white matter and a few islands of gray matter. The white matter consists of myelinated fibers that connect the cortical areas with each other and with other parts of the nervous system.

Basal nuclei, also called *basal ganglia*, are masses of gray matter located deep within each cerebral hemisphere. These groups of neurons work with the cerebral cortex to regulate body movement and the muscles of facial expression. The neurons of the basal nuclei secrete the neurotransmitter **dopamine** (DO-pah-mene).

The **corpus callosum** (kah-LO-sum) is an important band of white matter located at the bottom of the longitudinal fissure (see Fig. 9-1). This band is a bridge between the right and left hemispheres, permitting impulses to cross from one side of the brain to the other.

FUNCTIONS OF THE CEREBRAL CORTEX

It is within the cerebral cortex that nerve impulses are received and analyzed. These activities form the basis of knowledge. The brain "stores" information, much of which can be recalled on demand by means of the phenomenon called *memory*. It is in the cerebral cortex that thought processes such as association, judgment, and discrimination take place. Conscious deliberation and voluntary actions also arise from the cerebral cortex.

Although the various brain areas act in coordination to produce behavior, particular functions are localized in the cortex of each lobe (Fig. 9-6). Some of these are described below:

- The **frontal lobe,** which is relatively larger in humans than in any other organism, lies anterior to the central sulcus. The gyrus just anterior to the central sulcus in this lobe contains a **primary motor area,** which provides conscious control of skeletal muscles. Specific segments of the primary motor area control the muscles in

Box 9-1 *A Closer Look*

The Blood–Brain Barrier: Access Denied

Neurons in the central nervous system (CNS) function properly only if the composition of the extracellular fluid bathing them is carefully regulated. The semipermeable blood–brain barrier helps maintain this stable environment by allowing some substances to cross it while blocking others. Whereas it allows glucose, amino acids, and some electrolytes to cross, it prevents passage of hormones, drugs, neurotransmitters, and other substances that might adversely affect the brain.

Structural features of CNS capillaries create this barrier. In most parts of the body, capillaries are lined with simple squamous epithelial cells that are loosely attached to each other. The small spaces between cells let materials move between the bloodstream and the tissues. In CNS capillaries, the simple squamous epithelial cells are joined by tight junctions that limit passage of materials between them.

The blood–brain barrier excludes pathogens, although some viruses, including poliovirus and herpesvirus, can bypass it by traveling along peripheral nerves into the CNS. Some streptococci also can breach the tight junctions. Disease processes, such as hypertension, ischemia (lack of blood supply), and inflammation, can increase the blood–brain barrier's permeability.

The blood–brain barrier is an obstacle to delivering drugs to the brain. Some antibiotics can cross it, whereas others cannot. Neurotransmitters also pose problems. In Parkinson disease, the neurotransmitter dopamine is deficient in the brain. Dopamine itself will not cross the barrier, but a related compound, L-dopa, will. L-dopa crosses the blood–brain barrier and is then converted to dopamine. Mixing a drug with a concentrated sugar solution and injecting it into the bloodstream is another effective delivery method. The solution's high osmotic pressure causes water to osmose out of capillary cells, shrinking them and opening tight junctions through which the drug can pass.

different body regions. Relatively larger portions of the cortex are devoted to muscles requiring precise control, such as those of the hand. A large region of the frontal lobe is involved in planning and conscious thought. This lobe also contains two areas important in speech (the speech centers are discussed later).

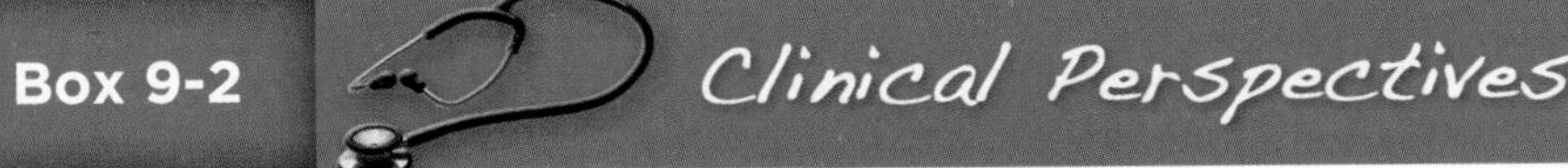

Brain Injury: A Heads-Up

Traumatic brain injury is a leading cause of death and disability in the United States. Each year, approximately 1.5 million Americans sustain a brain injury, of whom about 50,000 will die and 80,000 will suffer long-term or permanent disability. The leading causes of traumatic brain injury are motor vehicle accidents, gun shot wounds, sports injuries, and falls. Other causes include shaken baby syndrome (caused by violent shaking of an infant or toddler) and second impact syndrome (when a second head injury occurs before the first has fully healed).

Brain damage occurs either from penetrating head trauma or acceleration–deceleration events where a head in motion suddenly comes to a stop. Nervous tissue, blood vessels, and possibly the meninges may be bruised, torn, lacerated, or ruptured, which may lead to swelling, hemorrhage, and hematoma. The best protection from brain injury is to prevent it. The following is a list of safety tips:

- Always wear a seat belt and secure children in approved car seats.
- Never drive after using alcohol or drugs or ride with an impaired driver.
- Always wear a helmet during activities such as biking, motorcycling, in-line skating, horseback riding, football, ice hockey, and batting and running bases in baseball and softball.
- Inspect playground equipment and supervise children using it. Never swing children around to play "airplane," nor vigorously bounce or shake them.
- Allow adequate time for healing after a head injury before resuming potentially dangerous activities.
- Prevent falls by using a nonslip bathtub or shower mat and using a step stool to reach objects on high shelves. Use a safety gate at the bottom and top of stairs to protect young children (and adults with dementia or other disorienting conditions).
- Keep unloaded firearms in a locked cabinet or safe and store bullets in a separate location.

For more information, contact the Brain Injury Association of America.

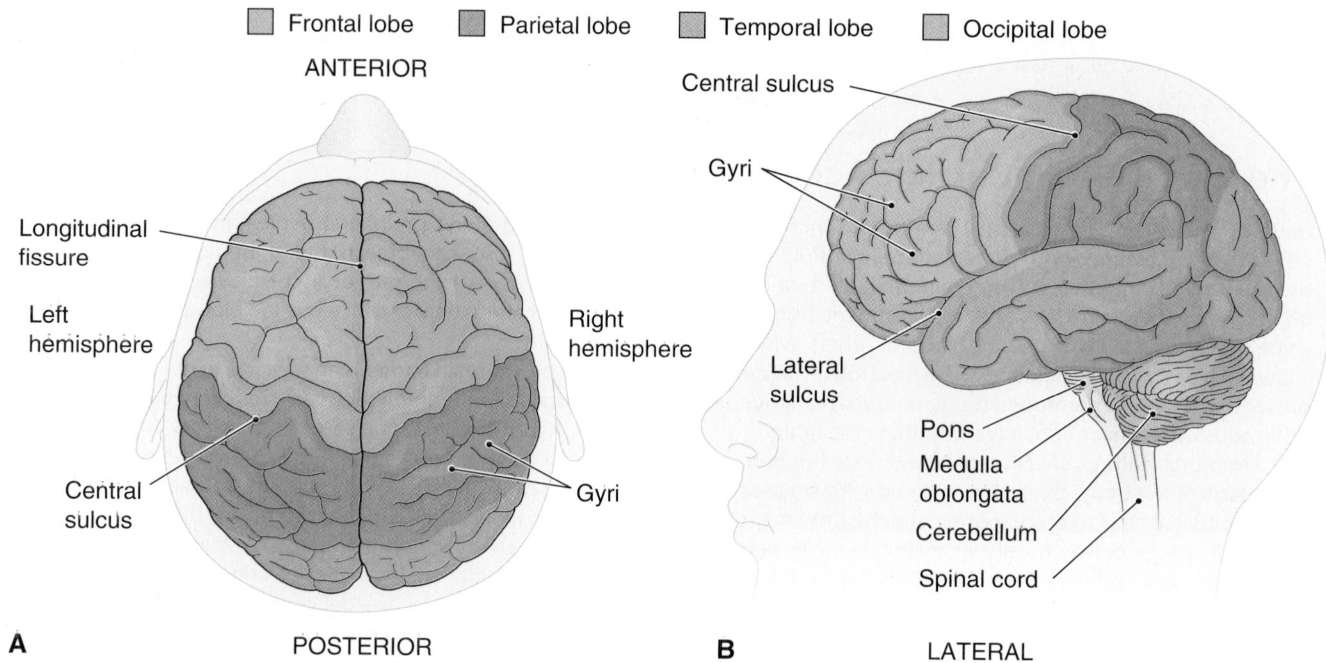

Figure 9-5 External surface of the brain. A. Superior view. **B.** Lateral view. KEY POINT The brain is divided into two hemispheres by the longitudinal fissure. Each hemisphere is subdivided into lobes. ZOOMING IN What structure separates the frontal from the parietal lobe? The temporal lobe from the frontal and parietal lobes?

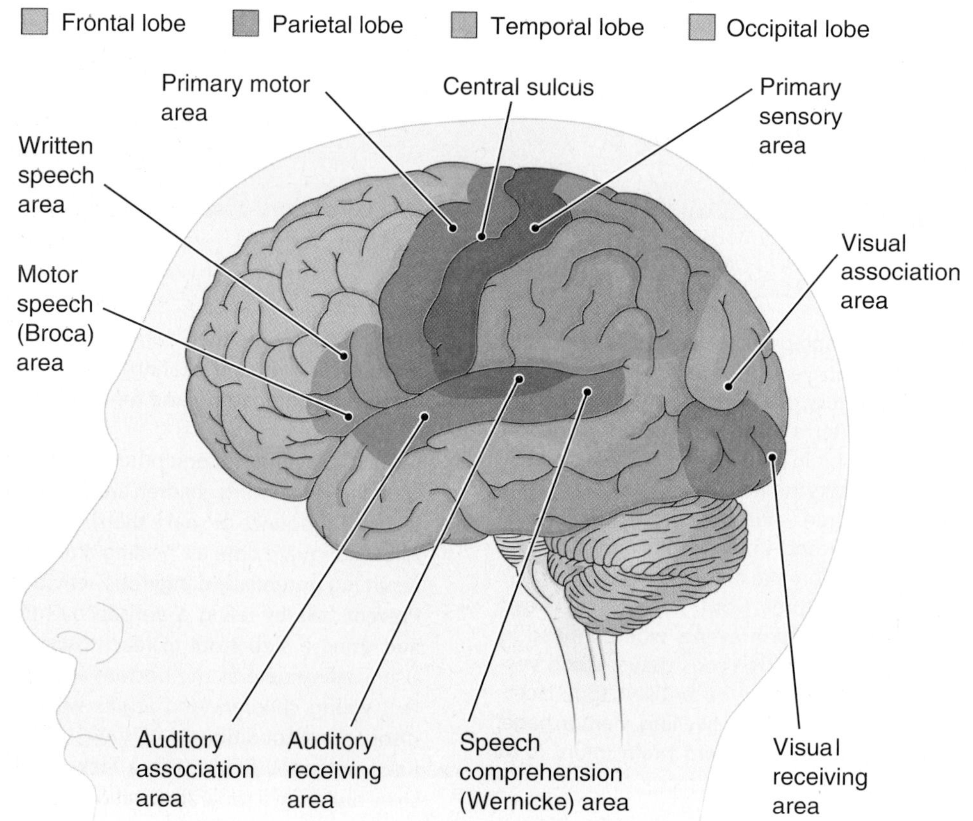

Figure 9-6 Functional areas of the cerebral cortex. KEY POINT Regions of the cerebral cortex are specialized for specific functions. ZOOMING IN What cortical area is posterior to the central sulcus? What area is anterior to the central sulcus?

- The **parietal lobe** occupies the superior part of each hemisphere and lies posterior to the central sulcus. A large region of the parietal lobe integrates information from all sensory areas. The estimation of distances, sizes, and shapes also takes place here. The gyrus just behind the central sulcus in this lobe contains the **primary sensory area**, where impulses from the skin, such as touch, pain, and temperature, are interpreted. As with the motor cortex, the greater the intensity of sensation from a particular area, the tongue or fingers, for example, the more area of the cortex is involved.
- The **temporal lobe** lies inferior to the lateral sulcus and folds under the hemisphere on each side. This lobe contains the auditory areas for receiving and interpreting impulses from the ear. The olfactory area, concerned with the sense of smell, is located in the medial part of the temporal lobe and is not visible from the surface; it is stimulated by impulses arising from receptors in the nose.
- The **occipital lobe** lies posterior to the parietal lobe and extends over the cerebellum. This lobe contains areas for interpreting impulses arising from the retina of the eye.

COMMUNICATION AREAS

The ability to communicate by written and verbal means is an interesting example of how areas of the cerebral cortex are interrelated (see Fig. 9-6). The development and use of these areas are closely connected with the learning process.

- One of the temporal auditory areas, the **auditory receiving area**, detects sound impulses transmitted from the environment, whereas the surrounding area, the **auditory association area**, interprets the sounds. Note that an association area integrates all of the input the cortex receives for a particular sense, such as integrating the pitch, loudness, and direction of sound. Another region of the auditory cortex, located on the left side in most people, is the *speech comprehension area*, or **Wernicke** (VER-nih-ke) **area**. This area functions in speech recognition and the meaning of words. Someone who suffers damage in this region of the brain, as by a stroke, will have difficulty in understanding the meaning of speech. The beginnings of language are learned by hearing; thus, the auditory areas for understanding sounds are near the auditory receiving area of the cortex. Babies often appear to understand what is being said long before they do any talking themselves. It is usually several years before children learn to read or write words.
- The visual areas of the occipital cortex are also involved in communication. Here, in the **visual receiving area**, visual images of language are collected. The **visual association area** that lies anterior to the visual receiving cortex then interprets these visual impulses as words. The ability to read with understanding also develops in this area. You might *see* writing in the Japanese language, for example, but this would involve only the visual receiving area in the occipital lobe unless you could also *understand* the words.
- The motor areas for spoken and written communication lie anterior to the most inferior part of the frontal lobe's motor cortex. The specialized cortical region known as the ***motor speech area***, or **Broca** (bro-KAH) **area**, plans the sequences of muscle contractions in the tongue, larynx, and soft palate required to form meaningful sentences. People with damage in this area can understand sentences but have trouble expressing their ideas in words. Similarly, the written speech center lies anterior to the cortical area that controls the arm and hand muscles. The ability to write words is usually one of the last phases in the development of learning words and their meanings.

There is a functional relation among areas of the brain. Many neurons must work together to enable a person to receive, interpret, and respond to verbal and written messages as well as to touch (tactile stimulus) and other sensory stimuli.

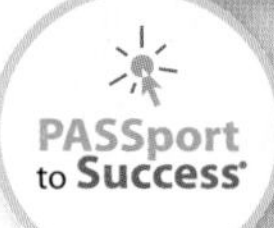

Speech therapists help to treat patients with language or communication problems from any cause. See the Student Resources on *thePoint* for more information on this career.

MEMORY AND THE LEARNING PROCESS

Memory is the mental faculty for recalling ideas. In the initial stage of the memory process, sensory signals (e.g., visual, auditory) are retained for a very short time, perhaps only fractions of a second. Nevertheless, they can be used for further processing. **Short-term memory** refers to the retention of bits of information for a few seconds or perhaps a few minutes, after which the information is lost unless reinforced. **Long-term memory** refers to the storage of information that can be recalled at a later time. There is a tendency for a memory to become more fixed the more often a person repeats the remembered experience; thus, short-term memory signals can lead to long-term memories. Furthermore, the more often a memory is recalled, the more indelible it becomes; such a memory can be so deeply fixed in the brain that it can be recalled immediately.

Physiologic studies show that rehearsal (repetition) of the same information again and again accelerates and potentiates the degree of short-term memory transfer into long-term memory. It has also been noted that the brain is able to organize information so that new ideas are stored in the same areas in which similar ones had been stored before.

Along the border between the cerebrum and the diencephalon is a region known as the **limbic system**. This system is involved in emotional states and behavior. It is also important for the formation of short-term memories and the consolidation of long-term memories, and thus is essential to learning. It includes the *hippocampus* (shaped like a sea horse), located under the lateral ventricles, and the *amygdala*, two clusters of nuclei deep in the temporal lobes.

The limbic system also includes regions that stimulate the *reticular formation*, a network of ascending and descending tracts that extends from the upper spinal cord through the brain stem to the diencephalon. This system includes the **reticular activating system** (**RAS**), which has sensory neurons that travel to the cerebral cortex to govern wakefulness and sleep. The limbic system thus links the conscious functions of the cerebral cortex and the autonomic functions of the brain stem.

CHECKPOINTS 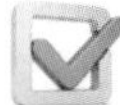

9-4 What are the four surface lobes of each cerebral hemisphere?

9-5 What is the name of the thin outer layer of gray matter where higher brain functions occur?

The Diencephalon

The **diencephalon**, or interbrain, is located between the cerebral hemispheres and the brain stem. One can see it by cutting into the central and inferior section of the brain. The diencephalon includes the **thalamus** (THAL-ah-mus) and the **hypothalamus** (Fig. 9-7).

The two parts of the thalamus form the lateral walls of the third ventricle (see Figs. 9-1 and 9-4). Nearly all sensory impulses travel through the masses of gray matter that form the thalamus. The role of the thalamus is to sort out the impulses and direct them to particular areas of the cerebral cortex.

The hypothalamus is located in the midline area inferior to the thalamus and forms the floor of the third ventricle. It helps to maintain homeostasis by controlling body temperature, water balance, sleep, appetite, and some emotions, such as fear and pleasure. Both the sympathetic and parasympathetic divisions of the autonomic nervous system are under hypothalamic control, as is the pituitary gland. The hypothalamus thus influences the heartbeat, the contraction and relaxation of blood vessels, hormone secretion, and other vital body functions.

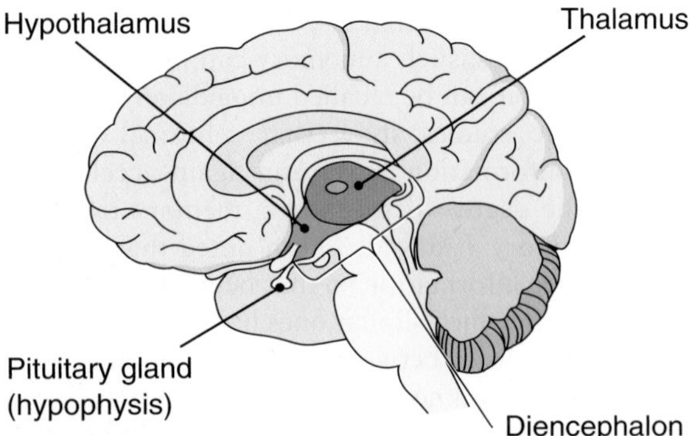

Figure 9-7 Regions of the diencephalon. KEY POINT The figure shows the relationship among the thalamus, hypothalamus, and pituitary gland (hypophysis). ZOOMING IN To what part of the brain is the pituitary gland attached?

CHECKPOINT 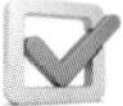

9-6 What are the two main portions of the diencephalon and what do they do?

The Brain Stem

The brain stem is composed of the midbrain, the pons, and the medulla oblongata (Fig. 9-8A). These structures connect the cerebrum and diencephalon with the spinal cord.

THE MIDBRAIN

The **midbrain**, inferior to the center of the cerebrum, forms the superior part of the brain stem (see Fig. 9-8A). Four rounded masses of gray matter that are hidden by the cerebral hemispheres form the superior part of the midbrain. These four bodies act as centers for certain reflexes involving the eye and the ear, for example, moving the eyes in order to track an image or to read. The white matter at the anterior of the midbrain conducts impulses between the higher centers of the cerebrum and the lower centers of the pons, medulla, cerebellum, and spinal cord.

THE PONS

The **pons** lies between the midbrain and the medulla, anterior to the cerebellum (see Fig. 9-8A). It is composed largely of myelinated nerve fibers, which connect the two halves of the cerebellum with the brain stem as well as with the cerebrum above and the spinal cord below. Its name means "bridge," and it is an important connecting link between the cerebellum and the rest of the nervous system. It also contains nerve fibers that carry impulses to and from the centers located above and below it. Certain reflex (involuntary) actions, such as some of those regulating respiration, are integrated in the pons.

THE MEDULLA OBLONGATA

The **medulla oblongata** of the brain stem is located between the pons and the spinal cord (see Fig. 9-8A). It appears white externally because, like the pons, it contains many myelinated nerve fibers. Internally, it contains collections of cell bodies (gray matter) called **nuclei**, or *centers*. Among these are vital centers, such as the following:

- The **respiratory center** controls the muscles of respiration in response to chemical and other stimuli.
- The **cardiac center** helps regulate the rate and force of the heartbeat.
- The **vasomotor** (vas-o-MO-tor) **center** regulates the contraction of smooth muscle in the blood vessel walls and thus controls blood flow and blood pressure.

The ascending sensory fibers that carry messages through the spinal cord up to the brain travel through the medulla,

ANTERIOR
Cerebral aqueduct
POSTERIOR
Midbrain
Pons
Fourth ventricle
Medulla oblongata
Central canal of spinal cord
White matter
Gray matter
Cerebellum
A

Vermis
Left hemisphere
Right hemisphere
POSTERIOR
B

Figure 9-8 The brain stem and cerebellum. A. Midsagittal section. KEY POINT The brain stem has three divisions: the midbrain, pons, and medulla oblongata. The white matter of the cerebellum is in a treelike pattern. **B.** Posterior view of the cerebellum. KEY POINT The cerebellum is divided into two hemispheres.

as do descending motor fibers. These groups of fibers form tracts (bundles) and are grouped together according to function.

The motor fibers from the motor cortex of the cerebral hemispheres extend down through the medulla, and most of them cross from one side to the other (decussate) while going through this part of the brain. The crossing of motor fibers in the medulla results in *contralateral* (opposite side) *control*—the right cerebral hemisphere controls muscles in the left side of the body and the left cerebral hemisphere controls muscles in the right side of the body. Read about this in the follow-up to Frank's case of stroke.

The medulla is an important reflex center; here, certain neurons end, and impulses are relayed to other neurons.

CHECKPOINT  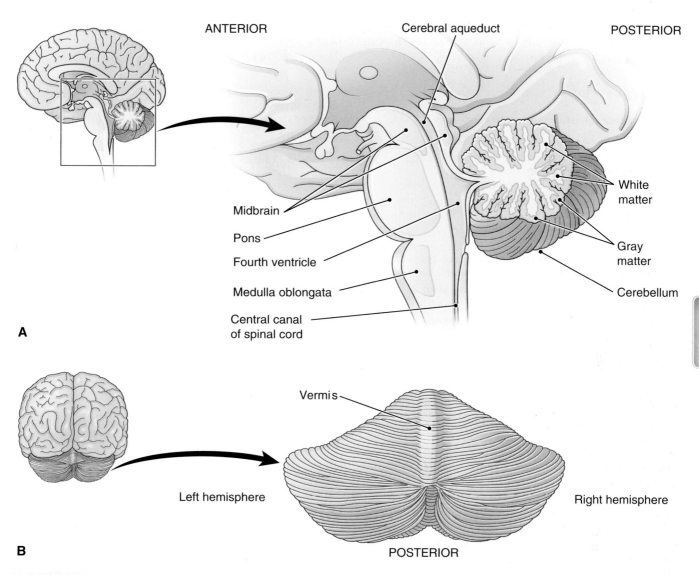

☐ 9-7 What are the three subdivisions of the brain stem?

The Cerebellum

The **cerebellum** is made up of three parts: the middle portion (vermis) and two lateral hemispheres, the left and right (see Fig. 9-8B). Like the cerebral hemispheres, the cerebellum has an outer area of gray matter and an inner portion that is largely white matter (see Fig. 9-8A). However, the white matter is distributed in a treelike pattern. The functions of the cerebellum are as follows:

- Help coordinate voluntary muscles to ensure smooth, orderly function. Disease of the cerebellum causes muscular jerkiness and tremors.
- Help maintain balance in standing, walking, and sitting as well as during more strenuous activities. Messages from the internal ear and from sensory receptors in tendons and muscles aid the cerebellum.

- Help maintain muscle tone so that all muscle fibers are slightly tensed and ready to produce changes in position as quickly as necessary.

CHECKPOINT 

9-8 What are some functions of the cerebellum?

Brain Studies

Some of the imaging techniques used to study the brain are described in **Box 1-2** in Chapter 1. These techniques include

- CT (computed tomography) scan, which provides photographs of the bone, soft tissue, and cavities of the brain **(Fig. 9-9A)**. Anatomic lesions, such as tumors or scar tissue accumulations, are readily seen. In Frank's case, a CT scan was used to diagnose a cerebral blood clot.
- MRI (magnetic resonance imaging), which gives more views of the brain than CT and may reveal tumors, scar tissue, and hemorrhaging not shown by CT **(see Fig. 9-9B)**.
- PET (positron emission tomography), which visualizes the brain in action **(see Fig. 9-9C)**.

The interactions of the brain's billions of nerve cells give rise to measurable electric currents. These may be recorded using an instrument called the **electroencephalograph** (e-lek-tro-en-SEF-ah-lo-graf). Electrodes placed on the head pick up the electrical signals produced as the brain functions. These signals are then amplified and recorded to produce the tracings, or brain waves, of an electroencephalogram (EEG).

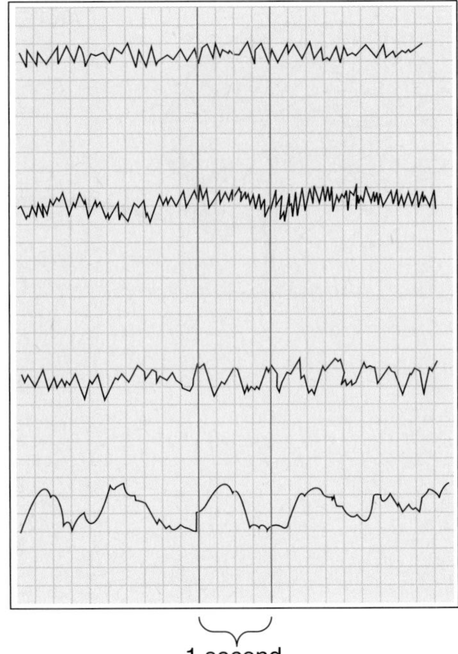

Figure 9-10 **Electroencephalography.** Normal brain waves.

The electroencephalograph is used to study sleep patterns, to diagnose disease, such as epilepsy, to locate tumors, to study the effects of drugs, and to determine brain death. **Figure 9-10** shows some typical normal tracings.

Cranial Nerves

There are 12 pairs of cranial nerves (in this discussion, when a cranial nerve is identified, a pair is meant). They are numbered, usually in Roman numerals, according to

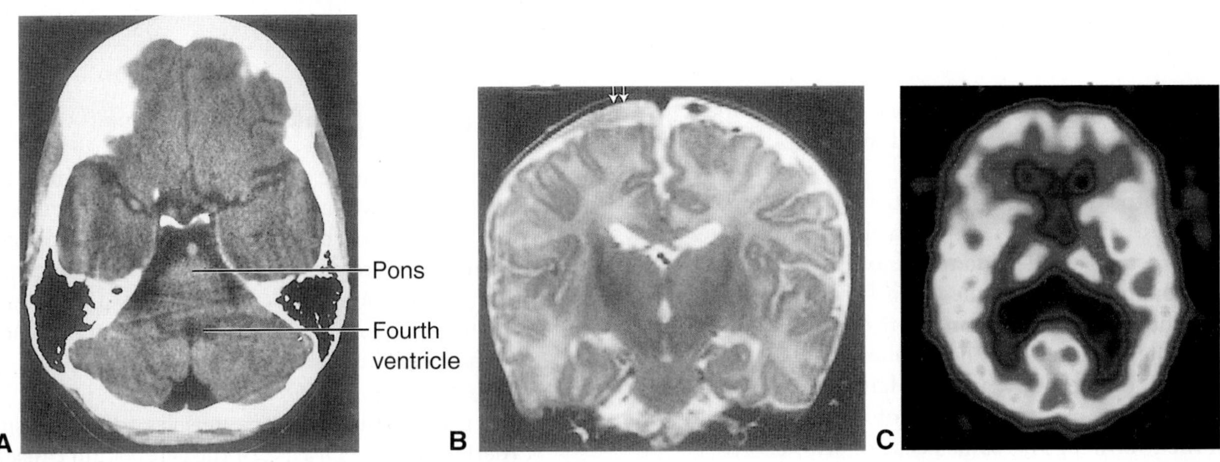

Figure 9-9 **Imaging the brain. A.** CT scan of a normal adult brain at the level of the fourth ventricle. **B.** MRI of the brain showing a point of injury (*arrows*). **C.** PET scan. (A and B, Reprinted with permission from Erkonen WE. *Radiology 101*. Philadelphia, PA: Lippincott Williams & Wilkins, 1998; C, Courtesy of Newport Diagnostic Center, Newport Beach, CA.)

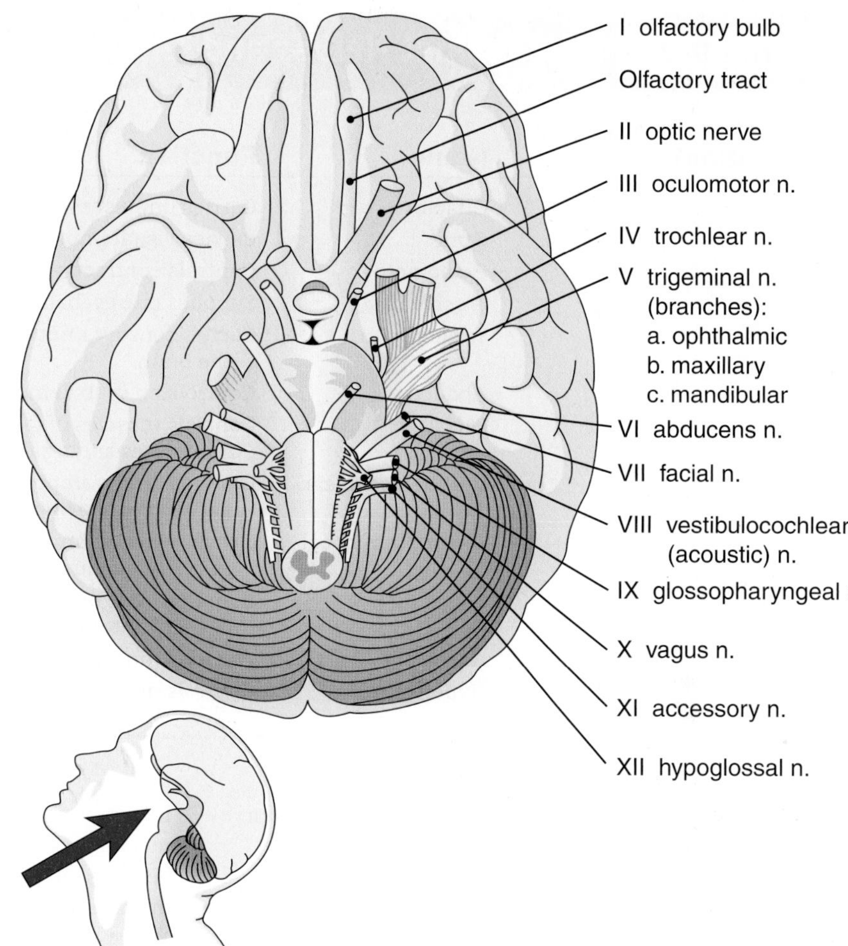

Figure 9-11 Cranial nerves. KEY POINT There are 12 pairs of cranial nerves, each designated by name and Roman numeral. They are shown here from the base of the brain.

9

their connection with the brain, beginning anteriorly and proceeding posteriorly (Fig. 9-11). Except for the first two pairs, which connect with the cerebrum and diencephalon, respectively, all the cranial nerves connect with the brain stem. Also note that anatomists now have found that cranial nerve XI connects with the cervical spinal cord. The first 9 pairs and the 12th pair supply structures in the head.

From a functional viewpoint, we may think of cranial nerve messages as belonging to one of four categories:

- **Special sensory impulses**, such as those for smell, taste, vision, and hearing, located in special sense organs in the head.
- **General sensory impulses**, such as those for pain, touch, temperature, deep muscle sense, pressure, and vibrations. These impulses come from receptors that are widely distributed throughout the body.
- **Somatic motor impulses** resulting in voluntary control of skeletal muscles.
- **Visceral motor impulses** producing involuntary control of glands and involuntary muscles (cardiac and smooth muscle). These motor pathways are part of the autonomic nervous system, parasympathetic division.

NAMES AND FUNCTIONS OF THE CRANIAL NERVES

A few of the cranial nerves (I, II, and VIII) contain only sensory fibers; some (III, IV, VI, XI, and XII) contain all or mostly motor fibers. The remainder (V, VII, IX, and X) contain both sensory and motor fibers; they are known as *mixed nerves*. All 12 nerves are listed below and summarized in Table 9-2:

I. The **olfactory nerve** carries smell impulses from receptors in the nasal mucosa to the brain.
II. The **optic nerve** carries visual impulses from the eye to the brain.
III. The **oculomotor nerve** is concerned with the contraction of most of the eye muscles.
IV. The **trochlear** (TROK-le-ar) **nerve** supplies one eyeball muscle.
V. The **trigeminal** (tri-JEM-in-al) **nerve** is the great sensory nerve of the face and head. It has three branches that transport general sense impulses (e.g., pain, touch, temperature) from the eye, the upper jaw, and the lower jaw. Motor fibers to the muscles of mastication (chewing) join the third branch. It is branches of the trigeminal nerve that a dentist anesthetizes to work on the teeth without causing pain.

Table 9-2 The Cranial Nerves and Their Functions

Nerve (Roman Numeral Designation)	Name	Function
I	Olfactory	Carries impulses for the sense of smell toward the brain
II	Optic	Carries visual impulses from the eye to the brain
III	Oculomotor	Controls contraction of eye muscles
IV	Trochlear	Supplies one eyeball muscle
V	Trigeminal	Carries sensory impulses from eye, upper jaw, and lower jaw toward the brain
VI	Abducens	Controls an eyeball muscle
VII	Facial	Controls muscles of facial expression; carries sensation of taste; stimulates small salivary glands and lacrimal (tear) gland
VIII	Vestibulocochlear	Carries sensory impulses for hearing and equilibrium from the inner ear toward the brain
IX	Glossopharyngeal	Carries sensory impulses from tongue and pharynx (throat); controls swallowing muscles and stimulates the parotid salivary gland
X	Vagus	Supplies most of the organs in the thoracic and abdominal cavities; carries motor impulses to the larynx (voice box) and pharynx
XI	Accessory	Controls muscles in the neck and larynx
XII	Hypoglossal	Controls muscles of the tongue

VI. The **abducens** (ab-DU-senz) **nerve** is another nerve sending controlling impulses to an eyeball muscle.

VII. The **facial nerve** is largely motor. The muscles of facial expression are all supplied by branches from the facial nerve. This nerve also includes special sensory fibers for taste (anterior two-thirds of the tongue), and it contains secretory fibers to the smaller salivary glands (the submandibular and sublingual) and to the lacrimal (tear) gland.

VIII. The **vestibulocochlear** (ves-tib-u-lo-KOK-le-ar) **nerve** carries sensory impulses for hearing and equilibrium from the inner ear. This nerve was formerly called the auditory or acoustic nerve.

IX. The **glossopharyngeal** (glos-o-fah-RIN-je-al) **nerve** contains general sensory fibers from the posterior tongue and the pharynx (throat). This nerve also contains sensory fibers for taste from the posterior third of the tongue, secretory fibers that supply the largest salivary gland (parotid), and motor nerve fibers to control the swallowing muscles in the pharynx.

X. The **vagus** (VA-gus) **nerve** is the longest cranial nerve. (Its name means "wanderer.") It supplies most of the organs in the thoracic and abdominal cavities. This nerve also contains motor fibers supplying the larynx (voice box) and pharynx and also glands that produce digestive juices and other secretions.

XI. The **accessory nerve** (also called the *spinal accessory nerve*) is a motor nerve with two branches. One branch controls two muscles of the neck, the trapezius and sternocleidomastoid; the other supplies muscles of the larynx.

XII. The **hypoglossal nerve**, the last of the 12 cranial nerves, carries impulses controlling the tongue muscles.

It has been traditional for students in medical fields to use mnemonics (ne-MON-iks), or memory devices, to remember lists of terms. These devices are usually words (real or made-up) or sayings formed from the first letter of each item. We've used the example SLUDD for the actions of the parasympathetic system; for the cranial nerves, students use "On Occasion Our Trusty Truck Acts Funny. Very Good Vehicle Any How." Can you and your classmates make up any other mnemonic phrases for the cranial nerves? You can also check the Internet for sites where medical mnemonics are shared, but be forewarned, students often enjoy making them raunchy!

CHECKPOINTS 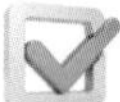

☐ **9-9** How many pairs of cranial nerves are there?

☐ **9-10** What are the three types of cranial nerves? What is a mixed nerve?

Effects of Aging on the Nervous System

The nervous system is one of the first systems to develop in the embryo. By the beginning of the third week of development, the rudiments of the central nervous system (CNS) have appeared. Beginning with maturity, the nervous system begins to undergo changes. The brain begins to decrease in size and weight due to a loss of cells, especially in the cerebral cortex, accompanied by decreases in synapses and neurotransmitters. The speed of processing information decreases, and movements are slowed. Memory diminishes, especially for recent events. Changes in the vascular system throughout the body with a narrowing of the arteries (atherosclerosis) reduce the brain's blood flow. Vascular degeneration increases the likelihood of stroke.

Much individual variation is possible, however, with regard to location and severity of changes. Although age might make it harder to acquire new skills, tests have shown that practice enhances skill retention. As with other body systems, the nervous system has vast reserves, and most elderly people are able to cope with life's demands.

A&P in Action Revisited

Frank's Stroke Recovery

"Good morning Mr. Carter. My name is Ross Baker and I'm a physiotherapist with the Brain Injury Team. My job is to assist your stroke recovery by helping you regain your strength, balance, and coordination. Before we continue, may I test your muscular and sensory functions?"

With Frank's permission, Ross began his assessment. He noted hemiplegia (muscle paralysis) in Frank's right arm and leg. Stroke damage to the primary motor area in the frontal lobe of Frank's *left* cerebral hemisphere had caused motor deficits in his *right* limbs. Loss of contralateral control is typical in stroke patients because most motor fibers from the cerebral cortex cross over (decussate) from one side of the medulla oblongata to the other before continuing down the spinal cord in descending tracts. For Frank, this meant that motor information from his damaged left cerebral hemisphere was not reaching the skeletal muscles of his right limbs.

Ross also noted a diminished sense of touch (hypesthesia) on Frank's right side, which suggested that the stroke had damaged the left parietal lobe's primary sensory area as well. Like motor deficits, contralateral sensory deficits are typical in stroke patients, because sensory fibers that enter one side of the spinal cord immediately cross over to the opposite side before continuing up the cord in ascending pathways. As a result, sensory information from Frank's right side was not processed in his left cerebral cortex.

Ross used his understanding of brain and spinal cord anatomy to make sense of Frank's symptoms. Based on his assessment of Frank's motor and sensory deficits, Ross will devise and implement a rehabilitation plan for him. Other allied health professionals like occupational and speech therapists will also help Frank recover from his stroke. See *thePoint* or see the Student Resource DVD in the back of this book for more information on these and other health professions careers.

Chapter Wrap-Up

Summary Overview

A detailed chapter outline with space for note-taking is on *thePoint*. The figure below illustrates the main topics covered in this chapter.

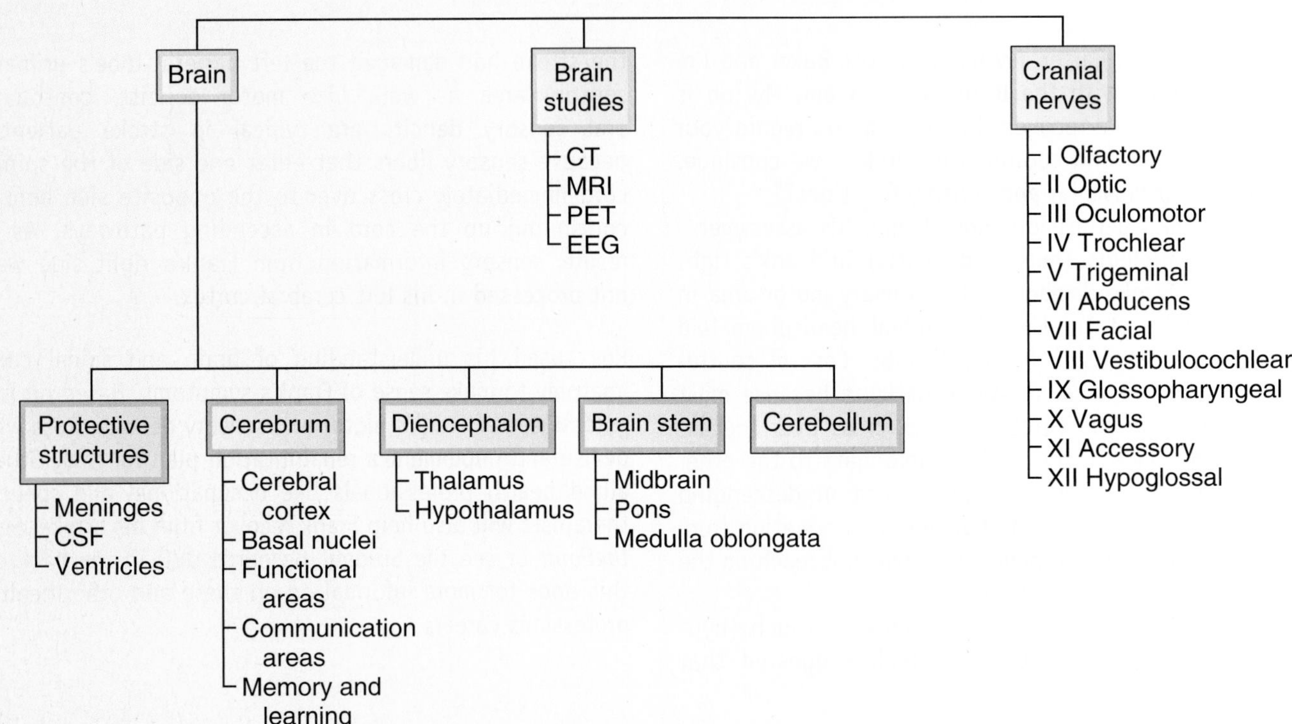

Key Terms

The terms listed below are emphasized in this chapter. Knowing them will help you organize and prioritize your learning. These and other boldface terms are defined in the Glossary with phonetic pronunciations.

basal nuclei
brain stem
cerebellum
cerebral cortex
cerebrospinal fluid (CSF)
cerebrum
corpus callosum
diencephalon
electroencephalograph (EEG)
gyrus (pl. gyri)
hypothalamus
limbic system
medulla oblongata
meninges
midbrain
pons
reticular activating system
sulcus (pl. sulci)
thalamus
ventricle

Word Anatomy

Scientific terms are built from standardized word parts (prefixes, roots, and suffixes). Learning the meanings of these parts can help you remember words and interpret unfamiliar terms.

WORD PART	MEANING	EXAMPLE
Protective structures of the brain and spinal cord		
cerebr/o	brain	*Cerebrospinal* fluid circulates around the brain and spinal cord.
chori/o	membrane	The *choroid* plexus is the vascular membrane in the ventricle that produces CSF.
gyr/o	circle	A *gyrus* is a circular raised area on the surface of the brain.
encephal/o	brain	The *diencephalon* is the part of the brain located between the cerebral hemispheres and the brain stem.
contra-	opposed, against	The cerebral cortex has *contralateral* control of motor function.
later/o	lateral, side	See preceding example.
Brain Studies		
tom/o	cut	*Tomography* is a method for viewing sections as if cut through the body.
Cranial Nerves		
gloss/o	tongue	The *hypoglossal* nerve controls muscles of the tongue.

Questions for Study and Review

BUILDING UNDERSTANDING

Fill in the blanks

1. The thickest and toughest layer of the meninges is the _____.
2. The third and fourth ventricles are connected by a small canal called the _____.
3. The muscles of speech are controlled by a region in the _____ lobe.
4. The band of white matter that permits impulses to cross from one hemisphere to the other is called the _____.
5. The thalamus and hypothalamus are parts of the division of the brain termed the _____.

Matching > Match each numbered item with the most closely related lettered item.

___ **6.** The sensory nerve of the face
___ **7.** The motor nerve of the muscles of facial expression
___ **8.** The sensory nerve for hearing and equilibrium
___ **9.** The motor nerve for swallowing
___ **10.** The motor nerve for digestion

a. trigeminal nerve
b. facial nerve
c. vestibulocochlear nerve
d. glossopharyngeal nerve
e. vagus nerve

Multiple Choice

___ **11.** What divides the cerebrum into left and right hemispheres?
a. central sulcus
b. insula
c. lateral sulcus
d. longitudinal fissure

___ **12.** Which lobe interprets impulses arising from the retina of the eye?
a. frontal
b. occipital
c. parietal
d. temporal

___ **13.** Which brain structure is associated with learning and memory?
a. hypothalamus
b. hippocampus
c. internal capsule
d. basal ganglia

___ **14.** Which imaging technique visualizes brain function?
a. computed tomography
b. electroencephalography
c. positron emission tomography
d. radiography

___ **15.** What type of impulse are pain messages?
a. special sensory
b. general sensory
c. somatic motor
d. visceral motor

UNDERSTANDING CONCEPTS

16. Briefly describe the effects of injury to the following brain areas:
a. cerebrum
b. diencephalon
c. brain stem
d. cerebellum

17. A neurosurgeon has drilled a hole through her patient's skull and is preparing to remove a cerebral glioma. List, in order, the membranes she must cut through to reach the cerebral cortex.

18. Compare and contrast the functions of the following structures:
a. frontal lobe and parietal lobe
b. temporal lobe and occipital lobe
c. thalamus and hypothalamus

19. What is the function of the limbic system? Describe the effect of damage to the hippocampus.

20. Compare and contrast short-term memory and long-term memory.

21. The term cerebellum means "little cerebrum." Why is this an appropriate term?

22. Make a table of the 12 cranial nerves and their functions. According to your table, which ones are sensory, motor, or mixed?

CONCEPTUAL THINKING

23. The parents of Molly R. (a 2-month-old girl) are informed that their daughter requires a shunt to drain excess CSF from her brain. What would happen to Molly if the shunt was not put in place?

24. In the case story, Frank suffered a stroke in his left cerebrum. Why were many of his symptoms isolated to the right side of his body?

25. In Frank's case, stroke damage was isolated to his cerebrum. Some strokes, though, can affect the brain stem. Why is damage to this part of the brain life threatening?

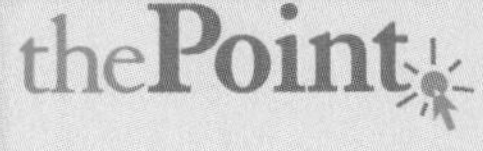

For more questions, see the learning activities on *thePoint.*

CHAPTER 10

The Sensory System

A&P in Action

Paul's Second Case: Seeing More of the Sun's Effects

Paul glanced at the postcard sitting on his entranceway table as he arrived home in the evening. It said he was due for a checkup with his ophthalmologist, but after his run-in with skin cancer a few months earlier, he was in no hurry to see the inside of a medical office. *Well, it's just routine, and I may need a slight change in my prescription, so I'll make the call,* he thought.

At the office, Dr. Gilbert greeted Paul and asked how he was feeling in general and if he thought there had been any change in his vision. "My vision sometimes seems a little blurry, especially when my eyes are tired, but no major changes," Paul replied. Dr. Gilbert proceeded with the eye exam, testing his visual acuity (sharpness of vision) and checking on his astigmatism (resulting in blurry vision due to an abnormally curved cornea).

"You're right; not much change," said the ophthalmologist. "But, we'll give you a new prescription for your glasses. At 42, you're a little young for presbyopia—far-sightedness that develops with age—but we'll do the routine check for glaucoma an eye disorder caused by increased pressure of the aqueous humor located in front of your lens. Left untreated, it could cause damage to your retina and result in blindness." The doctor dilated Paul's eyes with drops and examined the fundus of each eye with an ophthalmoscope. In answer to Paul's query, he explained that in this way he could examine the health of the retina and the optic nerve and also look at the vessels at the back of the eye for any signs of diabetes or circulatory problems. In addition, he used a tonometer to measure the pressure of Paul's aqueous humor. "I need to check on another patient," he told Paul. "Then I'll be back to explain what I've found. Just sit in the waiting room for a few minutes, please."

Dr. Gilbert uses his knowledge of the structure and function of the eye to diagnose medical conditions. In this chapter, you learn about the eye and other sensory organs. As well, we examine the consequences of Paul's sun-loving youth on his eyes and vision.

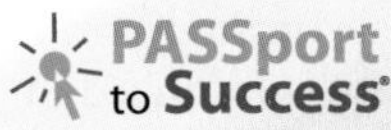

Ancillaries At-A-Glance

Visit *thePoint* to access the PASSport to Success and the following resources. For guidance in using these resources most effectively, see pp. ix–xviii.

Learning TOOLS

- Learning Style Self-Assessment
- Live Advise Online Student Tutoring
- Tips for Effective Studying

Learning RESOURCES

- E-book: Chapter 10
- Animation: The Retina
- Health Professions: Audiologist
- Detailed Chapter Outline
- Answers to Questions for Study and Review
- Audio Pronunciation Glossary

Learning ACTIVITIES

- Pre-Quiz
- Visual Activities
- Kinesthetic Activities
- Auditory Activities

Learning Outcomes

After careful study of this chapter, you should be able to:

1 Describe the function of the sensory system, ***p. 190***

2 Differentiate between the different types of sensory receptors and give examples of each, ***p. 190***

3 Describe sensory adaptation and explain its value, ***p. 190***

4 List and describe the structures that protect the eye, ***p. 191***

5 Identify the three tunics of the eye, ***p. 191***

6 Define *refraction* and list the refractive parts of the eye, ***p. 192***

7 Differentiate between the rods and the cones of the eye, ***p. 193***

8 Compare the functions of the extrinsic and intrinsic eye muscles, ***p. 194***

9 Describe the nerve supply to the eye, ***p. 196***

10 Describe the three divisions of the ear, ***p. 197***

11 Describe the receptor for hearing and explain how it functions, ***p. 200***

12 Compare the location and function of the equilibrium receptors, ***p. 201***

13 Discuss the location and function of the special sense organs for taste and smell, ***p. 202***

14 Explain the function of proprioceptors, ***p. 204***

15 Using the case, discuss changes in the anatomy and physiology of the eye resulting from chronic sun exposure, ***pp. 188, 205***

16 Show how word parts are used to build words related to the sensory system (see Word Anatomy at the end of the chapter), ***p. 207***

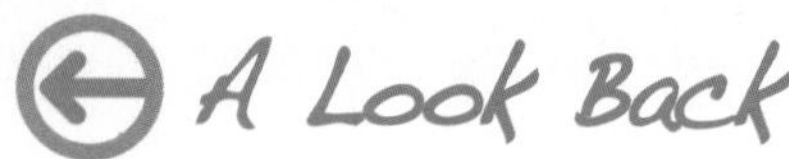

In describing the basic organization of the nervous system, we included both sensory and motor functions. Now we concentrate on just the sensory portion of the nervous system and the special receptors that respond to environmental changes. These specialized structures initiate the reflex pathways described in the previous chapters.

The Senses

The sensory system provides us with an awareness of our external and internal environments. An environmental change becomes a *stimulus* when it initiates a nerve impulse, which then travels to the central nervous system (CNS) by way of a sensory neuron. A stimulus becomes a sensation—something we experience—only when a specialized area of the cerebral cortex interprets the nerve impulse received. Many stimuli arrive from the external environment and are detected at or near the body surface. Others, such as stimuli from the viscera, originate internally and help to maintain homeostasis.

SENSORY RECEPTORS

The part of the nervous system that detects a stimulus is the **sensory receptor**. In structure, a sensory receptor may be one of the following:

- the free dendrite of a sensory neuron, such as the receptors for pain and temperature
- a modified ending on the dendrite of a sensory neuron, such as those for touch
- a specialized cell associated with an afferent neuron, such as the rods and cones of the eye's retina and the receptors in the other special sense organs (described shortly)

Receptors can be classified according to the type of stimulus to which they respond:

- Chemoreceptors, such as receptors for taste and smell, detect chemicals in solution.
- Photoreceptors, located in the retina of the eye, respond to light.
- Thermoreceptors detect changes in temperature. Many of these receptors are located in the skin.
- Mechanoreceptors respond to movement, such as stretch, pressure, or vibration. These include pressure receptors in the skin, receptors that monitor body position, and the receptors of hearing and equilibrium in the ear, which are activated by the movement of cilia on specialized receptor cells.

Any receptor must receive a stimulus of adequate intensity, that is, at least a **threshold stimulus**, in order to respond and generate a nerve impulse.

SPECIAL AND GENERAL SENSES

Another way of classifying the senses is according to the distribution of their receptors. A **special sense** is localized in a special sense organ; a **general sense** is widely distributed throughout the body.

- **Special senses**
  - **vision** from receptors in the eye
  - **hearing** from receptors in the inner ear
  - **equilibrium** from receptors in the inner ear
  - **taste** from receptors in the tongue
  - **smell** from receptors in the upper nasal cavities
- **General senses**
  - **pressure, temperature, pain,** and **touch** from receptors in the skin and internal organs
  - sense of **position** from receptors in the muscles, tendons, and joints

SENSORY ADAPTATION

When sensory receptors are exposed to a continuous and unimportant stimulus, they often adjust so that the sensation becomes less acute. The term for this phenomenon is **sensory adaptation.** For example, when you first put on a watch, you may be aware of its pressure on your wrist. Soon you do not notice it at all. If you are rinsing dishes in very warm water, you may be aware of the temperature at first, but you soon adapt and stop noticing the water's temperature. Similarly, when you step into sunlight after a day in class, the brightness is initially overwhelming, but rapidly becomes tolerable. As these examples show, both special and general senses are capable of adaptation. However, different receptors adapt at different rates. Those for warmth, cold, and light pressure adapt rapidly. In contrast, receptors for pain do not adapt. In fact, the sensations from receptors for slow, chronic pain tend to increase over time. This variation in receptors allows us to save energy by not responding to unimportant stimuli while always heeding the warnings of pain.

CHECKPOINTS 

- [ ] 10-1 What is a sensory receptor?
- [ ] 10-2 What are some categories of sensory receptors based on type of stimulus?
- [ ] 10-3 How do the special and general senses differ in location?
- [ ] 10-4 What happens when a sensory receptor adapts to a stimulus?

The Eye and Vision

In the embryo, the eye develops as an outpocketing of the brain, a process that begins at about 22 days of development. The eye is a complex organ with many receptors, but only about one-sixth of the eye is visible.

PROTECTIVE STRUCTURES OF THE EYE

The eye is a delicate organ and is protected by a number of structures:

- The skull bones form the walls of the eye orbit (cavity) and protect the posterior part of the eyeball.
- The upper and lower eyelids aid in protecting the eye's anterior portion (Fig. 10-1). The eyelids can be closed to keep harmful materials out of the eye, and blinking helps to lubricate the eye. A muscle, the levator palpebrae, is attached to the upper eyelid. When this muscle contracts, it keeps the eye open. If the muscle becomes weaker with age, the eyelids may droop and interfere with vision, a condition called *ptosis*.
- The eyelashes and eyebrow help to keep foreign matter out of the eye.
- A thin membrane, the **conjunctiva** (kon-junk-TI-vah), lines the inner surface of the eyelids and covers the visible portion of the white of the eye (sclera). Cells within the conjunctiva produce mucus that aids in lubricating the eye. Where the conjunctiva folds back from the eyelid to the eye's anterior surface, a sac is formed (Fig. 10-3). The lower portion of this conjunctival sac can be used to instill medication drops. With age, the conjunctiva often thins and dries, resulting in inflammation and enlarged blood vessels.
- Tears, produced by the **lacrimal** (LAK-rih-mal) **glands** (Fig. 10-2), lubricate the eye and contain an enzyme that protects against infection. As tears flow across the eye from the lacrimal gland, located in the orbit's upper lateral part, they carry away small particles that may have entered the eye. The tears then flow into ducts near the eye's nasal corner where they drain into the nose by way of the **nasolacrimal** (na-zo-LAK-rih-mal) **duct** (see Fig. 10-2). The lacrimal glands and ducts together make up the **lacrimal apparatus.** An excess of tears causes a "runny nose"; their overproduction causes tears to spill onto the cheeks. With age, the lacrimal glands secrete less, but tears still may overflow if the nasolacrimal ducts become plugged.

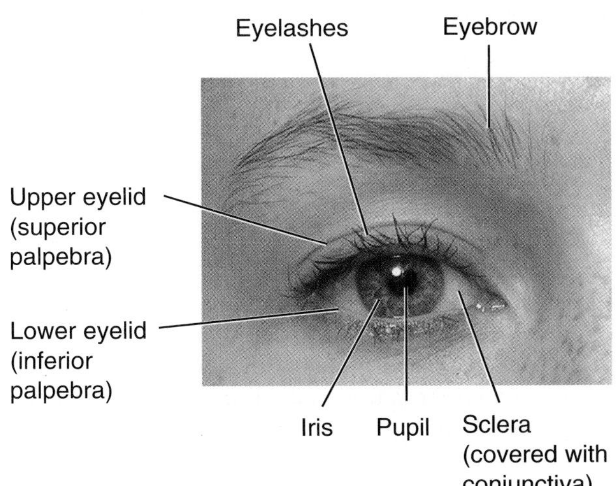

Figure 10-1 The eye's protective structures. KEY POINT The eye is a delicate organ well guarded by a bony socket and other protective structures. (Reprinted with permission from Bickley LS. *Bates' Guide to Physical Examination and History Taking*, 8th ed. Philadelphia, PA: Lippincott Williams & Wilkins, 2003.)

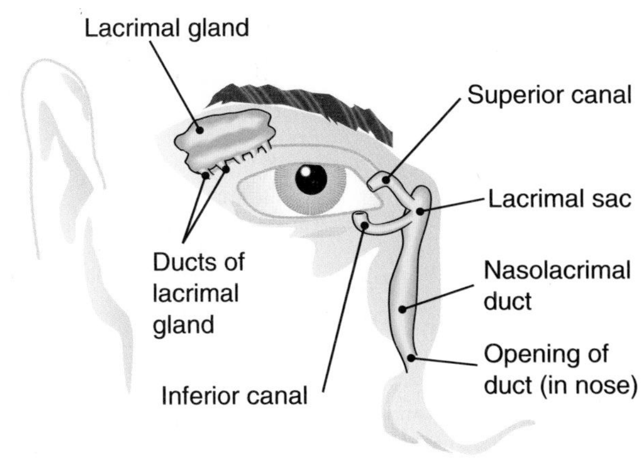

Figure 10-2 The lacrimal apparatus. KEY POINT Tears are produced in the lacrimal gland, located laterally, and flow across the eye to the nasolacrimal duct, located medially. The lacrimal (tear) gland and its associated ducts are shown.

STRUCTURE OF THE EYEBALL

The eyeball has three separate coats, or tunics. The components of these tunics are shown in Figure 10-3.

1. The outermost tunic is the fibrous tunic. It consists mainly of the **sclera** (SKLE-rah), which is made of tough connective tissue and is commonly referred to as the *white of the eye*. It appears white because of the collagen it contains and because it has no blood vessels to add color. (Reddened or "bloodshot" eyes result from inflammation and swelling of blood vessels in the conjunctiva.) The anterior portion of the fibrous tunic is the forward-curving, transparent, and colorless **cornea** (KOR-ne-ah).
2. The middle tunic is the vascular tunic, consisting mainly of the **choroid** (KO-royd). This layer is composed of a delicate network of connective tissue interlaced with many blood vessels. It also contains much dark brown pigment. The choroid may be compared to the dull black lining of a camera in that it prevents incoming light rays from scattering and reflecting off the eye's inner surface. At the eye's anterior, the vascular tunic continues as the **ciliary muscle** (SIL-e-ar-e) and **suspensory ligaments** (which control the shape of the **lens**, described shortly), and the **iris** (I-ris), the colored, ringlike portion of the eye.
3. The innermost coat is the nervous tunic, consisting of the **retina** (RET-ih-nah), the eye's actual receptor layer. The retina contains light-sensitive cells known as **rods** and **cones**, which generate the nerve impulses associated with vision.

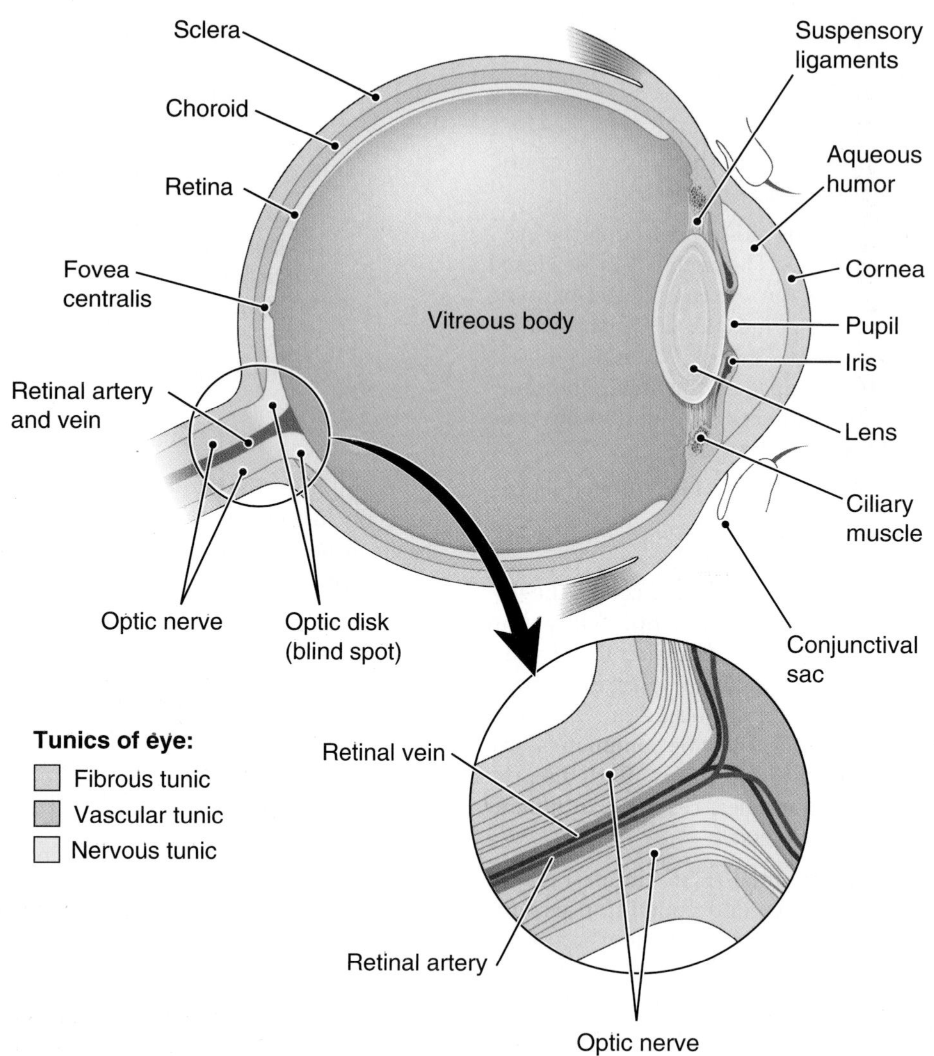

Figure 10-3 **The eye.** KEY POINT The eye has three tunics, or coats, the sclera, choroid, and retina. Its refractive parts are the cornea, aqueous humor, lens, and vitreous body. These and other structures involved in vision are shown. ZOOMING IN What anterior structure is continuous with the sclera?

PATHWAY OF LIGHT RAYS AND REFRACTION

As light rays pass through the eye toward the retina, they travel through a series of transparent, colorless parts described below and seen in Figure 10-3. On the way, they undergo a process known as **refraction**, which is the bending of light rays as they pass from one substance to another substance of different density. (For a simple demonstration of refraction, place a spoon into a glass of water and observe how the handle appears to bend at the surface of the water.) Because of refraction, light from a very large area can be focused on a very small area of the retina. The eye's transparent refracting parts are listed here, according to the pathway of light traveling from exterior to interior:

1. The transparent cornea curves forward slightly and is the eye's main refracting structure. The cornea has no blood vessels; it is nourished by the fluids that constantly bathe it.
2. The **aqueous** (A-kwe-us) **humor**, a watery fluid that fills much of the eyeball anterior to the lens, helps maintain the cornea's convex curve and refracts light. The aqueous humor is constantly produced and drained from the eye.
3. The lens, technically called the *crystalline lens*, is a clear, circular structure made of a firm, elastic material. The lens has two outward-curving surfaces and is thus described as biconvex. The lens is important in light refraction because its thickness can be adjusted to focus light for near or far vision.
4. The **vitreous** (VIT-re-us) **body** is a soft jelly-like substance that fills the entire space posterior to the lens (the adjective *vitreous* means "glasslike"). Like the aqueous humor, it is important in maintaining the shape of the eyeball as well as in aiding in refraction.

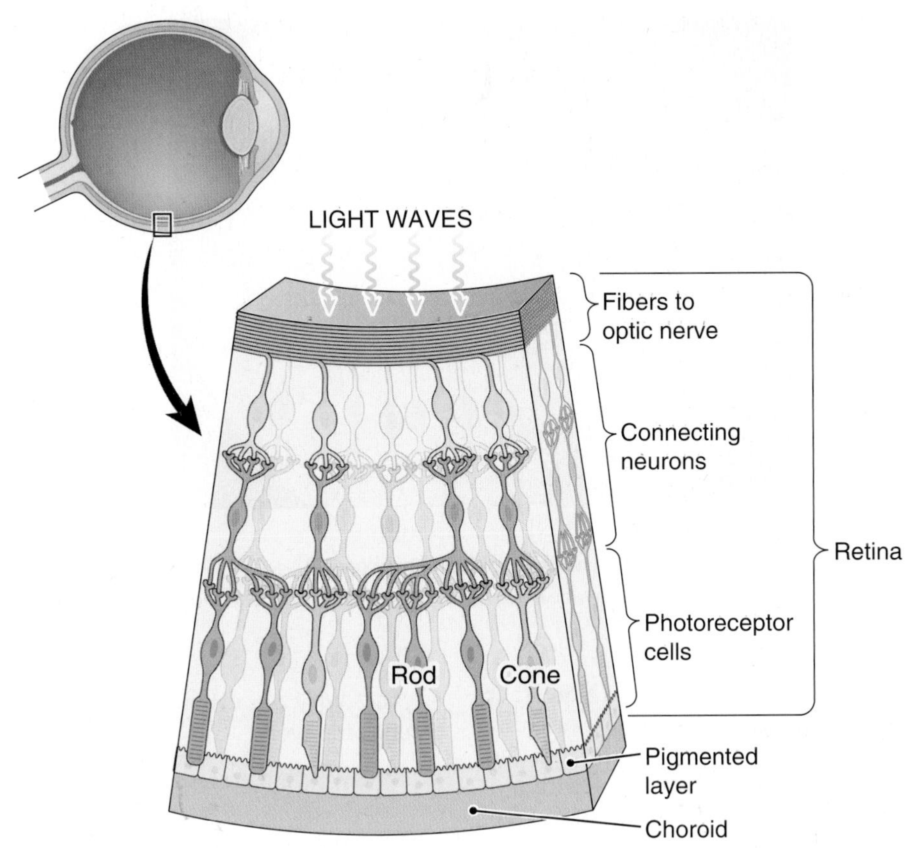

Figure 10-4 **Structure of the retina.** KEY POINT Rods and cones form a deep layer of the retina, near the choroid. Connecting neurons carry visual impulses toward the optic nerve.

10

FUNCTION OF THE RETINA

The retina has a complex structure with multiple layers of cells **(Fig. 10-4)**. The deepest layer is a pigmented layer just anterior to the choroid. Next are the rods and cones, the eye's receptor cells, named for their shape. Details on how these two types of cells differ are presented in **Table 10-1**. Anterior to the rods and cones are connecting neurons that carry impulses toward the optic nerve.

The rods are highly sensitive to light and thus function best in dim light, but they do not provide a sharp image. They are more numerous than the cones and are distributed more toward the periphery (anterior portion) of the retina. (If you visualize the retina as the inside of a bowl, the rods would be located toward the bowl's lip.) When you enter into dim light, such as a darkened movie theater, you cannot see for a short period. It is during this time that the rods are beginning to function well, a change that is described as **dark adaptation.** When you are able to see again, images are blurred and appear only in shades of gray, because the rods are unable to differentiate colors.

The cones function best in bright light, are sensitive to color, and give sharp images. The cones are localized at the retinal center, especially in a tiny depressed area near the optic nerve that is called the **fovea centralis** (FO-ve-ah

Table 10-1 Comparison of the Rods and Cones of the Retina

Characteristic	Rods	Cones
Shape	Cylindrical	Flask shaped
Number	About 120 million in each retina	About 6 million in each retina
Distribution	Toward the periphery (anterior) of the retina	Concentrated at the center of the retina
Stimulus	Dim light	Bright light
Visual acuity (sharpness)	Low	High
Pigments	Rhodopsin	Pigments sensitive to red, green, or blue
Color perception	None; shades of gray	Respond to color

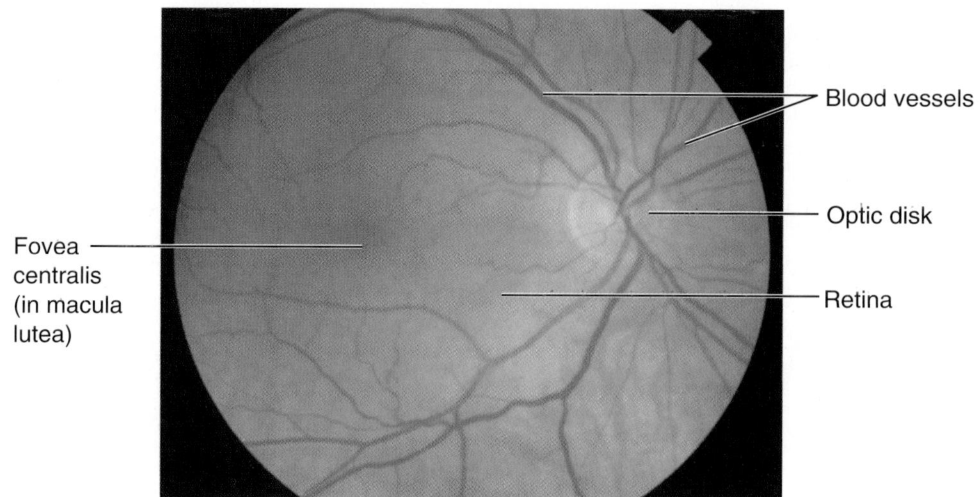

Figure 10-5 The fundus (back) of the eye as seen through an ophthalmoscope. KEY POINT An abnormal appearance of the fundus can indicate disease. (Reprinted with permission from Moore KL, Dalley AF. *Clinically Oriented Anatomy*, 5th ed. Baltimore, MD: Lippincott Williams & Wilkins, 2006.)

sen-TRA-lis) **(Fig. 10-5; see also Fig. 10-3)**. (Note that *fovea* is a general term for a pit or depression.) Because this area contains the highest concentration of cones, it is the point of sharpest vision. The fovea is contained within a yellowish spot, the **macula lutea** (MAK-u-lah LU-te-ah), an area that may show degenerative changes with age.

There are three types of cones, each sensitive to either red, green, or blue light. Color blindness results from a deficiency of retinal cones. People who completely lack cones are totally color blind; those who lack one type of cone are partially color blind. This disorder, because of its pattern of inheritance, occurs much more commonly in males.

The rods and cones function by means of pigments that are sensitive to light. The light-sensitive pigment in rods is **rhodopsin** (ro-DOP-sin). Vitamin A is needed for manufacture of these pigments. If a person lacks vitamin A, and thus rhodopsin, he or she may have difficulty seeing in dim light, because the rods cannot be activated; this condition is termed night blindness. Nerve impulses from the rods and cones flow into sensory neurons that eventually merge to form the optic nerve (cranial nerve II) at the eye's posterior **(see Figs. 10-3 and 10-5)**. The impulses travel to the visual center in the brain's occipital cortex.

When an **ophthalmologist** (of-thal-MOL-o-jist), a physician who specializes in treatment of the eye, examines the retina with an **ophthalmoscope** (of-THAL-mo-skope), he or she can see abnormalities in the retina and in the retinal blood vessels. This procedure was part of Paul's eye exam in the case study. Some of these changes may signal more widespread diseases that affect the eye, such as diabetes and high blood pressure (hypertension).

CHECKPOINTS 

☐ **10-5** What are some structures that protect the eye?

☐ **10-6** What are the components of the three tunics of the eyeball?

☐ **10-7** What are the structures that refract light as it passes through the eye?

☐ **10-8** What are the receptor cells of the retina?

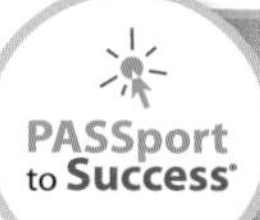

See the Student Resources on *thePoint* to view the animation *The Retina*, which illustrates the structure and function of this receptor.

MUSCLES OF THE EYE

Two groups of muscles are associated with the eye. Both groups are important in adjusting the eye so that a clear image can form on the retina.

The Extrinsic Muscles The voluntary muscles attached to the eyeball's outer surface are the **extrinsic** (eks-TRIN-sik) **muscles**. The six ribbon-like extrinsic muscles connected with each eye originate on the orbital bones and insert on the surface of the sclera **(Fig. 10-6)**. They are named for their location and the direction of the muscle fibers. These muscles pull on the eyeball in a coordinated fashion so that both eyes center on one visual field. This process of **convergence** is necessary to the production of a clear retinal image. Having the image come from a slightly different angle from each retina is believed to be important for three-dimensional (stereoscopic) vision, a characteristic of primates.

The Intrinsic Muscles The involuntary muscles located within the eyeball are the **intrinsic** (in-TRIN-sik) **muscles.** They form two circular structures within the eye, the iris and the ciliary muscle.

The **iris** (I-ris) is the visible pigmented (colored) part of the eye. It is composed of two sets of muscle fibers that govern the size of the iris's central opening, the

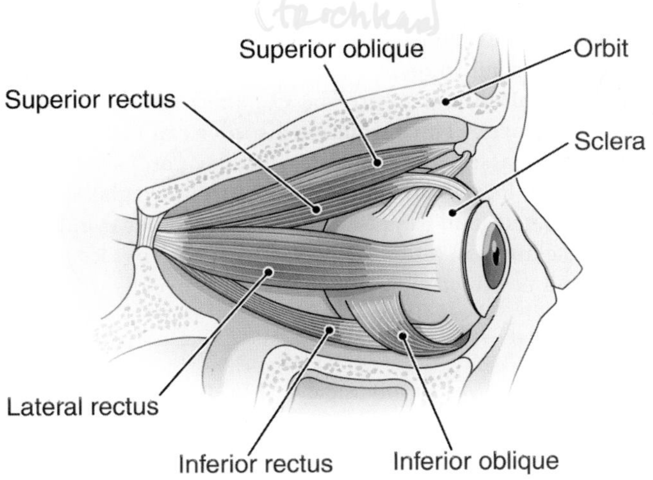

Figure 10-6 Extrinsic muscles of the eye. KEY POINT The extrinsic muscles coordinate eye movements for proper vision. The medial rectus is not shown. ZOOMING IN What characteristics are used in naming the extrinsic eye muscles?

pupil (PU-pil) (Fig. 10-7). One set of fibers is arranged in a circular fashion, and the other set extends radially like the spokes of a wheel. The iris regulates the amount of light entering the eye. In bright light, the iris's circular muscle fibers contract, reducing the size of the pupil. This narrowing is termed *constriction*. In contrast, in dim light, the radial muscles contract, pulling the opening outward and enlarging it. This enlargement of the pupil is known as *dilation*. In the case study, Paul has to wear dark glasses after his eye exam because the physician had dilated his pupils for the exam, allowing too much light to enter his eyes.

The **ciliary** (SIL-e-ar-e) **muscle** is shaped somewhat like a flattened ring with a central hole the size of the iris's outer edge. This muscle holds the lens in place by means of filaments, called **suspensory ligaments**, that project from the ciliary muscle to the edge of the lens around its entire circumference (Fig. 10-8). The ciliary muscle controls the lens' shape to allow for vision at near and far distances. This process of **accommodation** is necessary because the light rays from a close object diverge (separate) more than do the light rays from a distant object (Fig. 10-9). Consequently, when we view something close, the lens must become more rounded and bend the light rays more to focus them on the retina.

Accomodation occurs as follows. When the ciliary muscle is relaxed for distant vision, tension on the suspensory ligaments keeps the lens in a more flattened shape. For close vision, the ciliary muscle contracts, which draws the ciliary ring forward and relaxes tension on the suspensory ligaments. The elastic lens then recoils and becomes thicker, in much the same way that a rubber band thickens when we release the pull on it. When the ciliary muscle relaxes again, the lens flattens. These actions change the lens' refractive power to accommodate for near and far vision.

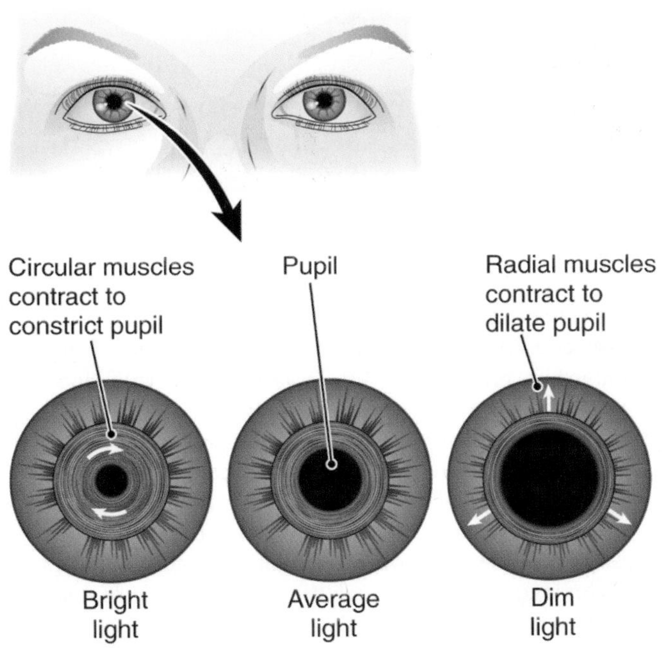

Figure 10-7 Function of the iris. KEY POINT In bright light, circular muscles contract and constrict the pupil, limiting the light that enters the eye. In dim light, the radial muscles contract and dilate the pupil, allowing more light to enter the eye. ZOOMING IN What muscles of the iris contract to make the pupil smaller? Larger?

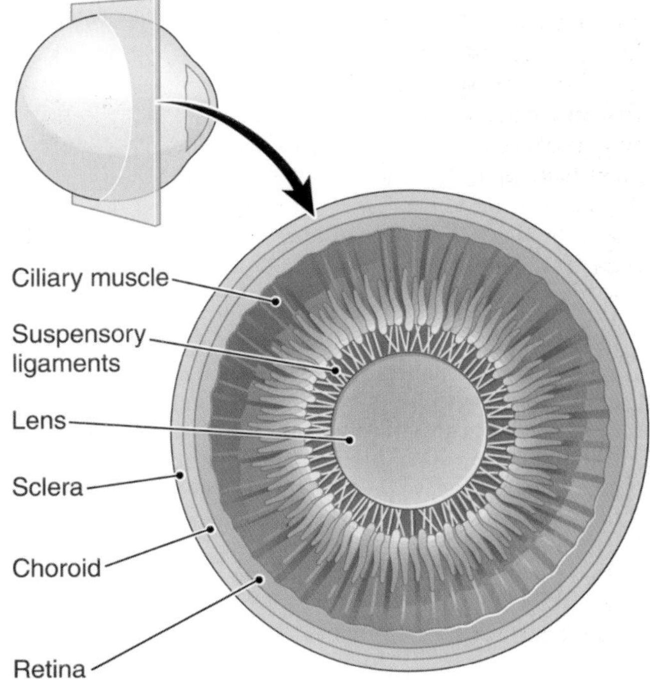

Figure 10-8 The ciliary muscle and lens (posterior view). KEY POINT Contraction of the ciliary muscle relaxes tension on the suspensory ligaments, allowing the lens to become more round for near vision. ZOOMING IN What structures hold the lens in place?

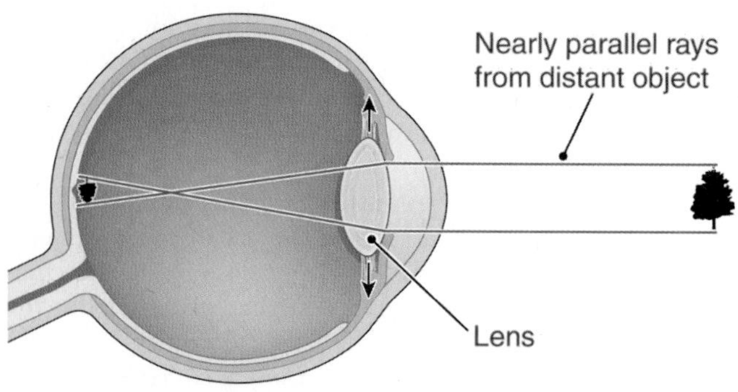

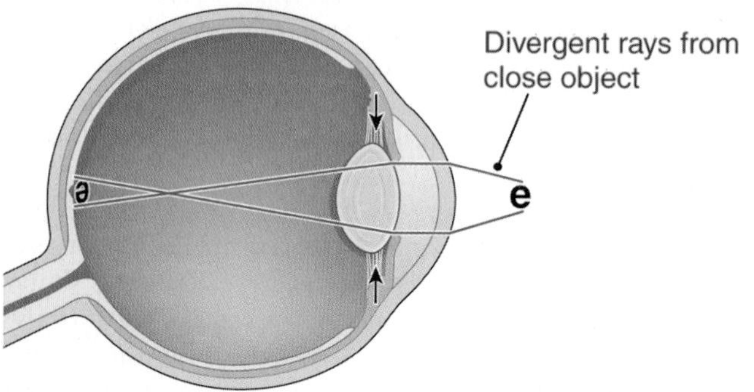

Figure 10-9 Accommodation for near vision. KEY POINT When viewing a close object, the lens must become more rounded to focus light rays on the retina.

In young people, the lens is elastic, and therefore its thickness can be readily adjusted according to the need for near or distance vision. With aging, the lens loses elasticity and therefore its ability to accommodate for near vision. It becomes difficult to focus clearly on close objects, a condition called **presbyopia** (pres-be-O-pe-ah), which literally means "old eye." This refractive disorder can be corrected using eye glasses and contacts. In the case study, Dr. Gilbert gave Paul a new prescription for his eyeglasses. He also examined Paul's eyes for evidence of other eye disorders like glaucoma and cataracts. Box 10-1 provides information on new methods of treating these eye disorders.

NERVE SUPPLY TO THE EYE

Two sensory nerves supply the eye (Fig. 10-10):

- The **optic nerve** (cranial nerve II) carries visual impulses from the retinal rods and cones to the brain.
- The **ophthalmic** (of-THAL-mik) **branch of the trigeminal nerve** (cranial nerve V) carries impulses of pain, touch, and temperature from the eye and surrounding parts to the brain.

The optic nerve arises from the retina a little toward the medial or nasal side of the eye. There are no retinal rods and cones in the area of the optic nerve. Consequently, no image can form on the retina at this point, which is known as the blind spot or **optic disk** (see Figs. 10-3 and 10-5).

The optic nerve transmits impulses from the retina to the thalamus (part of the diencephalon), from which they are directed to the occipital cortex. Note that the light rays passing through the eye are actually overrefracted (overly bent) so that an image falls on the retina upside down and backward (see Fig. 10-9). It is the job of the brain's visual centers to reverse the images.

Box 10-1 *Hot Topics*

Eye Surgery: A Glimpse of the Cutting Edge

Cataracts, glaucoma, and refractive errors are the most common eye disorders affecting Americans. In the past, cataract and glaucoma treatments concentrated on managing the diseases. Refractive errors were corrected using eyeglasses and, more recently, contact lenses. Today, laser and microsurgical techniques can remove cataracts, reduce glaucoma, and allow people with refractive errors to put their eyeglasses and contacts away. These cutting-edge procedures include

- *Laser in situ keratomileusis (LASIK)* to correct refractive errors. During this procedure, a surgeon uses a laser to reshape the cornea so that it refracts light directly onto the retina, rather than in front of or behind it. A microkeratome (surgical knife) is used to cut a flap in the cornea's outer layer. A computer-controlled laser sculpts the middle layer of the cornea and then the flap is replaced. The procedure takes only a few minutes and patients recover their vision quickly and usually with little postoperative pain.
- *Laser trabeculoplasty* to treat glaucoma. This procedure uses a laser to help drain fluid from the eye and lower intraocular pressure. The laser is aimed at drainage canals located between the cornea and iris and makes several burns that are believed to open the canals and allow fluid to drain better. The procedure is typically painless and takes only a few minutes.
- *Phacoemulsification* to remove cataracts. During this surgical procedure, a very small incision (approximately 3 mm long) is made through the sclera near the cornea's outer edge. An ultrasonic probe is inserted through this opening and into the center of the lens. The probe uses sound waves to emulsify the lens' central core, which is then suctioned out. Then, an artificial lens is permanently implanted in the lens capsule. The procedure is typically painless, although the patient may feel some discomfort for 1 to 2 days afterward.

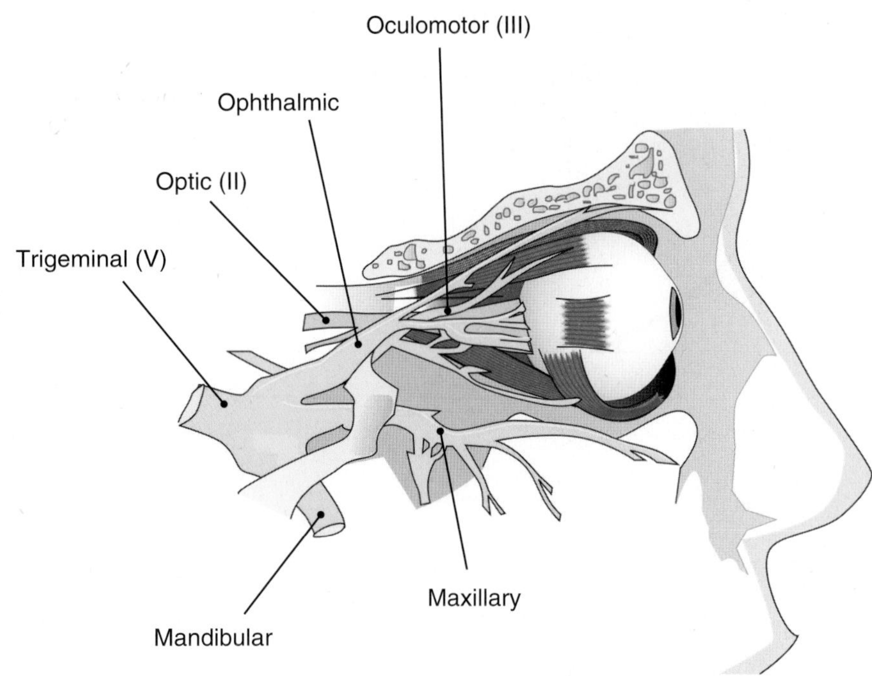

Figure 10-10 **Nerves of the eye.**
ZOOMING IN Which of the nerves shown controls eye movement?

10

Three nerves carry motor impulses to the eyeball muscles:

- The oculomotor nerve (cranial nerve III) is the largest; it supplies voluntary and involuntary motor impulses to all but two eye muscles **(see Fig. 10-10)**.
- The trochlear nerve (cranial nerve IV, not pictured) supplies the superior oblique extrinsic eye muscle **(see Fig. 10-6)**.
- The abducens nerve (cranial nerve VI, not pictured) supplies the lateral rectus extrinsic eye muscle.

To summarize, the events required for proper vision (some of which may be occurring simultaneously) are

- Light refracts through the cornea (and continues to refract through the aqueous humor, lens, and vitreous body).
- The muscles of the iris adjust the pupil.
- The ciliary muscle adjusts the lens (accommodation).
- The extrinsic eye muscles produce convergence.
- Light stimulates retinal receptor cells (rods and cones).
- The optic nerve transmits impulses to the brain.
- The occipital lobe cortex interprets the impulses.

Box 10-1 provides information on new methods of treating eye disorders.

CHECKPOINTS 

- 10-9 What is the function of the extrinsic eye muscles?
- 10-10 What is the function of the iris?
- 10-11 What is the function of the ciliary muscle?
- 10-12 What is cranial nerve II and what does it do?

The Ear

The ear is the sense organ for both hearing and equilibrium **(Fig. 10-11)**. It is divided into three main sections:

- The **outer ear** includes an outer projection and a canal ending at a membrane.
- The **middle ear** is an air space containing three small bones.
- The **inner ear** is the most complex and contains the sensory receptors for hearing and equilibrium.

THE OUTER EAR

The external portion of the ear consists of a visible projecting portion, the **pinna** (PIN-nah), also called the *auricle* (AW-rih-kl), and the **external auditory canal**, or *meatus* (me-A-tus), that leads into the ear's deeper parts. The pinna directs sound waves into the ear, but it is probably of little importance in humans. The external auditory canal extends medially from the pinna for about 2.5 cm or more, depending on which wall of the canal is measured. The skin lining this tube is thin and, in the first part of the canal, contains many wax-producing **ceruminous** (seh-RU-mih-nus) **glands**. The wax, or **cerumen** (seh-RU-men), may become dried and impacted in the canal and must then be removed.

The **tympanic** (tim-PAN-ik) **membrane**, or *eardrum*, is at the end of the external auditory canal and separates this canal from the middle ear cavity. The tympanic membrane vibrates freely when struck with sound waves that enter the ear.

THE MIDDLE EAR AND OSSICLES

The middle ear cavity is a small, flattened space that contains three small bones, or **ossicles** (OS-ih-klz) **(see Fig. 10-11)**. The three ossicles are joined in such a way that they amplify

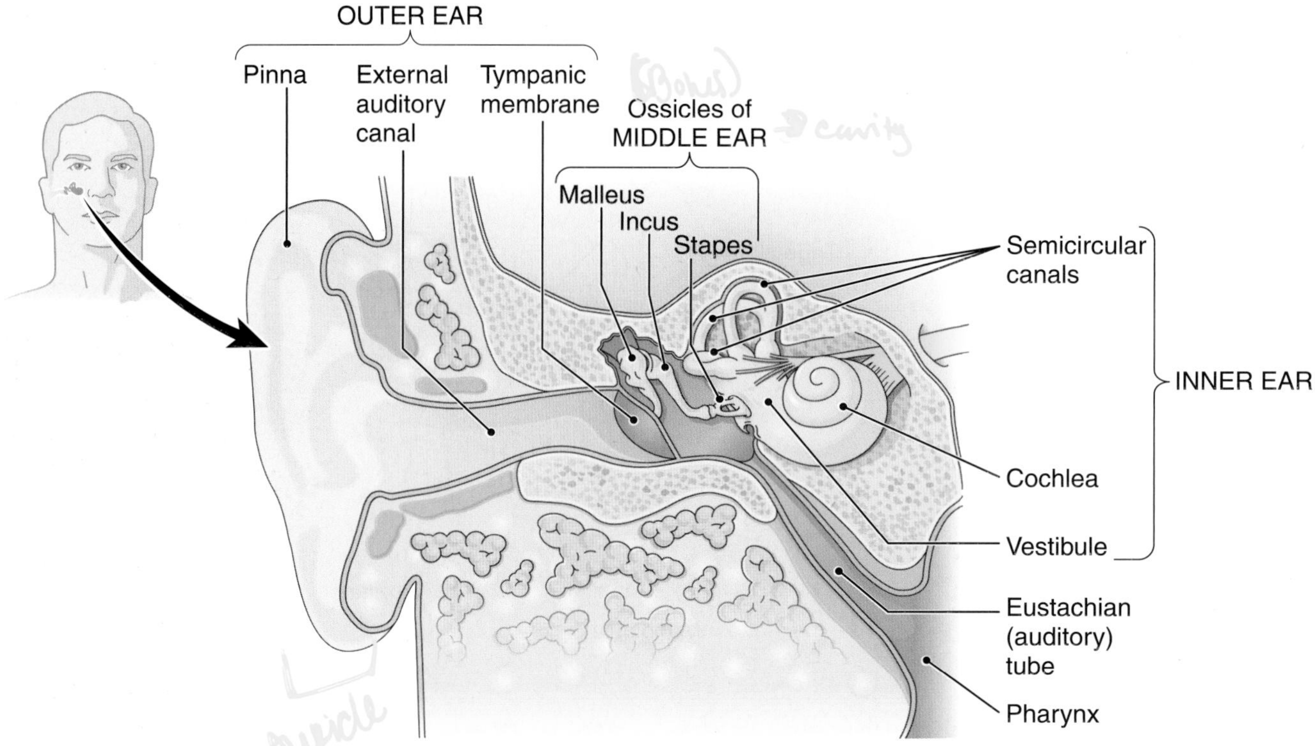

Figure 10-11 The ear. KEY POINT Structures in the outer, middle, and inner divisions are shown. ZOOMING IN What structure separates the outer ear from the middle ear?

the sound waves received by the tympanic membrane as they transmit the sounds to the inner ear. The first bone is shaped like a hammer (or mallet) and is called the **malleus** (MAL-e-us). The handle-like part of the malleus is attached to the tympanic membrane, whereas the headlike part is connected to the second bone, the **incus** (ING-kus). The incus is shaped like an anvil, an iron block used in shaping metal, as is used by a blacksmith. The innermost ossicle is

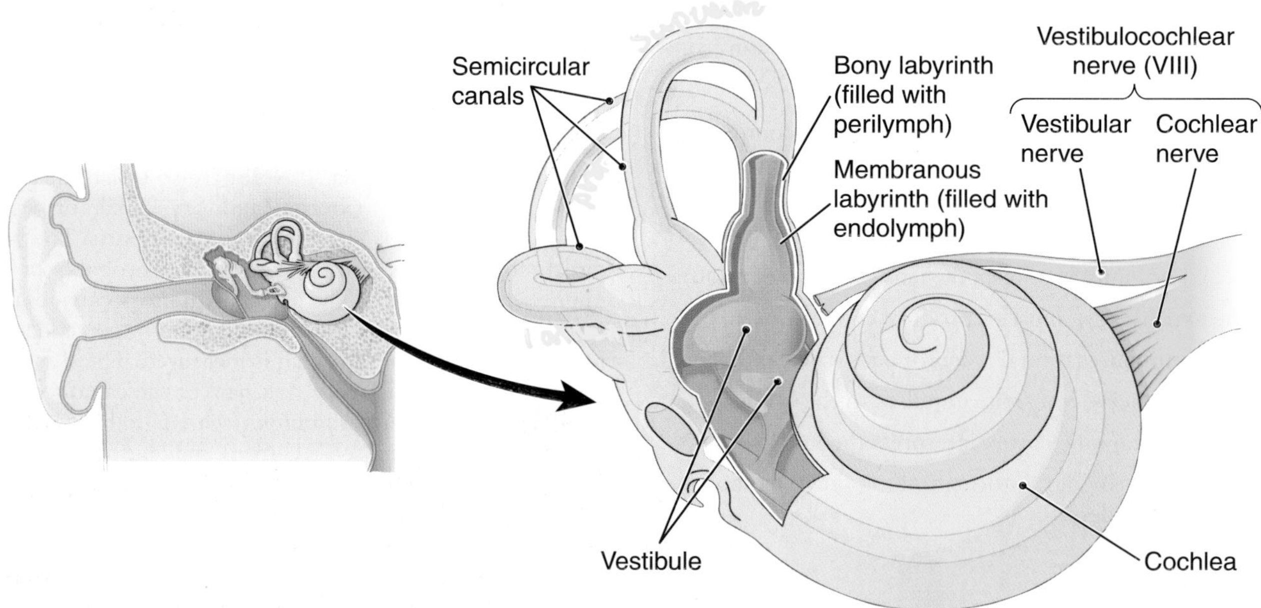

Figure 10-12 The inner ear. KEY POINT The vestibule, semicircular canals, and cochlea are made of a bony shell, described as a bony labyrinth, with an interior membranous labyrinth. Endolymph fills the membranous labyrinth and perilymph surrounds it in the bony labyrinth. The cochlea is the organ of hearing. The semicircular canals and vestibule are concerned with equilibrium. ZOOMING IN What nerve is formed by the merger of the nerves from the inner ear?

shaped somewhat like the stirrup of a saddle and is called the **stapes** (STA-peze), which is Latin for *stirrup*. The base of the stapes is in contact with the inner ear.

The **auditory tube**, also called the *eustachian* (u-STA-shu) *tube*, connects the middle ear cavity with the throat, or pharynx (FAR-inks) (see Fig. 10-11). This tube opens to allow pressure to equalize on the two sides of the tympanic membrane. A valve that closes the tube can be forced open by swallowing hard, yawning, or blowing with the nose and mouth sealed, as a person often does when experiencing pain from pressure changes in an airplane.

The mucous membrane of the pharynx is continuous through the auditory tube into the middle ear cavity. At the posterior of the middle ear cavity is an opening into the mastoid air cells, which are spaces inside the temporal bone's mastoid process (see Fig. 6-5B,C).

THE INNER EAR

The ear's most complicated and important part is the internal portion, which is described as a *labyrinth* (LAB-ih-rinth) because it has a complex, mazelike construction (Fig. 10-12). The outer shell of the inner ear is composed of hollow bone comprising the **bony labyrinth**. This outer portion is filled with a fluid called **perilymph** (PER-e-limf).

Within the bony labyrinth is an exact replica of this bony shell made of membrane, much like an inner tube within a tire. The tubes and chambers of this **membranous labyrinth** are filled with a fluid called **endolymph** (EN-do-limf) (see Fig. 10-12). Thus, the endolymph is within the membranous labyrinth, and the perilymph surrounds the membranous labyrinth. These fluids are important to the sensory functions of the inner ear. The inner ear has three divisions:

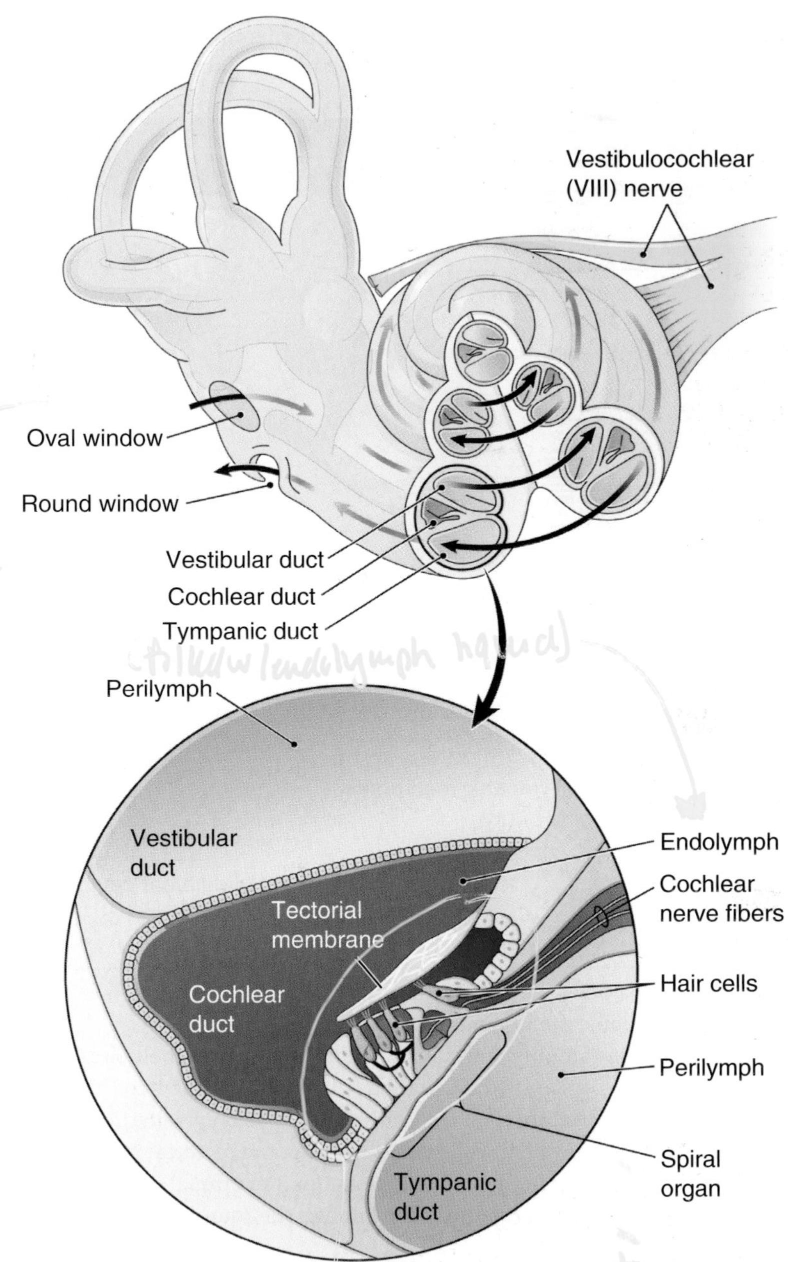

Figure 10-13 Cochlea and the spiral organ. KEY POINT The arrows show the direction of sound waves in the cochlea. ZOOMING IN Which part of the cochlea contains the spiral organ?

10

- The **vestibule** consists of two chambers that contain some of the receptors for equilibrium.
- The **semicircular canals** are three projecting tubes located toward the posterior. Areas at the bases of the semicircular canals also contain receptors for equilibrium.
- The **cochlea** (KOK-le-ah) is coiled like a snail shell (*cochlea* is Latin for "snail") and is located toward the anterior. It contains the receptors for hearing.

HEARING

In hearing, sound waves first enter the external auditory canal and set up vibrations in the tympanic membrane. The ossicles amplify these vibrations and finally transmit them from the stapes to a membrane covering the **oval window** of the inner ear **(Fig. 10-13)**.

The sound waves continue through the perilymph in the upper chamber of the bony cochlea, the **vestibular duct**, and then spiral into a lower chamber, the **tympanic duct** (*vestibular* refers to an entranceway; *tympanic* refers to a drum). As they travel, the sound waves set up vibrations within the cochlea's central membranous portion, the **cochlear duct**, where the organ of hearing, the **spiral organ** (*organ of Corti* [KOR-te]), is located. The vibrations cause tiny cilia on the spiral organ's receptor cells (hair cells) to move back and forth against the **tectorial membrane** located above them. (The membrane is named from a Latin word that means "roof.") This motion sets up nerve impulses that travel to the brain in the **cochlear nerve**, a branch of the eighth cranial nerve (formerly called the *auditory* or *acoustic nerve*). Sound waves ultimately leave the ear through another membrane-covered space in the bony labyrinth, the **round window** **(see Fig. 10-13)**. The steps in hearing are summarized and illustrated in **Table 10-2**. The cochlea is pictured as unrolled to show more easily how sound waves progress through the inner ear chambers.

Hearing receptors respond to both the pitch (tone) of sound and its intensity (loudness). The various pitches stimulate different regions of the spiral organ. Receptors

Table 10-2 The Steps in Hearing

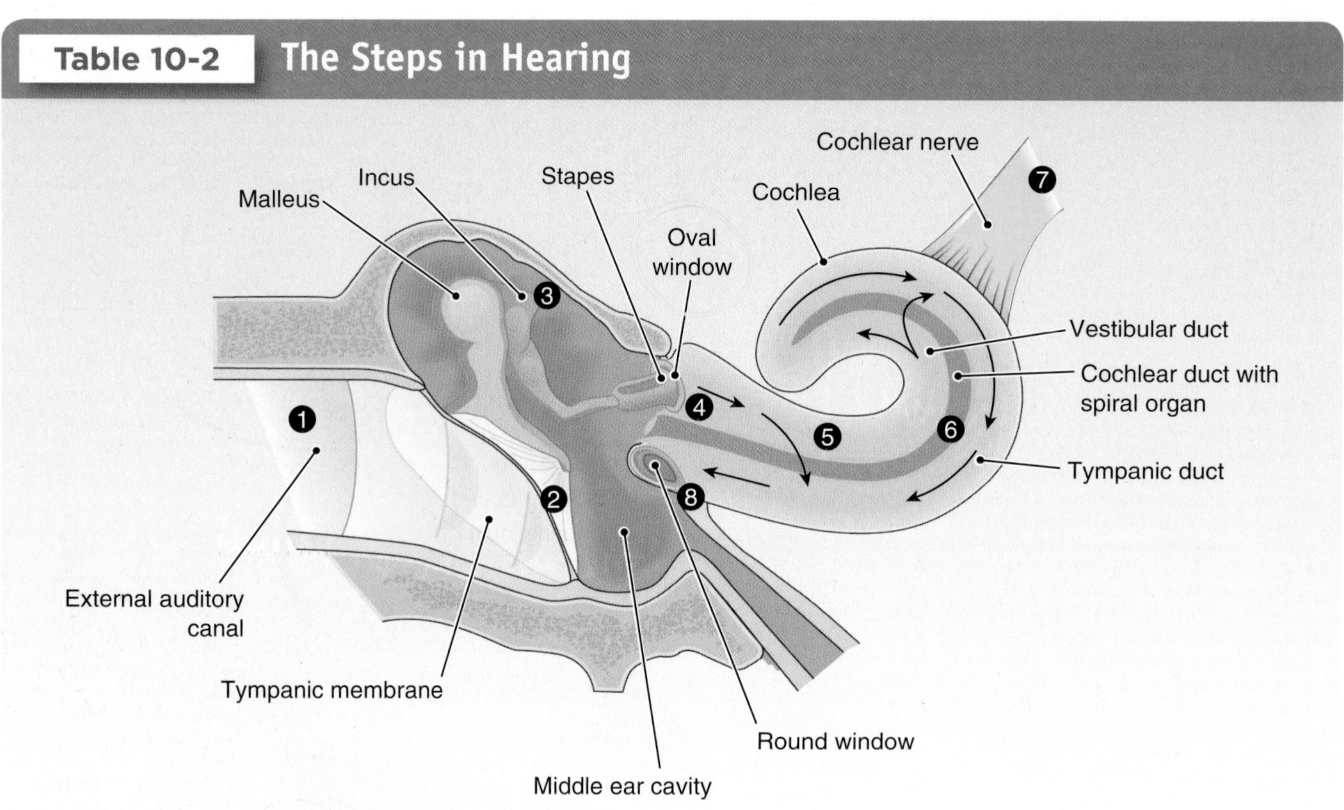

The steps in hearing are

1. Sound waves enter the external auditory canal.
2. The tympanic membrane vibrates.
3. The ossicles amplify and transmit vibrations across the middle ear cavity.
4. The stapes transmits the vibrations at the oval window to the inner ear fluid.
5. Vibrations travel through the perilymph of the bony labyrinth and start vibrations in the cochlear endolymph.
6. The spiral organ's hair cells vibrate against the tectorial membrane, generating nerve impulses.
7. Impulses travel via the cochlear nerve (part of cranial nerve VIII) to the temporal lobe cortex, where they are interpreted.
8. Sound waves leave the inner ear through the round window.

detect higher-pitched sounds near the base of the cochlea and lower-pitched sounds near the top. Loud sounds stimulate more cells and produce more vibrations, sending more nerve impulses to the brain. Exposure to loud noises, such as very loud music, jet plane noise, or industrial noises, can damage the receptors for particular pitches of sound and lead to hearing loss for those tones.

EQUILIBRIUM

The other sensory receptors in the inner ear are those related to equilibrium (balance). They are located in the vestibule and the semicircular canals. Receptors for the sense of equilibrium respond to acceleration and are, like the hearing receptors, ciliated hair cells. As the head moves, a shift in the position of the cilia within a thick material around them generates a nerve impulse.

Receptors located in the vestibule's two small chambers sense the position of the head relative to the force of gravity and also respond to acceleration in a straight line, as in a forward-moving vehicle or an elevator. Each receptor is called a **macula.** (There is also a macula in the eye, but *macula* is a general term that means "spot.") The macular hair cells are embedded in a gelatinous material, the **otolithic** (o-to-LITH-ik) **membrane**, which is weighted with small crystals of calcium carbonate, called **otoliths** (O-to-liths). The force of gravity pulls the membrane downward, which bends the cilia of the hair cells, generating a nerve impulse **(Fig. 10-14)**. In linear acceleration, the otolithic membrane lags behind the forward motion, bending the cilia in a direction opposite to the direction of acceleration. Picture sweeping mud off a garden path with a broom. As you move forward, the thick mud is dragging the broom straws in the opposite direction.

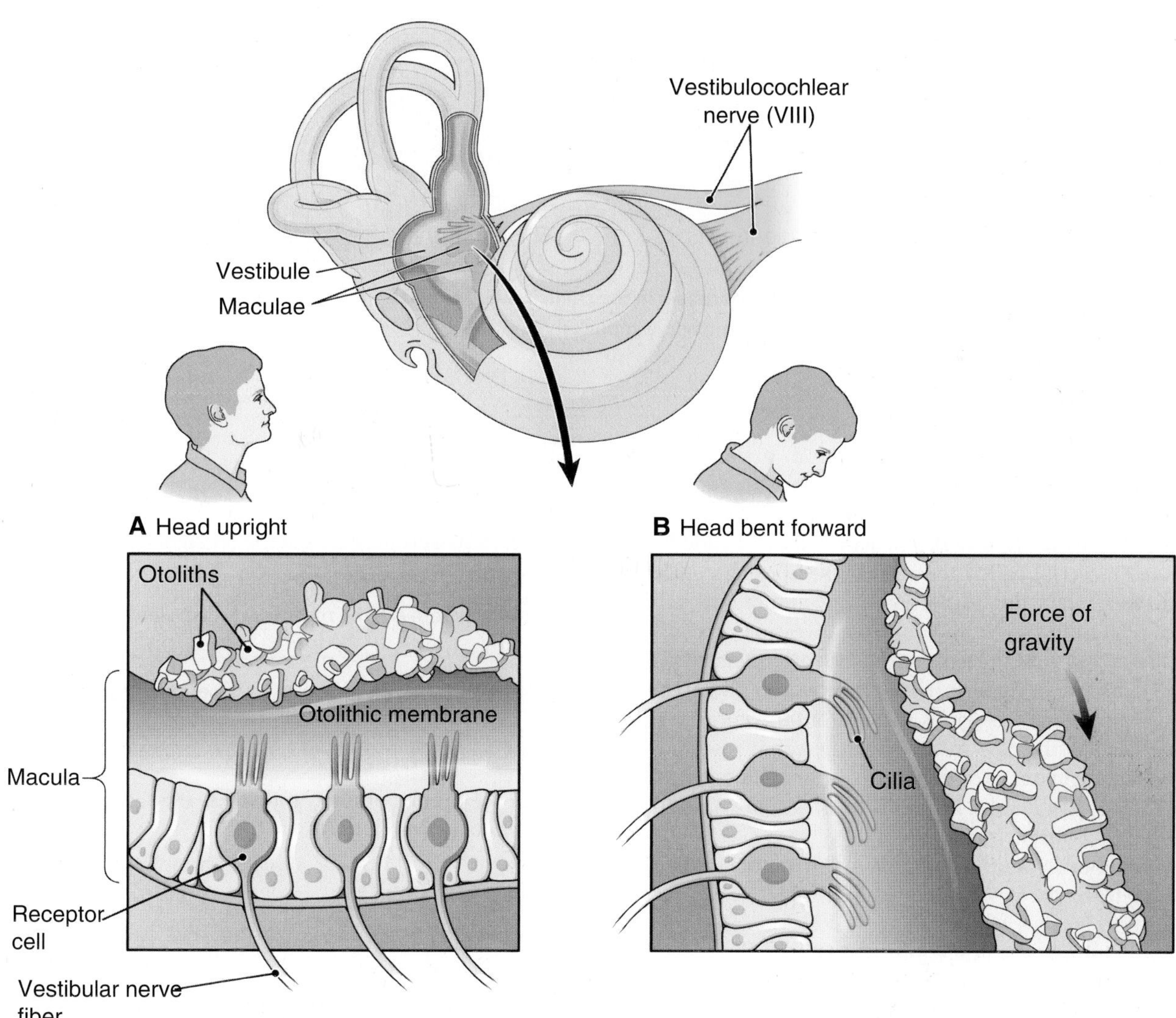

Figure 10-14 Action of the vestibular equilibrium receptors (maculae) KEY POINT As the head moves, the otolithic membrane, weighted with otoliths, pulls on the receptor cells' cilia, generating a nerve impulse. These receptors also function in linear acceleration. ZOOMING IN What happens to the cilia of the macular cells when the fluid around them moves?

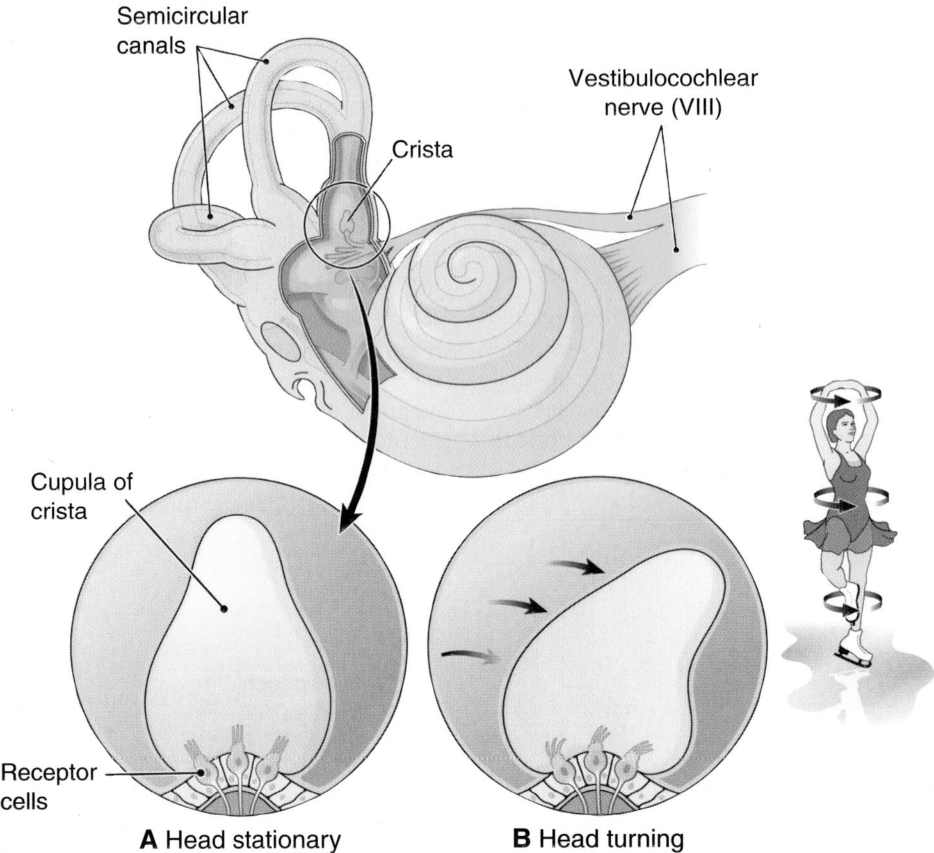

Figure 10-15 Action of the equilibrium receptors (cristae) in the semicircular canals. KEY POINT As the body spins or moves in different directions, the receptor cells' cilia bend, generating nerve impulses.

The receptors for detecting rotation, such as when you shake your head or twirl in a circle, are located at the bases of the semicircular canals (Fig. 10-15). These receptors, called **cristae** (KRIS-te), are hair cells embedded in a gelatinous material called the cupula (KU-pu-lah). As with the maculae, when the head moves, the cupula lags behind a bit, bending the cilia in the opposite direction. It's easy to remember what these receptors do, because the semicircular canals go off in three different directions. The crista in the horizontal canal responds to horizontal rotation, as in a dancer's spin; the one in the superior canal responds to forward and backward rotation, as in somersaulting; the one in the posterior canal responds to left–right rotation, as in doing a cartwheel.

Nerve fibers from the vestibule and from the semicircular canals form the **vestibular** (ves-TIB-u-lar) **nerve**, which joins the cochlear nerve to form the vestibulocochlear nerve, the eighth cranial nerve (see Fig. 10-14).

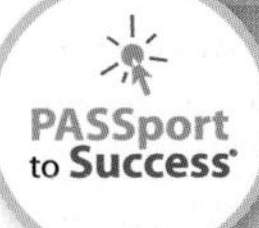

PASSport to Success

See the Student Resources on *thePoint* for information on how audiologists help to treat hearing disorders.

CHECKPOINTS 

- 10-13 What are the ossicles of the ear and what do they do?
- 10-14 What is the name of the organ of hearing and where is it located?
- 10-15 Where are the receptors for equilibrium located?

Other Special Sense Organs

The sense organs of taste and smell are designed to respond to chemical stimuli.

SENSE OF TASTE

The sense of taste, or **gustation** (gus-TA-shun), involves receptors in the tongue and two different nerves that carry taste impulses to the brain (Fig. 10-16). The taste receptors, known as **taste buds**, are located mainly on the superior surface of the tongue. Some are enclosed in raised projections called **papillae** (pah_PIL-e), which give the tongue's surface a rough texture and help to manipulate food when chewing. Taste buds are stimulated only if the

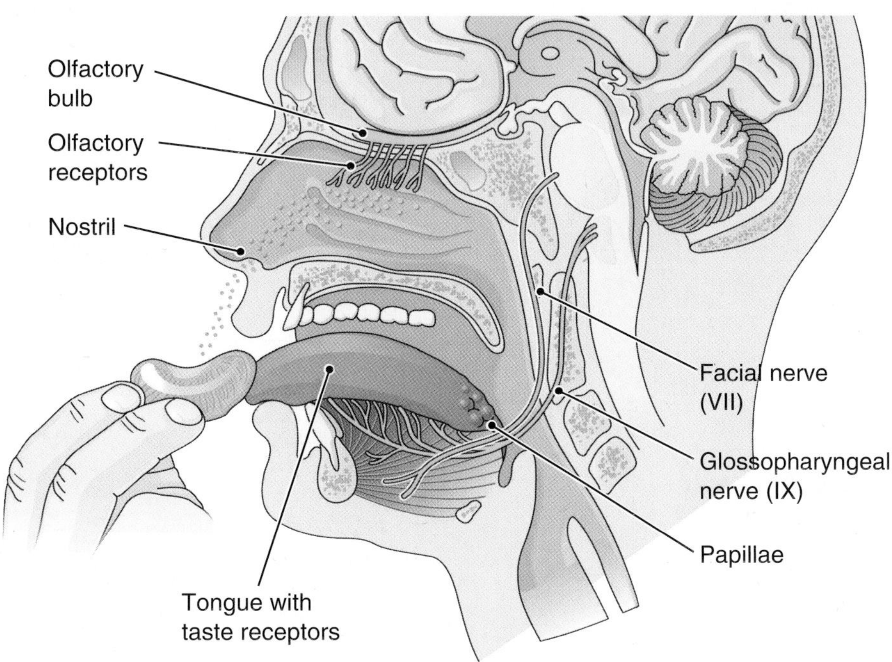

Figure 10-16 Special senses that respond to chemicals. KEY POINT Organs of taste (gustation) and smell (olfaction) work together in response to chemicals.

substance to be tasted is in solution or dissolves in the fluids of the mouth. Receptors for five basic tastes have been identified:

- **Sweet** receptors respond to sugar.
- **Salty** receptors respond to sodium.
- **Sour** receptors detect hydrogen ions.
- **Bitter** receptors respond to various organic compounds.
- **Umami** (u-MOM-e) is a pungent or savory taste based on a response to the amino acids glutamate and aspartate, which add to the meaty taste of protein. Glutamate is found in MSG (monosodium glutamate), a flavor enhancer used in some processed foods and some restaurants.

Other tastes are a combination of these five with additional smell sensations. More recently, researchers have identified two additional tastes: alkaline (basic) and metallic. The nerves of taste include the facial and the glossopharyngeal cranial nerves (VII and IX) **(see Fig. 10-16)**. The interpretation of taste impulses is probably accomplished by the brain's lower frontal cortex, although there may be no sharply separate gustatory center.

SENSE OF SMELL

The importance of the sense of smell, or **olfaction** (ol-FAK-shun), is often underestimated. This sense helps to detect gases and other harmful substances in the environment and helps to warn of spoiled food. Smells can trigger memories and other psychological responses. Smell is also important in sexual behavior.

The receptors for smell are located in the epithelium of the nasal cavity's superior region **(see Fig. 10-16)**. Again, the chemicals detected must be in solution in the fluids that line the nose. Because these receptors are high in the nasal cavity, you must "sniff" to bring odors upward in your nose.

The impulses from the smell receptors are carried by the olfactory nerve (I), which leads directly to the olfactory center in the brain's temporal cortex. The interpretation of smell is closely related to the sense of taste, but a greater variety of dissolved chemicals can be detected by smell than by taste. We have hundreds of different types of odor receptors. Different odors also can activate specific combinations of receptors, so that we can detect over 10,000 different smells. The smell of foods is just as important in stimulating appetite and the flow of digestive juices as is the sense of taste. When you have a cold, food often seems tasteless and unappetizing because nasal congestion reduces your ability to smell the food.

The olfactory receptors deteriorate with age and food may become less appealing. It is important when presenting food to elderly people that the food look inviting so as to stimulate their appetites.

CHECKPOINT 

☐ **10-16** What are the special senses that respond to chemical stimuli?

The General Senses

Unlike the special sensory receptors, which are localized within specific sense organs and are limited to a relatively small area, the general sensory receptors are scattered throughout the body. These include receptors for touch, pressure, heat, cold, position, and pain **(Fig. 10-17)**.

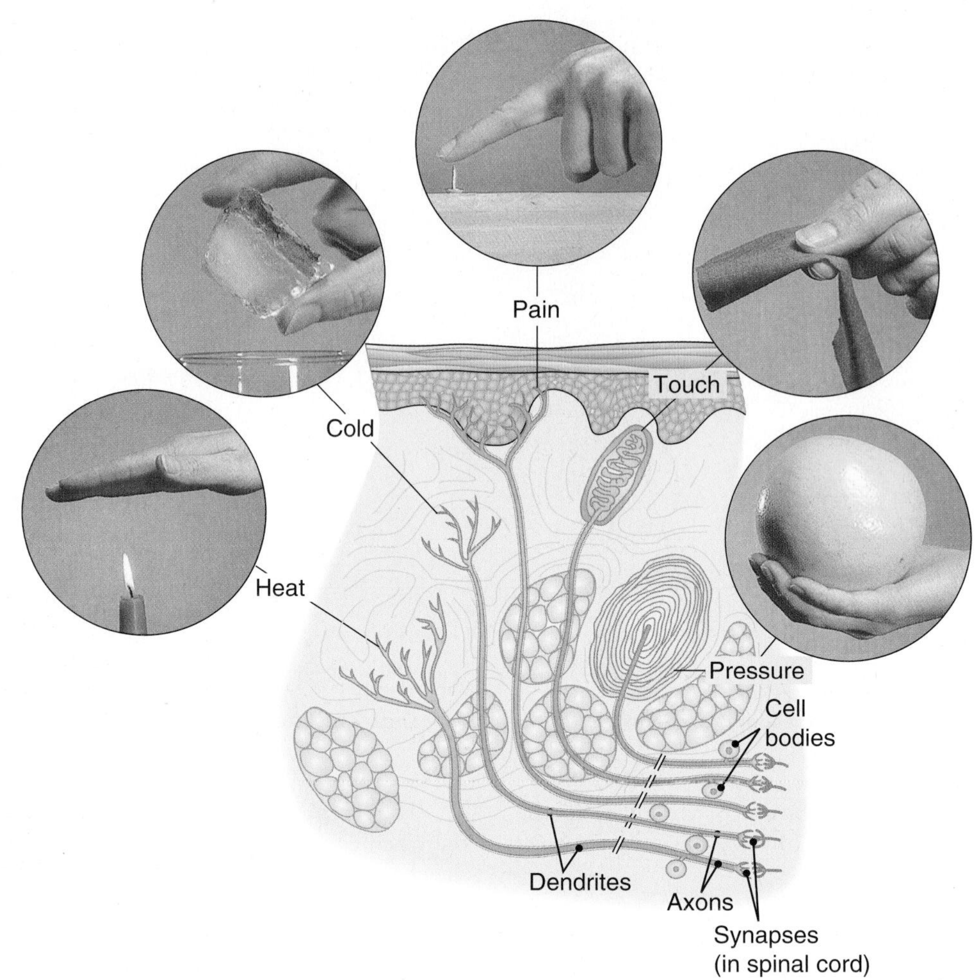

Figure 10-17 Sensory receptors in the skin. KEY POINT The skin has a variety of specialized sensory receptors. Synapses with interneurons are in the spinal cord.

SENSE OF TOUCH

The touch receptors, **tactile** (TAK-til) **corpuscles**, are found mostly in the dermis of the skin and around hair follicles. Touch sensitivity varies with the number of touch receptors in different areas. They are especially numerous and close together in the tips of the fingers and the toes. The lips and the tip of the tongue also contain many of these receptors and are very sensitive to touch. Other areas, such as the back of the hand and the back of the neck, have fewer receptors and are less sensitive to touch.

The sensation of tickle is related to the sense of touch, but is still something of a mystery. Tickle receptors are free nerve endings associated with the tactile mechanoreceptors. No one knows the value of tickling, but it may be a form of social interaction. Oddly, we experience tickling only when touched by someone else. Apparently, the brain inhibits these sensations when you are trying to tickle yourself and know the tickling site, eliminating the element of surprise.

SENSE OF PRESSURE

Even when the skin is anesthetized, it can still respond to pressure stimuli. These sensory receptors for deep pressure are located in the subcutaneous tissues beneath the skin and also near joints, muscles, and other deep tissues. They are sometimes referred to as *receptors for deep touch*.

SENSE OF TEMPERATURE

The temperature receptors are **free nerve endings**, receptors that are not enclosed in capsules but are simply branchings of nerve fibers. Temperature receptors are widely distributed in the skin, and there are separate receptors for heat and cold. A warm object stimulates only the heat receptors, and a cool object affects only the cold receptors. Internally, there are temperature receptors in the brain's hypothalamus, which help to adjust body temperature according to the temperature of the circulating blood.

SENSE OF POSITION

Receptors located in muscles, tendons, and joints relay impulses that aid in judging body position and changes in the locations of body parts in relation to each other. They also inform the brain of the amount of muscle contraction and tendon tension. These rather widespread receptors, known as **proprioceptors** (pro-pre-o-SEP-tors), are aided in this function by the internal ear's equilibrium receptors.

Information received by proprioceptors is needed for muscle coordination and is important in such activities as walking, running, and many more complicated skills, such as playing a musical instrument. They help to provide a sense of body movement, known as **kinesthesia** (kin-es-THE-ze-ah). Proprioceptors play an important part in maintaining muscle tone and good posture. They also help to assess the weight of an object to be lifted so that the right amount of muscle force is used.

The nerve fibers that carry impulses from these receptors enter the spinal cord and ascend to the brain in the posterior part of the cord. The cerebellum is a main coordinating center for these impulses.

SENSE OF PAIN

Pain is the most important protective sense. The receptors for pain are widely distributed free nerve endings. They are found in the skin, muscles, and joints and to a lesser extent in most internal organs (including the blood vessels and viscera). Two pathways transmit pain to the CNS. One is for acute, sharp pain, and the other is for slow, chronic pain. Thus, a single strong stimulus can produce an immediate sharp pain, followed in a second or so by a slow, diffuse pain that increases in severity with time.

Referred Pain Sometimes, pain that originates in an internal organ is experienced as coming from a more superficial part of the body, particularly the skin. This phenomenon is known as *referred pain*. Liver and gallbladder disease often cause referred pain in the skin over the right shoulder. Spasm of the coronary arteries that supply the heart may cause pain in the left shoulder and arm. Infection of the appendix can be felt as pain of the skin covering the lower right abdominal quadrant.

Apparently, some neurons in the spinal cord have the twofold duty of conducting impulses from visceral pain receptors in the chest and abdomen and from somatic pain receptors in neighboring areas of the skin, resulting in referred pain. The brain cannot differentiate between these two possible sources, but because most pain sensations originate in the skin, the brain automatically assigns the pain to this more likely place of origin.

Itch Itch receptors are free nerve endings that may be specific for that sensation or may share pathways with other receptors, such as those for pain. There are multiple causes for itching, including skin disorders, allergies, kidney disease, infection, and a host of chemicals. Usually, itching is a mild, short-lived annoyance, but for some, it can be chronic and debilitating. No one knows why scratching helps alleviate itch. It may replace the itch sensation with pain or send signals to the brain to relieve the sensation. 10

CHECKPOINTS

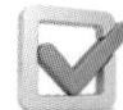

- ☐ **10-17** What are examples of general senses?
- ☐ **10-18** What are proprioceptors and where are they located?

A&P in Action Revisited

Early Signs of Cataract

Dr. Gilbert's assistant called Paul back to the consultation room after his eye examination. "You seem to be doing fine, Paul," the ophthalmologist reported. "No signs of glaucoma. I am a little concerned about some early signs of cataract, though. A cataract is a clouding of the eye's lens. Normally, the lens is clear, like the lens in a camera, but as we age, proteins in the lens break down, making the lens cloudy and resulting in blurry vision. Cataracts are a normal part of aging, but chronic sun exposure can speed this process up."

"Yikes!" Paul exploded. "Another run-in with the sun! I've already heard about the sun's unfriendly rays with my skin cancer, and I thought that's where it would end."

"Cataracts can be dealt with pretty effectively," said Dr. Gilbert, "but there's more. Sunlight is also a factor in a more serious condition, macular degeneration, which affects central vision and can lead to blindness. Your macula, located in the center of your retina, is the point of sharpest vision. With age, and over-exposure to the sun, the macula degenerates, resulting in a loss of vision in the center of the visual field. That's not as easily treatable at present. I don't see any signs of that right now, but you need to wear good quality sunglasses with a UV filter. Wearing dark glasses without the filter is worse than nothing, because they dilate your pupils and allow more harmful UV rays to enter your eyes."

"Great! One more thing to worry about as I get older," Paul complained.

"Not a worry if you take precautions," Dr. Gilbert responded. "Pick up your glasses prescription at the desk, and Paul, also take a pair of the dark disposable glasses we have there to protect your dilated eyes. They will be extra-sensitive to the sun for a while."

During this case, we learned that structural damage leads to functional changes. We also learned that some changes develop with age. Later chapters include information on age-related changes that affect other systems.

Chapter Wrap-Up

Summary Overview

A detailed chapter outline with space for note-taking is on *thePoint*. The figure below illustrates the main topics covered in this chapter.

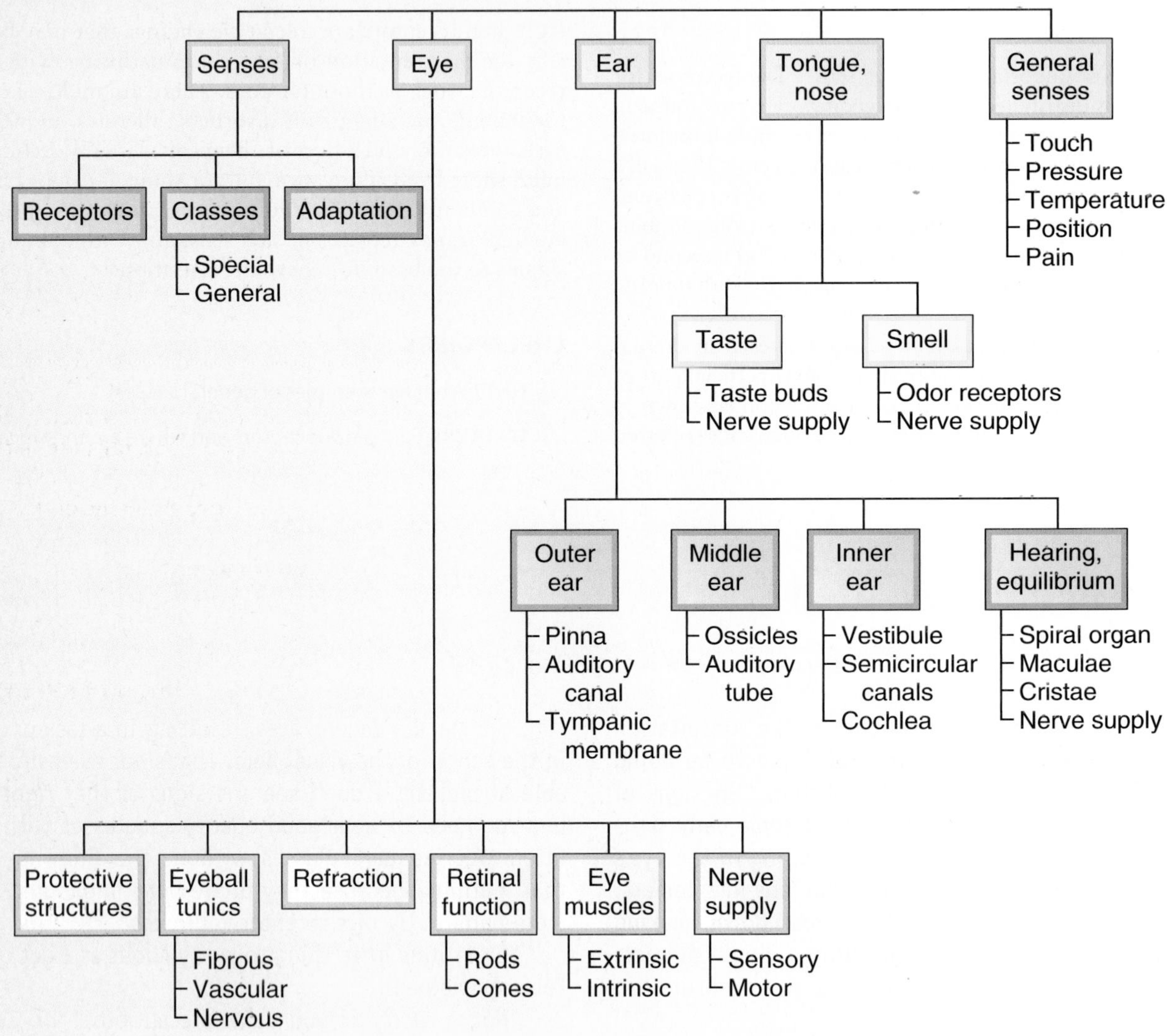

Key Terms

The terms listed below are emphasized in this chapter. Knowing them will help you organize and prioritize your learning. These and other boldface terms are defined in the Glossary with phonetic pronunciations.

accommodation
adaptation
auditory tube
aqueous humor
choroid
cochlea
conjunctiva
convergence
cornea
gustation
iris
lacrimal apparatus
lens (crystalline lens)
macula
olfaction
ossicle
proprioceptor
refraction
retina
sclera
semicircular canal
sensory adaptation
sensory receptor
spiral organ
tympanic membrane
vestibule
vitreous body

Word Anatomy

Medical terms are built from standardized word parts (prefixes, roots, and suffixes). Learning the meanings of these parts can help you remember words and interpret unfamiliar terms.

WORD PART	MEANING	EXAMPLE
The Eye and Vision		
ophthalm/o	eye	An *ophthalmologist* is a physician who specializes in treatment of the eye.
-scope	instrument for examination	An *ophthalmoscope* is an instrument used to examine the posterior of the eye.
lute/o	yellow	The macula *lutea* is a yellowish spot in the retina that contains the fovea centralis.
presby-	old	*Presbyopia* is farsightedness that occurs with age.
The Ear		
tympan/o	drum	The *tympanic* membrane is the eardrum.
equi-	equal	*Equilibrium* is balance (*equi-* combined with the Latin word *libra* meaning "balance").
ot/o	ear	*Otology* is the study of the ear.
lith	stone	*Otoliths* are small crystals in the inner ear that aid in static equilibrium.
-cusis	hearing	*Presbycusis* is hearing loss associated with age.
The General Senses		
propri/o-	own	*Proprioception* is perception of one's own body position.
kine	movement	*Kinesthesia* is a sense of body movement.
-esthesia	sensation	*Anesthesia* is loss of sensation, as of pain.

Questions for Study and Review

BUILDING UNDERSTANDING

Fill in the Blanks

1. The part of the nervous system that detects a stimulus is the ______.
2. The bending of light rays as they pass from air to fluid is called ______.
3. Nerve impulses are carried from the ear to the brain by the ______ nerve.
4. A receptor that senses knee joint position is a ______.
5. A receptor's ability to decrease its sensitivity to a continuous stimulus is called ______.

Matching > Match each numbered item with the most closely related lettered item.

___ **6.** Contains ciliated receptors sensitive to vibration
___ **7.** Contains receptors sensitive to light
___ **8.** An equilibrium receptor
___ **9.** A touch receptor
___ **10.** A pain receptor

a. retina
b. free nerve ending
c. macula
d. spiral organ
e. touch corpuscle

Multiple Choice

___ **11.** Which sense is not categorized as *special*?
a. smell
b. taste
c. equilibrium
d. pain

___ **12.** From superficial to deep, what is the order of the eyeball's tunics?
a. nervous, vascular, fibrous
b. fibrous, nervous, vascular
c. vascular, nervous, fibrous
d. fibrous, vascular, nervous

___ **13.** Which eye structure is most responsible for light refraction?
a. cornea
b. lens
c. vitreous body
d. retina

___ **14.** Which nerve carries sensory signals from the retina?
a. ophthalmic
b. optic
c. oculomotor
d. abducens

___ **15.** What do receptors in the vestibule sense?
a. muscle tension
b. sound
c. light
d. acceleration

UNDERSTANDING CONCEPTS

___ **16.** Differentiate between the terms in each of the following pairs:
a. special sense and general sense
b. aqueous humor and vitreous body
c. rods and cones
d. endolymph and perilymph
e. maculae and cristae

17. Trace the path of a light ray from the outside of the eye to the retina.

18. Define *convergence* and *accommodation* and describe several disorders associated with them.

19. List in order the structures that sound waves pass through in traveling through the ear to the receptors for hearing.

20. Name the five basic tastes. Where are the taste receptors? Name the nerves of taste.

21. Trace the pathway of a nerve impulse from the olfactory receptors to the olfactory center in the brain.

CONCEPTUAL THINKING

22. Why can you taste eyedrops after applying them to your eyeball?

23. You and a friend have just finished riding the roller coaster at the amusement park. As you walk away from the ride, your friend stumbles and comments that the ride has affected her balance. How do you explain this?

24. In the case story, Paul discovered he might be developing an age-related eye disorder. What is a cataract? What are some other age-related disorders of the sensory system?

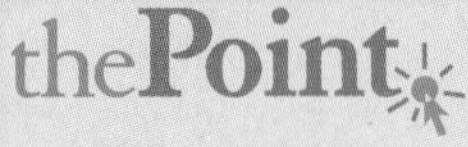

For more questions, see the learning activities on *thePoint*.

CHAPTER 11

The Endocrine System: Glands and Hormones

A&P in Action

Becky's Case: When an Endocrine Organ Fails

Becky stumbled down the stairs, wiping the sleep from her eyes, and hoping that Max hadn't finished all the pancakes that she could smell from the kitchen. "How was your sleep last night?" asked Becky's mother, who slid a plate across the table toward her. "Awful," sighed Becky, drowning her pancakes in a lake of syrup. "I woke up a bunch of times to go to the bathroom."

"Were you actually able to make it this time?" chimed Becky's little brother. Becky wished Max hadn't brought *that* up. She hoped he wasn't blabbing to his friends that she was wetting the bed again. "You know, if you didn't drink so much, you wouldn't have to pee so much," explained Max, as his sister gulped down her third glass of orange juice. Becky ate her pancakes and pretended that she didn't care about Max's comment. But he was right. She was so thirsty—and hungry!

It was a long day when the bell finally rang and Becky boarded the bus for the ride home. Math class had been a disaster because she couldn't concentrate. During gym, she was tired and had a stomach ache. And she had to keep asking for permission to go to the bathroom! Now, she was exhausted and her head hurt. Fighting tears, she remembered that during breakfast, her mom had mentioned that she'd made an appointment for Becky to see her doctor. She hadn't been too keen on the idea, but now she was relieved.

Later that week, Becky's pediatrician weighed her, measured her height, and asked her a bunch of questions. "So, let me see if I've got this right, Becky," said Dr. Carter. "For the past couple of weeks, you've felt lethargic and sick to your stomach. You've been really thirsty and have needed to go to the bathroom a lot. You've also been really hungry. You've had headaches and some difficulty concentrating at school, and have felt tired when playing sports." Becky wasn't too sure what lethargic meant, but other than that he seemed to have gotten the facts right. So, Becky nodded her head yes.

Turning to Becky's mother, Dr. Carter said, "Checking her chart, it appears that she's lost several pounds since her last appointment—despite her appetite. I'm going to order a urine test and blood test. I'd like to see what her glucose levels are." Becky didn't enjoy the tests one bit. Having to pee in a cup was gross and as for the blood test, that was the worst!

The next day, Dr. Carter called Becky's mother. "The urinalysis was positive for glucose and ketones, suggesting that Becky is not metabolizing glucose correctly. Her blood test revealed that she's hyperglycemic. In other words, her blood sugar is too high. We need to run a few more tests, but my diagnosis so far is that Becky has type 1 diabetes mellitus and needs insulin."

Dr. Carter suspects that Becky's pancreas, an important endocrine organ, does not produce sufficient amounts of the hormone insulin. Without insulin, Becky's cells cannot convert glucose into energy. As we will see later, type 1 diabetes has a dramatic effect on Becky's health.

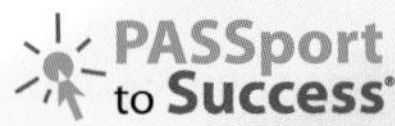

Ancillaries At-A-Glance

Visit *thePoint* to access the PASSport to Success and the following resources. For guidance in using these resources most effectively, see pp. ix–xviii.

Learning TOOLS

- Learning Style Self Assessment
- Live Advise Online Student Tutoring
- Tips for Effective Studying

Learning RESOURCES

- E-book: Chapter 11
- Animation: Hormonal Control of Glucose
- Health Professions: Exercise and Fitness Specialist
- Detailed Chapter Outline
- Answers to Questions for Study and Review
- Audio Pronunciation Glossary

Learning ACTIVITIES

- Pre-Quiz
- Visual Activities
- Kinesthetic Activities
- Auditory Activities

Learning Outcomes

After careful study of this chapter, you should be able to:

1. Compare the effects of the nervous system and the endocrine system in controlling the body, ***p. 212***
2. Describe the functions of hormones, ***p. 214***
3. Discuss the chemical composition of hormones, ***p. 212***
4. Explain how hormones are regulated, ***p. 212***
5. Identify the glands of the endocrine system on a diagram, ***p. 213***
6. List the hormones produced by each endocrine gland and describe the effects of each on the body, ***p. 214***
7. Describe how the hypothalamus controls the anterior and posterior pituitary, ***p. 213***
8. List tissues other than the endocrine glands that produce hormones, ***p. 220***
9. List some medical uses of hormones, ***p. 221***
10. Explain how the endocrine system responds to stress, ***p. 222***
11. Referring to the case study, discuss the effects of insulin deficiency on body function, ***pp. 210, 223***
12. Show how word parts are used to build words related to the endocrine system (see Word Anatomy at the end of the chapter), ***p. 225***

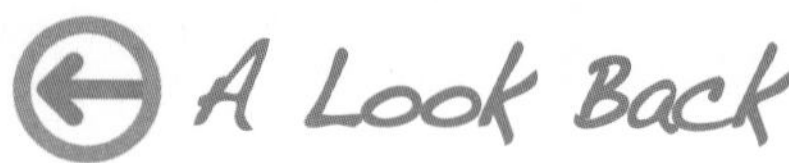

The past several chapters have described the nervous system and its role in regulating body responses. The endocrine system is also viewed as a controlling system, exercising its effects through hormones. The endocrine glands differ from the exocrine glands described in Chapter 4, because they secrete directly into body fluids and not through ducts. Control of the endocrine system relies mainly on negative feedback, described in Chapter 1.

The endocrine system consists of a group of glands that produces regulatory chemicals called **hormones**. The endocrine system and the nervous system work together to control and coordinate all other body systems. The nervous system controls such rapid actions as muscle movement and intestinal activity by means of electrical and chemical stimuli. The effects of the endocrine system occur more slowly and over a longer period. They involve chemical stimuli only, and these chemical messengers have widespread effects on the body.

Although the nervous and endocrine systems differ in some respects, the two systems are closely related. For example, the activity of the pituitary gland, which in turn regulates other glands, is controlled by the brain's hypothalamus. The connections between the nervous system and the endocrine system enable endocrine function to adjust to the demands of a changing environment.

Hormones

Hormones are chemical messengers that have specific regulatory effects on certain cells or organs. Hormones from the endocrine glands are released, not through ducts, but directly into surrounding tissue fluids. Most then diffuse into the bloodstream, which carries them throughout the body. They regulate growth, metabolism, reproduction, and behavior. Some hormones affect many tissues. These include, for example, growth hormone, thyroid hormone, and insulin. Others affect only specific tissues. For example, one pituitary hormone, thyroid-stimulating hormone (TSH), acts only on the thyroid gland; another, adrenocorticotropic hormone (ACTH), stimulates only the outer portion of the adrenal gland. Others act more locally, close to where they are secreted.

The specific tissue acted on by each hormone is the **target tissue**. The cells that make up these tissues have receptors in the plasma membrane or within the cytoplasm to which the hormone attaches. Once a hormone binds to a receptor on or in a target cell, it affects cell activities, regulating the manufacture of proteins; changing the membrane's permeability to specific substances; or affecting metabolic reactions.

HORMONE CHEMISTRY

Chemically, hormones fall into two main categories:

- **Amino acid compounds**. These hormones are proteins or related compounds also made of amino acids. All hormones except those of the adrenal cortex and the sex glands fall into this category.
- **Steroids**. These hormones are derived from the steroid cholesterol, a type of lipid **(see Fig. 2-9)**. Steroid hormones are produced by the adrenal cortex and the sex glands. Most can be recognized by the ending *-sterone*, as in progesterone and testosterone.

HORMONE REGULATION

The amount of each hormone that is secreted is normally kept within a specific range. Negative feedback is the method most commonly used to regulate these levels. That is, the hormone itself (or the result of its action) controls further hormone secretion. When the target tissue becomes too active, there is a negative effect on the endocrine gland, which then decreases its secretory activity.

We can use as an example the secretion of thyroid hormones **(Fig. 11-1)**. As described in more detail later in the chapter, a pituitary hormone, called *thyroid-stimulating hormone* (TSH), triggers hormone secretion from the thyroid gland located in the neck. As blood levels of these hormones rise under the effects of TSH, they act as negative feedback messengers to inhibit further TSH release from the

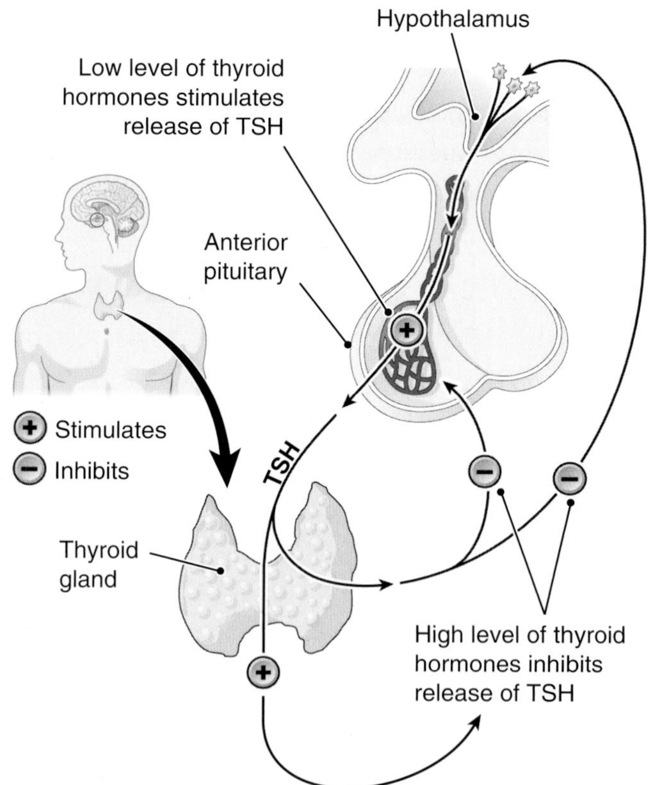

Figure 11-1 Negative feedback control of thyroid hormones. KEY POINT The anterior pituitary releases thyroid-stimulating hormone (TSH) when the blood level of thyroid hormones is low. A high level of thyroid hormones inhibits release of TSH and thyroid hormone levels fall. ZOOMING IN What gland controls the thyroid gland?

pituitary. With less TSH, the thyroid releases less hormone and blood levels decline. When hormone levels fall below the normal range, the pituitary can again begin to release TSH. This is a typical example of the kind of self-regulating system that keeps hormone levels within a set normal range.

Hormone release may fall into a rhythmic pattern. Hormones of the adrenal cortex follow a 24-hour cycle related to a person's sleeping pattern, with the secretion level greatest just before arising and least at bedtime. Hormones of the female menstrual cycle follow a monthly pattern.

CHECKPOINTS 

11-1 What are hormones and what are some effects of hormones?

11-2 What is the most common mechanism used to regulate hormone secretion?

The Endocrine Glands and Their Hormones

The remainder of this chapter discusses hormones and the tissues that produce them. Refer to **Figure 11-2** to locate each of the endocrine glands as you study them. **Table 11-1** summarizes the information on the endocrine glands and their hormones.

Although most of the discussion centers on the endocrine glands, which specialize in hormone production, it is important to note that many tissues—other than the endocrine glands—also secrete hormones. These tissues include the brain, digestive organs, and kidney. Some of these other tissues are discussed later in the chapter.

THE PITUITARY

The **pituitary** (pih-TU-ih-tar-e), or *hypophysis* (hi-POF-ih-sis), is a gland about the size of a cherry. It is located in a saddle-like depression of the sphenoid bone just posterior to the point where the optic nerves cross. It is surrounded by bone except where it connects with the brain's hypothalamus by a stalk called the **infundibulum** (in-fun-DIB-u-lum). The gland is divided into two parts: the **anterior lobe** and the **posterior lobe** (Fig. 11-3).

The anterior pituitary is often called the *master gland* because it releases hormones that affect the working of other glands, such as the thyroid, gonads (ovaries and testes), and adrenal glands. (Hormones that stimulate other glands may be recognized by the ending *tropin*, as in *thyrotropin*, which means "acting on the thyroid gland.") However, the pituitary itself is controlled by the hypothalamus, by means of secretions and nerve impulses sent to the pituitary through the infundibulum (see Fig. 11-3).

Control of the Pituitary The hormones produced in the anterior pituitary are not released until chemical messengers called **releasing hormones** arrive from the hypothalamus. These releasing hormones travel to the anterior pituitary by way of a special type of circulatory pathway called a **portal system**. By this circulatory "detour," some of the blood that leaves the hypothalamus travels to capillaries in the anterior pituitary before returning to the heart. As the

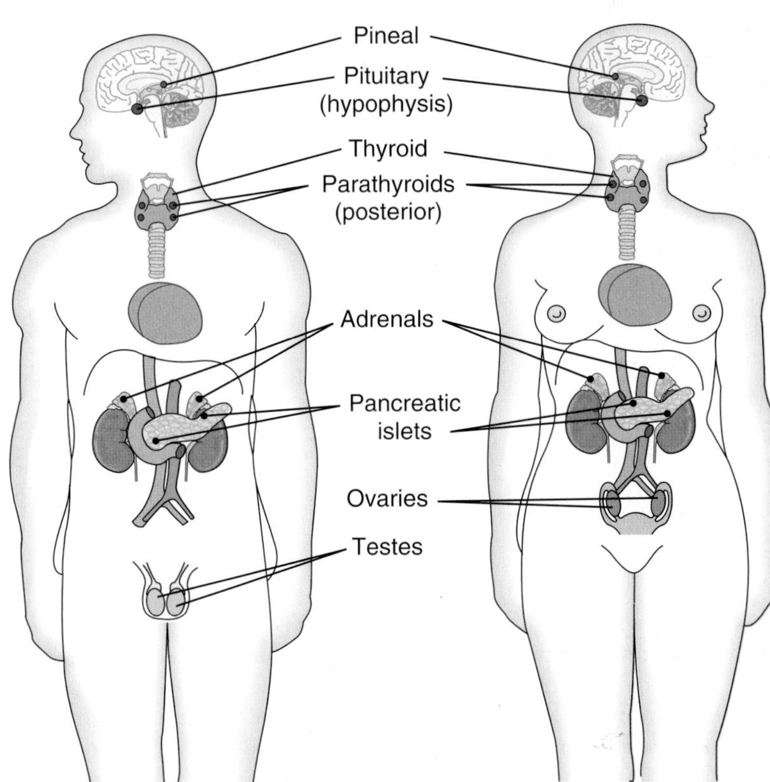

Figure 11-2 The endocrine glands. KEY POINT The endocrine system is comprised of glands with a primary function of hormone secretion.

11

Table 11-1 The Endocrine Glands and Their Hormones

Gland	Hormone	Principal Functions
Anterior pituitary	GH (growth hormone)	Promotes growth of all body tissues
	TSH (thyroid-stimulating hormone)	Stimulates thyroid gland to produce thyroid hormones
	ACTH (adrenocorticotropic hormone)	Stimulates adrenal cortex to produce glucocorticoids (cortisol) and androgens; aids in protecting body in stress situations (injury and pain)
	PRL (prolactin)	Stimulates milk production by mammary glands
	FSH (follicle-stimulating hormone)	Stimulates growth and hormonal activity of ovarian follicles; stimulates growth of testes; promotes sperm cell development
	LH (luteinizing hormone)	Initiates ovulation, corpus luteum formation, and progesterone production in the female; stimulates testosterone secretion in male
Posterior pituitary	ADH (antidiuretic hormone)	Promotes water reabsorption in kidney tubules; at high concentration stimulates constriction of blood vessels
	Oxytocin	Causes uterine muscle contraction; causes milk ejection from mammary glands
Thyroid	Thyroxine (T_4) and triiodothyronine (T_3)	Increase metabolic rate, influencing both physical and mental activities; required for normal growth
Parathyroids	PTH (parathyroid hormone)	Regulates exchange of calcium between blood and bones; increases calcium level in blood
Adrenal medulla	Epinephrine	Increases blood pressure and heart rate; activates cells influenced by sympathetic nervous system plus many not supplied by sympathetic nerves
Adrenal cortex	Cortisol (95% of glucocorticoids)	Increases blood glucose concentration in response to stress
	Aldosterone (95% of mineralocorticoids)	Promotes salt (and thus water) retention and potassium excretion
	Sex hormones	May influence secondary sexual characteristics
Pancreatic islets	Insulin	Reduces blood glucose concentrations by promoting glucose uptake into cells and glucose storage; promotes fat and protein synthesis
	Glucagon	Stimulates liver to release glucose, thereby increasing blood glucose levels
Testes	Testosterone	Stimulates growth and development of sexual organs (testes and penis) plus development of secondary sexual characteristics, such as hair growth on body and face and deepening of voice; stimulates sperm cell maturation
Ovaries	Estrogens (e.g., estradiol)	Stimulates growth of primary sexual organs (uterus and tubes) and development of secondary sexual organs, such as breasts; stimulates development of ovarian follicles
	Progesterone	Stimulates development of mammary glands' secretory tissue; prepares uterine lining for implantation of fertilized ovum; aids in maintaining pregnancy
Pineal	Melatonin	Regulates mood, sexual development, and daily cycles in response to the amount of light in the environment

blood circulates through the capillaries, it delivers the hormones that stimulate the release of anterior pituitary secretions. Hypothalamic releasing hormones are indicated with the abbreviation *RH* added to an abbreviation for the name of the hormone stimulated. For example, the releasing hormone (RH) that controls growth hormone (GH) is GH-RH. All of the anterior pituitary hormones are also regulated by inhibitory hormones from the hypothalamus.

The two hormones of the posterior pituitary (antidiuretic hormone, or ADH, and oxytocin) are actually produced in the hypothalamus and only stored in the posterior pituitary. Their release is controlled by nerve impulses that

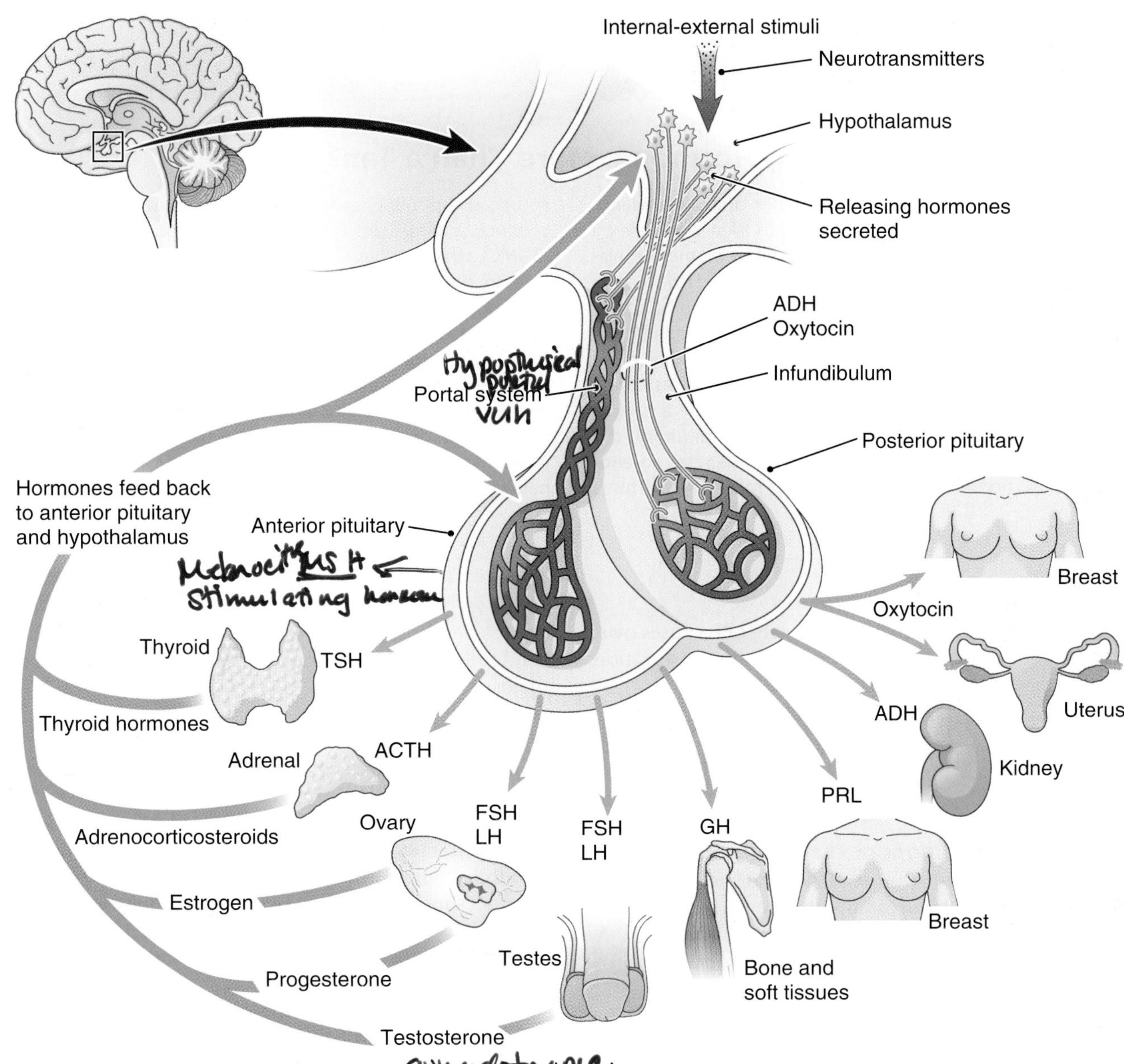

Figure 11-3 The hypothalamus, pituitary gland, and target tissues. KEY POINT Hormone secretion is regulated mainly by negative feedback. *Arrows* indicate the hormones' target tissues and feedback pathways. ZOOMING IN What two structures does the infundibulum connect?

travel over pathways (tracts) between the hypothalamus and the posterior pituitary.

Anterior Lobe Hormones

- **Growth hormone (GH)**, or *somatotropin* (so-mah-to-TRO-pin), acts directly on most body tissues, promoting protein manufacture that is essential for growth. GH causes increases in size and height to occur in youth, before the closure of long bone epiphyses. GH is produced throughout life. It stimulates protein synthesis and is needed for cellular maintenance and repair. It also stimulates the liver to release fatty acids and glucose for energy in time of stress.
- **Thyroid-stimulating hormone** (TSH), or *thyrotropin* (thi-ro-TRO-pin), stimulates the thyroid gland to produce thyroid hormones.
- **Adrenocorticotropic** (ad-re-no-kor-tih-ko-TRO-pik) **hormone** (ACTH) stimulates hormone production in the cortex of the adrenal glands.
- **Prolactin** (pro-LAK-tin) (**PRL**) stimulates milk production in the breasts.
- **Follicle-stimulating hormone** (**FSH**) stimulates the development of ovarian follicles in which egg cells mature and the development of sperm cells in the testes.

Box 11-1 A Closer Look

Melanocyte-Stimulating Hormone: More Than a Tan?

In amphibians, reptiles, and certain other animals, melanocyte-stimulating hormone (MSH) darkens skin and hair by stimulating melanocytes to manufacture the pigment melanin. In humans, though, MSH levels are usually so low that its role as a primary regulator of skin pigmentation and hair color is questionable. What, then, is its function in the human body?

Recent research suggests that MSH is probably more important as a neurotransmitter in the brain than as a hormone in the rest of the body. MSH is produced by a narrow region between the anterior and posterior pituitary, the intermediate lobe. When the pituitary gland secretes adrenocorticotropic hormone (ACTH), it secretes MSH as well. This is so because pituitary cells do not produce ACTH directly but produce a large precursor molecule, proopiomelanocortin (POMC), which enzymes cut into ACTH and MSH. In Addison disease, the pituitary tries to compensate for decreased glucocorticoid levels by increasing POMC production. The resulting increased levels of ACTH and MSH appear to cause the blotchy skin pigmentation that characterizes the disease.

MSH's other roles include helping the brain to regulate food intake, fertility, and even the immune response. Interestingly, despite MSH's relatively small role in regulating pigmentation, women do produce more MSH during pregnancy and often have darker skin.

- **Luteinizing** (LU-te-in-i-zing) **hormone** (**LH**) causes ovulation in females and promotes progesterone secretion in females and testosterone secretion in males.

FSH and LH are classified as **gonadotropins** (gon-ah-do-TRO-pinz), hormones that act on the gonads to regulate growth, development, and reproductive function in both males and females.

Posterior Lobe Hormones

- **Antidiuretic** (an-ti-di-u-RET-ik) **hormone** (**ADH**) promotes the reabsorption of water from the kidney tubules and thus decreases water excretion. A large amount of this hormone causes contraction of smooth muscle in blood vessel walls and raises blood pressure.
- **Oxytocin** (ok-se-TO-sin) causes uterine contractions and triggers milk ejection from the breasts. Under certain circumstances, commercial preparations of this hormone are administered during childbirth to promote uterine contraction.

Box 11-1 offers information on melanocyte-stimulating hormone, another hormone produced by the pituitary gland.

CHECKPOINTS

- 11-3 What part of the brain controls the pituitary?
- 11-4 What are the hormones from the anterior pituitary?
- 11-5 What hormones are released from the posterior pituitary?

THE THYROID GLAND

The **thyroid**, located in the neck, is the largest of the endocrine glands (Fig. 11-4) (see also Fig. A3-5 in the dissection atlas). The thyroid has two roughly oval lateral lobes on either side of the larynx (voice box) connected by a narrow band called an *isthmus* (IS-mus). A connective tissue capsule encloses the entire gland.

Thyroid Hormones The thyroid produces two hormones that regulate metabolism. The principal hormone is **thyroxine** (thi-ROK-sin), which is symbolized as T_4, based on the four iodine atoms contained in each molecule. The other hormone, which contains three atoms of iodine, is **triiodothyronine** (tri-i-o-do-THI-ro-nene), or T_3. These hormones increase the metabolic rate in body cells. That is, they increase the rate at which cells use nutrients to generate ATP and heat. Both thyroid hormones and growth hormone are needed for normal growth.

The thyroid also produces a hormone called **calcitonin** (kal-sih-TO-nin), which was named for the belief that it helped to control calcium balance. In fact, the effects of this

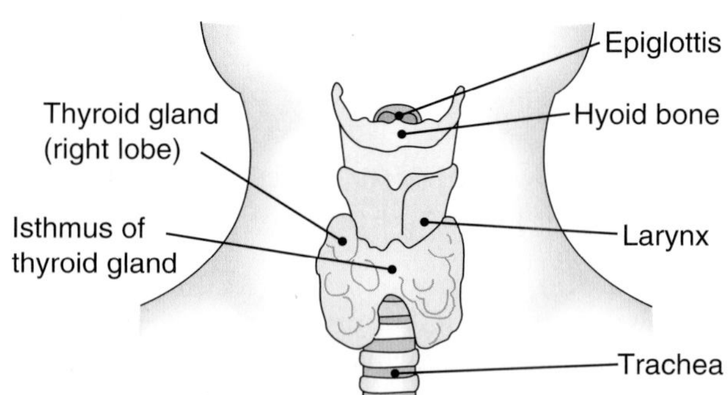

Figure 11-4 Thyroid gland (anterior view). KEY POINT The thyroid has two lobes connected by an isthmus. These are shown here in relation to other structures in the throat. The epiglottis is a cartilage of the larynx. ZOOMING IN What structure is superior to the thyroid? Inferior to the thyroid?

hormone in humans are minimal. Its ability to lower blood calcium levels was first described in animals, but in humans, there is no evidence that it is important.

THE PARATHYROID GLANDS

The four tiny **parathyroid glands** are embedded in the thyroid's posterior capsule **(Fig. 11-5)**. The secretion of these glands, **parathyroid hormone** (PTH), promotes calcium release from bone tissue, thus increasing the amount of calcium circulating in the bloodstream. PTH also causes the kidney to conserve calcium. PTH levels are controlled by negative feedback based on the amount of calcium in the blood; when calcium is low, PTH is produced.

Calcium Metabolism Calcium balance is required not only for the health of bones and teeth but also for the proper function of the nervous system and muscles. Another hormone, in addition to PTH, is needed for calcium balance. This hormone is **calcitriol** (kal-sih-TRI-ol), technically called dihydroxycholecalciferol (di-hi-drok-se-ko-le-kal-SIF-eh-rol), the active form of vitamin D. Calcitriol is produced by modification of vitamin D in the liver and then the kidney, a process stimulated by PTH. Calcitriol increases intestinal absorption of calcium to raise blood calcium levels.

PTH and calcitriol work together to regulate the amount of calcium in the blood and provide calcium for bone maintenance and other functions.

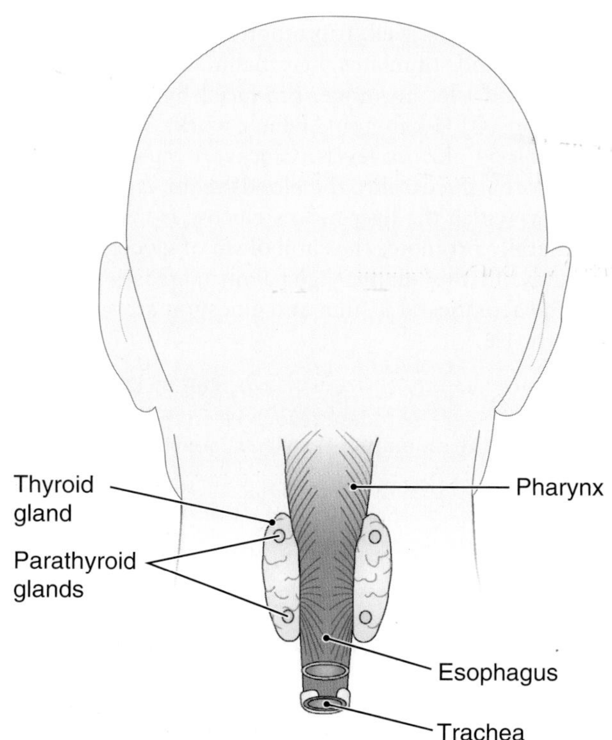

Figure 11-5 Parathyroid glands (posterior view).
KEY POINT The four small parathyroid glands are embedded in the posterior surface of the thyroid.

CHECKPOINTS 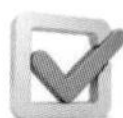

- 11-6 What is the effect of thyroid hormones on cells?
- 11-7 What mineral is needed to produce thyroid hormones?
- 11-8 What mineral is regulated by parathyroid hormone (PTH) and calcitriol?

THE ADRENAL GLANDS

The **adrenals**, also called the *suprarenal glands*, are two small glands located atop the kidneys (see Fig. A3.8 in the dissection atlas). Each adrenal gland has two parts that act as separate glands. The inner area is called the **medulla**, and the outer portion is called the **cortex (Fig. 11-6)**.

Hormones from the Adrenal Medulla The hormones of the adrenal medulla are released in response to

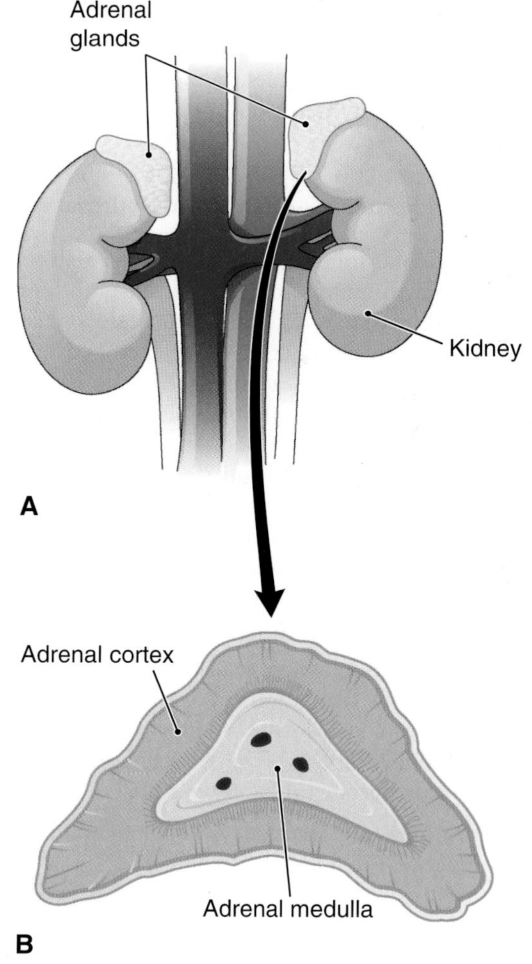

Figure 11-6 The adrenal gland. KEY POINT The medulla secretes epinephrine. The cortex secretes steroid hormones. (Reprinted with permission from Cohen BJ, *Medical Terminology*, 6th ed. Philadelphia, PA: Lippincott Williams & Wilkins, 2011.)
ZOOMING IN What is the outer region of the adrenal gland called? The inner region?

stimulation by the sympathetic nervous system. The principal hormone produced by the medulla is **epinephrine**, also called *adrenaline*. Epinephrine is chemically and functionally similar to norepinephrine, the neurotransmitter active in the sympathetic nervous system, as described in Chapter 8. However, epinephrine is generally considered to be a hormone because it is released into the bloodstream instead of being released locally at synapses. Both epinephrine and norepinephrine are responsible for *fight-or-flight* responses during emergency situations. Some of their effects are as follows:

- Stimulation of smooth muscle contraction in the walls of some arterioles, causing them to constrict and blood pressure to rise accordingly
- Conversion of glycogen stored in the liver into glucose. The glucose pours into the blood and travels throughout the body, allowing the voluntary muscles and other tissues to do an extraordinary amount of work
- Increase in the heart rate
- Increase in the metabolic rate of body cells
- Dilation of the bronchioles, through relaxation of the smooth muscle in their walls

Hormones from the Adrenal Cortex There are three main groups of hormones secreted by the adrenal cortex:

- **Glucocorticoids** (glu-ko-KOR-tih-koyds) help the body to respond to unfavorable conditions and promote tissue healing. They maintain blood glucose levels in time of stress by stimulating the liver to convert amino acids into glucose instead of protein (as indicated by *gluco* in the name). In addition, they raise the level of other nutrients in the blood, including amino acids from tissue proteins and fatty acids from fats stored in adipose tissue. Glucocorticoids also have the ability to suppress the inflammatory response and are often administered as medication for this purpose. The major hormone of this group is **cortisol**, which is also called *hydrocortisone*.
- **Mineralocorticoids** (min-er-al-o-KOR-tih-koyds) are important in the regulation of electrolyte balance. They control sodium reabsorption and potassium secretion by the kidney tubules. The major hormone of this group is **aldosterone** (al-DOS-ter-one).
- **Sex hormones** are secreted in small amounts, having little effect on the body.

CHECKPOINTS 

11-9 What is the main hormone produced by the adrenal medulla?

11-10 What three categories of hormones are released by the adrenal cortex?

11-11 What effect does cortisol have on blood glucose levels?

THE ENDOCRINE PANCREAS

The **pancreas** is located in the left upper quadrant of the abdomen, inferior to the liver and gallbladder and lateral to the first portion of the small intestine, the duodenum (Fig. 11-7). It has two main types of cells that perform very different functions. One type forms small clusters called *acini* (AS-ih-ni) (singular *acinus*) that resemble blackberries (*acinus* comes from a Latin word meaning "berry.") Acini secrete digestive enzymes through ducts directly into the small intestine (see Chapter 17), thus making up the exocrine portion of the pancreas. In addition, scattered throughout the pancreas are specialized cells that form "little islands" called **islets** (I-lets), originally the *islets of Langerhans* (LAHNG-er-hanz) (see Fig. 11-7). These cells produce hormones that diffuse into the bloodstream, thus making up the endocrine portion of the pancreas, which we discuss further here.

Pancreatic Hormones

The most important hormone secreted by the islets is **insulin** (IN-su-lin), which is produced by beta (β) cells. Insulin promotes the transport of glucose across plasma membranes, thus increasing cellular glucose uptake. Once inside a cell, glucose is metabolized for energy. Insulin also increases the rate at which the liver and skeletal muscles convert glucose into glycogen (the storage form of glucose) and the rate at which the liver changes excess glucose into fatty acids. These fatty acids can then be converted to fats and stored in adipose tissue or the liver. Through these actions, insulin has the effect of lowering the blood glucose level. Insulin has other metabolic effects as well. It promotes the cellular uptake of amino acids and stimulates their manufacture into proteins.

A second islet hormone, produced by alpha (α) cells, is **glucagon** (GLU-kah-gon), which works with insulin to regulate blood glucose levels. Glucagon causes the liver to release stored glucose into the bloodstream. It also increases the rate at which the liver makes glucose from amino acids and generally promotes the catabolism of glycogen and fats for energy. In this manner, glucagon increases blood glucose. The activities of insulin and glucagon are summarized in Figure 11-8.

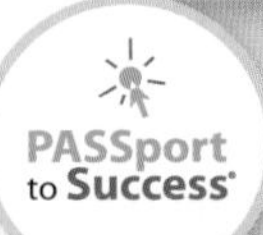

See the student resources on *thePoint* to view the animation *Hormonal Control of Glucose*.

THE SEX GLANDS

The sex glands, the female ovaries and the male testes, not only produce the sex cells but also are important endocrine organs. The hormones produced by these organs are needed in the development of the sexual characteristics, which usually appear in the early teens, and for the maintenance of the reproductive organs once full development has been attained. Those features that typify a male or female other than the structures directly concerned with reproduction are termed

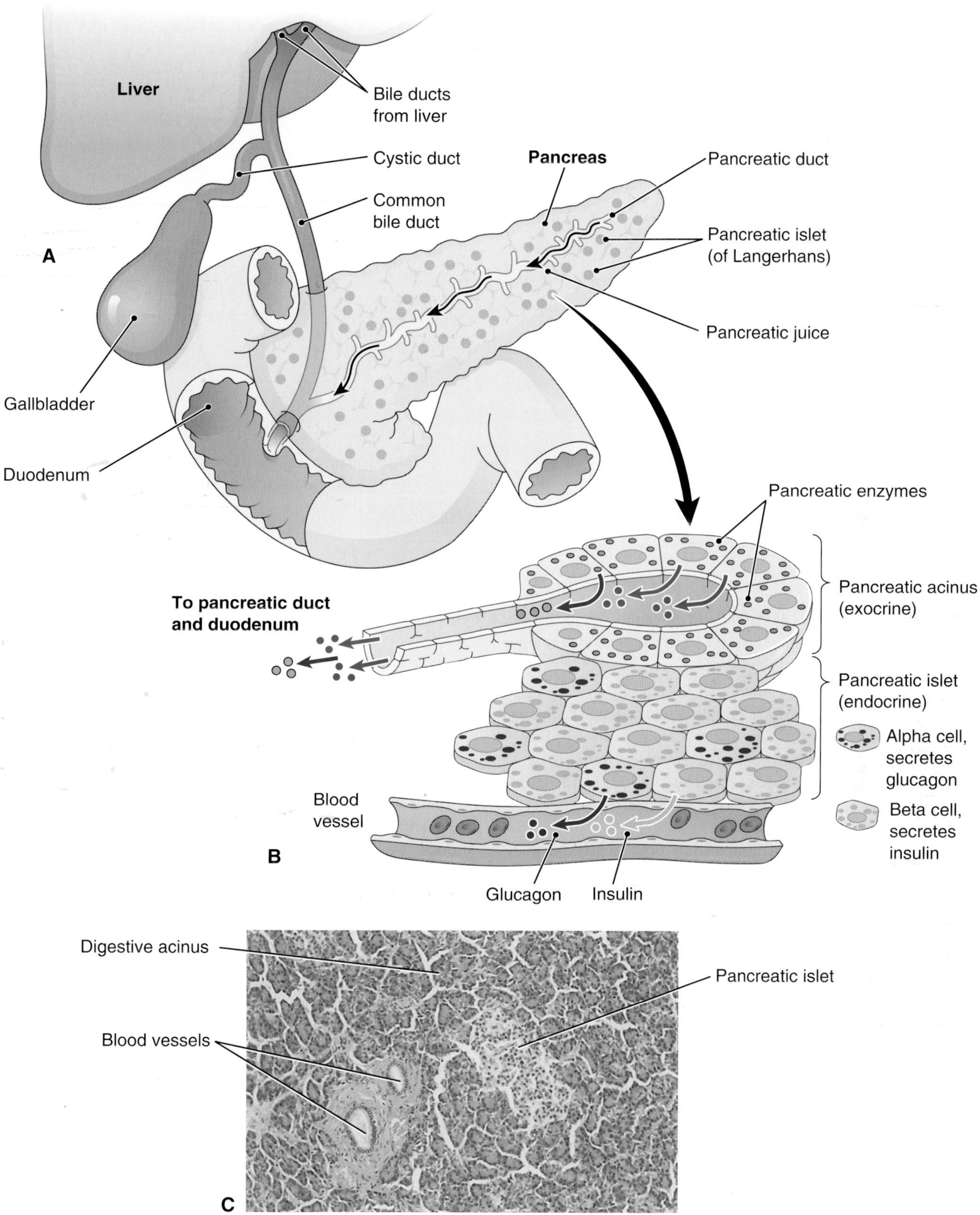

Figure 11-7 The pancreas and its functions. KEY POINT The pancreas has both exocrine and endocrine functions. **A.** The pancreas in relation to the liver, gallbladder, and duodenum (small intestine). **B.** Diagram of an acinus, which secretes digestive juices into ducts, and an islet, which secretes hormones into the bloodstream. **C.** Photomicrograph of pancreatic cells. Light-staining islets are visible among the many acini that produce digestive juices. (A and B, Reprinted with permission from McConnell TH. *The Nature of Disease*: Philadelphia, PA: Lippincott Williams & Wilkins, 2007; C, Courtesy of Dana Morse Bittus and B. J. Cohen)

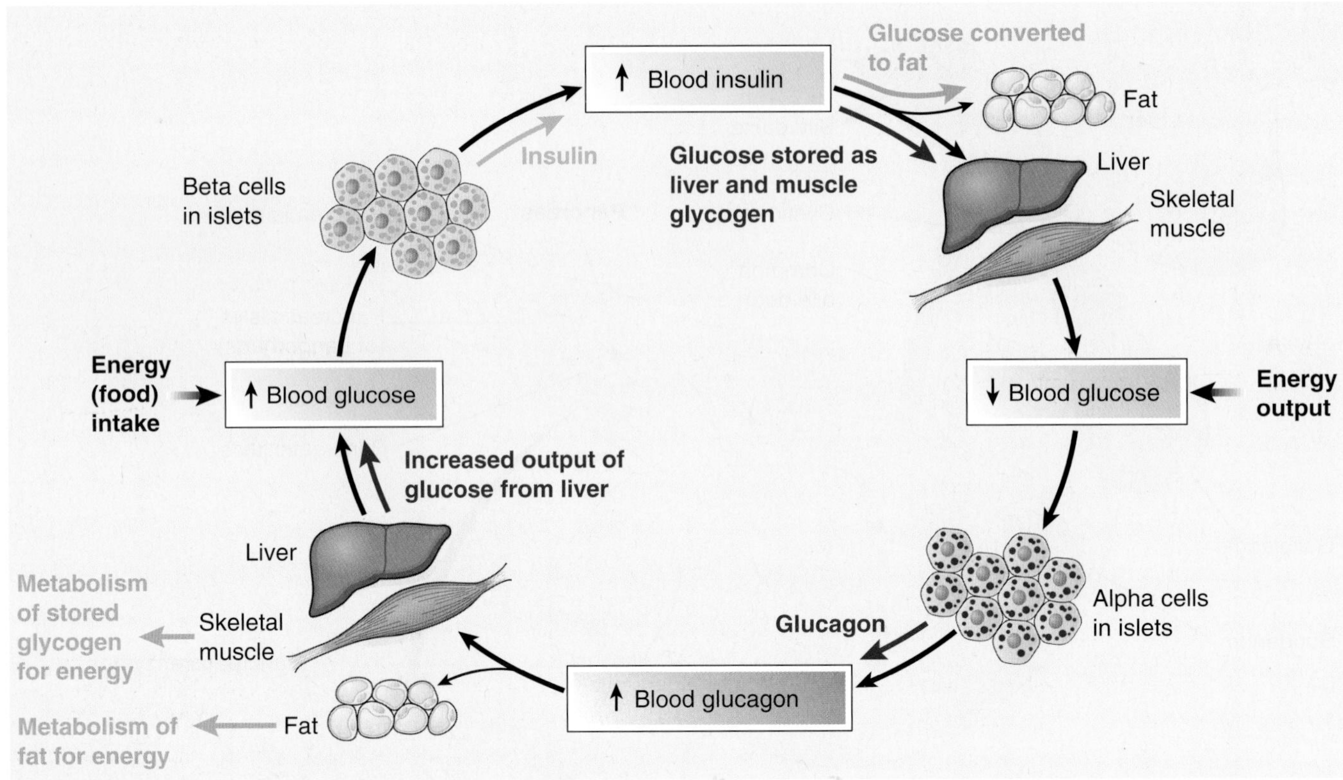

Figure 11-8 The effects of insulin and glucagon. KEY POINT These two hormones work together to regulate blood glucose levels. ZOOMING IN What organs do insulin and glucagon mainly influence?

secondary sex characteristics. They include a deep voice and facial and body hair in males, and wider hips, breast development, and a greater ratio of fat to muscle in females.

All male sex hormones are classified as **androgens** (AN-dro-jens). The main androgen produced by the testes is testosterone (tes-TOS-ter-one).

In the female, the hormones that most nearly parallel testosterone in their actions are the **estrogens** (ES-tro-jens), produced by the ovaries. Estrogens contribute to the development of the female secondary sex characteristics and stimulate mammary gland development, the onset of menstruation, and the development and functioning of the reproductive organs.

The other hormone produced by the ovaries, called **progesterone** (pro-JES-ter-one), assists in the normal development of pregnancy (gestation). All the sex hormones are discussed in more detail in Chapter 20.

THE PINEAL GLAND

The **pineal** (PIN-e-al) **gland** is a small, flattened, cone-shaped structure located posterior to the midbrain and connected to the roof of the third ventricle (see Fig. 11-2).

The pineal gland produces the hormone **melatonin** (mel-ah-TO-nin) during dark periods; little hormone is produced during daylight hours. This pattern of hormone secretion influences the regulation of sleep–wake cycles (see Box 11-2). Melatonin also appears to delay the onset of puberty.

CHECKPOINTS 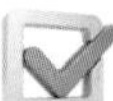

☐ **11-12** What two hormones produced by the islets of the pancreas regulate blood glucose levels?

☐ **11-13** Sex hormones confer certain features associated with male and female gender. What are these features called as a group?

Other Hormone-Producing Tissues

Originally, the word *hormone* applied to the secretions of the endocrine glands only. The term now includes various body substances that have regulatory actions, either locally or at a distance from where they are produced. Many body organs and tissues produce such regulatory substances.

HORMONE-PRODUCING ORGANS

Some body organs that produce hormones include the following:

- The stomach secretes a hormone called gastrin that stimulates its own digestive activity.

Box 11-2 *Clinical Perspectives*

Seasonal Affective Disorder: Seeing the Light

Most of us find that long, dark days make us blue and sap our motivation. Are these learned responses or is there a physical basis for them? Studies have shown that the amount of light in the environment does have a physical effect on behavior. Evidence that light alters mood comes from people who are intensely affected by the dark days of winter—people who suffer from **seasonal affective disorder**, aptly abbreviated SAD. When days shorten, these people feel sleepy, depressed, and anxious. They tend to overeat, especially carbohydrates. Research suggests that SAD has a genetic basis and may be associated with decreased levels of the neurotransmitter serotonin.

As light strikes the retina of the eye, it sends impulses that decrease the amount of melatonin produced by the pineal gland in the brain. Because melatonin depresses mood, the final effect of light is to elevate mood. Daily exposure to bright lights has been found to improve the mood of most people with SAD. Exposure for 15 minutes after rising in the morning may be enough, but some people require longer sessions both morning and evening. Other aids include aerobic exercise, stress management techniques, and antidepressant medications.

- The small intestine secretes hormones that stimulate the production of digestive juices and help regulate the digestive process.
- The kidneys produce a hormone called **erythropoietin** (e-rith-ro-POY-eh-tin) (EPO), which stimulates red blood cell production in the bone marrow. This hormone is produced when there is a decreased oxygen supply in the blood.
- The brain, as noted, secretes releasing hormones and release-inhibiting hormones that control the anterior pituitary, as well as ADH and oxytocin that are released from the posterior pituitary.
- The atria (upper chambers) of the heart produce a substance called **atrial natriuretic** (na-tre-u-RET-ik) **peptide** (**ANP**) in response to their increased filling with blood. ANP increases sodium excretion by the kidneys and lowers blood pressure.
- The thymus is a mass of lymphoid tissue that lies in the upper part of the chest superior to the heart (see Fig. A5-7 in the dissection atlas). This organ is important in the development of immunity early in life, but it shrinks and becomes less important in adulthood. Its hormone, thymosin (THI-mo-sin), assists in the maturation of certain white blood cells known as T cells (T lymphocytes) after they have left the thymus gland and taken up residence in lymph nodes throughout the body. The immune system is discussed in Chapter 15.
- The **placenta** (plah-SEN-tah) produces several hormones during pregnancy. These cause changes in the uterine lining and, later in pregnancy, help to prepare the breasts for lactation. Pregnancy tests are based on the presence of placental hormones (see Chapter 21).

PROSTAGLANDINS

Prostaglandins (pros-tah-GLAN-dins) are a group of hormone-like substances derived from fatty acids. The name *prostaglandin* comes from the fact that they were first discovered in semen and thought to be derived from the male prostate gland. We now know that prostaglandins are synthesized by almost all body cells. One reason that they are not strictly classified as hormones is that they are produced, act, and are rapidly inactivated in or close to where they are produced. In addition, they are not produced at a defined location, but throughout the body.

A bewildering array of functions has been ascribed to prostaglandins. Some cause constriction of blood vessels, bronchial tubes, and the intestine, whereas others cause dilation of these same structures. Prostaglandins are active in promoting inflammation; certain anti-inflammatory drugs, such as aspirin, act by blocking prostaglandin production. Some prostaglandins have been used to induce labor or abortion and have been recommended as possible contraceptive agents. Much has been written about these substances, and extensive research on them continues.

Hormones and Treatment

Hormones used for medical treatment are obtained from several different sources. Some are extracted from animal tissues. Some hormones and hormone-like substances are available in synthetic form, meaning that they are manufactured in commercial laboratories. A few hormones are produced by the genetic engineering technique of recombinant DNA. In this method, a gene for the cellular manufacture of a given product is introduced in the laboratory into a harmless strain of the common bacterium *Escherichia coli*. The organisms are then grown in quantity, and the desired substance is harvested and purified.

A few examples of natural and synthetic hormones used in treatment are:

- **Growth hormone** is used for the treatment of children and adults with a deficiency of this hormone. Adequate supplies are produced by recombinant DNA techniques.

- **Insulin** is used in the treatment of diabetes mellitus. Pharmaceutical companies now produce "human" insulin by recombinant DNA methods.
- **Adrenal steroids**, primarily the glucocorticoids, are used for the relief of inflammation in such diseases as rheumatoid arthritis, lupus erythematosus, asthma, and cerebral edema; for immunosuppression after organ transplantation; and for relief of symptoms associated with circulatory shock.
- **Epinephrine** (adrenaline) has many uses, including stimulation of the heart muscle when rapid response is required; treatment of asthmatic attacks by relaxation of the small bronchial tubes; and treatment of the acute allergic reaction called anaphylaxis (an-ah-fi-LAK-sis).
- **Thyroid hormones** are used in the treatment of hypothyroidism and as replacement therapy after surgical removal of the thyroid gland.
- **Oxytocin** is used to cause uterine contractions and induce labor.
- **Androgens**, including testosterone and androsterone, are used in severe chronic illness to aid tissue building and promote healing.
- **Estrogen and progesterone** are used as oral contraceptives (e.g., birth control pills; "the pill"). They are highly effective in preventing pregnancy. Occasionally, they give rise to unpleasant side effects, such as nausea. More rarely, they cause serious complications, such as thrombosis (blood clots) or hypertension (high blood pressure). These adverse side effects are more common among women who smoke. Any woman taking birth control pills should have a yearly medical examination.

In women experiencing menopause, levels of estrogen and progesterone begin to decline. Thus, preparations of synthetic estrogen and progesterone, called *hormone replacement therapy* (*HRT*), have been developed to treat the symptoms associated with this decline and to protect against the adverse changes—such as decreased bone density—that typically occur in the years after menopause. Recent studies on the most popular forms of HRT have raised questions about their benefits and revealed some risks associated with their use. This issue is still under study.

Hormones and Stress

Stress in the form of physical injury, disease, emotional anxiety, and even pleasure calls forth a specific physiologic response that involves both the nervous system and the endocrine system. The nervous system response, the "fight-or-flight" response, is mediated by parts of the brain, especially the hypothalamus, and by the sympathetic nervous system, which releases norepinephrine. During stress, the hypothalamus also triggers the release of ACTH from the anterior pituitary. The hormones released from the adrenal cortex as a result of ACTH stimulation raise the levels of glucose and other nutrients in the blood and inhibit inflammation. Growth hormone, thyroid hormones, sex hormones, and insulin are also released.

These hormones help the body meet stressful situations. Unchecked, however, they are harmful and may lead to such stress-related disorders as high blood pressure, heart disease, ulcers, insomnia, back pain, and headaches. Cortisones decrease the immune response, leaving the body more susceptible to infection.

Although no one would enjoy a life totally free of stress in the form of stimulation and challenge, unmanaged stress, or "distress," has negative physical effects. For this reason, techniques such as biofeedback and meditation to control stress are useful. The simple measures of setting priorities, getting adequate periods of relaxation, and getting regular physical exercise are important in maintaining total health.

CHECKPOINTS 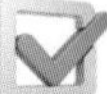

☐ **11-14** What are some organs other than the endocrine glands that produce hormones or hormone-like substances?

☐ **11-15** What are some hormones released in times of stress?

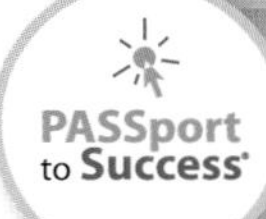

See the student resources on *thePoint* for information on careers in exercise and fitness.

Effects of Aging on the Endocrine System

Some of the changes associated with aging, such as loss of muscle and bone tissue, can be linked to changes in the endocrine system. The main clinical conditions associated with the endocrine system involve the pancreas and the thyroid. Many elderly people develop type 2 diabetes mellitus as a result of decreased insulin secretion, which is made worse by poor diet, inactivity, and increased body fat. Some elderly people also show the effects of decreased thyroid hormone secretion.

There are other hormonal changes with age as well. GH declines, accounting for some losses in strength, immunity, skin thickness, and healing. There is also diminished activity of the adrenal cortex. Sex hormones decline during the middle-age years in both males and females. These changes come from decreased activity of the gonads and also decreased anterior pituitary activity, resulting in decline of gonadotropic hormone secretion. Decrease in bone mass leading to osteoporosis is one result of these declines. HRT has shown some beneficial effects on mucous membranes and bone mass, but as noted above, its use is controversial.

A&P in Action Revisited

Becky's New "Normal"

Becky stumbled down the stairs wiping the sleep from her eyes as she made her way to the kitchen, hoping that Max hadn't finished all the pancakes that she could smell from down the hallway. "Good morning, sleepy-head," greeted her mother as she handed Becky the glucose monitor and lancet. "How was your sleep last night?"

"Great," yawned Becky as she lanced the side of her finger and squeezed a tiny drop of blood onto the monitor's test strip. After a few seconds, the monitor beeped and displayed her blood glucose concentration. "I'm normal," said Becky, half-expecting a wisecrack from her little brother, but he kept on eating.

Since Dr. Carter's diagnosis, Becky had been getting used to her new "normal." It wasn't easy being diabetic. She had to be really careful about what she ate and when. She had to measure her glucose before meals and inject herself with insulin after. Monitoring her glucose wasn't too bad, but Becky didn't think she would ever get used to the needles. She was also a little worried about what the kids at school were saying about her and her disease. One unexpected benefit was that Max seemed to have a newfound respect for her and her ability to inject herself. "What a weirdo!" she thought as she carefully poured a little bit of syrup on her pancakes.

During this case, we saw that the lack of the hormone insulin had negative effects on Becky's whole body. In later chapters, we learn more about the endocrine system's role in regulating body function. We also check on how Becky is managing her diabetes in Chapter 18: Metabolism, Nutrition, and Body Temperature.

Chapter Wrap-Up

Summary Overview

A detailed chapter outline with space for note-taking is on *thePoint*. The figure below illustrates the main topics covered in this chapter.

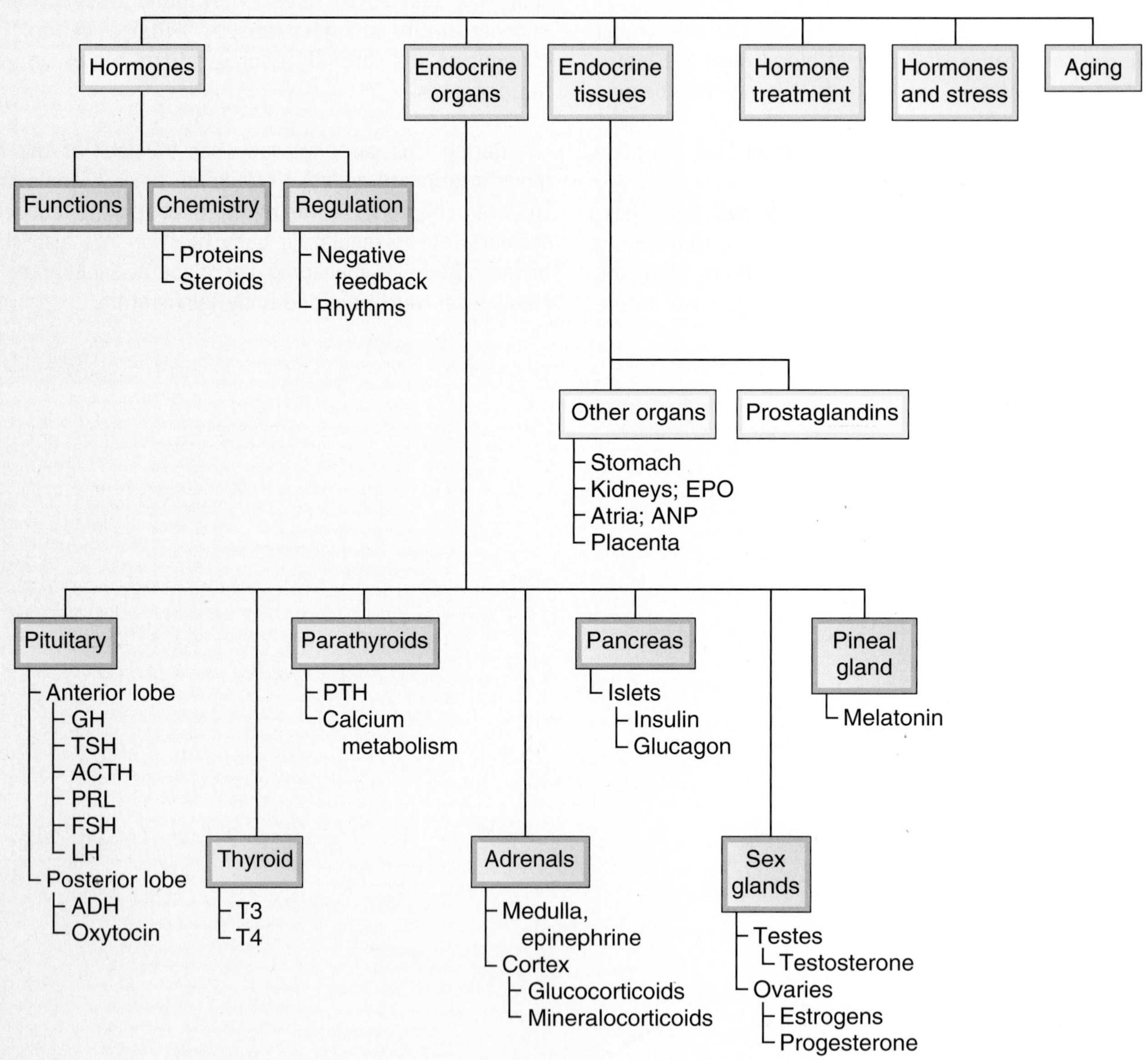

Key Terms

The terms listed below are emphasized in this chapter. Knowing them will help you organize and prioritize your learning. These and other boldface terms are defined in the Glossary with phonetic pronunciations.

endocrine	hypothalamus	prostaglandin	steroid
hormone	pituitary (hypophysis)	receptor	target tissue

Word Anatomy

Scientific terms are built from standardized word parts (prefixes, roots, and suffixes). Learning the meanings of these parts can help you remember words and interpret unfamiliar terms.

WORD PART	MEANING	EXAMPLE
The Endocrine Glands and Their Hormones		
-sterone	steroid hormone	*Testosterone* is a steroid hormone from the testes.
trop/o	acting on, influencing	*Somatotropin* stimulates growth in most body tissues.
cortic/o	cortex	*Adrenocorticotropic* hormone acts on the adrenal cortex.
lact/o	milk	*Prolactin* stimulates milk production in the breasts.
ur/o	urine	*Antidiuretic* hormone promotes reabsorption of water in the kidneys and decreases excretion of urine.
oxy	sharp, acute	*Oxytocin* stimulates uterine contractions during labor.
toc/o	labor	See preceding example.
ren/o	kidney	The *adrenal* glands are near (ad-) the kidneys.
nephr/o	kidney	*Epinephrine* (adrenaline) is secreted by the adrenal gland near the kidney.
insul/o	pancreatic islet, island	*Insulin* is a hormone produced by the pancreatic islets.
glyc/o	glucose, sugar	*Glycolysis* is the conversion of glucose into carbon dioxide and water.
andr/o	male	An *androgen* is any male sex hormone.
Other Hormone-Producing Tissues		
-poiesis	making, forming	*Erythropoietin* is a hormone from the kidneys that stimulates production of red blood cells.
natri	sodium (*L. natrium*)	Atrial *natriuretic* peptide stimulates release of sodium in the urine.

Questions for Study and Review

BUILDING UNDERSTANDING

Fill in the blanks

1. Chemical messengers carried by the blood are called ______.
2. The part of the brain that regulates pituitary gland activity is the ______.
3. Red blood cell production in the bone marrow is stimulated by the hormone ______.
4. The main androgen produced by the testes is ______.
5. A hormone produced by the heart is ______.

Matching > Match each numbered item with the most closely related lettered item.

___ **6.** An anterior pituitary lobe hormone
___ **7.** An adrenal cortex hormone
___ **8.** A pancreatic hormone
___ **9.** A posterior pituitary lobe hormone
___ **10.** An ovarian hormone

a. aldosterone
b. estrogen
c. glucagon
d. growth hormone
e. oxytocin

Multiple Choice

___ **11.** What do hormones bind to?

a. lipid bilayer
b. transporters
c. ion channels
d. receptors

___ **12.** Which hormone promotes uterine contractions and milk ejection?

a. prolactin
b. oxytocin
c. estrogen
d. luteinizing hormone

___ **13.** Choose the principal hormonal regulator of metabolism.

a. thyroxine
b. triiodothyronine
c. aldosterone
d. progesterone

___ **14.** Which structure secretes epinephrine?

a. adrenal cortex
b. adrenal medulla
c. kidneys
d. pancreas

___ **15.** Which organ regulates sleep–wake cycles?

a. pituitary
b. thyroid
c. thymus
d. pineal

UNDERSTANDING CONCEPTS

16. With regard to regulation, what are the main differences between the nervous system and the endocrine system?

17. Explain how the hypothalamus and pituitary gland regulate certain endocrine glands. Use the thyroid as an example.

18. Name the two divisions of the pituitary gland. List the hormones released from each division and describe the effects of each.

19. Compare and contrast the following hormones:

a. thyroxine and triiodothyronine
b. cortisol and aldosterone
c. insulin and glucagon
d. testosterone and estrogen

20. Describe the anatomy of the following endocrine glands:

a. thyroid
b. pancreas
c. adrenals

21. Name the hormones released by the kidneys and by the pineal body. What are the effects of each?

22. List several hormones released during stress. What is the relationship between prolonged stress and disease?

CONCEPTUAL THINKING

23. One consequence of decreased blood levels of thyroid hormone is increased blood levels of thyroid stimulating hormone. Why?

24. In the case story, Dr. Carter noted that Becky presented with the three cardinal signs of diabetes—weight loss, glucose and ketones in the urine, and hyperglycemia. How does a lack of insulin cause these signs?

thePoint For more questions, see the learning activities on *thePoint.*

UNIT IV

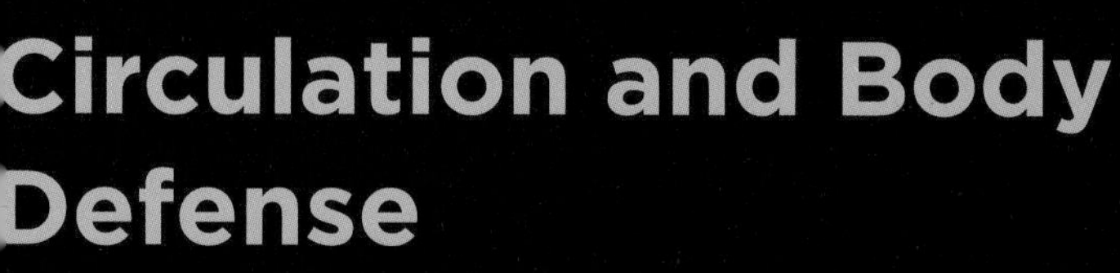

Circulation and Body Defense

The chapters in this unit discuss the systems that move materials through the body. The blood is the main transport medium. It circulates through the cardiovascular system, consisting of the heart and the blood vessels. The lymphatic system, in addition to other functions, helps to balance body fluids by bringing substances from the tissues back to the heart. Components of the blood and the lymphatic system are also involved in body defenses against infection as part of the immune system.

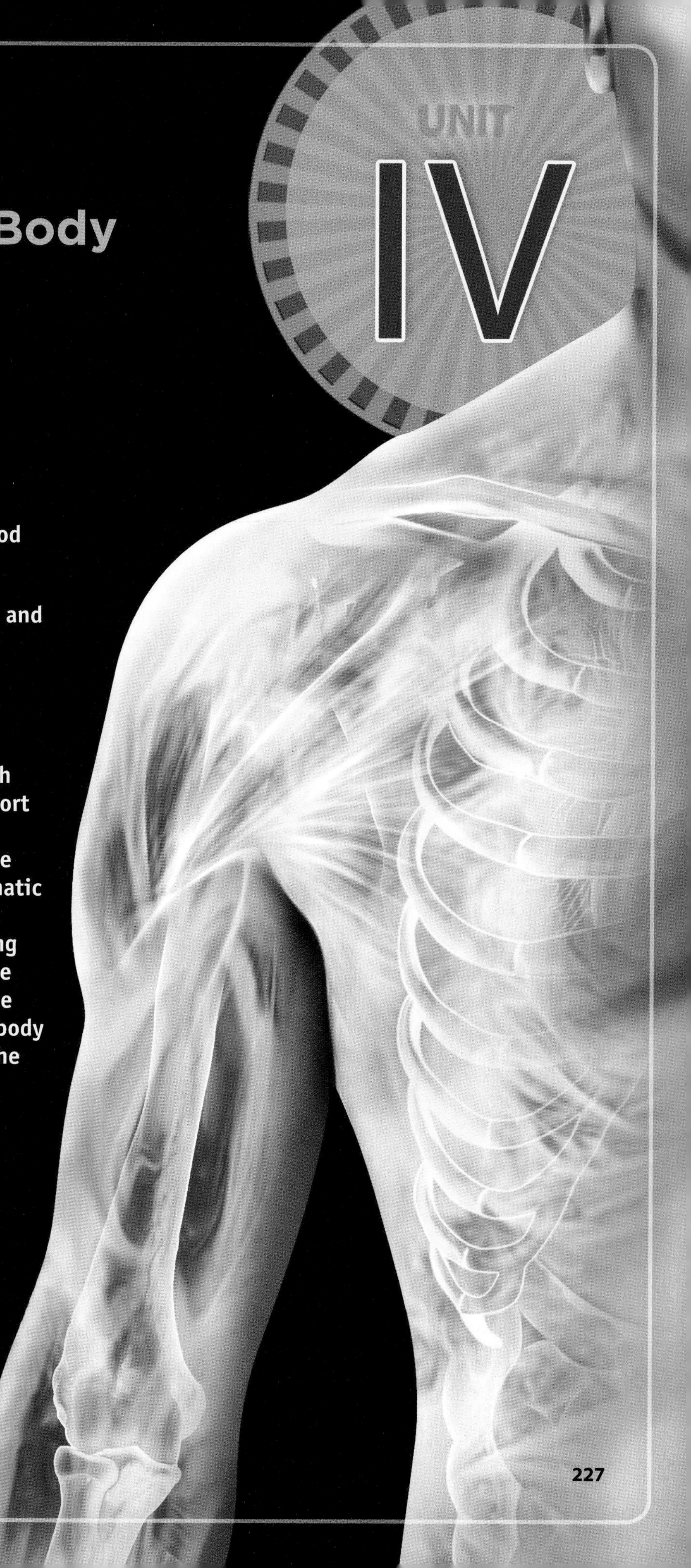

CHAPTER 12 The Blood

A&P in Context

Cole's Case: A Hemoglobin Abnormality

Both baby Cole and his mother Jada were resting comfortably in the maternity ward. Although Cole was only a few hours old, he had already been bathed, fed, and thoroughly examined by his pediatrician. As part of the hospital's routine neonatal procedures, a sample of Cole's blood was collected and sent to the hematology laboratory.

When Cole's blood sample arrived in the laboratory, a technologist divided it into several portions for analysis. First, she tested for Cole's blood type. When she added anti-B serum to his blood, the erythrocytes in the sample clumped together. There was no reaction to the anti-A serum. Since the antibodies in the sera showed only B antigens on the red blood cells, the medical laboratory technologist knew that Cole's blood was type B. Next, she performed a blood cell count using an automated machine. Cole's platelet count was normal, suggesting that he did not suffer from thrombocytopenia, the most common clotting disorder. His leukocyte count was normal too, signifying that his immune system was healthy. His erythrocyte count was also within normal limits, indicating that his red bone marrow (the site of erythrocyte production) was functioning as well. As required by many hospitals in the United States, the technologist screened Cole's blood for the presence of abnormal hemoglobin in his erythrocytes. When the test result came back positive for abnormal hemoglobin, the technologist requested that a blood sample be drawn from both of Cole's parents. She needed to run some more sensitive blood tests to determine whether or not the infant suffered from sickle cell disease.

The medical laboratory technologist performed several tests on Cole's blood. In this chapter, you study blood and learn about its constituents and functions. Later, we find out more about Cole's abnormal hemoglobin.

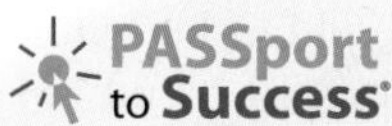

Ancillaries At-A-Glance

Visit *thePoint* to access the PASSport to Success and the following resources. For guidance in using these resources most effectively, see pp. ix–xviii.

Learning TOOLS

- Learning Style Self-Assessment
- Live Advise Online Student Tutoring
- Tips for Effective Studying

Learning RESOURCES

- E-book: Chapter 12
- Web Figure: Hemostasis
- Web Figure: Production, circulation, and death of red blood cells
- Web Chart: Hematopoiesis
- Animation: Hemostasis
- Health Professions: Hematology specialist
- Detailed Chapter Outline
- Answers to Questions for Study and Review
- Audio Pronunciation Glossary

Learning ACTIVITIES

- Pre-Quiz
- Visual Activities
- Kinesthetic Activities
- Auditory Activities

Learning Outcomes

After careful study of this chapter, you should be able to:

1. List the functions of the blood, ***p. 230***
2. Identify the main components of plasma, ***p. 231***
3. Describe the formation of blood cells, ***p. 232***
4. Name and describe the three types of formed elements in the blood and give the function of each, ***p. 232***
5. Characterize the five types of leukocytes, ***p. 233***
6. Define *hemostasis* and cite three steps in hemostasis, ***p. 236***
7. Briefly describe the steps in blood clotting, ***p. 236***
8. Define *blood type* and explain the relation between blood type and transfusions, ***p. 237***
9. Explain the basis of Rh incompatibility and its possible consequences, ***p. 238***
10. List the possible reasons for transfusions of whole blood and blood components, ***p. 238***
11. Identify six types of tests used to study blood, ***p. 240***
12. Referring to the case study, describe the genetic basis and potential complications of sickle cell anemia, ***pp. 228, 243***
13. Show how word parts are used to build words related to the blood (see Word Anatomy at the end of the chapter), ***p. 245***

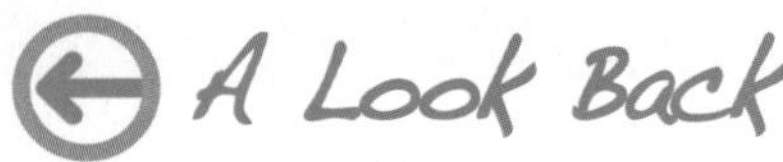

Blood is one of the two types of circulating connective tissue introduced in Chapter 4. The other is lymph, discussed more fully in Chapter 15. The various highly specialized blood cells illustrate once again the cellular diversity noted in Chapter 3. The circulating blood is of fundamental importance in maintaining homeostasis.

Blood is a life-giving fluid that brings nutrients and oxygen to the cells and carries away waste. The heart pumps blood continuously through a closed system of vessels. The heart and blood vessels are described in Chapters 13 and 14, respectively.

Blood is classified as a connective tissue because it consists of cells suspended in an extracellular background material, or matrix. Blood cells share many characteristics of origination and development with other connective tissues. However, blood differs from other connective tissues in that its cells are not fixed in position; instead, they move freely in the plasma, the blood's liquid matrix.

Whole blood is a viscous (thick) fluid that varies in color from bright scarlet to dark red, depending on how much oxygen it is carrying. (It is customary in drawings to color blood high in oxygen as red and blood low in oxygen as blue.) The blood volume accounts for approximately 8% of total body weight. The actual quantity of circulating blood differs with a person's size; the average adult male, weighing 70 kg (154 lb), has about 5 L (5.2 quarts) of blood.

Functions of the Blood

The circulating blood serves the body in three ways: transportation, regulation, and protection.

TRANSPORTATION

- **Gases.** Oxygen from inhaled air diffuses into the blood through thin membranes in the lungs and is carried by the circulation to all body tissues. Carbon dioxide, a waste product of cellular metabolism, is carried from the tissues to the lungs, where it is breathed out.
- **Nutrients.** The blood transports nutrients, including the by-products of food digestion, water, vitamins, and electrolytes, to the cells. These materials enter the blood from the digestive system or are released into the blood from body reserves.
- **Waste.** The blood transports the waste products from the cells to sites where they are removed. For example, the kidney removes excess water, acid, electrolytes, and urea (a nitrogen-containing waste). The liver removes blood pigments, hormones, and drugs, and the lungs eliminate carbon dioxide.
- **Hormones.** The blood carries hormones from their sites of origin to the organs they affect.

REGULATION

- **pH.** Buffers in the blood help keep the pH of body fluids steady at about 7.4. (The actual range of blood pH is 7.35 to 7.45.) Recall that pH is a measure of a solution's acidity or alkalinity. At an average pH of 7.4, blood is slightly alkaline (basic).
- **Fluid balance.** The blood regulates the amount of fluid in the tissues by means of substances (mainly proteins) that maintain the proper osmotic pressure. Recall that osmotic pressure is related to the concentration of dissolved and suspended materials in a solution; as their concentration increases, osmotic pressure increases. Proper osmotic pressure is needed for fluid balance, as described in Chapter 14.
- **Heat.** The blood transports heat that is generated in the muscles to other parts of the body, thus aiding in the regulation of body temperature.

PROTECTION

- **Disease.** The blood is important in defense against disease. It carries the substances and cells active in the immune system that protects against pathogens.
- **Blood loss.** The blood contains substances called *clotting factors* that protect against blood loss from the site of an injury. The process of blood coagulation, needed to prevent blood loss, is described later in this chapter.

CHECKPOINTS 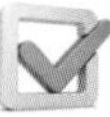

- 12-1 What are some substances transported in the blood?
- 12-2 What is the pH range of the blood?

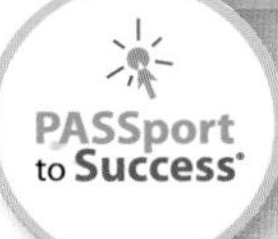

See the Student Resources for information on careers in hematology, the study of blood.

Blood Constituents

The blood is divided into two main components (Fig. 12-1). The liquid portion is the **plasma**. The **formed elements**, which include cells and cell fragments, fall into three categories, as follows:

- **Erythrocytes** (eh-RITH-ro-sites), from *erythro*, meaning "red," are the red blood cells, which transport oxygen.
- **Leukocytes** (LU-ko-sites), from *leuko*, meaning "white," are the several types of white blood cells (WBCs), which protect against infection.
- **Platelets**, also called **thrombocytes** (THROM-bo-sites), are cell fragments that participate in blood clotting.

Table 12-1 summarizes information on the different types of formed elements. Figure 12-2 shows all the categories of

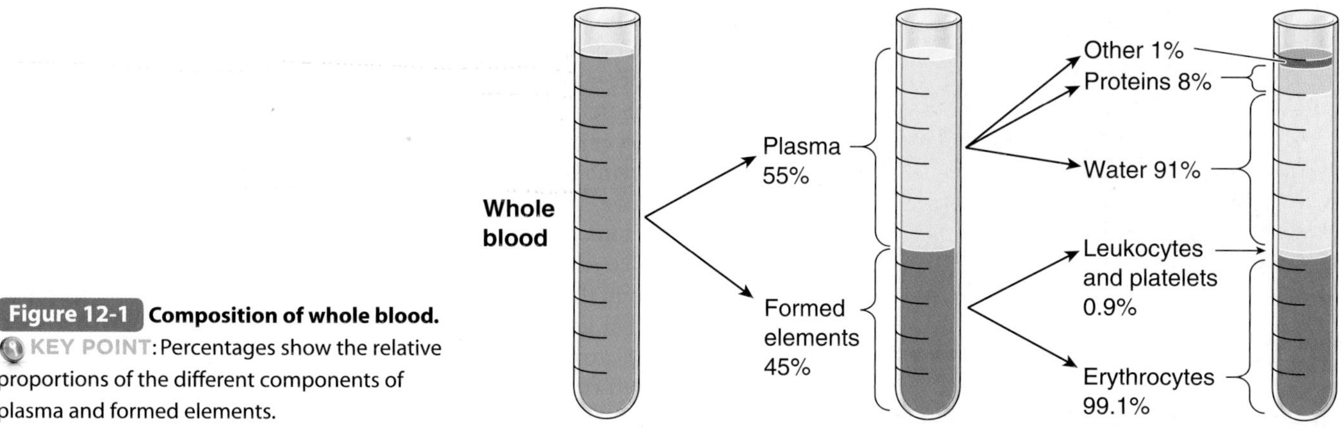

Figure 12-1 Composition of whole blood. KEY POINT: Percentages show the relative proportions of the different components of plasma and formed elements.

formed elements in a blood smear, that is, a blood sample spread thinly over the surface of a glass slide, as viewed under a microscope.

BLOOD PLASMA

About 55% of the total blood volume is plasma. The plasma itself is 91% water. Many different substances, dissolved or suspended in the water, make up the other 9% by weight (see Fig. 12-1). The plasma content may vary somewhat because substances are removed and added as the blood circulates to and from the tissues. However, the body tends to maintain a fairly constant level of most substances. For example, the level of glucose, a simple sugar, is maintained at a remarkably constant level of about one-tenth of one percent (0.1%) in solution.

After water, the next largest percentage (about 8%) of material in the plasma is protein. The plasma proteins include the following:

- **Albumin** (al-BU-min), the most abundant protein in plasma, is important for maintaining the blood's osmotic pressure. This protein is manufactured in the liver.
- **Clotting factors,** necessary for blood coagulation, are also manufactured in the liver.
- **Antibodies,** substances that combat infection and are made by certain WBCs involved in immunity.
- **Complement** consists of a group of enzymes that helps antibodies in their fight against pathogens (see Chapter 15).

The remaining 1% of the plasma consists of nutrients, electrolytes, and other materials that must be transported. With regard to the nutrients, glucose is the principal carbohydrate found in the plasma. This simple sugar is absorbed from digested foods in the intestine. It also can be released from the liver, where it is stored as glycogen. Amino acids, the products of protein digestion, also circulate in the plasma. Lipids constitute a small percentage of blood plasma. Lipid components include cholesterol and fats. As lipids are not soluble in plasma, they combine with proteins to form lipoproteins. The electrolytes in the plasma include sodium, potassium, calcium, magnesium, chloride, carbonate, and phosphate. These electrolytes have a variety of functions, including the formation of bone (calcium and phosphorus); the production of certain hormones (such as iodine for the production of thyroid hormones); and maintenance of the acid–base balance (such as sodium and potassium carbonates and phosphates present in buffers). 12

Other materials transported in plasma include hormones, waste products, drugs, and dissolved gases, primarily oxygen and carbon dioxide.

Table 12-1 Formed Elements of Blood

Formed Elements	Number per mcL of Blood	Description	Function
Erythrocytes (red blood cells)	5 million	Tiny (7 mcm diameter), biconcave disks without nucleus (anuclear)	Carry oxygen bound to hemoglobin; also carry some carbon dioxide and buffer blood
Leukocytes (white blood cells)	5,000–10,000	Larger than red cells with prominent nucleus that may be segmented (granulocyte) or unsegmented (agranulocyte); vary in staining properties	Active in immunity; located in blood, tissues, and lymphatic system
Platelets	150,000–450,000	Fragments of large cells (megakaryocyte)	Hemostasis; form a platelet plug and start blood clotting (coagulation)

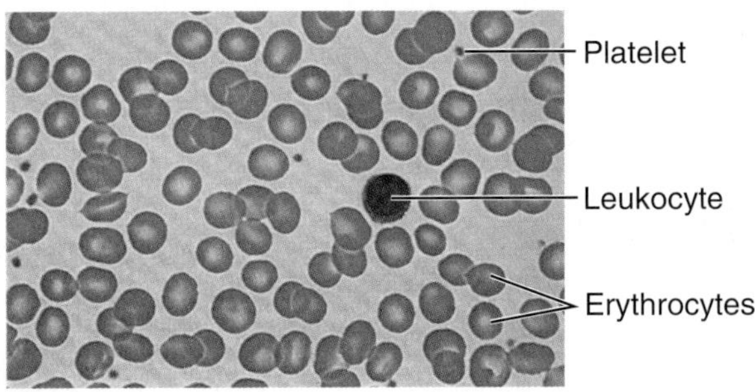

Figure 12-2 Blood cells as viewed under the microscope. KEY POINT: All three types of formed elements are visible. ZOOMING IN Which cells are the most numerous in the blood?

THE FORMED ELEMENTS

All of the blood's formed elements are produced in red bone marrow, which is located in the ends of long bones and in the inner portion of all other bones. The ancestors of all the blood cells are called **hematopoietic** (blood-forming) **stem cells.** These cells have the potential to develop into any of the blood cell types produced within the red bone marrow.

In comparison with other cells, most blood cells are short lived. The need for constant blood cell replacement means that normal activity of the red bone marrow is absolutely essential to life.

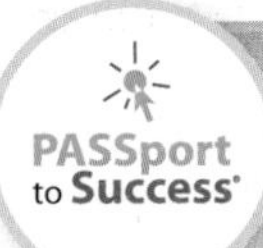

See the Student Resources on *thePoint* for a chart on hematopoiesis detailing the development of all the formed elements and a figure on the life cycle of red cells.

Erythrocytes Erythrocytes, the red blood cells (RBCs, or red cells), measure about 7 mcm (micrometers) in diameter. They are disk-shaped bodies with a depression on both sides. This biconcave shape creates a central area that is thinner than the edges (Fig. 12-3). Erythrocytes are different from other cells in that the mature form found in the circulating blood lacks a nucleus (is anuclear) and also lacks most of the other organelles commonly found in cells. As red cells mature, these components are lost, providing more space for the cells to carry oxygen. This vital gas is bound in the red cells to **hemoglobin** (he-mo-GLO-bin), a protein that contains iron. (See Box 12-1 on the structure and function of hemoglobin.) Hemoglobin, combined with oxygen, gives the blood its characteristic red color. The more oxygen carried by the hemoglobin, the brighter is the blood's red color. Therefore, the blood that goes from the lungs to the tissues is a bright red because it carries a great supply of oxygen; in contrast, the blood that returns to the lungs is a much darker red because it has given up some of its oxygen to the tissues.

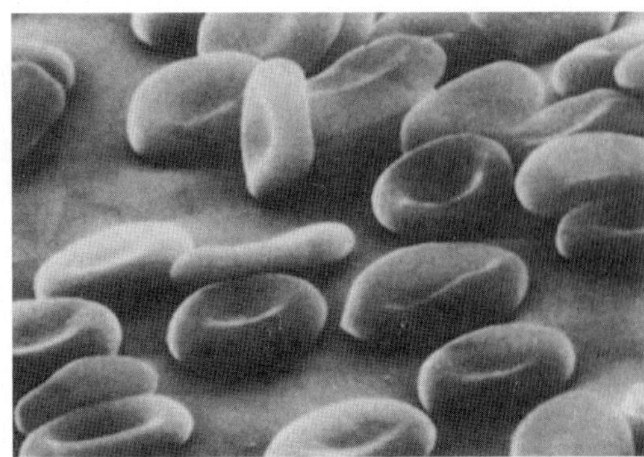

Figure 12-3 Red blood cells as seen under a scanning electron microscope. KEY POINT: This type of microscope provides a three-dimensional view of the cells, revealing their shape. ZOOMING IN Why are these cells described as biconcave?

Hemoglobin has two lesser functions in addition to the transport of oxygen. Hemoglobin that has given up its oxygen is able to carry hydrogen ions. In this way, hemoglobin acts as a buffer and plays an important role in acid–base balance (see Chapter 19). Hemoglobin also carries some carbon dioxide from the tissues to the lungs for elimination. The carbon dioxide is bound to a different part of the molecule than the part that holds oxygen, so that a hemoglobin molecule can carry both oxygen and carbon dioxide.

Hemoglobin's ability to carry oxygen can be blocked by carbon monoxide. This odorless and colorless but harmful gas combines with hemoglobin to form a stable compound that can severely restrict the erythrocytes' ability to carry oxygen. Carbon monoxide is a by-product of the incomplete burning of fuels, such as gasoline and other petroleum products and coal, wood, and other carbon-containing materials. It also occurs in cigarette smoke and automobile exhaust.

Erythrocytes are by far the most numerous of the blood cells, averaging from 4.5 to 5 million per microliter (mcL) of blood. (A microliter is one millionth of a liter.) Because mature red cells have no nucleus and cannot divide or repair themselves, they must be replaced constantly. After leaving the bone marrow, they circulate in the bloodstream for about 120 days before their membranes deteriorate and they are destroyed by the liver and spleen. Red cell production is stimulated by the hormone **erythropoietin** (eh-rith-ro-POY-eh-tin) (**EPO**), which is released from the kidney in response to decreased oxygen. Constant red cell production requires an adequate supply of nutrients, particularly protein; the vitamins B_{12} and folic acid, required for the production of DNA; and the minerals iron and copper for the production of hemoglobin. Vitamin C is also important for the proper absorption of iron from the small intestine.

CHECKPOINTS 

- 12-3 What are the two main components of blood?
- 12-4 Next to water, what is the most abundant type of substance in plasma?
- 12-5 Where do blood cells form?
- 12-6 What type of cell gives rise to all blood cells?
- 12-7 What is the main function of hemoglobin?

Box 12-1 *A Closer Look*

Hemoglobin: Door-to-Door Oxygen Delivery

The hemoglobin molecule is a protein made of four amino acid chains (the globin part of the molecule), each of which holds an iron-containing heme group. Each of the four hemes can bind one molecule of oxygen.

Hemoglobin allows the blood to carry much more oxygen than it could were the oxygen simply dissolved in the plasma. A red blood cell contains about 250 million hemoglobins, each capable of binding four molecules of oxygen. So, a single red blood cell can carry about one billion oxygen molecules! Hemoglobin reversibly binds oxygen, picking it up in the lungs and releasing it in the body tissues. Active cells need more oxygen and also generate heat and acidity. These changing conditions promote the release of oxygen from hemoglobin into metabolically active tissues.

Immature red blood cells (erythroblasts) produce hemoglobin as they mature into erythrocytes in the red bone marrow. When the liver and spleen destroy old erythrocytes, they break down the released hemoglobin. Some of its components are recycled, and the remainder leaves the body as a brown fecal pigment called stercobilin. In spite of some conservation, dietary protein and iron are still essential to maintain hemoglobin supplies.

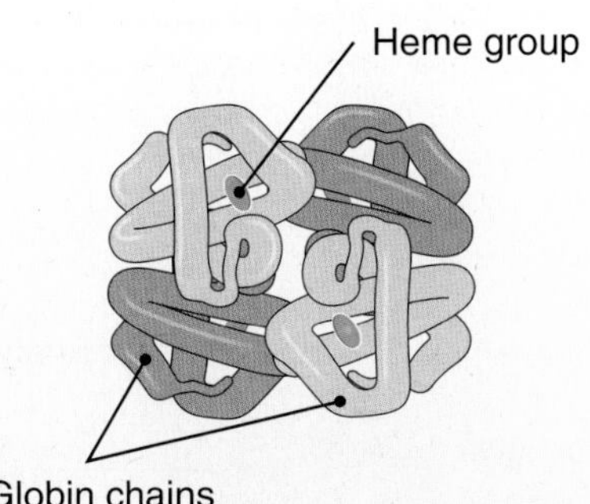

Hemoglobin. This protein in red blood cells consists of four amino acid chains (globins), each with an oxygen-binding heme group.

12

Leukocytes The **leukocytes**, or white blood cells (WBCs, or white cells), differ from the erythrocytes in appearance, quantity, and function. The cells themselves are round, but they contain prominent nuclei of varying shapes and sizes. Occurring at a concentration of 5,000 to 10,000/mcL of blood, leukocytes are outnumbered by red cells by about 700 to 1. Although the red cells have a definite color, the leukocytes are colorless and must be stained if we are to study them under the microscope.

Types of Leukocytes The different types of white cells are identified by their size, the shape of the nucleus, and the appearance of granules in the cytoplasm when the cells are stained (Table 12-2). The stain commonly used for blood is Wright stain, which is a mixture of dyes that differentiates the various blood cells. The "granules" in the white cells are actually lysosomes and secretory vesicles. They are present in all WBCs, but they are more easily stained and more visible in some cells than in others. Leukocytes are active in immunity. As we discuss later in this chapter, the relative percentage of the different types of leukocytes is a valuable clue in arriving at a medical diagnosis.

The granular leukocytes, or **granulocytes** (GRAN-u-lo-sites), are so named because they show visible granules in the cytoplasm when stained. Each has a very distinctive, highly segmented nucleus (see Table 12-2). The different types of granulocytes are named for the type of dyes they take up when stained. They include the following:

- **Neutrophils** (NU-tro-fils) stain with either acidic or basic dyes.
- **Eosinophils** (e-o-SIN-o-fils) stain with acidic dyes (eosin is one).
- **Basophils** (BA-so-fils) stain with basic dyes.

Neutrophils are the most numerous of the white cells, constituting approximately 60% of all leukocytes. Because the nuclei of the neutrophils have various shapes, these cells are also called **polymorphs** (meaning "many forms") or simply *polys*. Other nicknames are *segs*, referring to the segmented nucleus, and *PMNs*, an abbreviation of **p**oly**m**orphonuclear **n**eutrophils. Before reaching full maturity and becoming segmented, a neutrophil's nucleus looks like a thick, curved band (Fig. 12-4). An increase in the number of these **band cells** (also called *stab* or *staff cells*) is a sign of infection and active neutrophil production. Eosinophils and basophils make up a small percentage of the white cells but increase in number during allergic reactions.

The agranular leukocytes, or **agranulocytes**, are so named because they lack easily visible granules (see Table 12-2). Their nuclei are round or curved and are not segmented. There are two types of agranular leukocytes:

- **Lymphocytes** (LIM-fo-sites) are the second most numerous of the white cells. Although lymphocytes originate in the red bone marrow, they develop to maturity in lymphoid tissue and can multiply in this tissue as well. They circulate in the lymphatic system (see Chapter 16).
- **Monocytes** (MON-o-sites) are the largest in size. They average about 5% of the leukocytes.

Table 12-2 Leukocytes (White Blood Cells)

Cell Type		Relative Percentage (Adult)	Description	Function
Granulocytes (have segmented nucleus)				
Neutrophils	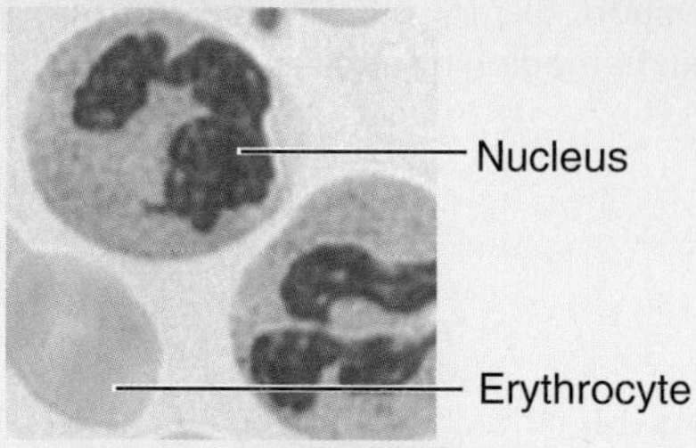	54%–62%	Stain with either acidic or basic dyes; show lavender granules when stained	Phagocytosis
Eosinophils	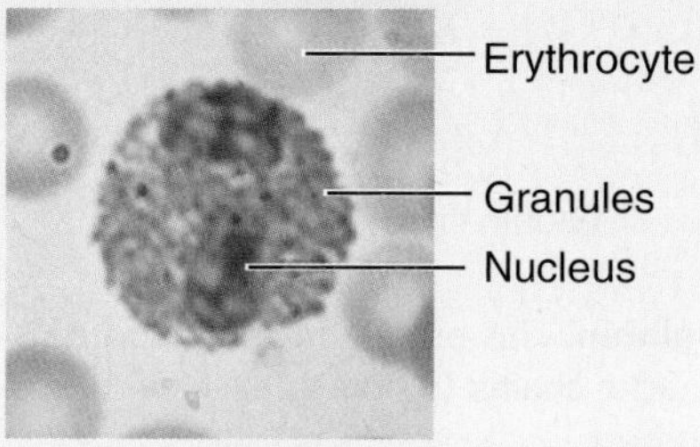	1%–3%	Stain with acidic dyes; show beadlike, bright pink granules when stained	Allergic reactions; defense against parasites
Basophils	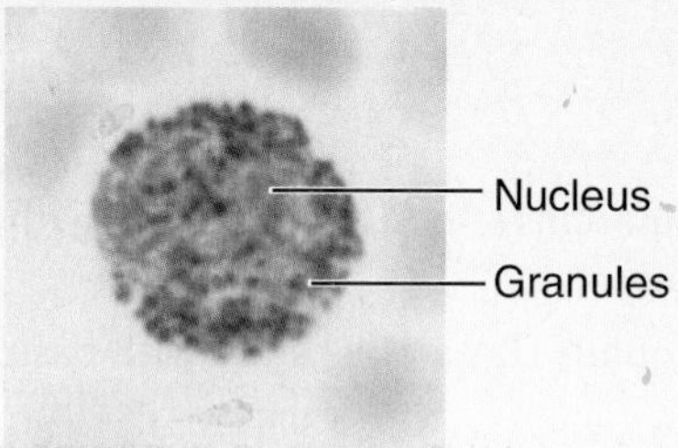	<1%	Stain with basic dyes; have large, dark blue granules that can obscure the nucleus	Allergic reactions; inflammatory reactions
Agranulocytes (have unsegmented nucleus)				
Lymphocytes	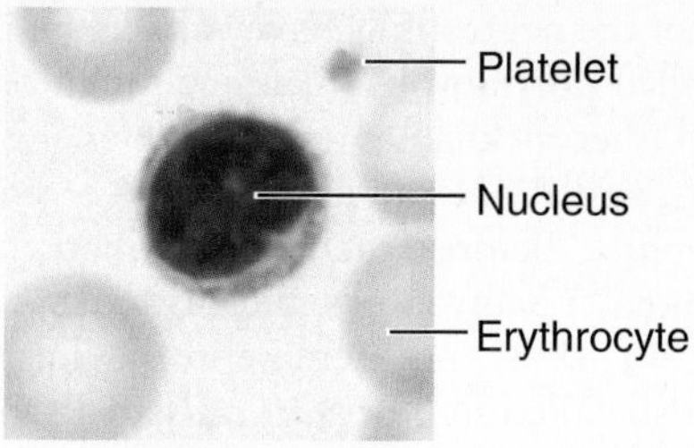	25%–38%	Mature and can multiple in lymphoid tissue	Immunity (T cells and B cells)
Monocytes	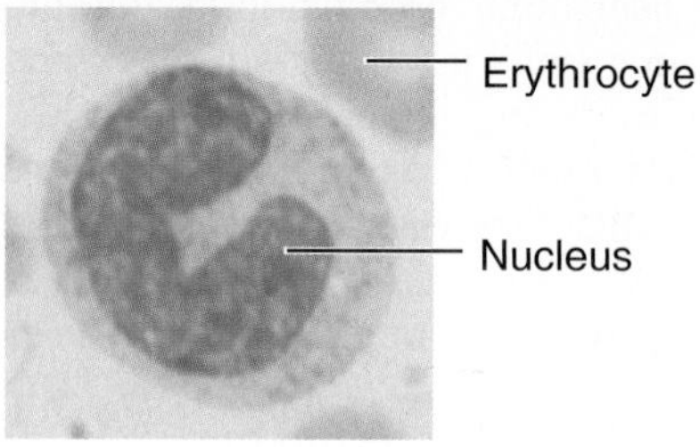	3%–7%	Largest of leukocytes	Phagocytosis

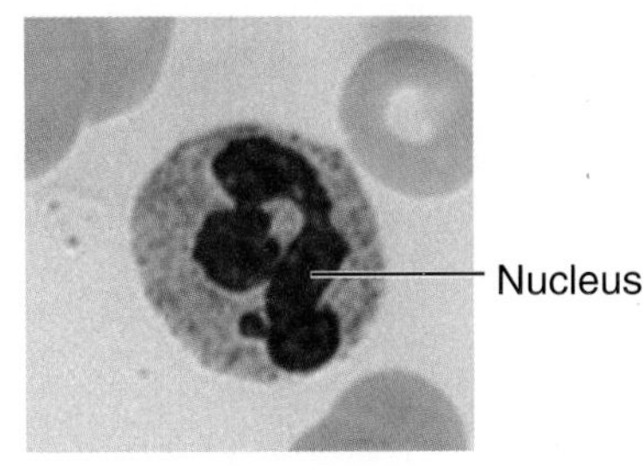

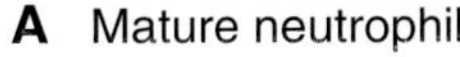

A Mature neutrophil

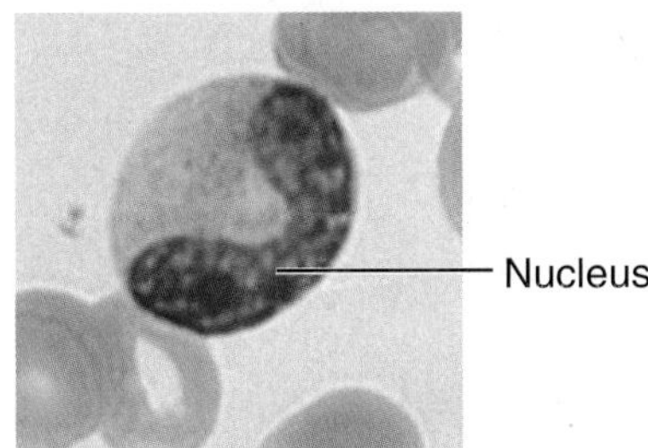

B Band cell (immature neutrophil)

Figure 12-4 Stages in neutrophil development. KEY POINT: **A.** A mature neutrophil has a segmented nucleus. **B.** An immature neutrophil is called a band cell because the nucleus is shaped like a thick, curved band (×1325). (Reprinted with permission from Gartner LP, Hiatt JL. *Color Atlas of Histology*, 5th ed. Philadelphia, PA: Lippincott Williams & Wilkins, 2009.)

Functions of Leukocytes Leukocytes clear the body of foreign material and cellular debris. Most importantly, they destroy pathogens that may invade the body. Neutrophils and monocytes engage in **phagocytosis** (fag-o-si-TO-sis), the engulfing of foreign matter (Fig. 12-5). Whenever pathogens enter the tissues, as through a wound, phagocytes are attracted to the area. They squeeze between the cells of the capillary walls and proceed by ameboid (ah-ME-boyd), or ameba-like, motion to the area of infection where they engulf the invaders. Lysosomes in the cytoplasm then digest the foreign organisms and the cells eliminate the waste products.

When foreign organisms invade, the bone marrow and lymphoid tissue go into emergency production of white cells, and their number increases enormously as a result. Detection of an abnormally large number of white cells in the blood is an indication of infection. In battling pathogens, leukocytes themselves may be destroyed. A mixture of dead and living bacteria, together with dead and living leukocytes, forms **pus**.

Some monocytes enter the tissues, enlarge, and mature into **macrophages** (MAK-ro-faj-ez), which are highly active in disposing of invaders and foreign material. Although most circulating lymphocytes live only 6 to 8 hours, those that enter the tissues may survive for longer periods—days, months, or even years.

Some lymphocytes become **plasma cells**, active in the production of circulating antibodies needed for immunity. The activities of the various white cells are further discussed in Chapter 15.

Platelets **Blood platelets** (thrombocytes) are the smallest of all the formed elements (Fig. 12-6A). These tiny structures are not cells in themselves but rather fragments constantly released from giant bone marrow cells called **megakaryocytes** (meg-ah-KAR-e-o-sites) (see Fig. 12-6B). Platelets do not have nuclei or DNA, but they do contain active enzymes and mitochondria. The number of platelets in the circulating blood has been estimated to range from 150,000 to 450,000/mcL. They have a life span of about 10 days.

12

Platelets are essential for the prevention of blood loss (hemostasis) and blood coagulation (clotting), discussed next. When blood comes in contact with any tissue other than the smooth lining of the blood vessels, as in the case of injury, the platelets stick together and

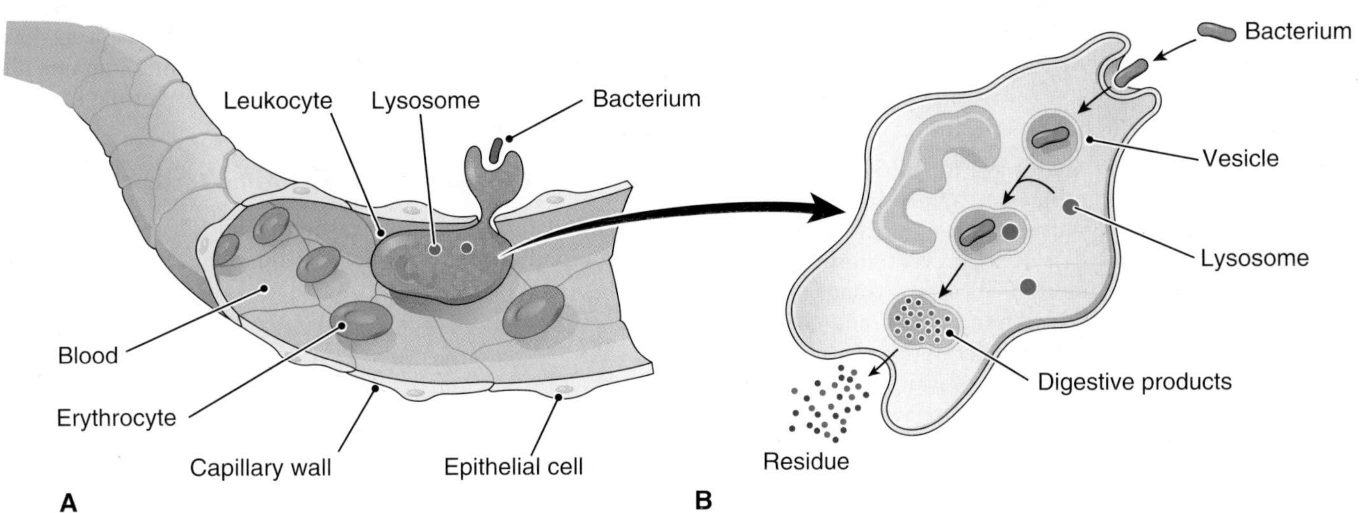

Figure 12-5 Phagocytosis. KEY POINT: Phagocytosis is the engulfing of foreign matter by white cells. **A.** A phagocytic leukocyte (white blood cell) squeezes through a capillary wall in the region of an infection and engulfs a bacterium. **B.** The bacterium is enclosed in a vesicle and digested by a lysosome. ZOOMING IN What type of epithelium makes up the capillary wall?

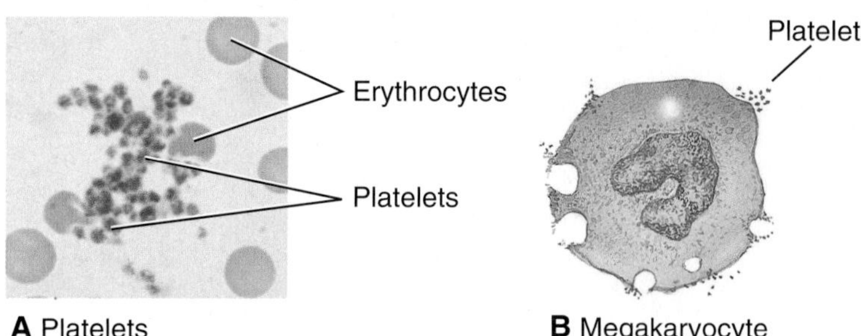

Figure 12-6 Platelets (thrombocytes). KEY POINT: Platelets are fragments of larger cells **A.** Platelets in a blood smear. **B.** A megakaryocyte releases platelets. (B, Reprinted with permission from Gartner LP, Hiatt JL. *Color Atlas of Histology*, 5th ed. Philadelphia, PA: Lippincott Williams & Wilkins, 2009.)

form a plug that seals the wound. The platelets then release chemicals that participate in the formation of a clot to stop blood loss. More details on these reactions follow.

CHECKPOINTS 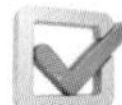

- 12-8 What are the types of granular leukocytes? Of agranular leukocytes?
- 12-9 What is the most important function of leukocytes?
- 12-10 What is the function of blood platelets?

Hemostasis and Coagulation

Hemostasis (he-mo-STA-sis) is the process that prevents blood loss from the circulation when a blood vessel is ruptured by an injury. Events in hemostasis include the following:

1. **Contraction** of the smooth muscles in the blood vessel wall. This reduces blood flow and loss from the defect in the vessel. The term for this reduction in a vessel's diameter is *vasoconstriction*.
2. Formation of a **platelet plug**. Activated platelets become sticky and adhere to the defect to form a temporary plug.
3. Formation of a **blood clot**, by the process of **coagulation** (ko-ag-u-LA-shun).

The many substances necessary for blood clotting are normally inactive in the bloodstream. A balance is maintained between compounds that promote clotting, known as **procoagulants**, and those that prevent clotting, known as **anticoagulants**. In addition, there are chemicals in the circulation that dissolve any unnecessary and potentially harmful clots that may form. Under normal conditions, the substances that prevent clotting prevail. When an injury occurs, however, the procoagulants are activated and a clot is formed (**Fig. 12-7**).

The clotting process is a well-controlled series of separate events involving 12 different clotting factors, each designated by a Roman numeral. Calcium ion (Ca^{2+}) is one such factor. Others are released from damaged tissue and sticky platelets formed in hemostasis. Still others are enzyme precursors, made in the liver and released into the bloodstream, which can be activated in the clotting process. To manufacture these enzymes, the liver requires vitamin K. We obtain some of this vitamin in food from green vegetables and grains, but a large proportion is made by bacteria living symbiotically in the large intestine. The final step in the clotting reactions is the conversion of a plasma protein called **fibrinogen** (fi-BRIN-o-jen) into solid threads of **fibrin**, in which blood cells are trapped to form the clot. The final steps involved in blood clot formation are described below and illustrated in **Figure 12-7**.

1. Substances released from damaged tissue and sticky platelets initiate a reaction sequence that leads to the formation of an active enzyme called **prothrombinase** (pro-THROM-bih-nase).
2. Prothrombinase converts prothrombin in the blood to **thrombin**. Calcium is needed for this step.
3. Thrombin, in turn, converts soluble fibrinogen into insoluble **fibrin**. Threads of fibrin form a meshwork that entraps plasma and blood cells to form a clot.

Blood clotting occurs in response to injury. Blood also clots when it comes into contact with some surface other than the lining of a blood vessel, for example, a glass or plastic tube used for a blood specimen. In this case, the preliminary steps of clotting are somewhat different and require more time, but the final steps are the same as those illustrated in **Figure 12-7**. The fluid that remains after clotting has occurred is called **serum** (plural, *sera*). Serum contains all the components of blood plasma *except* the clotting factors, as expressed in the formula:

Plasma = serum + clotting factors

Several methods used to measure the body's ability to coagulate blood are described later in this chapter.

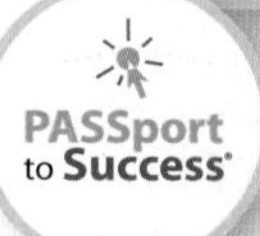

See the Student Resources on *thePoint* for a summary diagram and an animation on hemostasis.

CHECKPOINTS 

- 12-11 What happens when fibrinogen converts to fibrin?
- 12-12 What does plasma contain that is missing in serum?

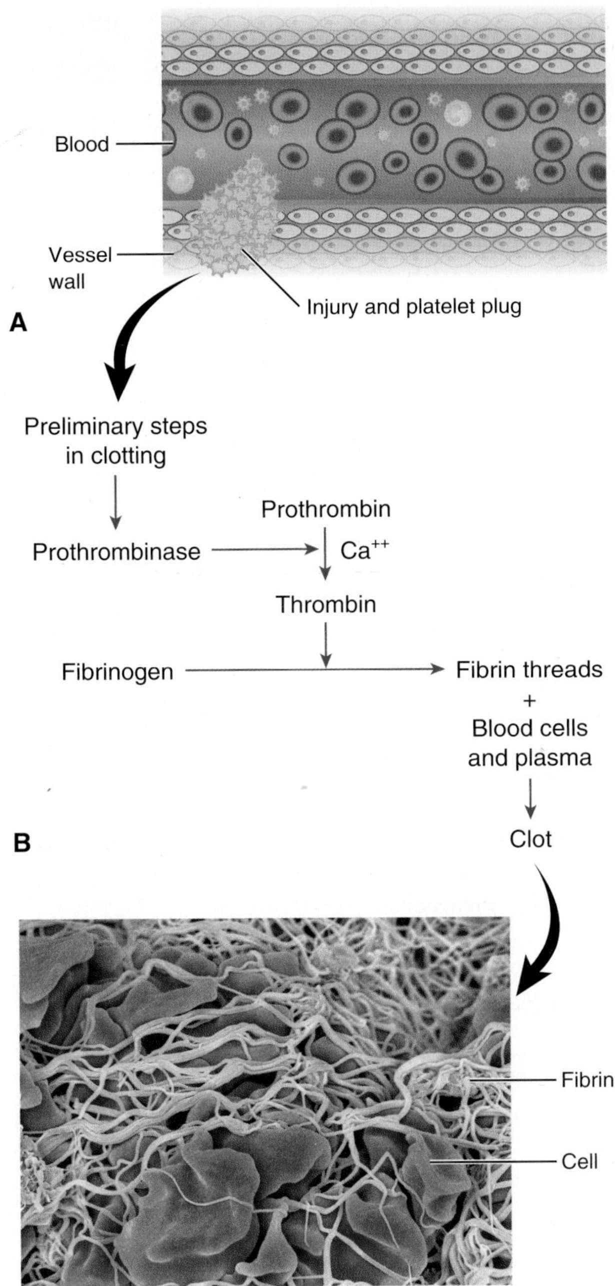

Figure 12-7 Blood clotting (coagulation). KEY POINT: Blood coagulation requires a complex series of reactions that lead to the formation of fibrin, an insoluble protein. Fibrin threads trap blood cells to form a clot. **A.** Substances released from damaged tissue and sticky platelets initiate the preliminary steps in clotting. **B.** The final coagulation reactions lead to formation of a fibrin clot. **C.** Scanning electron micrograph of blood cells trapped in fibrin. (C, Reprinted with permission from McConnell TH, Hull KH, *Human Form Human Function*, Baltimore, MD: Lippincott Williams & Wilkins, 2011.) ZOOMING IN What part of the word *prothrombinase* indicates that it is an enzyme? What part of the word *prothrombin* indicates that it is a precursor?

Blood Types

If for some reason the amount of blood in the body is severely reduced, through hemorrhage (HEM-eh-rij) (excessive bleeding) or disease, the body cells suffer from lack of oxygen and nutrients. One possible measure to take in such an emergency is to administer blood from another person into the veins of the patient, a procedure called *transfusion*. Care must be taken in transferring blood from one person to another, however, because the patient's plasma may contain antibodies in these reactions called *agglutinins*, that can cause the red cells of the donor's blood to undergo **agglutination** (ah-GLU-tih-NA-shun) (clumping). The cells then rupture and release their hemoglobin by a process called *hemolysis* (he-MOL-ih-sis). The resulting condition can be dangerous to the patient.

Proteins, called **antigens** (AN-ti-jens), stimulate antibody production. We learn more about antigen–antibody reactions in Chapter 15, but for now, it's important to know that the presence of certain antigens on the surface of red cells causes the incompatibility reactions just described. There are many types of red blood cell antigens, but only two groups are particularly likely to cause a transfusion reaction: the so-called A and B antigens and the Rh factor.

THE ABO BLOOD TYPE GROUP

12

There are four blood types involving the A and B antigens: A, B, AB, and O (Table 12-3). These letters indicate the type of antigen present on the red cells. If only the A antigen is present, the person has type A blood; if only the B antigen is present, he or she has type B blood. Type AB red cells have both antigens, and type O has neither. Of course, no one has antibodies to his or her own blood type antigens, or their plasma would destroy their own cells. Each person does, however, develop antibodies that react with the AB antigens he or she is lacking. (These antibodies develop early in life from exposure to A and B antigens in the environment.) It is these antibodies in the patient's plasma that can react with antigens on the donor's red cells to cause a transfusion reaction.

Testing for Blood Type Blood sera containing antibodies to the A or B antigens are used to test for blood type. These **antisera** are prepared in animals using either the A or the B antigens to induce a response. Blood serum containing antibodies that can agglutinate and destroy red cells with A antigen is called **anti-A serum**; blood serum containing antibodies that can destroy red cells with B antigen is called **anti-B serum.** When combined with a blood sample in the laboratory, each antiserum causes the corresponding red cells to agglutinate. The blood's agglutination pattern when mixed with these two sera *one at a time* reveals its blood type (Fig. 12-8). Type A reacts with anti-A serum only; type B reacts with anti-B serum only. Type AB agglutinates with both, and type O agglutinates with neither A nor B. In the

Table 12-3 The ABO Blood Group System

Blood Type	Red Blood Cell Antigen	Reacts with Antiserum	Plasma Antibodies	Can Take From	Can Donate To
A	A	Anti-A	Anti-B	A, O	A, AB
B	B	Anti-B	Anti-A	B, O	B, AB
AB	A, B	Anti-A, Anti-B	None	AB, A, B, O	AB
O	None	None	Anti-A, Anti-B	O	O, A, B, AB

case study, Cole's blood reacted with anti-B serum only, indicating that his blood was type B.

A blood specimen from any person who has had a prior blood transfusion or a pregnancy is tested further for the presence of any less common antibodies. Both the red cells and the serum are tested separately for any possible cross-reactions with donor blood.

Blood Compatibility Heredity determines a person's blood type, and the percentage of people with each of the different blood types varies in different populations. For example, about 45% of the white population of the United States have type O blood, 40% have A, 11% have B, and only 4% have AB. The percentages vary within other population groups.

In an emergency, type O blood can be given to any ABO type because the cells lack both A and B antigens and will not react with either A or B antibodies (see Table 12-3). People with type O blood are called *universal donors*. Conversely, type AB blood contains no antibodies to agglutinate red cells, and people with this blood type can therefore receive blood from any ABO type donor. Those with AB blood are described as *universal recipients*. Whenever possible, it is safest to give the same blood type as the recipient's blood.

THE Rh FACTOR

More than 85% of the United States' population has another red cell antigen group called the **Rh factor**, named for *Rh*esus monkeys, in which it was first found. Rh is also known as the *D antigen*. People with this antigen are said to be **Rh positive**; those who lack this protein are said to be **Rh negative**. If Rh-positive blood is given to an Rh-negative person, he or she may produce antibodies to the "foreign" Rh antigens. The blood of this "Rh-sensitized" person will then destroy any Rh-positive cells received in a later transfusion.

Rh incompatibility is a potential problem in certain pregnancies (Fig. 12-9). A mother who is Rh negative may develop antibodies to the Rh protein of an Rh-positive fetus (the fetus having inherited this factor from the father). Red cells from the fetus that enter the mother's circulation during pregnancy and childbirth evoke the response. In a subsequent pregnancy with an Rh-positive fetus, some of the anti-Rh antibodies may pass from the mother's blood into the blood of her fetus and destroy the fetus's red cells. This condition is called **hemolytic disease of the newborn** (HDN). An older name is *erythroblastosis fetalis*. HDN is now prevented by administration of immune globulin Rh_0(D), trade name RhoGAM, to the mother during pregnancy and shortly after delivery. These preformed antibodies clear the mother's circulation of Rh antigens and prevent stimulation of an immune response. In many cases, a baby born with HDN could be saved by a transfusion that replaces much of the baby's blood with Rh-negative blood.

CHECKPOINTS 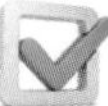

- 12-13 What are the four ABO blood type groups?
- 12-14 What are the blood antigens most often involved in incompatibility reactions?

Uses of Blood and Blood Components

Blood can be packaged and kept in blood banks for emergencies. To keep the blood from clotting, a solution such as citrate–phosphate–dextrose–adenine (CPDA-1) is added. The blood may then be stored for up to 35 days. The blood supplies in the bank are dated with an expiration date to prevent the use of blood in which red cells may have disintegrated. Blood banks usually have all types of blood and blood products available. It is important that there be an extra supply of type O, Rh-negative blood because in an emergency this type can be used for any patient. It is normal procedure, however, to test the recipient and give blood of the same type.

A person can donate his or her own blood before undergoing elective (planned) surgery to be used during surgery if needed. This practice eliminates the possibility of incompatibility and of disease transfer as well. Such **autologous** (aw-TOL-o-gus) (self-originating) blood is stored in a blood bank only until the surgery is completed.

WHOLE BLOOD TRANSFUSIONS

The transfer of whole human blood from a healthy person to a patient is often a life-saving process. Whole blood

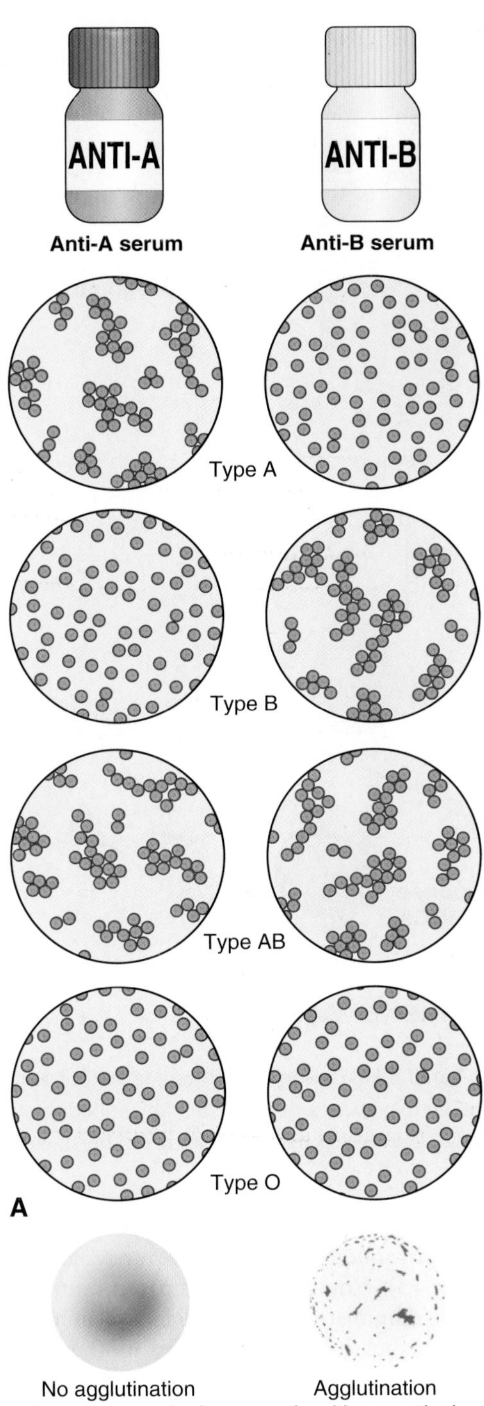

Figure 12-8 Blood typing KEY POINT: Blood type can be determined by mixing the blood, one at a time, with antisera prepared against the different red cell antigens (proteins). Agglutination (clumping) with an antiserum indicates the presence of the corresponding antigen **A.** Labels at the top of each column denote the kind of antiserum added to the blood samples. Anti-A serum agglutinates red cells in type A blood, but anti-B serum does not. Anti-B serum agglutinates red cells in type B blood, but anti-A serum does not. Both sera agglutinate type AB blood cells, and neither serum agglutinates type O blood. **B.** Photographs of blood typing reactions. ZOOMING IN Can you tell from these reactions whether these cells are Rh positive or Rh negative?

transfusions may be used for any condition in which there is loss of a large volume of blood, for example:

- In the treatment of massive hemorrhage from serious mechanical injuries
- For blood loss during internal bleeding, as from bleeding ulcers
- During or after an operation that causes considerable blood loss
- For blood replacement in the treatment of HDN

Caution and careful evaluation of the need for a blood transfusion is the rule, however, because of the risk for transfusion reactions and the possible transmission of viral diseases, particularly hepatitis and AIDS. (In developed countries, careful screening has virtually eliminated transmission of these viruses in donated blood.)

USE OF BLOOD COMPONENTS

Most often, when some blood ingredient is needed, it is not whole blood but a blood component that is given. Blood can be broken down into its various parts, which may be used for different purposes.

A common method for separating the blood plasma from the formed elements is by use of a **centrifuge** (SEN-trih-fuje), a machine that spins in a circle at high speed to separate a mixture's components according to density. When a container of blood is spun rapidly, all the blood's heavier formed elements are pulled to the bottom of the container. They are thus separated from the plasma, which is less dense. The formed elements may be further separated and used for specific purposes, for example, packed red cells alone or platelets alone.

12

Blood losses to the donor can be minimized if the blood is removed, the desired components are separated, and the remainder is returned to the donor. The general term for this procedure is **hemapheresis** (hem-ah-fer-E-sis) (from the Greek word *apheresis* meaning "removal"). If the plasma is removed and the formed elements returned to the donor, the procedure is called **plasmapheresis** (plas-mah-fer-E-sis).

Blood plasma alone may be given in an emergency to replace blood volume and prevent circulatory failure (shock). Plasma is especially useful when blood typing and the use of whole blood are not possible, such as in natural disasters or in emergency rescues. Because the red cells have been removed from the plasma, there are no incompatibility problems; plasma can be given to anyone. Plasma separated from the cellular elements is usually further separated by chemical means into various components, such as plasma protein fraction, serum albumin, immune serum, and clotting factors.

The packaged plasma that is currently available is actually plasma protein fraction. Further separation yields serum albumin that is available in solutions of 5% or 25% concentration. In addition to its use in treatment of circulatory shock, these solutions are given when plasma proteins are deficient. They increase the blood's osmotic pressure

Figure 12-9 **Rh** incompatibility. KEY POINT: An Rh-negative mother can form antibodies (become sensitized) to an Rh-positive fetus' red cells when exposed to the antigen during delivery. Unless she is treated with RhoGam to prevent a response, her Rh antibodies can cross the placenta in a subsequent pregnancy and destroy fetal red cells if they are Rh positive. The result is hemolytic disease of the newborn.

and thus draw fluids back into circulation. The use of plasma proteins and serum albumin has increased because these blood components can be treated with heat to prevent transmission of viral diseases.

In emergency situations, health care workers may administer fluids known as *plasma expanders*. These are cell-free isotonic solutions used to maintain blood fluid volume to prevent circulatory shock.

Fresh plasma may be frozen and saved. Plasma frozen when it is less than 6 hours old contains all the factors needed for clotting. When frozen plasma is thawed, a white precipitate called **cryoprecipitate** (kri-o-pre-SIP-ih-tate) forms in the bottom of the container. Cryoprecipitate is especially rich in fibrinogen and clotting factors. It may be given when there is a special need for these substances.

A portion of the plasma called the *gamma globulin fraction* contains antibodies produced by lymphocytes when they come in contact with foreign agents, such as bacteria and viruses. Antibodies play an important role in immunity (see Chapter 15). Commercially prepared immune sera are available for administration to patients in immediate need of antibodies, such as infants born to mothers with active hepatitis.

CHECKPOINT  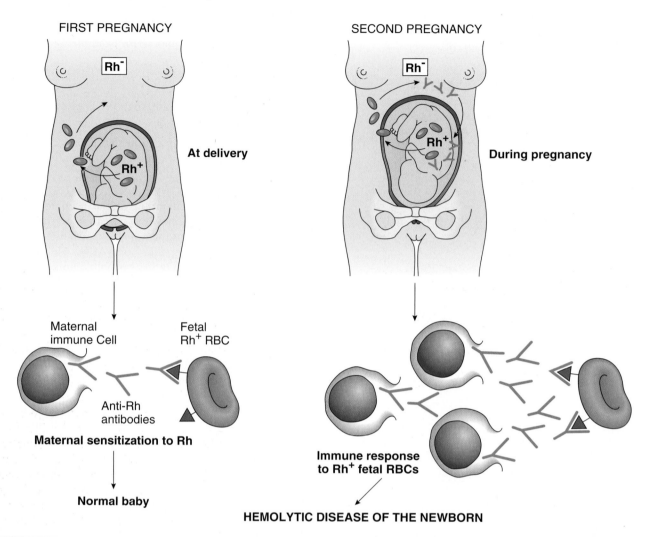

☐ **12-15** How is blood commonly separated into its component parts?

Blood Studies

Many kinds of studies can be done on blood, and some of these have become a standard part of a routine physical examination. Machines that are able to perform several tests at the same time have largely replaced manual procedures, particularly in large institutions.

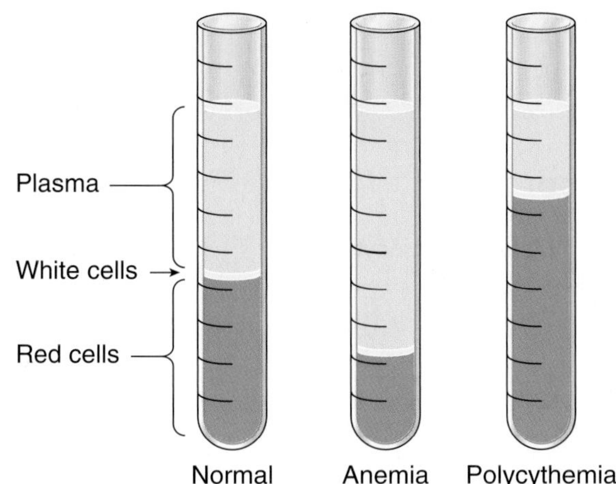

Figure 12-10 **Hematocrit.** KEY POINT: The hematocrit tests the volume percentage of red cells in whole blood. The tube on the left shows a normal hematocrit. The middle tube shows that the percentage of red blood cells is low, indicating anemia. The tube on the right shows an excessively high percentage of red cells, as seen in polycythemia. (Reprinted with permission from Cohen BJ. *Medical Terminology*, 6th ed. Philadelphia, PA: Lippincott Williams & Wilkins, 2011.)

THE HEMATOCRIT

The **hematocrit** (he-MAT-o-krit) (Hct), the volume percentage of red cells in whole blood, is determined by spinning a blood sample in a high-speed centrifuge for 3 to 5 minutes to separate the cellular elements from the plasma **(Fig. 12-10)**.

The hematocrit is expressed as the volume of packed red cells per unit volume of whole blood. For example, "hematocrit, 38%" in a laboratory report means that the patient has 38 mL red cells/dL (deciliter; 100 mL) of blood; red cells comprise 38% of the total blood volume. For adult men, the normal range is 42% to 54%, whereas for adult women the range is slightly lower, 36% to 46%. These normal ranges, like all normal ranges for humans, may vary depending on the method used and the interpretation of the results by an individual laboratory. Hematocrit values much below or much above these figures point to an abnormality requiring further study.

HEMOGLOBIN TESTS

A sufficient amount of hemoglobin in red cells is required for adequate oxygen delivery to the tissues. To measure its level, the hemoglobin is released from the red cells, and the color of the blood is compared with a known color scale. Hemoglobin (Hb) is expressed in grams per dL of whole blood. Normal hemoglobin concentrations for adult males range from 14 to 17 g/dL blood. Values for adult women are in a somewhat lower range, at 12 to 15 g/dL blood. The hemoglobin reading can also be expressed as a percentage of a given standard, usually the average male normal of 15.6 g Hb/dL. Thus, a reading of 90% would mean 90% of 15.6 or 14 g Hb/dL. A decrease in hemoglobin to below normal levels signifies anemia.

Normal and abnormal types of hemoglobin can be separated and measured by the process of **electrophoresis** (e-lek-tro-fo-RE-sis). In this procedure, an electric current is passed through the liquid that contains the hemoglobin to separate different components based on their electrical charge. This test is useful in the diagnosis of sickle cell anemia and other disorders caused by abnormal types of hemoglobin.

BLOOD CELL COUNTS

Most laboratories use automated methods for obtaining the data for blood counts. Visual counts are sometimes done using a **hemocytometer** (he-mo-si-TOM-eh-ter), a ruled slide used to count the cells in a given volume of blood under the microscope.

Red Cell Counts The normal red cell count varies from 4.5 to 5.5 million cells/mcL of blood. An increase in the red cell count is called **polycythemia** (pol-e-si-THE-me-ah). People who live at high altitudes develop polycythemia, as do patients with the disease **polycythemia vera**, a disorder of the bone marrow that causes red cell proliferation.

White Cell Counts The leukocyte count varies from 5,000 to 10,000 cells/mcL of blood. In **leukopenia**, the white count is below 5,000 cells/mcL. This condition indicates depressed bone marrow or a bone marrow neoplasm. In **leukocytosis** (lu-ko-si-TO-sis), the white cell count exceeds 10,000 cells/mcL. This condition is characteristic of most bacterial infections. It may also occur after hemorrhage, in cases of gout (a type of arthritis), and in uremia, the presence of nitrogenous waste in the blood as a result of kidney disease.

Platelet Counts It is difficult to count platelets visually because they are so small. Laboratories can obtain more accurate counts with automated methods. These counts are necessary for the evaluation of platelet loss (thrombocytopenia) such as occurs after radiation therapy or cancer chemotherapy. The normal platelet count ranges from 150,000 to 450,000/mcL of blood, but counts may fall to 100,000 or less without causing serious bleeding problems. If a count is very low, a platelet transfusion may be given.

THE BLOOD SLIDE (SMEAR)

In addition to the above tests, blood studies include the examination of a stained blood slide **(see Fig. 12-2)**. In this procedure, a drop of blood is spread thinly and evenly over a glass slide, and a special stain (Wright) is applied to differentiate the otherwise colorless white cells. The slide is then studied under the microscope. The red cells are examined for abnormalities in size, color, or shape and for variations in the percentage of immature forms, known as reticulocytes. (See **Box 12-2** to learn about reticulocytes and how their counts are used to diagnose disease.) The number of platelets is estimated. Parasites, such as the malarial organism and others, may be found.

Box 12-2 *Clinical Perspectives*

Counting Reticulocytes to Diagnose Disease

As erythrocytes mature in the red bone marrow, they go through a series of stages in which they lose their nucleus and most other organelles, maximizing the space available to hold hemoglobin. In one of the last stages of development, small numbers of ribosomes and some rough endoplasmic reticulum remain in the cell. These appear as a network (or reticulum) when stained. Cells at this stage are therefore called **reticulocytes.** Reticulocytes leave the red bone marrow and enter the bloodstream where they become fully mature erythrocytes in about 24 to 48 hours. The average number of red cells maturing through the reticulocyte stage at any given time is about 1% to 2%. Changes in these numbers can be used in diagnosing certain blood disorders.

When erythrocytes are lost or destroyed, as from chronic bleeding or some form of hemolytic anemia, red blood cell production is "stepped up" to compensate for the loss. Greater numbers of reticulocytes are then released into the blood before reaching full maturity, and counts increase above normal. On the other hand, a decrease in the number of circulating reticulocytes suggests a problem with red blood cell production, as in cases of deficiency anemias or suppression of bone marrow activity.

Reticulocytes. Some ribosomes and rough ER appear as a network in a late stage of erythrocyte development. (Reprinted with permission from Cormack DH. *Essential Histology*, 2nd ed. Philadelphia, PA: Lippincott Williams & Wilkins, 2001.)

In addition, a **differential white count** is done. This is an estimation of the percentage of each white cell type in the smear. Because each type has a specific function, changes in their proportions can be a valuable diagnostic aid (see Table 12-2).

BLOOD CHEMISTRY TESTS

Batteries of tests on blood serum are often done by machine. One machine, the Sequential Multiple Analyzer, can run some 20 tests/min. Tests for electrolytes, such as sodium, potassium, chloride, and bicarbonate, may be performed at the same time along with tests for blood glucose, and nitrogenous waste products, such as blood urea nitrogen, and **creatinine** (kre-AT-in-in).

Other tests check for enzymes. Increased levels of **CK** (creatine kinase), **LDH** (lactic dehydrogenase), and other enzymes indicate tissue damage, such as damage that may occur in heart disease. An excess of **alkaline phosphatase** (FOS-fah-tase) could indicate a liver disorder or metastatic cancer involving bone.

Blood can be tested for amounts of lipids, such as cholesterol, triglycerides (fats), and lipoproteins, or for amounts of plasma proteins. These tests help to diagnose and evaluate diseases. For example, the presence of more than the normal amount of glucose in the blood indicates unregulated diabetes mellitus. The list of blood chemistry tests is extensive and is constantly increasing. We may now obtain values for various hormones, vitamins, antibodies, and toxic or therapeutic drug levels.

COAGULATION STUDIES

Before surgery and during treatment of certain diseases, hemophilia for example, it is important to know that coagulation will take place within normal time limits. Because clotting is a complex process involving many reactants, a delay may result from a number of different causes, including lack of certain hormones, calcium, or vitamin K. The amounts of the various clotting factors are measured to aid in the diagnosis and treatment of bleeding disorders.

Additional tests for coagulation include tests for bleeding time, clotting time, capillary strength, and platelet function.

CHECKPOINTS 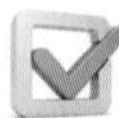

- ☐ 12-16 What is a hematocrit?
- ☐ 12-17 What are two ways of expressing hemoglobin level?

A&P in Action Revisited

Sickle Cell Anemia

Dr. Kepron, a pediatric hematologist, carefully read Cole Armstrong's medical chart. Cole, now 2 days old, was positive for the presence of Hemoglobin S. Blood tests from his parents, Jada and Darryl, confirmed Cole's diagnosis—sickle cell anemia.

Later that afternoon, Dr. Kepron met with Cole's parents and shared with them the news of their son's diagnosis. She explained, "The disease is caused by a mutation in the gene that directs the manufacture of a blood protein called hemoglobin." Dr. Kepron told Darryl and Jada that they each carried two versions of the gene, one normal and one abnormal, but they did not express the disease because the normal gene masked the effect of the abnormal one. Cole had inherited a copy of the abnormal hemoglobin gene from each of his parents and thus expressed the disease.

"Hemoglobin is found in red blood cells," she continued. "It's the protein that transports oxygen from the lungs to other tissues in the body. Normally, the red blood cells are round and flexible, which lets them bend and twist as they pass through the narrow capillaries in the body. Cole's abnormal hemoglobin causes the red blood cells to become stiff and sickle-shaped. As a result, the cells can become stuck in the capillaries, blocking blood flow and the delivery of oxygen to tissues and organs. This can be painful." However, Dr. Kepron assured them, "I'm going to work with you to manage Cole's disease—if we monitor him carefully we should be able to minimize organ and tissue damage as well as pain."

During this case, we saw that sickle cell anemia is an inherited disease. To learn more about heredity, see Chapter 21.

Chapter Wrap-Up

Summary Overview

A detailed chapter outline with space for note-taking is on *thePoint*. The figure below illustrates the main topics covered in this chapter.

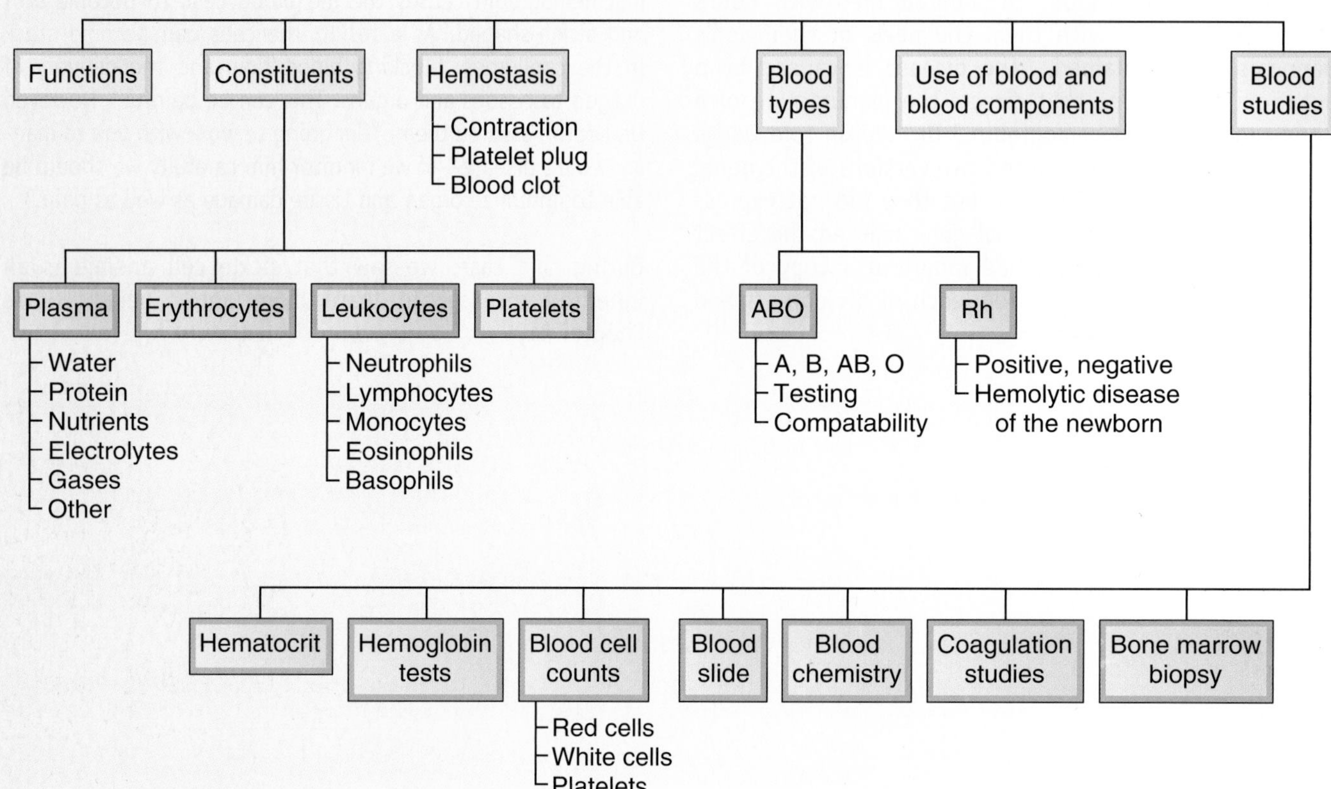

Key Terms

The terms listed below are emphasized in this chapter. Knowing them helps you organize and prioritize your learning. These and other boldface terms are defined in the Glossary with phonetic pronunciations.

agglutination	cryoprecipitate	hemolysis	plasma
albumin	eosinophil	hemostasis	platelet (thrombocyte)
antigen	erythrocyte	leukocyte	serum
antiserum	fibrin	lymphocyte	thrombin
basophil	hematocrit	megakaryocyte	transfusion
centrifuge	hematopoietic	monocyte	
coagulation	hemoglobin	neutrophil	

Word Anatomy

Scientific terms are built from standardized word parts (prefixes, roots, and suffixes). Learning the meanings of these parts can help you remember words and interpret unfamiliar terms.

WORD PART	MEANING	EXAMPLE
Blood Constituents		
erythr/o	red, red blood cell	An *erythrocyte* is a red blood cell.
leuk/o	white, colorless	A *leukocyte* is a white blood cell.
thromb/o	blood clot	A *thrombocyte* is a cell fragment that is active in blood clotting.
hemat/o	blood	*Hematopoietic* stem cells form (-poiesis) all of the blood cells.
hemo	blood	*Hemoglobin* is a protein the carries oxygen in the blood.
morph/o	shape	The nuclei of *polymorphs* have many shapes.
lymph/o	lymph, lymphatic system	*Lymphocytes* are white blood cells that circulate in the lymphatic system.
mon/o	single, one	A *monocyte* has a single, unsegmented nucleus.
phag/o	eat, ingest	Certain leukocytes take in foreign matter by the process of *phagocytosis*.
macr/o	large	A *macrophage* takes in large amounts of foreign matter by phagocytosis.
kary/o	nucleus	A *megakaryocyte* has a very large nucleus.
Hemostasis and Coagulation		
-gen	producing, originating	*Fibrinogen* converts to fibrin in the formation of a blood clot.
pro-	before, in front of	Prothrombinase is an enzyme (-ase) that converts *prothrombin* to thrombin.
Blood Types		
-lysis	loosening, dissolving, separating	A recipient's antibodies to donated red cells can cause *hemolysis* of the cells.
Uses of Blood and Blood Components		
cry/o		*Cryoprecipitate* forms when blood plasma is frozen and then thawed.

Questions for Study and Review

BUILDING UNDERSTANDING

Fill in the blanks

1. The liquid portion of blood is called ______.
2. The ancestors of all blood cells are called ______cells.
3. Platelets are produced by certain giant cells called ______.
4. Some monocytes enter the tissues and mature into phagocytes called ______.
5. Erythrocytes have a life span of approximately ______ days.

Matching > Match each numbered item with the most closely related lettered item:

___ **6.** Type A blood
___ **7.** Type B blood
___ **8.** Type O blood
___ **9.** Type AB blood
___ **10.** Rh positive blood

a. its plasma contains anti-A antibody only
b. it's considered the universal donor
c. only A antigen is present on its erythrocytes
d. it's considered the universal recipient
e. Rh antigens are present on its erythrocytes

Multiple choice

___ **11.** What iron-containing protein transports oxygen?

a. erythropoietin
b. complement
c. hemoglobin
d. thrombin

___ **12.** Which cells are agranulocytes?

a. lymphocytes
b. neutrophils
c. eosinophils
d. basophils

___ **13.** What is the correct sequence for hemostasis?

a. vessel contraction, plug formation, blood clot
b. blood clot, plug formation, vessel contraction
c. plug formation, blood clot, vessel contraction
d. vessel contraction, blood clot, plug formation

___ **14.** The hematology specialist needs to measure the number of eosinophils in a blood sample. Which test should she conduct?

a. hematocrit
b. electrophoresis
c. bone marrow biopsy
d. differential white blood cell count

UNDERSTANDING CONCEPTS

15. List the three main functions of blood. What is the average volume of circulating blood in the body?
16. Compare and contrast the following:
    - **a.** formed elements and plasma
    - **b.** erythrocyte and leukocyte
    - **c.** hemorrhage and transfusion
    - **d.** hemapheresis and plasmapheresis
17. List four main types of proteins in blood plasma and state their functions. What are some other substances carried in blood plasma?
18. Describe the structure and function of erythrocytes. State the normal blood cell count for erythrocytes.
19. Construct a chart that compares the structure and function of the five types of leukocytes. State the normal blood cell count for leukocytes.
20. Diagram the three final steps in blood clot formation.
21. Name the four blood types in the ABO system. What antigens and antibodies (if any) are found in each type?
22. Is an Rh-negative fetus of an Rh-negative mother in any danger of HDN? Explain.

CONCEPTUAL THINKING

23. J. Regan, a 40-year-old firefighter, has just had his annual physical. He is in excellent health, except for his red blood cell count, which is elevated. How might Mr. Regan's job explain his test results?

24. Nikki has type A blood. Why can she receive a transfusion of type A or type O blood, but not a transfusion of type B or type AB blood?

25. In Cole's case, he was diagnosed with sickle cell disease. A slow growth rate is one consequence of the disease. Explain why a hemoglobin abnormality is associated with delayed growth.

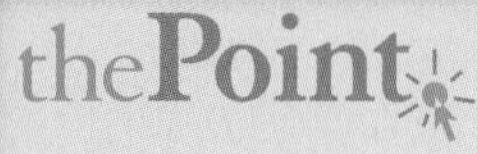
For more questions, see the learning activities on *thePoint*.

CHAPTER 13

The Heart

A&P in Action

Jim's Second Case: A Coronary Emergency

The emergency room's dispatch radio echoed from the triage desk. "This is Medic 5 en route with Jim, a 46-year-old Caucasian male. Suspected acute myocardial infarction while playing basketball. Cardiopulmonary resuscitation was initiated on scene. Patient was defibrillated in ambulance twice. Portable electrocardiography (ECG) indicates S-T interval depression and an inverted T wave. Patient is receiving oxygen through nasal cannulae. ETA approximately 10 minutes."

When Jim arrived at the ER, the emergency team rushed to stabilize him. A trauma nurse measured Jim's vital signs—he was hypertensive with tachycardia—while another inserted an IV needle into Jim's arm and placed an oxygen mask over his nose and mouth. Meanwhile, a phlebotomist drew blood from Jim's other arm for testing in the lab. A cardiology technician attached ECG leads to Jim's chest and began to record his cardiac muscle's electrical activity. The emergency doctor looked at the printout from the electrocardiograph and confirmed that Jim was having a heart attack, technically called an acute myocardia infarction. The doctor knew that one or more of the coronary arteries feeding Jim's heart muscle was blocked with a thrombus (blood clot). He administered several medications in an attempt to restore blood flow to the heart and minimize myocardial damage. Aspirin, which prevents platelets from adhering to each other, was given to inhibit the formation of any more thrombi. Nitroglycerin, a potent vasodilator, was given to widen Jim's coronary arteries and thus increase blood flow to the heart. Morphine was given to manage Jim's pain and lower his cardiac output in order to reduce the heart's workload. Finally, tissue plasminogen activator was administered to dissolve the thrombi present in Jim's coronary arteries.

Thanks to the quick action of the paramedics and emergency team, Jim was resting comfortably in the intensive care unit a few hours after thrombolytic treatment—he was lucky to be alive! Later in the chapter, we will visit Jim again and learn how cardiac surgeons repair coronary arteries to prevent future infarctions.

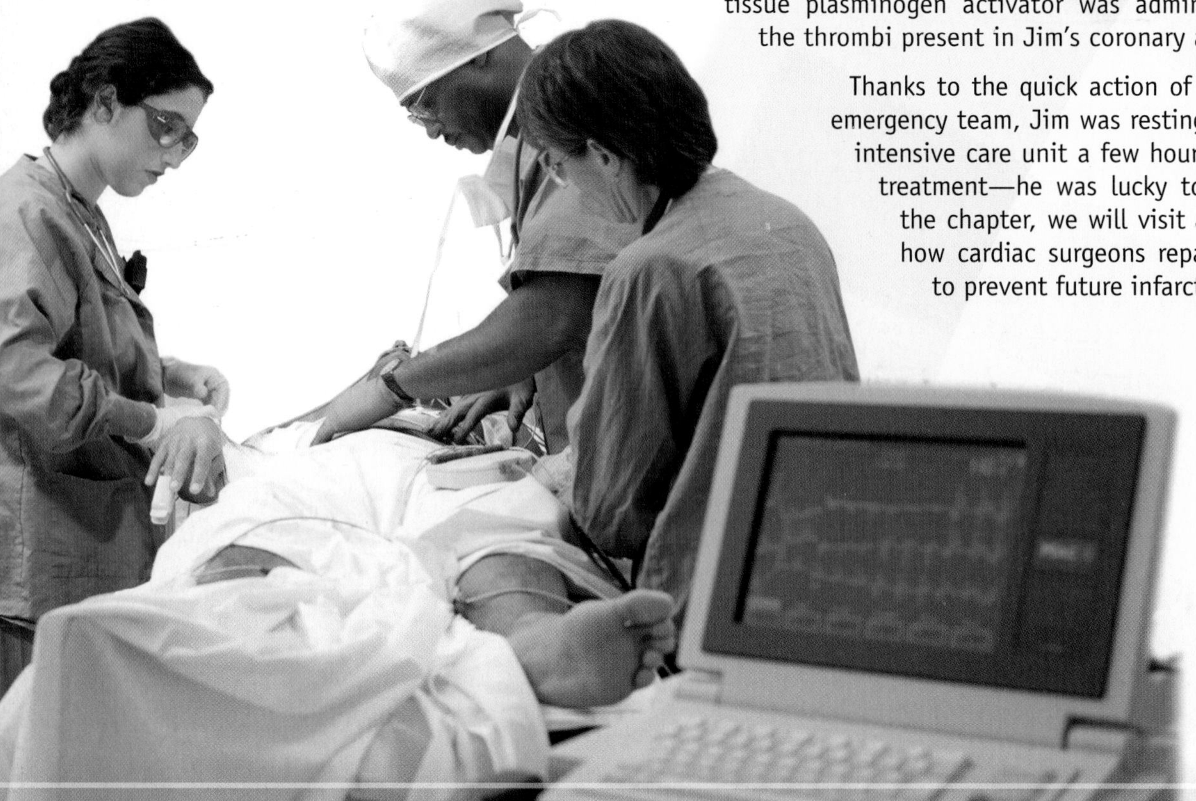

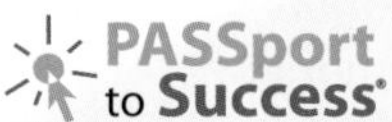

Ancillaries At-A-Glance

Visit *thePoint* to access the PASSport to Success and the following resources. For guidance in using these resources most effectively, see pp. ix–xviii.

Learning TOOLS

- Learning Style Self-Assessment
- Live Advise Online Student Tutoring
- Tips for Effective Studying

Learning RESOURCES

- E-book: Chapter 13
- Web Figure: Interior view of the left atrium and ventricle
- Web Figure: Pathway of blood through the heart
- Web Chart: Layers of the heart wall
- Web Chart: Layers of the pericardium
- Web Chart: Chambers of the heart
- Web Chart: Valves of the heart
- Animation: Blood Circulation
- Animation: Cardiac Cycle
- Animation: Myocardial Blood Flow
- Health Professions: Surgical Technologist
- Detailed Chapter Outline
- Answers to Questions for Study and Review
- Audio Pronunciation Glossary

Learning ACTIVITIES

- Pre-Quiz
- Visual Activities
- Kinesthetic Activities
- Auditory Activities

Learning Outcomes

After careful study of this chapter, you should be able to:

1. Describe the three tissue layers of the heart wall, ***p. 250***
2. Describe the location and structure of the pericardium and cite its functions, ***p. 250***
3. Compare the functions of the right and left chambers of the heart, ***p. 251***
4. Name the valves at the entrance and exit of each ventricle and identify the function of each, ***p. 252***
5. Briefly describe blood circulation through the myocardium, ***p. 253***
6. Briefly describe the cardiac cycle, ***p. 255***
7. Name and locate the components of the heart's conduction system, ***p. 255***
8. Explain the effects of the autonomic nervous system (ANS) on the heart rate, ***p. 256***
9. List and define several terms that describe variations in heart rates, ***p. 257***
10. Explain what produces each of the two normal heart sounds and identify the usual cause of a murmur, ***p. 257***
11. Describe several lifestyle choices that can help maintain heart health, ***p. 258***
12. Briefly describe methods used to study the heart, ***p. 259***
13. Referring to the case study, list the emergency and surgical procedures commonly performed following a myocardial infarction and explain why they are done, ***pp. 248, 260***
14. Show how word parts are used to build words related to the heart (see Word Anatomy at the end of the chapter). ***p. 262***

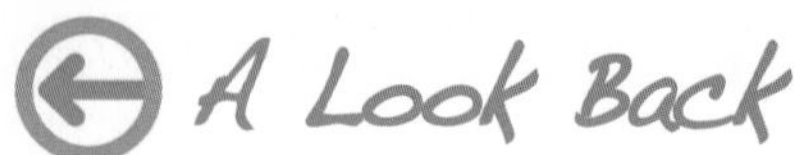

In Chapter 4, we learned that cardiac muscle is one of the three types of muscle in the body. Now it is time to study this tissue and the organ it makes up—the heart. We will also see that, even though the heart is self-stimulated, the nervous and endocrine systems influence its actions.

The next two chapters investigate how the blood delivers oxygen and nutrients to the cells and carries away the waste products of cellular metabolism. The continuous one-way circuit of blood through the blood vessels is known as the **circulation.** The prime mover that propels blood throughout the body is the **heart.** This chapter examines the heart's structure and function as a foundation for the detailed discussion of blood vessels that follows.

The heart's importance has been recognized for centuries. Strokes (contractions) of this pump average about 72 per minute and are carried on unceasingly for a lifetime. The beating of the heart is affected by the emotions, which may explain the frequent references to it in song and poetry. However, the heart's vital functions and its disorders are of more practical concern.

Structure of the Heart

The heart is slightly bigger than a person's fist. It is located between the lungs in the center and a bit to the left of the body's midline **(Fig. 13-1)**. It occupies most of the mediastinum, the central region of the thorax. The heart's **apex,** the pointed, inferior portion, is directed toward the left. The broad, superior **base,** directed toward the right, is the area of attachment for the large vessels carrying blood into and out of the heart. See Dissection Atlas **Figure A3-5** for a photograph of the heart in position in the thorax.

TISSUE LAYERS OF THE HEART WALL

The heart is a hollow organ, with walls formed of three different layers. Just as a warm coat might have a smooth lining, a thick interlining, and an outer covering of a third fabric, so the heart wall has three tissue layers **(Fig. 13-2)**. Starting with the innermost layer, these are as follows:

1. The **endocardium** (en-do-KAR-de-um) is a thin, smooth layer of epithelial cells that lines the heart's interior. The endocardium provides a smooth surface for easy flow as blood travels through the heart. Extensions of this membrane cover the flaps (cusps) of the heart valves.
2. The **myocardium** (mi-o-KAR-de-um), the heart muscle, is the thickest layer and pumps blood through the vessels. The cardiac muscle's unique structure will be described in more detail shortly.
3. The **epicardium** (ep-ih-KAR-de-um) is a serous membrane that forms the thin, outermost layer of the heart wall. It is also considered the visceral layer of the pericardium, discussed next.

THE PERICARDIUM

The **pericardium** (per-ih-KAR-de-um) is the sac that encloses the heart **(see Fig. 13-2)**. The formation of the pericardial sac was described and illustrated in Chapter 4 under the discussion of membranes **(see Fig. 4-8)**. This sac's outermost and heaviest layer is the fibrous pericardium. Connective tissue anchors this pericardial layer to the diaphragm, located inferiorly; the sternum, located anteriorly; and to other structures surrounding the heart, thus holding the heart in place. A serous membrane lines this fibrous sac and folds back at the base of the heart to cover the heart's surface.

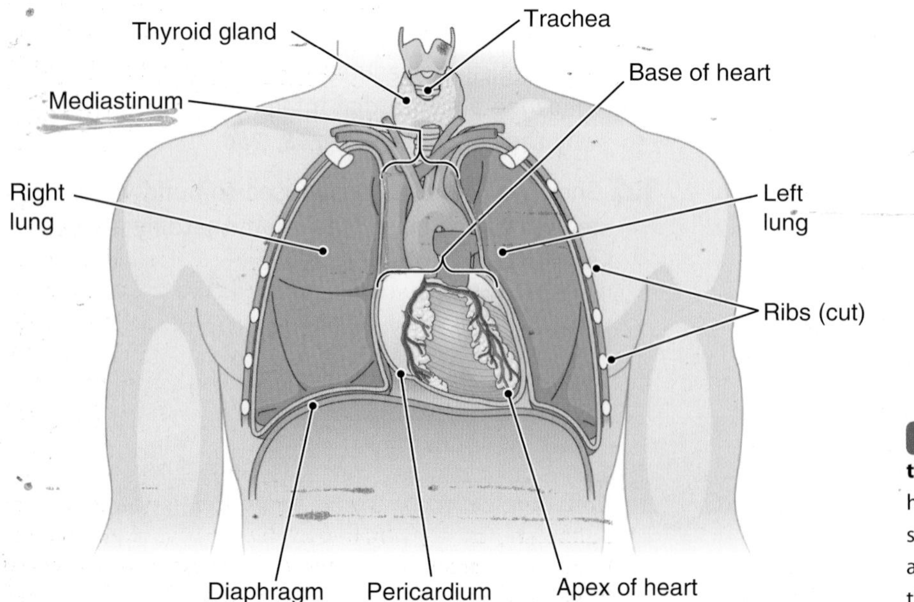

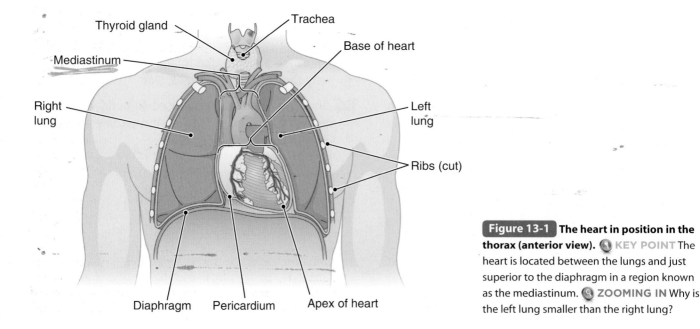

Figure 13-1 The heart in position in the thorax (anterior view). KEY POINT The heart is located between the lungs and just superior to the diaphragm in a region known as the mediastinum. ZOOMING IN Why is the left lung smaller than the right lung?

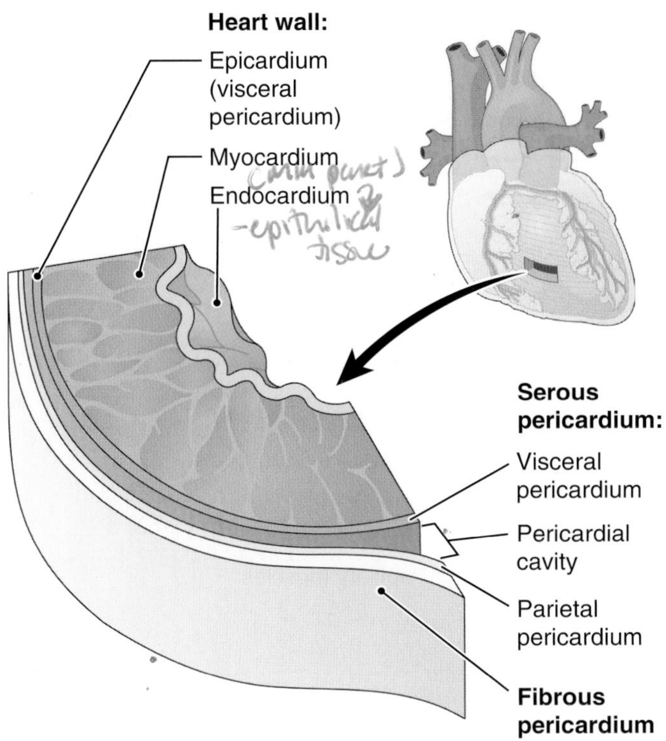

Figure 13-2 Layers of the heart wall and pericardium. KEY POINT The serous pericardium covers the heart and lines the fibrous pericardium. ZOOMING IN Which layer of the heart wall is the thickest?

Anatomically, the outer layer of this serous membrane is called the parietal layer, and the inner layer is the visceral layer, also known as the epicardium, as previously noted. A thin film of fluid between these two layers reduces friction as the heart moves within the pericardium. Normally, the visceral and parietal layers are very close together, but fluid may accumulate in the region between them, the pericardial cavity, under certain disease conditions.

SPECIAL FEATURES OF THE MYOCARDIUM

Cardiac muscle cells are lightly striated (striped) based on alternating actin and myosin filaments, as seen in skeletal muscle cells (see Chapter 7). Unlike skeletal muscle cells, however, cardiac muscle cells have a single nucleus instead of multiple nuclei. Also, cardiac muscle tissue is involuntarily controlled; it typically contracts independently of conscious thought. There are specialized partitions between cardiac muscle cells that show faintly under a microscope (Fig. 13-3). These **intercalated** (in-TER-cah-la-ted) **disks** are actually modified plasma membranes that firmly attach adjacent cells to each other but allow for rapid transfer of electric impulses between them. The adjective *intercalated* is from Latin and means "inserted between." Such electrical synapses, mentioned in Chapter 8, provide rapid and coordinated communication between cells.

Another feature of cardiac muscle tissue is the branching of the muscle fibers (cells). These branched fibers are

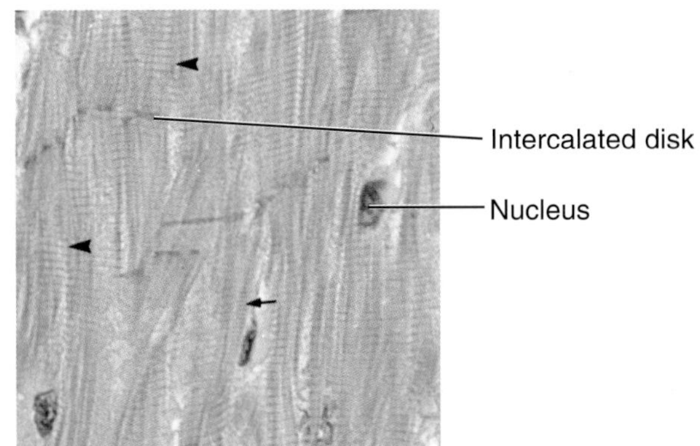

Figure 13-3 Cardiac muscle tissue viewed under the microscope (×540). KEY POINT The sample shows light striations (see the *arrowheads*), intercalated disks, and branching fibers (*arrow*). (Reprinted with permission from Gartner LP, Hiatt JL. *Color Atlas of Histology*, 5th ed. Philadelphia, PA: Lippincott Williams & Wilkins, 2009.)

interwoven so that the stimulation that causes the contraction of one fiber results in the contraction of a whole group. The intercalated disks between the fibers and the branching cellular networks allow cardiac muscle cells to contract in a coordinated manner for effective pumping.

DIVISIONS OF THE HEART

Healthcare professionals often refer to the *right heart* and the *left heart*, because the human heart is really a double pump (Fig. 13-4). The right side pumps blood low in oxygen content to the lungs through the pulmonary circuit. The left side pumps highly oxygenated blood to the remainder of the body through the systemic circuit. Each side of the heart is divided into two chambers. See Figure A3-6 in the Dissection Atlas for a photograph of the human heart showing the chambers and the vessels that connect to the heart.

Four Chambers The upper chambers on the right and left sides, the **atria** (A-tre-ah), are mainly blood-receiving chambers (see Fig. 13-4). The lower chambers on the right and left side, the **ventricles** (VEN-trih-klz) are forceful pumps. The chambers, listed in the order in which blood flows through them, are as follows:

1. The **right atrium** (A-tre-um) is a thin-walled chamber that receives the blood returning from the body tissues. This blood, which is low in oxygen, is carried in veins, the blood vessels leading back to the heart. The superior vena cava brings blood from the head, chest, and arms; the inferior vena cava delivers blood from the trunk and legs. A third vessel that opens into the right atrium brings blood from the heart muscle itself, as described later in this chapter.
2. The **right ventricle** pumps the venous blood received from the right atrium to the lungs. It pumps into a large pulmonary trunk, which then divides into right and left pulmonary arteries. Branches of these arteries carry blood to the lungs. An artery is a vessel that takes blood

13

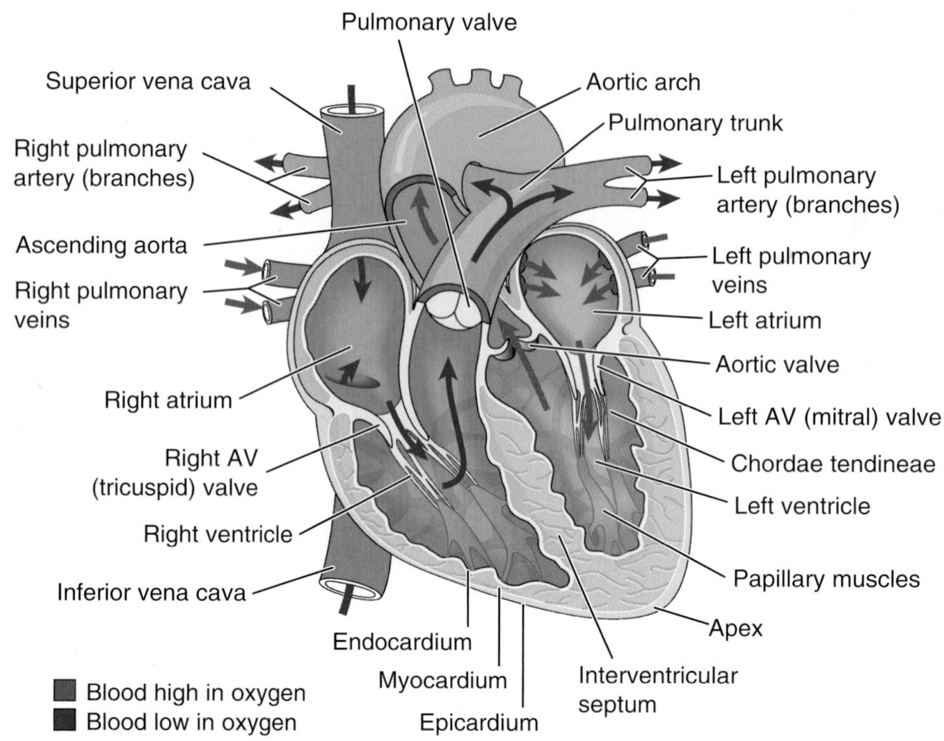

Figure 13-4 The heart and great vessels. KEY POINT The right heart has blood low in oxygen; the left heart has blood high in oxygen. The *arrows* show the direction of blood flow through the heart. The abbreviation AV means atrioventricular. ZOOMING IN Which heart chamber has the thickest wall?

from the heart to the tissues. Note that the pulmonary arteries in **Figure 13-4** are colored blue because they are carrying blood low in oxygen, unlike other arteries, which carry blood high in oxygen.

3. The **left atrium** receives blood high in oxygen content as it returns from the lungs in pulmonary veins. Note that the pulmonary veins in **Figure 13-4** are colored red because they are carrying blood high in oxygen content, unlike other veins, which carry blood low in oxygen.
4. The **left ventricle**, which is the chamber with the thickest wall, pumps highly oxygenated blood to all parts of the body. This blood goes first into the aorta (a-OR-tah), the largest artery, and then into the branching systemic arteries that take blood to the tissues. The heart's apex, the lower pointed region, is formed by the wall of the left ventricle.

The heart's right and left chambers are completely separated from each other by partitions, each of which is called a **septum**. The **interatrial** (in-ter-A-tre-al) **septum** separates the two atria, and the **interventricular** (in-ter-ven-TRIK-u-lar) **septum** separates the two ventricles. The septa, like the heart wall, consist largely of myocardium.

Four Valves One-way valves that direct blood flow through the heart are located at the entrance and exit of each ventricle **(see Fig. 13-4)**. The entrance valves are the **atrioventricular** (a-tre-o-ven-TRIK-u-lar) (AV) **valves**, so named because they are between the atria and ventricles. The exit valves are the **semilunar** (sem-e-LU-nar) **valves**, so named because each flap of these valves resembles a half-moon. Each valve has a specific name, as follows:

- The **right atrioventricular** (AV) **valve** is also known as the **tricuspid** (tri-KUS-pid) **valve** because it has three cusps, or flaps, that open and close **(Fig. 13-5)**. When this valve is open, blood flows freely from the right atrium into the right ventricle. When the right ventricle begins to contract, however, the valve is closed by blood squeezed backward against the cusps. With the valve closed, blood cannot return to the right atrium but must flow forward into the pulmonary arterial trunk.
- The **left atrioventricular** (AV) **valve** is the bicuspid valve, but it is commonly referred to as the **mitral** (MI-tral) **valve** (named for a miter, the pointed, two-sided hat worn by bishops). It has two heavy cusps that permit blood to flow freely from the left atrium into the left ventricle. The cusps close when the left ventricle begins to contract; this closure prevents blood from returning to the left atrium and ensures the forward flow of blood into the aorta. Both the right and left AV valves are attached by means of thin fibrous threads to columnar muscles, called **papillary** (PAP-ih-lar-e) **muscles**, arising from the walls of the ventricles. The function of these threads, called the **chordae tendineae** (KOR-de ten-DIN-e-e) **(see Fig. 13-4)**, is to stabilize the valve

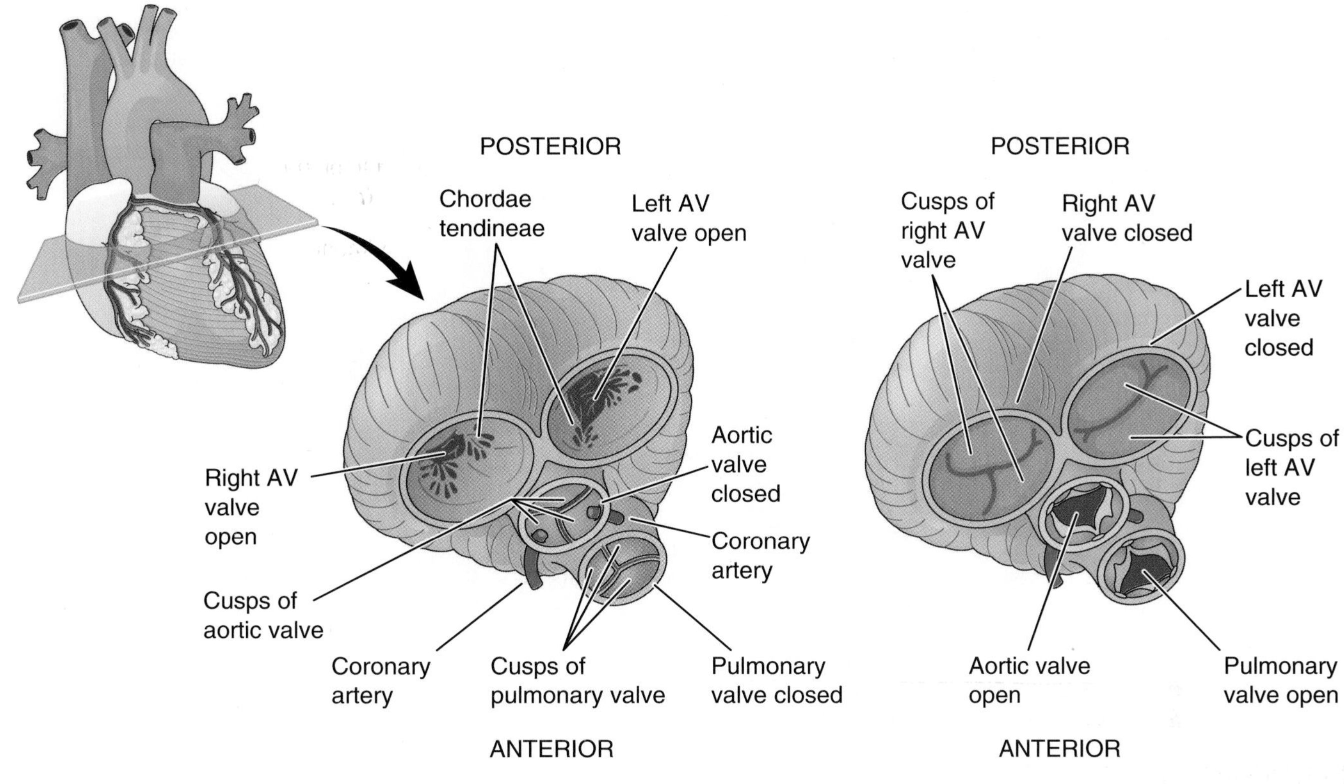

Figure 13-5 **Heart valves (superior view from anterior, atria removed).** KEY POINT Valves keep blood flowing in a forward direction through the heart. **A.** When the heart is relaxed (diastole), the AV valves are open and blood flows freely from the atria to the ventricles. The pulmonary and aortic valves are closed. **B.** When the ventricles contract (systole), the AV valves close and blood pumped out of the ventricles opens the pulmonary and aortic valves. ZOOMING IN How many cusps does the right AV valve have? The left?

flaps when the ventricles contract so that the blood's force will not push the valves up into the atria. In this manner, they help to prevent a backflow of blood when the heart beats.

- The **pulmonary** (PUL-mon-ar-e) **valve**, also called the *pulmonic valve*, is a semilunar valve located between the right ventricle and the pulmonary trunk that leads to the lungs. As soon as the right ventricle begins to relax from a contraction, pressure in that chamber drops. The higher pressure in the pulmonary artery, described as *back pressure*, closes the valve and prevents blood from returning to the ventricle.
- The **aortic** (a-OR-tik) **valve** is a semilunar valve located between the left ventricle and the aorta. After contraction of the left ventricle, back pressure closes the aortic valve and prevents the back flow of blood from the aorta into the ventricle.

Note that blood passes through the heart twice in making a trip from the heart's right side through the pulmonary circuit to the lungs and back to the heart's left side to start on its way through the systemic circuit. However, it is important to bear in mind that the heart's two sides function in unison to pump blood through both circuits at the same time.

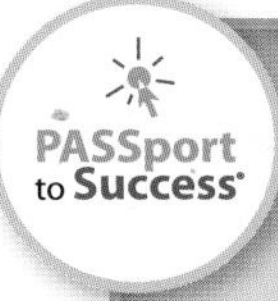

See the student resources on *thePoint* for charts summarizing the structure of the heart and pericardium and for a detailed picture of the heart's interior. See also the animation *Blood Circulation* and a numbered diagram showing blood flow through the heart.

BLOOD SUPPLY TO THE MYOCARDIUM

Only the endocardium comes into contact with the blood that flows through the heart chambers. Therefore, the myocardium must have its own blood vessels to provide oxygen and nourishment and to remove waste products. Together, these blood vessels provide the **coronary** (KOR-o-na-re) **circulation.** It is the coronary circulation that is involved in Jim's case study. The main arteries that supply blood to the heart muscle are the right and left coronary arteries (Fig. 13-6), named because they encircle the heart like a crown. These arteries, which are the first to branch off the aorta, arise just above the cusps of the aortic valve and branch to all regions of the heart muscle. They receive blood only when the ventricles relax because the aortic valve must be closed to expose the entrance to these vessels (Fig. 13-7). After passing through the capillaries in the

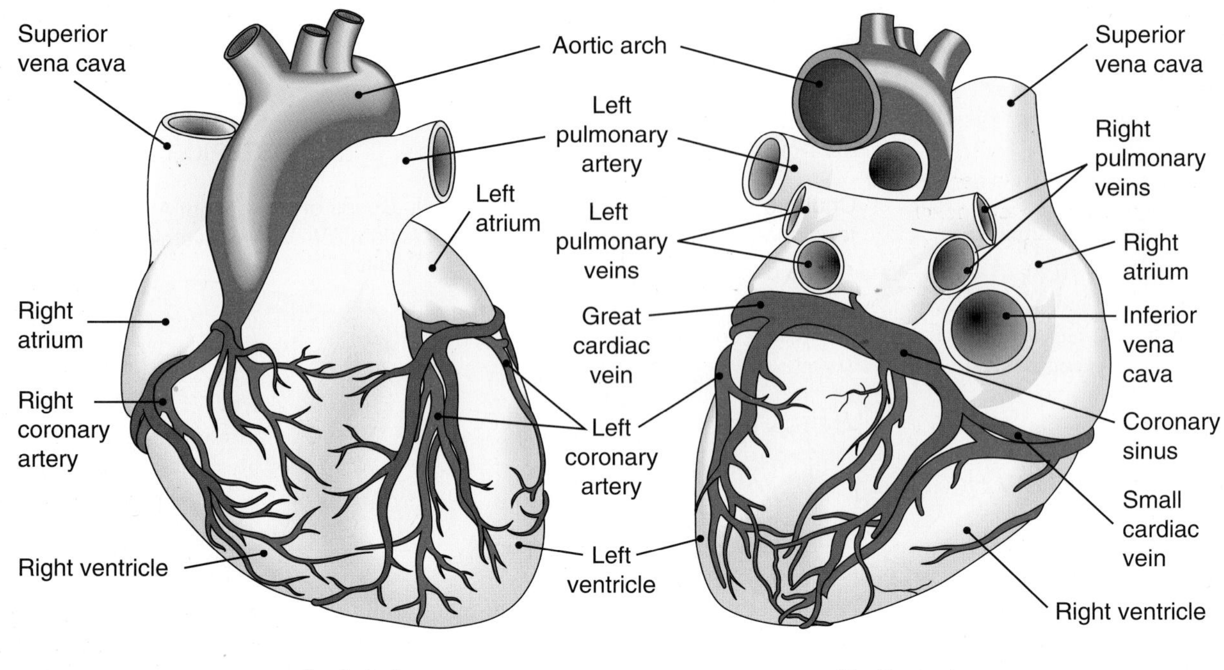

Figure 13-6 Blood vessels that supply the myocardium. KEY POINT Coronary arteries and cardiac veins comprise the heart's circulatory pathways. **A.** Anterior view. **B.** Posterior view. ZOOMING IN What is the largest cardiac vein and where does it lead?

myocardium, blood drains into a system of cardiac veins that brings blood back toward the right atrium. Blood finally collects in the **coronary sinus**, a dilated vein that opens into the right atrium near the inferior vena cava (see Fig. 13-6).

CHECKPOINTS 

☐ **13-1** What are the names of the innermost, middle, and outermost layers of the heart wall?

☐ **13-2** What is the name of the sac that encloses the heart?

☐ **13-3** What is the heart's upper receiving chamber on each side called? What is the lower pumping chamber called?

☐ **13-4** What is the purpose of each of the four valves in the heart?

☐ **13-5** What is the name of the system that supplies blood to the myocardium?

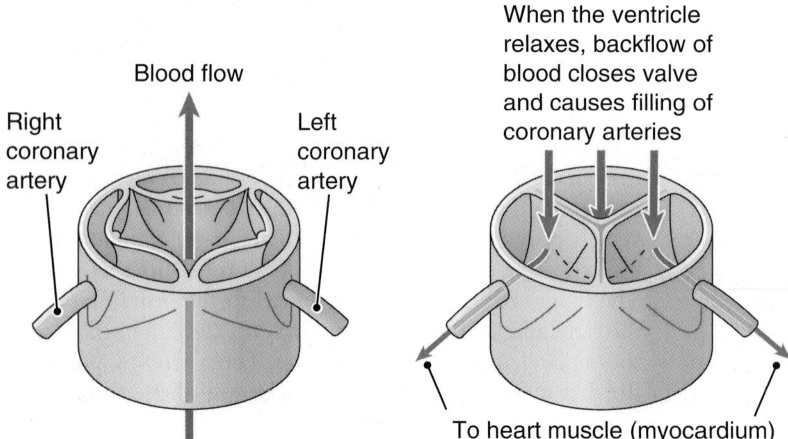

Figure 13-7 Opening of coronary arteries in the aortic valve (anterior view). KEY POINT **A.** When the left ventricle contracts, the aortic valve opens. The valve cusps prevent filling of the coronary arteries. **B.** When the left ventricle relaxes, backflow of blood closes the aortic valve and the coronary arteries fill. (Modified with permission from Moore KL, Dalley AF. *Clinically Oriented Anatomy*, 5th ed. Baltimore, MD: Lippincott Williams & Wilkins, 2006.)

Heart Function

Although the heart's right and left sides are separated from each other, they work together. Blood is squeezed through the chambers by a heart muscle contraction that begins in the thin-walled upper chambers, the atria, and is followed by a contraction of the thick muscle of the lower chambers, the ventricles. In each case, the active phase, called **systole** (SIS-to-le), is followed by a resting phase known as **diastole** (di-AS-to-le). One complete sequence of heart contraction and relaxation is called the **cardiac cycle** (Fig. 13-8). Each cardiac cycle represents a single heartbeat. At rest, one cycle takes an average of 0.8 seconds.

The cardiac cycle begins with contraction of both atria, which forces blood through the AV valves into the ventricles. The atrial walls are thin, and their contractions are not very powerful. However, they do improve the heart's efficiency by forcing blood into the ventricles before these lower chambers contract. Atrial contraction is completed at the time ventricular contraction begins. Thus, a resting phase (diastole) begins in the atria at the same time that a contraction (systole) begins in the ventricles. While the ventricles are contracting, forcing blood through the semilunar valves, the atria are relaxed and again are filling with blood (see Fig. 13-8).

After the ventricles have contracted, all the chambers are relaxed for a short period as they passively fill with blood. Then another cycle begins with an atrial contraction followed by a ventricular contraction. Although both upper and lower chambers have a systolic and diastolic phase in each cardiac cycle, discussions of heart function usually refer to these phases as they occur in the ventricles, because these chambers contract more forcefully and drive blood into the arteries.

CARDIAC OUTPUT

A unique property of heart muscle is its ability to adjust the strength of contraction to the amount of blood received. When the heart chamber is filled and the wall stretched (within limits), the contraction is strong. As less blood enters the heart, contractions become less forceful. Thus, as more blood enters the heart, the muscle contracts with greater strength to push the larger volume of blood out into the blood vessels (see Box 13-1). The heart's ability to pump out all of the blood it receives prevents blood from pooling in the chambers.

The volume of blood pumped by each ventricle in 1 minute is termed the **cardiac output** (CO). It is the product of the **stroke volume** (SV)—the volume of blood ejected from the ventricle with each beat—and the **heart rate** (HR)—the number of times the heart beats per minute. To summarize:

$$CO = HR \times SV$$

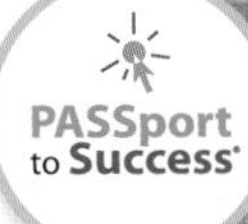

See the student resources on *thePoint* for the animations *Myocardial Blood Flow* and *The Cardiac Cycle.*

THE HEART'S CONDUCTION SYSTEM

Like other muscles, the heart muscle is stimulated to contract by a wave of electric energy that passes along the cells. This action potential is generated by specialized tissue within the heart and spreads over structures that form the heart's conduction system (Fig. 13-9). Two of these

13

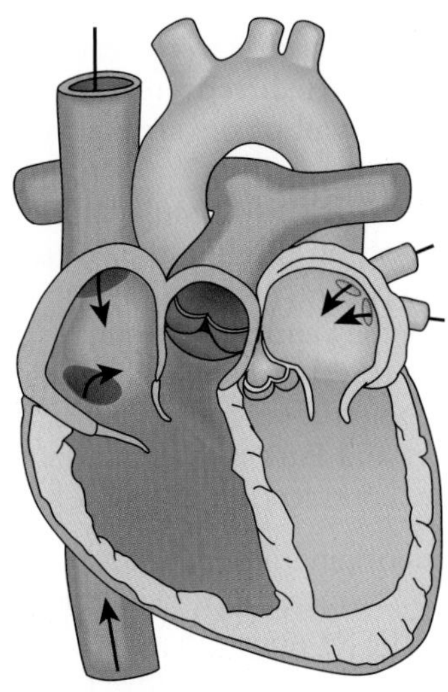

Diastole
Atria fill with blood, which flows directly into the relaxed ventricles.

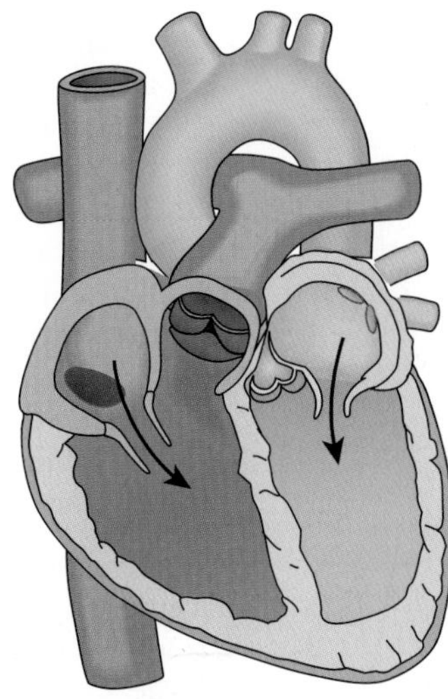

Atrial systole
Contraction of atria pumps additional blood into the ventricles.

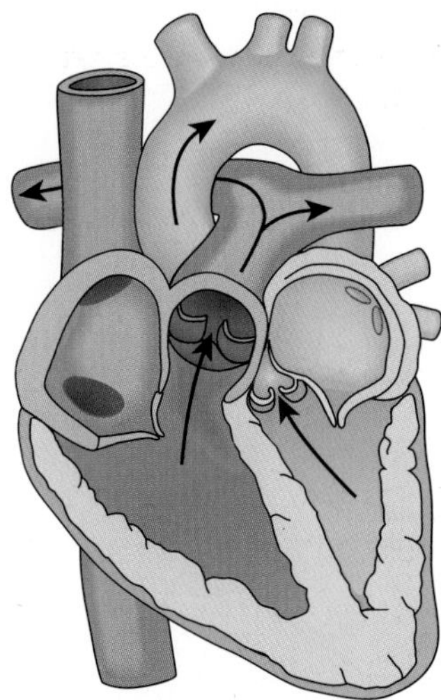

Ventricular systole
Contraction of ventricles pumps blood into aorta and pulmonary arteries.

Figure 13-8 The cardiac cycle. KEY POINT In one cardiac cycle, contraction of both atria is followed by contraction of both ventricles. ZOOMING IN When the ventricles contract, what valves close? What valves open?

Box 13-1 A Closer Look

Cardiac Reserve: Extra Output When Needed

Based on a heart rate of 75 beats/min and a stroke volume of 70 mL/beat, the average cardiac output for an adult at rest is about 5 L/min. This means that at rest, the heart pumps the equivalent of the total blood volume each minute. But like many other organs, the heart has great reserves of strength. The cardiac reserve is a measure of how many times more than resting output the heart can produce when needed.

During mild exercise, cardiac output might double. During strenuous exercise, it might double again. In other words, for most people, the cardiac reserve is 4 to 5 times the resting output. This increase is achieved by an increase in stroke volume and heart rate. In athletes exercising vigorously, the ratio may reach 6 to 7 times the resting volume. In contrast, those with heart disease may have little or no cardiac reserve. They may be fine at rest but quickly become short of breath or fatigued when exercising or even when carrying out the simple tasks of daily living.

Cardiac reserve can be evaluated using an exercise stress test that measures cardiac output while the patient walks on a treadmill or pedals an exercise bicycle. The exercise becomes more and more strenuous until the patient's peak cardiac output (cardiac reserve) is reached.

structures are tissue masses called nodes, and the remainder consists of specialized fibers that branch through the myocardium.

The **sinoatrial** (SA) **node** is located in the upper wall of the right atrium in a small depression described as a sinus. This node initiates the heartbeats by generating an action potential at regular intervals. Because the SA node sets the rate of heart contractions, it is commonly called the **pacemaker**. The second node, located in the interatrial septum at the bottom of the right atrium, is called the **atrioventricular** (AV) **node**.

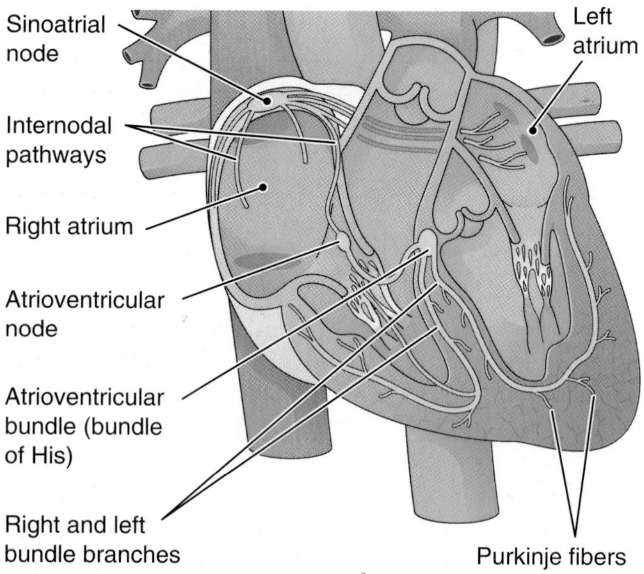

Figure 13-9 Conduction system of the heart. KEY POINT The sinoatrial (SA) node, the atrioventricular (AV) node, and specialized fibers conduct the electric energy that stimulates the heart muscle to contract. ZOOMING IN What parts of the conduction system do the internodal pathways connect?

The **atrioventricular** (AV) **bundle**, also known as the *bundle of His*, is located at the top of the interventricular septum. It has branches that extend to all parts of the ventricular walls. Fibers travel first down both sides of the interventricular septum in groups called the right and left bundle branches. Smaller **Purkinje** (pur-KIN-je) **fibers** then travel in a branching network throughout the myocardium of the ventricles. Intercalated disks allow the rapid flow of impulses throughout the heart muscle.

The order in which impulses travel through the heart is as follows:

1. The SA generates the electric impulse that begins the heartbeat (see Fig. 13-9).
2. The excitation wave travels throughout the myocardium of each atrium, causing the atria to contract. At the same time, impulses also travel directly to the AV node by means of fibers in the wall of the atrium that make up the **internodal pathways**.
3. The atrioventricular node is stimulated. A relatively slower rate of conduction through the AV node allows time for the atria to contract and complete the filling of the ventricles before the ventricles contract.
4. The excitation wave travels rapidly through the AV bundle and then throughout the ventricular walls by means of the bundle branches and Purkinje fibers. The entire ventricular musculature contracts almost at the same time.

A normal heart rhythm originating at the SA node is termed a **sinus rhythm**. As a safety measure, a region of the conduction system other than the SA node can generate a heartbeat if the SA node fails, but it does so at a slower rate.

CONTROL OF THE HEART RATE

Although the heart's fundamental beat originates within the heart itself, the heart rate can be influenced by the nervous system, hormones, and other factors in the internal environment.

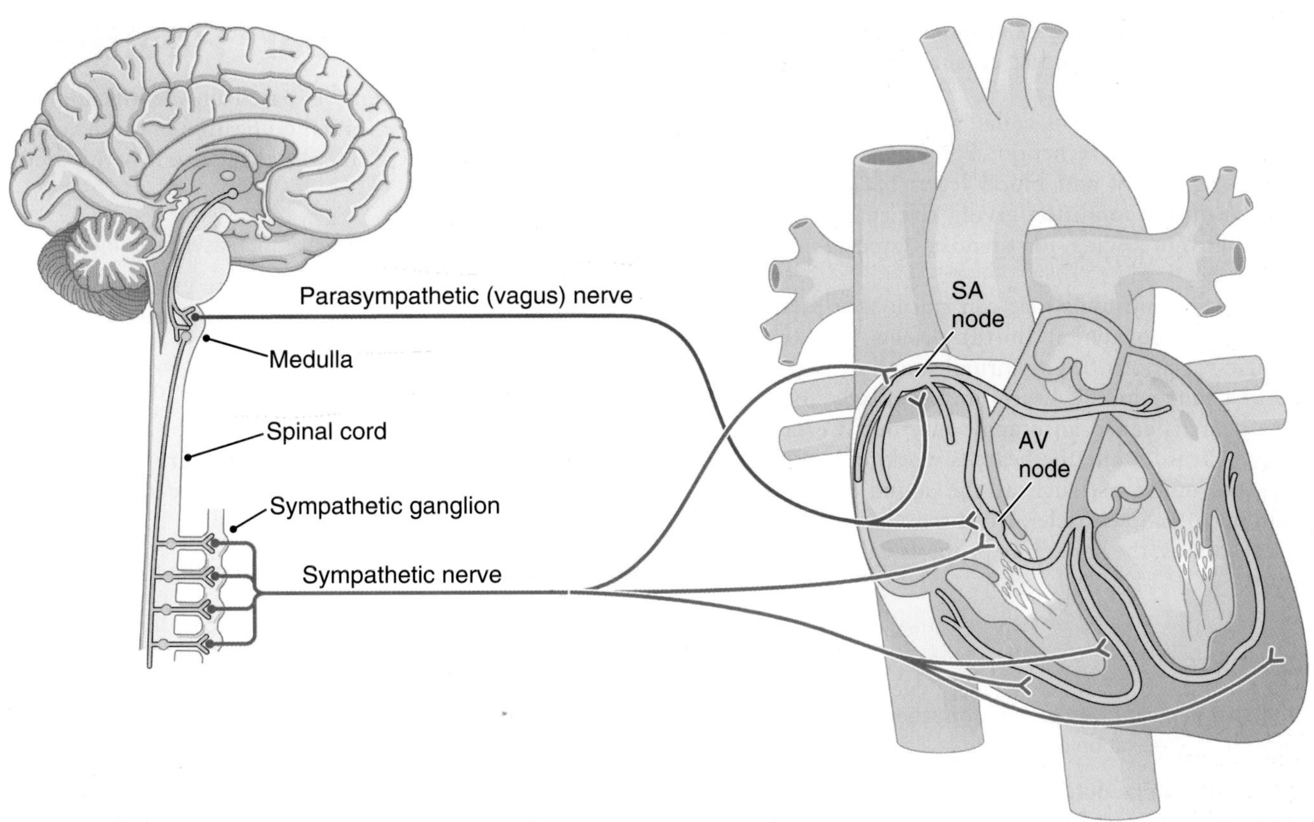

Figure 13-10 **Autonomic nervous system (ANS) regulation of the heart.** KEY POINT The ANS affects the rate and force of heart contractions by acting on the SA and AV nodes and the myocardium itself. ZOOMING IN Which cranial nerve carries parasympathetic impulses to the heart?

The ANS plays a major role in modifying the heart rate according to the need (Fig. 13-10). Sympathetic nervous system stimulation increases the heart rate in response to increased activity. During a fight-or-flight response, the sympathetic nerves can boost the cardiac output on average four to five times the resting value. Sympathetic fibers increase the contraction rate by stimulating the SA and AV nodes. They also increase the contraction force by acting directly on the fibers of the myocardium. These actions translate into increased cardiac output. Parasympathetic stimulation decreases the heart rate to restore homeostasis. The parasympathetic nerve that supplies the heart is the vagus nerve (cranial nerve X). It slows the heart rate by acting on the SA and AV nodes (see Fig. 13-10).

These ANS influences allow the heart to meet changing needs rapidly. The heart rate is also affected by substances circulating in the blood, including hormones, such as epinephrine and thyroxine; ions, primarily K^+, Na^+, and Ca^{2+}; and drugs. Regular exercise strengthens the heart and increases the amount of blood ejected with each beat. Consequently, the body's circulatory needs at rest can be met with a lower heart rate. Trained athletes usually have a low resting heart rate.

The following variations in heart rate occur commonly. Note that these variations do not necessarily indicate pathology:

- **Bradycardia** (brad-e-KAR-de-ah) is a relatively slow heart rate of less than 60 beats/min. During rest and sleep, the heart may beat less than 60 beats/min, but the rate usually does not fall below 50 beats/min.
- **Tachycardia** (tak-e-KAR-de-ah) refers to a heart rate of more than 100 beats/min. Tachycardia is normal during exercise or stress, or with excessive caffeine intake, but may also occur with certain disorders.
- **Sinus arrhythmia** (ah-RITH-me-ah) is a regular variation in heart rate caused by changes in the rate and depth of breathing. It is a normal phenomenon.
- **Premature beat**, also called *extrasystole*, is a beat that comes before the expected normal beat. In healthy people, premature beats may be initiated by caffeine, nicotine, or psychologic stresses. They are also common in people with heart disease.

NORMAL AND ABNORMAL HEART SOUNDS

The normal heart sounds are usually described by the syllables "lub" and "dup." The first heart sound (S_1), the "lub," is a longer, lower-pitched sound that occurs at the start of ventricular systole. It is caused by a combination of events, mainly closure of the AV valves. This action causes vibrations in the blood passing through the valves and in the tissue surrounding the valves. The second heart sound (S_2), the "dup," is shorter and sharper.

It occurs at the beginning of ventricular relaxation and is caused largely by sudden closure of the semilunar valves.

An abnormal sound is called a **murmur** and is usually due to faulty valve action. For example, if a valve fails to close tightly and blood leaks back, a murmur is heard. Another condition giving rise to an abnormal sound is the narrowing, or **stenosis** (sten-O-sis), of a valve opening.

The many conditions that can cause abnormal heart sounds include congenital (birth) defects, disease, and physiologic variations. An abnormal sound caused by any structural change in the heart or the vessels connected with the heart is called an **organic murmur**. Certain normal sounds heard while the heart is working may also be described as murmurs, such as the sound heard during rapid filling of the ventricles. To differentiate these from abnormal sounds, they are more properly called **functional murmurs.**

CHECKPOINTS 

☐ 13-6 What name is given to the contraction phase of the cardiac cycle? To the relaxation phase?

☐ 13-7 What is cardiac output? What two factors determine cardiac output?

☐ 13-8 What is the scientific name of the heart's pacemaker?

☐ 13-9 What system exerts the main influence on the rate and strength of heart contractions?

☐ 13-10 What is a heart murmur?

Maintaining Heart Health

Prevention of heart ailments is based on identification of cardiovascular risk factors and modification of those factors that can be changed. Risk factors that cannot be modified include the following:

- Age. The risk of heart disease increases with age.
- Gender. Until middle age, men have greater risk than women. Women older than 50 years or past menopause have risk equal to that of men.
- Heredity. Those with immediate family members with heart disease are at greater risk.
- Body type. In particular, the hereditary tendency to deposit fat in the abdomen or on the chest surface increases risk.

Risk factors that can be modified include the following:

- Smoking and other forms of tobacco use, which lead to spasm and hardening of the arteries. These arterial changes result in decreased blood flow and poor supply of oxygen and nutrients to the myocardium.
- Physical inactivity. Lack of exercise weakens the heart muscle and decreases the heart's efficiency. It also decreases the efficiency of the skeletal muscles, which further taxes the heart.
- Weight over the ideal increases risk.
- Saturated fat in the diet. Elevated fat levels in the blood lead to blockage of the coronary arteries by plaque **(see Box 13-2).**

Box 13-2 *Clinical Perspectives*

Lipoproteins: What's the Big DL?

Although cholesterol has received a lot of bad press in recent years, it is a necessary substance in the body. It is found in bile salts needed for digestion of fats, in hormones, and in the cell's plasma membrane. However, high levels of cholesterol in the blood have been associated with atherosclerosis and heart disease.

It now appears that the total amount of blood cholesterol is not as important as the form in which it occurs. Cholesterol is transported in the blood in combination with other lipids and with protein, forming compounds called lipoproteins. These compounds are distinguished by their relative density. High-density lipoprotein (HDL) is composed of a high proportion of protein and relatively little cholesterol. HDLs remove cholesterol from the tissues, including the arterial walls, and carry it back to the liver for reuse or disposal. In contrast, low-density lipoprotein (LDL) contains less protein and a higher proportion of cholesterol. LDLs carry cholesterol from the liver to the tissues, making it available for membrane or hormone synthesis. However, excess LDLs can deposit cholesterol along the lining of arterial walls. Thus, high levels of HDLs (60 mg/dL and above) indicate efficient removal of arterial plaques, whereas high levels of LDLs (130 mg/dL and above) suggest that arteries will become clogged.

Diet is an important factor in regulating lipoprotein levels. Saturated fatty acids (found primarily in animal fats) raise LDL levels, while unsaturated fatty acids (found in most vegetable oils) lower LDL levels and stimulate cholesterol excretion. Thus, a diet lower in saturated fat and higher in unsaturated fat may reduce the risk of atherosclerosis and heart disease. Other factors that affect lipoprotein levels include cigarette smoking, caffeine, and stress, which raise LDL levels, and exercise, which lowers LDL levels.

- High blood pressure (hypertension) damages heart muscle. Smoking cessation, regular physical activity, and a healthful, low-sodium diet, and appropriate medication, if needed, are all important in reducing this risk factor.
- Diabetes causes damage to small blood vessels. Type 2 diabetes can be managed with diet, exercise, and proper medication, if needed.

Efforts to prevent heart disease should include having regular physical examinations and minimizing the controllable risk factors.

In recent years, researchers have identified several substances circulating in the blood that, at high levels, are associated with a risk of heart disease. These so-called *markers* include the following:

- C-reactive protein (CRP), a protein produced in the liver in response to inflammation. Chronic inflammation appears to promote atherosclerosis. Some of its possible sources include infection, arthritis, and periodontal (gum) disease. CRP can predict a risk of myocardial infarction (MI), even when blood cholesterol is low, and testing for CRP is recommended for people with normal cholesterol levels and moderate risk of MI.
- Homocysteine (ho-mo-SIS-tene), an amino acid. Higher than average levels of this amino acid in the blood are linked to cardiovascular disease.
- Lipoprotein(a), a type of low-density lipoprotein (LDL) (see Box 13-2). A high level of lipoprotein(a) promotes atherosclerosis.

Heart Studies

Experienced listeners can gain important information about the heart using a **stethoscope** (STETH-o-skope). This relatively simple instrument is used to convey sounds from within the patient's body to an examiner's ear.

The **electrocardiograph** (**ECG** or **EKG**) is used to record the electrical activity of the heart as it functions. (The abbreviation EKG comes from the German spelling of the word.) This activity corresponds to the depolarization and repolarization that occur during an action potential, as described in Chapters 8 and 9. The ECG may reveal certain myocardial injuries. Electrodes (leads) placed on the skin surface pick up electric activity, and the ECG tracing, or electrocardiogram, represents this activity as waves (Fig. 13-11). These waves are identified by consecutive letters of the alphabet. The P wave corresponds to depolarization of the atria; the QRS wave corresponds to depolarization of the ventricles. The T wave shows ventricular repolarization, but atrial repolariation is hidden by the QRS wave. Cardiologists use changes in the waves and the intervals between them to diagnose heart damage and arrhythmias.

Many people with heart disease undergo **catheterization** (kath-eh-ter-i-ZA-shun). In right heart catheterization, an extremely thin tube (catheter) is passed through the veins of the right arm or right groin and then into the right side of heart. This procedure gives diagnostic information and monitors heart

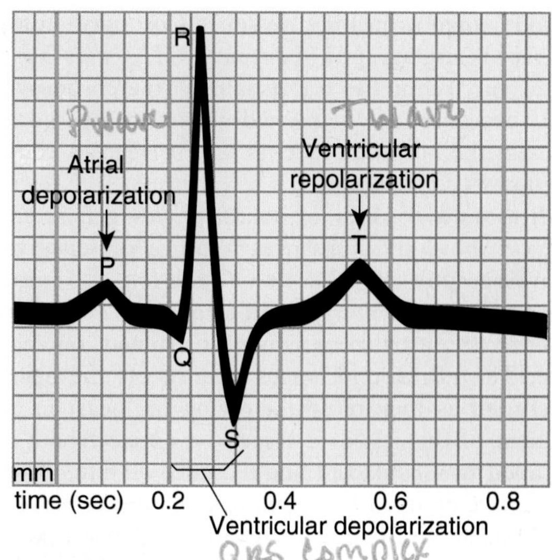

Figure 13-11 Normal Electrocardiography(ECG) tracing. KEY POINT Electric activity in the myocardium produces ECG waves. Changes in the wave patterns indicate a disorder. The tracing shows one cardiac cycle. ZOOMING IN What is the length of the cardiac cycle shown in this diagram?

function. A **fluoroscope** (flu-OR-o-scope), an instrument for examining deep structures with x-rays, is used to show the route taken by the catheter. The tube is passed all the way through the pulmonary valve into the large lung arteries. Blood samples are obtained along the way for testing, and pressure readings are taken. In left heart catheterization, a catheter is passed through an artery in the left groin or arm to the heart. The tube may be passed through the aortic valve into the left ventricle for studies of pressure and volume in that chamber.

During catheterization, dye can be injected into the coronary arteries to map vascular damage, a procedure known as **coronary angiography** (an-je-OG-rah-fe) (Fig. 13-12).

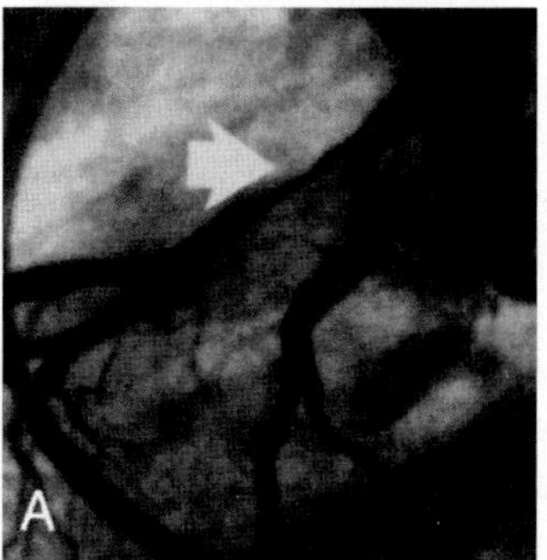

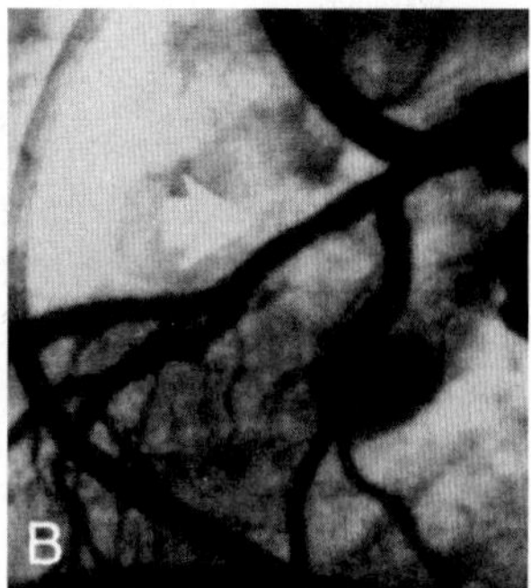

Figure 13-12 Coronary angiography. KEY POINT The coronary vessels are imaged following administration of a dye. **A.** Coronary angiography shows narrowing in the mid-left anterior descending (LAD) artery (*arrow*) **(B)** The same vessel after a procedure to remove plaque. Note the improved blood flow through the artery. (Reprinted with permission from Baim DS. *Grossman's Cardiac Catheterization, Angiography, and Intervention*, 7th ed. Philadelphia, PA: Lippincott Williams & Wilkins, 2006.)

The root *angi/o* means "vessel." **Coronary computed tomography angiography** (coronary CTA) uses advanced radiographic techniques for visualizing the coronary arteries. The necessary dye is injected intravenously and abnormalities in the coronary arteries can be seen in computed tomography (CT) scans.

Ultrasound consists of sound waves generated at a frequency above the human ear's range of sensitivity. In **echocardiography** (ek-o-kar-de-OG-rah-fe), also known as *ultrasound cardiography*, high-frequency sound waves are sent to the heart from a small instrument on the chest surface. The ultrasound waves bounce off the heart and are recorded as they return, showing the heart in action. Movement of the echoes is traced on an electronic instrument called an *oscilloscope* and recorded on film. (The same principle is employed by submarines to detect ships.) The method is safe and painless, and it does not use x-rays. It provides information on the size and shape of heart structures, on cardiac function, and on possible heart defects.

CHECKPOINTS 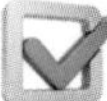

- [ ] 13-11 What do ECG and EKG stand for?
- [ ] 13-12 What is the general term for using a thin tube threaded through a vessel for diagnosis or repair?

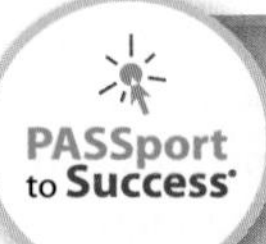

See the Student Resources on *thePoint* for career information on surgical technologists, who assist in all types of surgical operations.

Effects of Aging on the Heart

There is a great deal of individual variation in the way the heart ages, depending on heredity, environmental factors, diseases, and personal habits such as diet, exercise patterns, and tobacco use. However, some of the changes that commonly occur with age are as follows. The heart becomes smaller, and there is a decrease in the strength of heart muscle contraction. The valves become less flexible, and incomplete closure may produce an audible murmur. By 70 years of age, the cardiac output may decrease by as much as 35%. Damage within the conduction system can produce abnormal rhythms, including extra beats, rapid atrial beats, and slowing of ventricular contraction rate. Temporary failure of the conduction system (heart block) can cause periodic loss of consciousness. Because of the decrease in the heart's reserve strength, elderly people may be less able to respond efficiently to physical or emotional stress.

A&P in Action Revisited

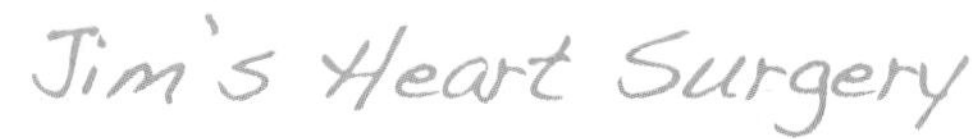

Several weeks after his heart attack, Jim was back in the hospital for his coronary bypass surgery. Even though his cardiologist had fully explained the procedure to him, Jim was still nervous—in a couple of hours a surgeon would literally have Jim's heart in his hands!

Jim was brought to the operating room and given general anesthesia. While the cardiac surgeon sawed through Jim's sternum, the saphenous vein was harvested from Jim's leg. Having split the sternum and retracted the ribs, the cardiac surgeon made an incision through the tough fibrous pericardium surrounding Jim's heart. Next, the surgeon inserted a cannula into Jim's right atrium and another one into his aorta. The doctor connected the cannulae to the heart–lung machine and stopped Jim's heart from beating. Now, venous blood from Jim's right atrium flowed through the heart–lung machine where it was oxygenated before being pumped into Jim's aorta. Then the surgeon prepared the left coronary artery for bypass. He made a small incision through the arterial wall and carefully sutured the cut end of the harvested vein to the opening. Next, he sutured the other end of the vein to a small opening that he made in the aorta, bypassing the occluded portion of the coronary artery. He repeated this procedure two more times in different parts of Jim's obstructed coronary arteries—giving Jim a "triple bypass." The surgeon disconnected Jim from the heart–lung machine and restarted his heart. Blood flowed through the vein grafts to Jim's myocardium, bypassing the diseased parts of Jim's coronary arteries. Jim's surgery was a success!

Jim's surgical team saved his life. See the Student Resources on *thePoint* for career information on surgical technologists, who assist in all types of surgical operations. Although this chapter concentrates on scientific terms related to the heart, Jim's case also contains terminology about blood vessels. In Chapter 14, Blood Vessels and Blood Circulation, you will examine these terms in more detail.

Chapter Wrap-Up

Summary Overview

A detailed chapter outline with space for note-taking is on *thePoint*. The figure below illustrates the main topics covered in this chapter.

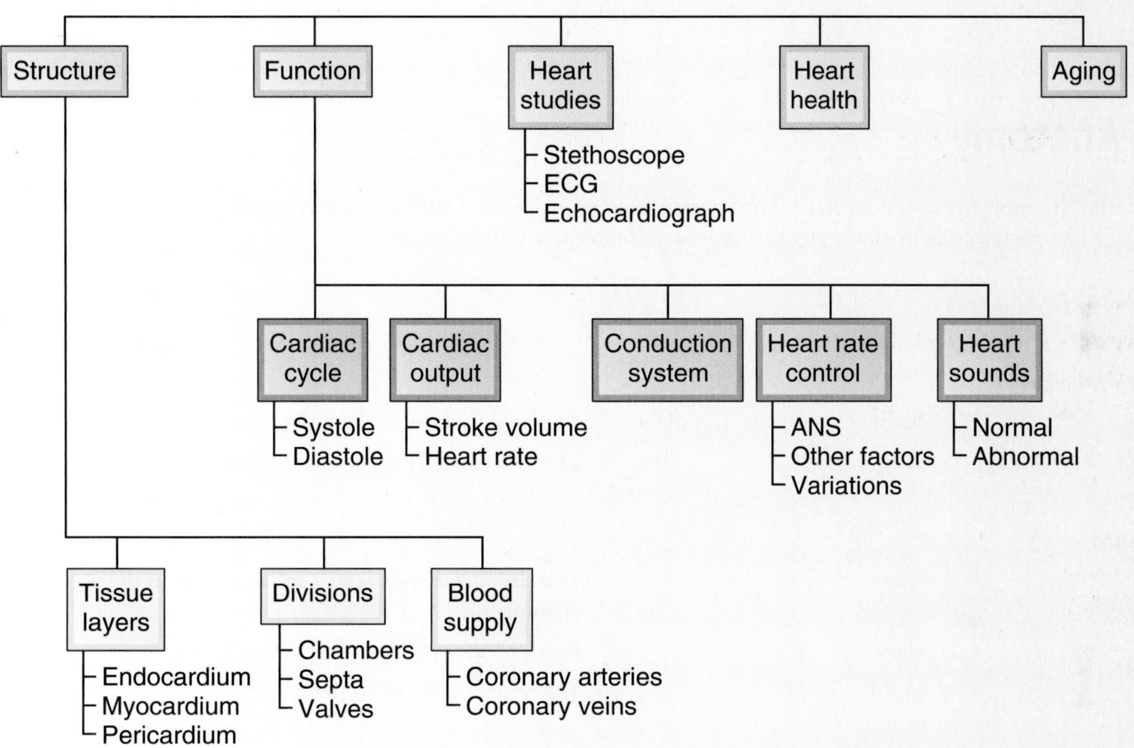

Key Terms

The terms listed below are emphasized in this chapter. Knowing them will help you organize and prioritize your learning. These and other boldface terms are defined in the Glossary with phonetic pronunciations.

angiography	diastole	myocardium	tachycardia
atrium	electrocardiograph	pacemaker	valve
bradycardia	endocardium	pericardium	ventricle
cardiac output	epicardium	septum	
coronary	murmur	systole	

Word Anatomy

Scientific terms are built from standardized word parts (prefixes, roots, and suffixes). Learning the meanings of these parts can help you remember words and interpret unfamiliar terms.

WORD PART	MEANING	EXAMPLE
Structure of the Heart		
cardi/o	heart	The *myocardium* is the heart muscle.
pulmon/o	lung	The *pulmonary* circuit carries blood to the lungs.
Heart Function		
sin/o	sinus	The *sinoatrial* node is in a space (sinus) in the wall of the right atrium.
brady-	slow	*Bradycardia* is a slow heart rate.
tachy-	rapid	*Tachycardia* is a rapid heart rate.
Heart Studies		
steth/o	chest	A *stethoscope* is used to listen to body sounds
angi/o	vessel	*Angiography* is radiographic study of vessels.

Questions for Study and Review

BUILDING UNDERSTANDING

Fill in the Blanks

1. The heart's pointed inferior portion is the _____.
2. The layer of the heart wall that pumps blood is the_____.
3. The heart beat is initiated by electrical impulses from the____.
4. Adjacent cardiac muscle cells are firmly attached to each other by modified plasma membranes called _____.
5. The partition that separates the left ventricle from the right ventricle is called the _____.

Matching > Match each numbered item with the most closely related lettered item.

______**6.** receives blood low in oxygen from the body	**a.** right atrium
______**7.** receives blood high in oxygen from the lungs	**b.** left atrium
______**8.** sends blood low in oxygen to the lungs	**c.** right ventricle
______**9.** sends blood high in oxygen to the body	**d.** left ventricle

Multiple Choice

_____**10.** Which structural characteristic promotes rapid transfer of electrical signals between cardiac muscle cells?

a. the striated nature of the cells
b. branching of the cells
c. the abundance of mitochondria within the cells
d. intercalated disks between the cells

_____**11.** What separates the upper chambers of the heart from each other?

a. intercalated disk
b. interatrial septum
c. interventricular septum
d. ductus arteriosus

_____**12.** Which term describes one complete sequence of heart contraction and relaxation?

a. systole
b. diastole
c. cardiac cycle
d. cardiac output

_____**13.** Which vessel supplies blood directly to the myocardium?

a. superior vena cava
b. pulmonary artery
c. aorta
d. coronary artery

_____**14.** Which structure initiates the heartbeat?

a. Purkinje fibers
b. bundle of His
c. atrioventricular node
d. sinoatrial node

_____**15.** Which variation in heart rate is due to changes in the rate and depth of breathing?

a. murmur
b. cyanosis
c. sinus arrhythmia
d. stent

UNDERSTANDING CONCEPTS

16. Differentiate between the terms in each of the following pairs:

a. serous pericardium and fibrous pericardium
b. atrium and ventricle
c. coronary artery and coronary sinus
d. systole and diastole
e. bradycardia and tachycardia

17. Explain the purpose of the four heart valves and describe their structure and location. What prevents the valves from opening backward?

18. Trace a drop of blood from the superior vena cava to the lungs and then from the lungs to the aorta.

19. Describe the order in which electrical impulses travel through the heart. What is an interruption of these impulses in the heart's conduction system called?

20. Compare the effects of the sympathetic and parasympathetic nervous systems on heart function.

21. List some age-related changes to the heart.

CONCEPTUAL THINKING

22. In the case story, Jim suffered a massive myocardial infarction. What can Jim do to lower his risk of having it happen again? What risk factors can he not change? Apply your knowledge of these factors to your own life or the life of someone you know.

23. Three-month-old Hannah R. is brought to the doctor by her parents. They have noticed that when she cries she becomes breathless and turns blue. The doctor examines Hannah and notices that she is lethargic, small for her age, and has a loud mitral valve murmur. With this information, explain the cause of Hannah's symptoms.

thePoint For more questions, see the learning activities on *thePoint.*

CHAPTER 14

Blood Vessels and Blood Circulation

A&P in Action

Reggie's Second Case: Embolytic Emergency

"And now, news from the Sports Desk. Yesterday, wide receiver Reggie Wilson was side-lined with a femoral fracture. Team doctors do not expect him to return until later in the season." Reggie pressed the off button on the hospital's television remote and closed his eyes for a moment. The last 24 hours had been a whirlwind—first the injury, then the surgery, and now the prospect of a long road to recovery. "Well, I've made it through tough situations before," Reggie thought as he fell asleep.

Inside Reggie's thigh, his femur was beginning to repair itself, but a more dangerous situation lurked in the femoral vein that lay beside the fractured bone. During the accident, the vein's thin inner wall had been injured. Even though Reggie had received heparin (an anticoagulant) after his surgery, blood platelets had adhered to the damaged vein and formed a tiny clot on the inner lining of the vessel. Now that Reggie's thigh was immobile, blood flowed much more slowly through the femoral vein. This venous stasis allowed more and more platelets to stick together at the site of the clot until finally his vein was completely obstructed. Reggie had developed deep vein thrombosis. Blood continued to flow into Reggie's thigh through his femoral artery, but now, it could not flow out through the vein. Reggie's thigh began to swell and turn red because of the build up of blood within it. Although still asleep, Reggie felt some discomfort from the swelling in his leg and shifted his weight to relieve it. That slight movement caused a small piece of the clot to break away from the thrombus and be carried away toward his heart. Reggie had developed an embolism!

A blood clot is traveling through Reggie's systemic veins toward his heart and lungs. In this chapter, we will examine the important role the vascular system plays in carrying blood to and from the tissues. Later in the chapter, we will see how Reggie's medical team manages his new emergency.

PASSport to Success®

Ancillaries At-A-Glance

Visit *thePoint* to access the PASSport to Success and the following resources. For guidance in using these resources most effectively, see pp. ix–xviii.

Learning TOOLS

- Learning Style Self-Assessment
- Live Advise Online Student Tutoring
- Tips for Effective Studying

Learning RESOURCES

- E-book: Chapter 14
- Web Figure: Capillary Micrograph
- Animation: Blood Circulation
- Health Professions: Vascular Technologist
- Detailed Chapter Outline
- Answers to Questions for Study and Review
- Audio Pronunciation Glossary

Learning ACTIVITIES

- Pre-Quiz
- Visual Activities
- Kinesthetic Activities
- Auditory Activities

Learning Outcomes

After careful study of this chapter, you should be able to:

1. Differentiate among the five types of blood vessels with regard to structure and function, ***p. 266***
2. Compare the pulmonary and systemic circuits relative to location and function, ***p. 267***
3. Name the four sections of the aorta and list the main branches of each section, ***p. 269***
4. Trace the pathway of blood through the main arteries of the upper and lower limbs, ***p. 269***
5. Define *anastomosis*, cite its function, and give several examples, ***p. 272***
6. Compare superficial and deep veins and give examples of each type, ***p. 273***
7. Name the main vessels that drain into the superior and inferior venae cavae, ***p. 274***
8. Define *venous sinus* and give several examples of venous sinuses, ***p. 274***
9. Describe the structure and function of the hepatic portal system, ***p. 275***
10. Explain the forces that affect exchange across the capillary wall, ***p. 276***
11. Describe the factors that regulate blood flow, ***p. 277***
12. Define *pulse* and list the factors that affect pulse rate, ***p. 277***
13. List the factors that affect blood pressure, ***p. 278***
14. Explain how blood pressure is commonly measured, ***p. 280***
15. Trace the pathway of a blood clot from the femoral vein to the pulmonary artery, referring to the case study, ***pp. 264, 281***
16. Show how word parts are used to build words related to the blood vessels and circulation (see Word Anatomy at the end of the chapter), ***p. 283***

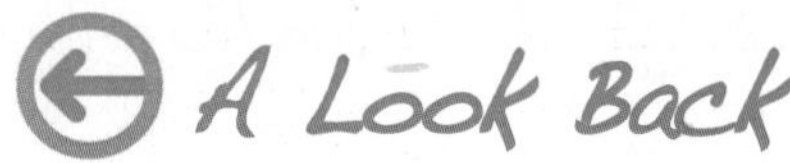

The story of circulation continues with a discussion of the vessels that carry blood away from and then back to the heart. In describing how materials flow between the tissues and the bloodstream, we return to discussions of diffusion, filtration, osmosis, and osmotic pressure introduced in Chapter 3.

The blood vessels, together with the four chambers of the heart, form a closed system in which blood is carried to and from the tissues. Although whole blood does not leave the vessels, components of the plasma and tissue fluids can be exchanged through the walls of the tiniest vessels—the capillaries (Fig. 14-1).

The vascular system is easier to understand if you refer to the appropriate illustrations in this chapter as the vessels are described. When this information is added to what you already know about the blood and the heart, a picture of the cardiovascular system as a whole will emerge.

Overview of Blood Vessels

Blood vessels may be divided into five groups, named below according to the sequence of blood flow from the heart:

1. **Arteries** carry blood away from the heart and toward the tissues. The heart's ventricles pump blood into the arteries (see Fig. 14-1).
2. **Arterioles** (ar-TE-re-olz) are small subdivisions of the arteries. They carry blood into the capillaries.
3. **Capillaries** are tiny, thin-walled vessels that allow for exchanges between systems. These exchanges occur between the blood and the body cells and between the blood and the air in the lung tissues. The capillaries connect the arterioles and venules.

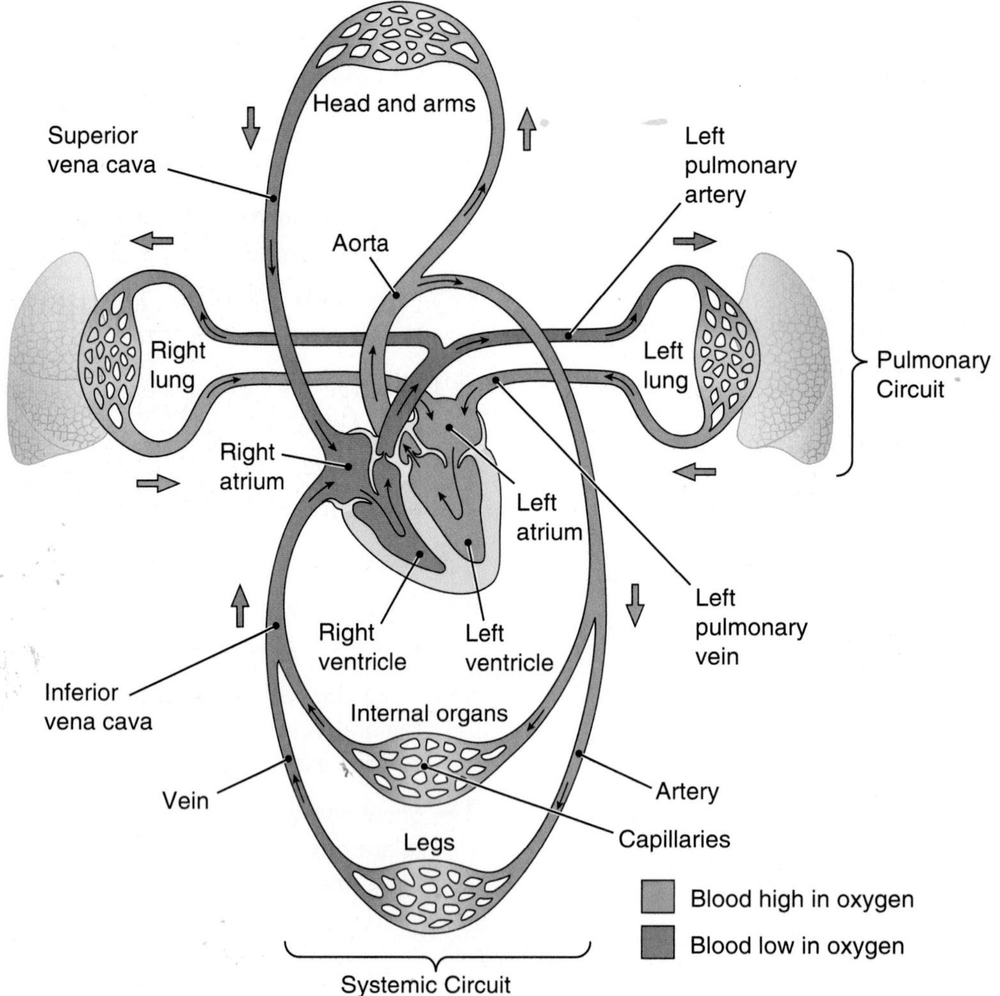

Figure 14-1 The cardiovascular system. KEY POINT Blood flows in a closed system with exchanges of material between the blood and tissues through the capillary walls. There are two circuits, pulmonary and systemic. ZOOMING IN Which vessels carry blood away from the heart? Which carry blood toward the heart?

4. **Venules** (VEN-ulz) are small vessels that receive blood from the capillaries and begin its transport back toward the heart.
5. **Veins** are vessels formed by the merger of venules. They continue blood's transport until it is returned to the heart.

BLOOD CIRCUITS

The vessels together may be subdivided into two groups, or circuits: pulmonary and systemic. Figure 14-1 diagrams blood flow through these two circuits.

The Pulmonary Circuit The **pulmonary circuit** delivers blood to the lungs, where some carbon dioxide is eliminated and oxygen is replenished. The pulmonary vessels that carry blood to and from the lungs include the following:

1. The pulmonary trunk and its arterial branches, which carry blood low in oxygen from the right ventricle to the lungs.
2. The capillaries in the lungs, through which gases, nutrients, and wastes are exchanged.
3. The pulmonary veins, which carry freshly oxygenated blood back to the left atrium.

Note that the pulmonary vessels differ from those in the systemic circuit in that the pulmonary arteries carry blood that is *low* in oxygen content, and the pulmonary veins carry blood that is *high* in oxygen content. In contrast, the systemic arteries carry highly oxygenated blood, and the systemic veins carry blood that is low in oxygen.

The Systemic Circuit The **systemic** (sis-TEM-ik) **circuit** serves the rest of the body. These vessels supply nutrients and oxygen to all the tissues and carry waste materials away from the tissues for disposal. The systemic vessels include the following:

1. The **aorta** (a-OR-tah) receives freshly oxygenated blood from the left ventricle and then branches into the systemic arteries carrying blood to the tissues.
2. The systemic capillaries are the blood vessels through which materials are exchanged.
3. The systemic veins carry blood low in oxygen back toward the heart. The venous blood flows into the right atrium of the heart through the superior vena cava and inferior vena cava.

VESSEL STRUCTURE

The arteries have thick walls because they must be strong enough to receive blood pumped under pressure from the heart's ventricles (Fig. 14-2). The three tunics (coats) of the

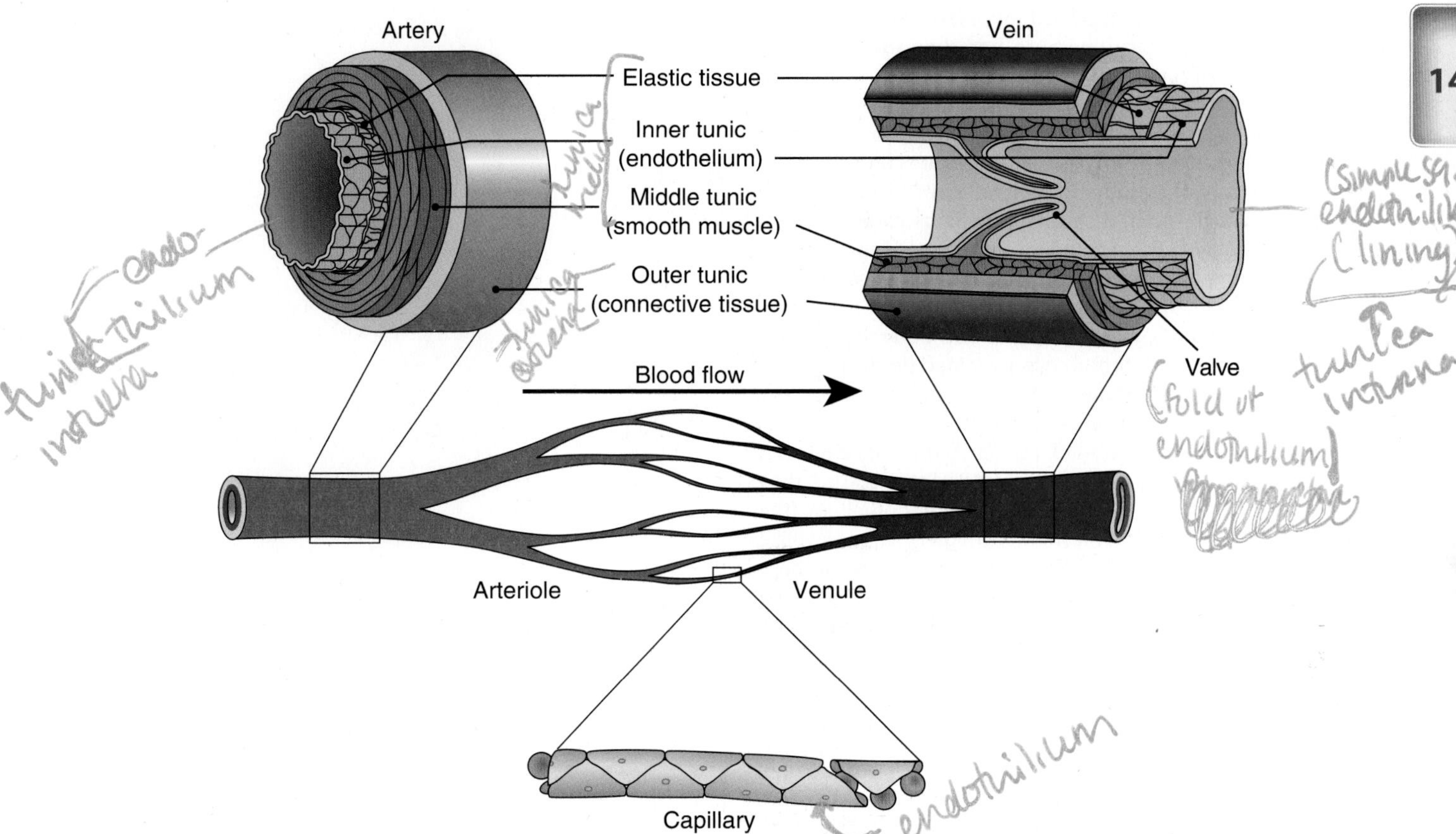

Figure 14-2 **Sections of small blood vessels.** KEY POINT Drawings show the thick wall of an artery, the thin wall of a vein, and the single-layered wall of a capillary. A valve is also shown. The *arrow* indicates the direction of blood flow. ZOOMING IN Which vessels have valves that control blood flow?

arteries resemble the heart's three tissue layers. Named from internal to external, they are:

1. The inner tunic, a membrane of simple, squamous epithelial cells making up the **endothelium** (en-do-THE-le-um), forms a smooth surface over which the blood flows easily.
2. The middle tunic, the thickest layer, is made up of smooth (involuntary) muscle, which is under the control of the autonomic nervous system.
3. The outer tunic is made of supporting connective tissue.

Elastic tissue between the layers of the arterial wall allows these vessels to stretch when receiving blood and then return to their original size. The amount of elastic tissue diminishes as the arteries branch and become smaller.

The small subdivisions of the arteries, the arterioles, have thinner walls in which there is little elastic connective tissue but relatively more smooth muscle. The autonomic nervous system controls this involuntary muscle. The vessel lumens (openings) become narrower (constrict) when the muscle contracts and widen (dilate) when the muscle relaxes. In this manner, the arterioles regulate the amount of blood that enters the various tissues at a given time. Change in the arterioles' diameter is also a major factor in blood pressure control.

The microscopic capillaries that connect arterioles and venules reach a maximum diameter of 10 mcm, just about wide enough for a blood cell to pass through. They have the thinnest walls of any vessels: one cell layer (see Fig. 14-2). The transparent capillary walls are a continuation of the smooth endothelium that lines the arteries. The thinness of these walls allows for exchanges between the blood and the body cells and between the lung tissue and the outside air. The capillary boundaries are the most important center of activity for the entire circulatory system. Their function is explained later in this chapter. Capillary structure varies according to function, as described in Box 14-1.

Box 14-1 *A Closer Look*

Capillaries: The Body's Free Trade Zones

The exchange of substances between body cells and the blood occurs along about 50,000 miles (80,000 km) of capillaries. Exchange rates vary because, based on their structure, different types of capillaries vary in permeability.

Continuous capillaries (top) are the most common type and are found in muscle, connective tissue, the lungs, and the central nervous system (CNS). These capillaries are composed of a continuous layer of endothelial cells. Adjacent cells are loosely attached to each other, with small openings called intercellular clefts between them. Although continuous capillaries are the least permeable, water and small molecules can diffuse easily through their walls. Large molecules, such as plasma proteins and blood cells, cannot. In certain body regions, like the CNS, adjacent endothelial cells are joined tightly together, making the capillaries impermeable to many substances (see Box 9-1, The Blood–Brain Barrier, in Chapter 9).

Fenestrated (FEN-es-tra-ted) *capillaries* (middle) are much more permeable than continuous capillaries, because they have many holes, or fenestrations, in the endothelium (the word is derived from Latin meaning "window"). These sievelike capillaries are permeable to water and solutes as large as peptides. In the digestive tract, fenestrated capillaries permit rapid absorption of water and nutrients into the bloodstream. In the kidneys, they permit rapid filtration of blood plasma, the first step in urine formation.

Sinusoidal capillaries (bottom) are the most permeable. In addition to fenestrations, they have large spaces between endothelial cells that allow the exchange of water, large solutes, such as plasma proteins, and even blood cells. Sinusoidal capillaries, also called *sinusoids*, are found in the liver and red bone marrow, for example. Albumin, clotting factors, and other proteins formed in the liver enter the bloodstream through sinusoidal capillaries. In red bone marrow, newly formed blood cells travel through sinusoidal capillary walls to join the bloodstream.

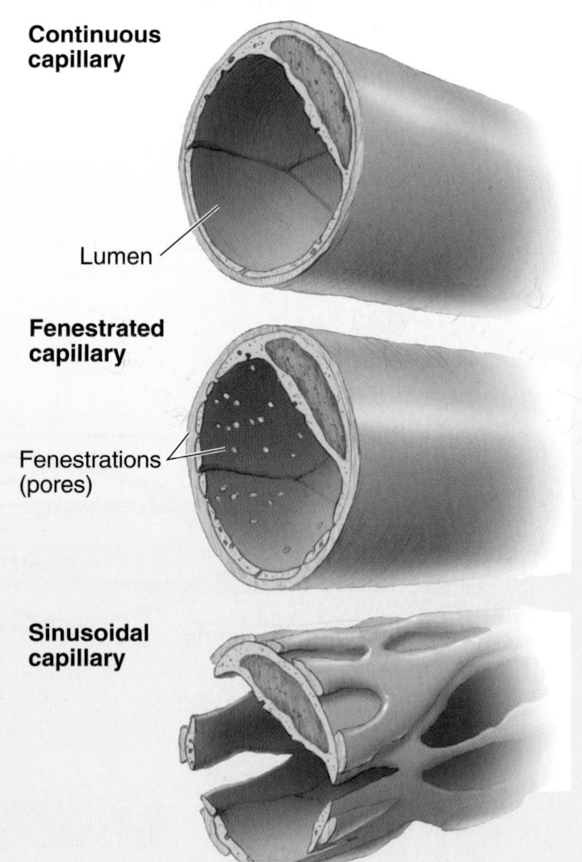

Types of capillaries. (Reprinted with permission from *The Massage Connection Anatomy and Physiology*, Philadelphia, PA: Lippincott Williams & Wilkins, 2004.)

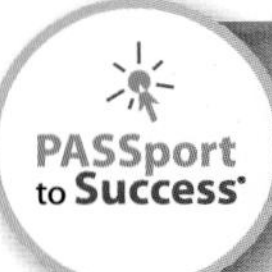

See the Student Resources on *thePoint* to review the animation *Blood Circulation* and for a micrograph of a capillary in cross section.

The smallest veins, the venules, are formed by the union of capillaries, and their walls are only slightly thicker than those of the capillaries. As the venules merge to form veins, the smooth muscle in the vessel walls becomes thicker and the venules begin to acquire the additional layers found in the larger vessels.

The walls of the veins have the same three layers as those of the arteries. However, the middle smooth muscle tunic is relatively thin in the veins. A vein wall is much thinner than the wall of a comparably sized artery (see Fig. 14-2). These vessels also have less elastic tissue between the layers, so they expand easily and carry blood under much lower pressure. Because of their thinner walls, the veins collapse easily. Even a slight pressure on a vein by a tumor or other mass may interfere with blood flow.

Most veins are equipped with one-way valves that permit blood to flow in only one direction: toward the heart (see Fig. 14-2). Such valves are most numerous in the veins of the extremities. Figure 14-3 is a cross section of an artery and a vein as seen through a microscope.

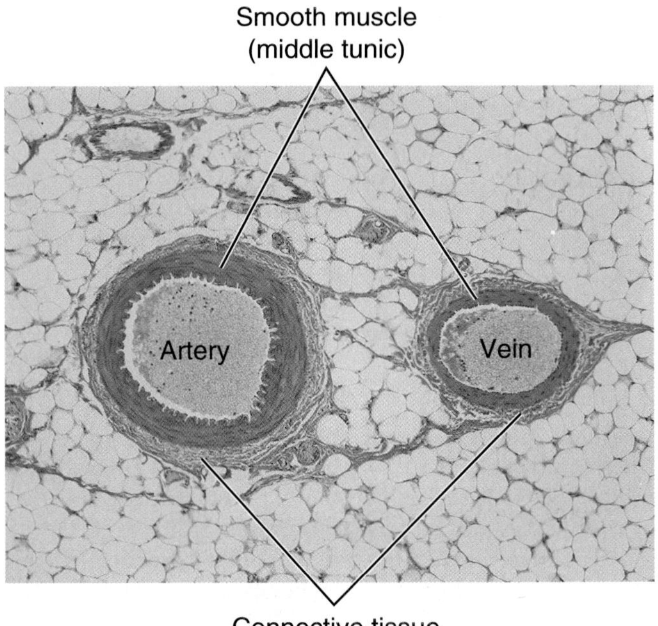

Figure 14-3 Cross section of an artery and vein. The smooth muscle and connective tissue of the vessels are visible in this photomicrograph. (Reprinted with permission from Cormac k DH. *Essential Histology*, 2nd ed. Philadelphia, PA: Lippincott Williams & Wilkins, 2001.) ZOOMING IN Which type of vessel shown has a thicker wall?

CHECKPOINTS 

- 14-1 What are the five types of blood vessels?
- 14-2 What are the two blood circuits and what areas does each serve?
- 14-3 What type of tissue makes up the middle tunic of arteries and veins, and how is this tissue controlled?
- 14-4 How many cell layers make up the wall of a capillary?

Systemic Arteries

The systemic arteries begin with the aorta, the largest artery, which measures about 2.5 cm (1 in.) in diameter. This vessel receives blood from the left ventricle, ascends from the heart, and then arches back to travel downward through the body, branching to all organs. (See Dissection Atlas Figure A3-4 for a photograph showing the major vessels of the trunk.)

THE AORTA AND ITS PARTS

The aorta ascends toward the right from the left ventricle (Fig. 14-4). Then it curves posteriorly and to the left. It continues downward posterior to the heart and just anterior to the vertebral column, through the diaphragm, and into the abdomen. The aorta is one continuous artery, but its regions are named as follows:

1. The **ascending aorta** is near the heart and inside the pericardial sac.
2. The **aortic arch** curves from the right to the left and also extends posteriorly.
3. The **thoracic aorta** lies just anterior to the vertebral column posterior to the heart in the mediastinum.
4. The **abdominal aorta** is the longest section of the aorta, beginning at the diaphragm and spanning the abdominal cavity.

The thoracic and abdominal aorta together make up the descending aorta.

Branches of the Ascending Aorta and Aortic Arch The aorta's ascending part has two branches near the heart, called the **left** and **right coronary arteries**, which supply the heart muscle (see Figs. 13-6 and 13-7). As noted in Chapter 13, these arteries form a crown around the heart's base and give off branches to all parts of the myocardium.

The aortic arch, located immediately past the ascending aorta, gives rise to three large branches.

1. The first, the **brachiocephalic** (brak-e-o-seh-FAL-ik) **artery**, is a short vessel that supplies the arm and the head on the right side (see Fig. 14-4). After extending upward about 5 cm (2 in.), it divides into the **right subclavian** (sub-KLA-ve-an) **artery**, which extends under the

14

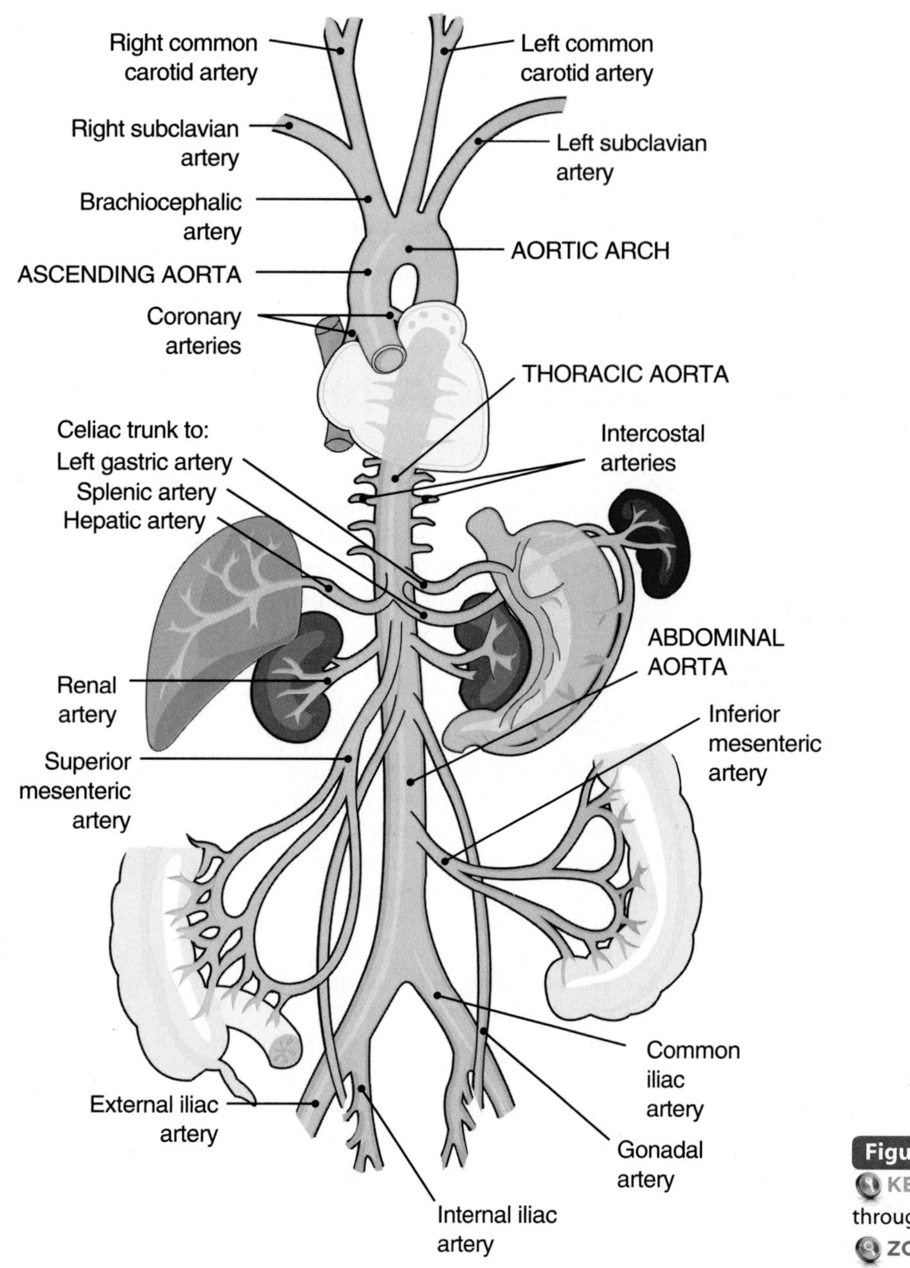

Figure 14-4 The aorta and its branches. KEY POINT As the aorta travels from the heart through the body, it branches to all tissues. ZOOMING IN How many brachiocephalic arteries are there?

right clavicle (collar bone) and supplies the right upper extremity (arm), and the **right common carotid** (kah-ROT-id) **artery,** which supplies the right side of the neck, head, and brain. Note that the brachiocephalic artery is unpaired.

2. The second, the **left common carotid artery,** extends upward from the highest part of the aortic arch. It supplies the left side of the neck and the head.
3. The third, the **left subclavian artery,** extends under the left clavicle and supplies the left upper extremity. This is the aortic arch's last branch.

Branches of the Descending Aorta The thoracic aorta supplies branches to the chest wall and esophagus (e-SOF-ah-gus), the bronchi (subdivisions of the trachea), the lungs, and the muscles of the chest wall **(Fig. 14-5)**. There are usually 9 to 10 pairs of **intercostal** (in-ter-KOS-tal) **arteries** that extend between the ribs, sending branches to the muscles and other structures of the chest wall.

The abdominal aorta has unpaired branches extending anteriorly and paired branches extending laterally. The unpaired vessels are large arteries that supply the abdominal viscera. The most important of these visceral branches are as follows:

1. The **celiac** (SE-le-ak) **trunk** is a short artery, about 1.25 cm (1/2 in.) long, that subdivides into three branches: the **left gastric artery** goes to the stomach, the **splenic** (SPLEN-ik) **artery** goes to the spleen, and the **hepatic** (heh-PAT-ik) **artery** goes to the liver **(see Fig. 14-4)**.

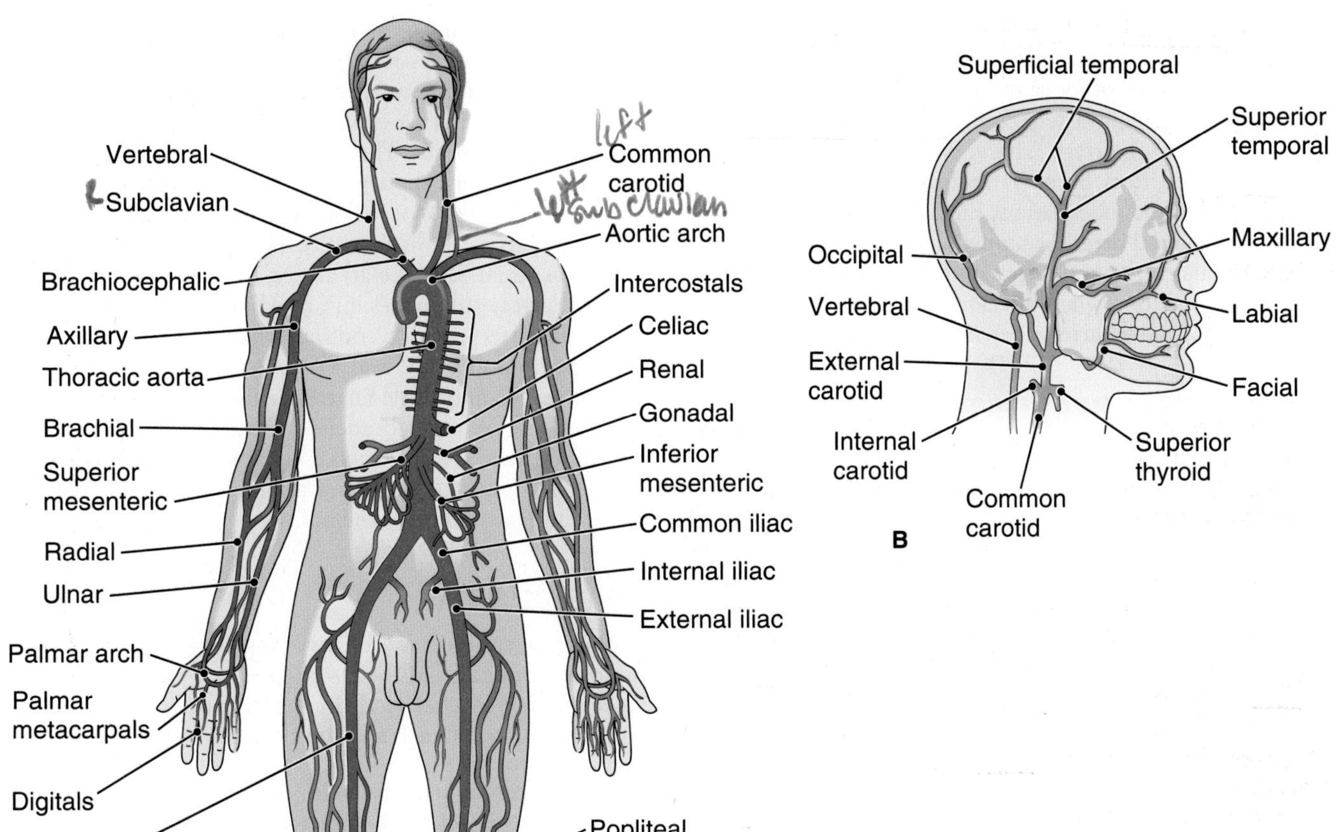

Figure 14-5 **Principal systemic arteries.** ZOOMING IN What large vessels branch from the terminal aorta?

2. The **superior mesenteric** (mes-en-TER-ik) **artery**, the largest of these branches, carries blood to most of the small intestine and to the first half of the large intestine.
3. The much smaller **inferior mesenteric artery**, located below the superior mesenteric artery and near the end of the abdominal aorta, supplies the second half of the large intestine.

The abdominal aorta's paired lateral branches include the following right and left vessels:

1. The **superior and inferior phrenic** (FREN-ik) **arteries** supply the diaphragm. (These are not shown in the figures.)
2. The **renal** (RE-nal) **arteries**, the largest in this group, carry blood to the kidneys.
3. The **gonadal** (go-NAD-al) **arteries**—the **ovarian** (o-VAR-e-an) **arteries** in females and **testicular** (tes-TIK-u-lar) **arteries** in males—supply the sex glands.
4. Four pairs of **lumbar** (LUM-bar) **arteries** extend into the musculature of the abdominal wall. (These are not shown in the figures.)

THE ILIAC ARTERIES AND THEIR SUBDIVISIONS

The abdominal aorta finally divides into two **common iliac** (IL-e-ak) **arteries** (see Fig. 14-5). These vessels, which are about 5 cm (2 in.) long, extend into the pelvis, where each subdivides into an **internal** and an **external iliac artery**.

The internal iliac vessels then send branches to the pelvic organs, including the urinary bladder, the rectum, and reproductive organs other than the gonads.

Each external iliac artery continues into the thigh as the **femoral** (FEM-or-al) **artery.** This vessel gives rise to branches in the thigh and then becomes the **popliteal** (pop-LIT-e-al) **artery,** which subdivides below the knee into the anterior and posterior **tibial arteries,** supplying the leg and foot. The anterior tibial artery terminates as the **dorsalis pedis** (dor-SA-lis PE-dis) at the foot. The posterior tibial artery gives rise to the **fibular** (FIB-u-lar) **artery** (peroneal artery) in the leg.

ARTERIES THAT BRANCH TO THE ARM AND HEAD

Each common carotid artery travels along the trachea enclosed in a sheath with the internal jugular vein and the vagus nerve. Just anterior to the angle of the mandible (lower jaw) it branches into the **external** and **internal carotid arteries** (see Fig. 14-5B). You can feel the pulse of the carotid artery just anterior to the large sternocleidomastoid muscle in the neck and below the jaw. The internal carotid artery travels into the head and branches to supply the eye, the anterior portion of the brain, and other structures in the cranium. The external carotid artery branches to the thyroid gland and to other structures in the head and upper part of the neck.

The **subclavian** (sub-KLA-ve-an) **artery** supplies blood to the arm and hand. Its first branch, however, is the **vertebral** (VER-te-bral) **artery,** which passes through the transverse processes of the first six cervical vertebrae and supplies blood to the posterior brain. The subclavian artery changes names as it travels through the arm and branches to the forearm and hand (see Fig. 14-5A). It first becomes the **axillary** (AK-sil-ar-e) **artery** in the axilla (armpit). The longest part of this vessel, the **brachial** (BRA-ke-al) **artery,** is in the arm proper. The brachial artery subdivides into two branches near the elbow: the **radial artery,** which continues down the thumb side of the forearm and wrist, and the **ulnar artery,** which extends along the medial or little finger side into the hand.

Just as the larger branches of a tree divide into limbs of varying sizes, so the arterial tree has a multitude of subdivisions. Hundreds of names might be included. We have mentioned only some of them.

ANASTOMOSES

A communication between two vessels is called an **anastomosis** (ah-nas-to-MO-sis). By means of arterial anastomoses, blood reaches vital organs by more than one route. Some examples of such end-artery unions are as follows:

- The **cerebral arterial circle** (circle of Willis) (Fig. 14-6) receives blood from the two internal carotid arteries

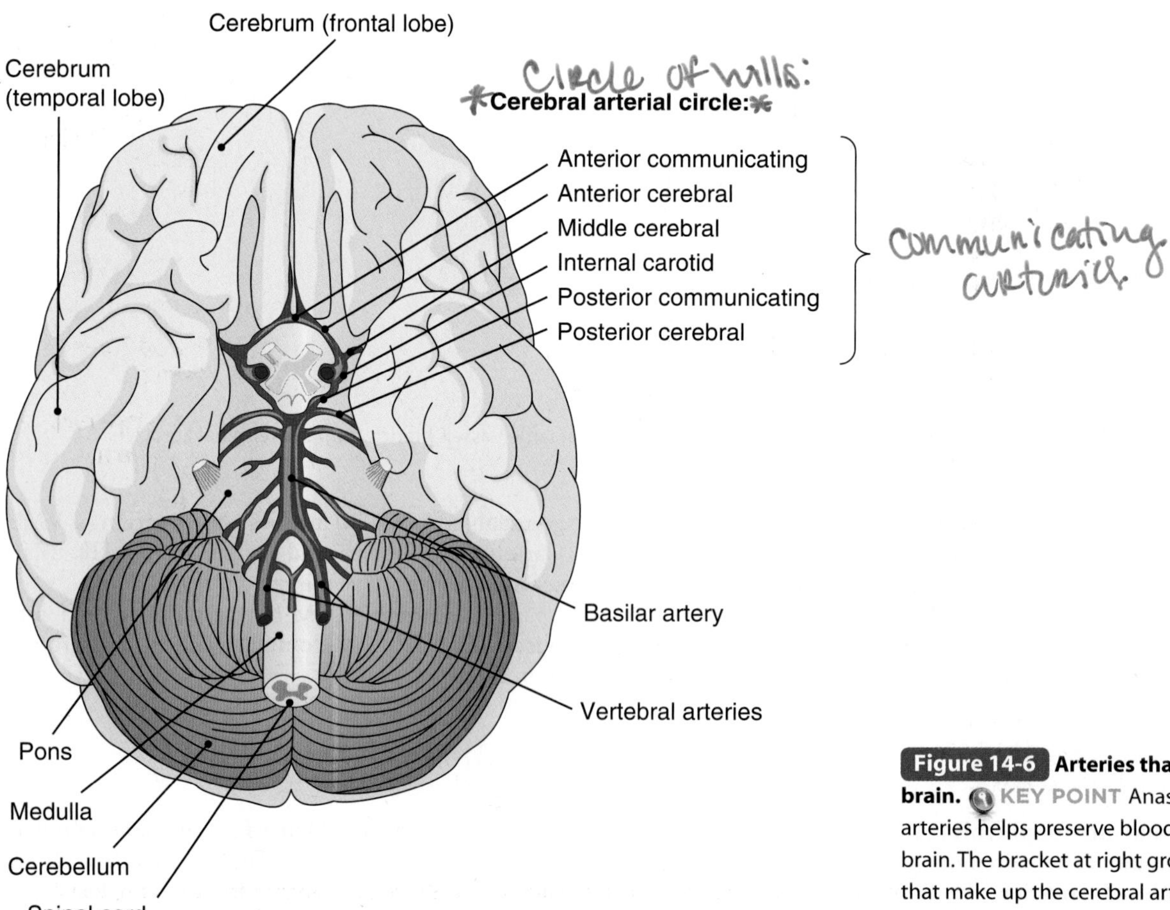

Figure 14-6 Arteries that supply the brain. KEY POINT Anastomosis of arteries helps preserve blood supply to the brain. The bracket at right groups the arteries that make up the cerebral arterial circle (circle of Willis).

and from the **basilar** (BAS-il-ar) **artery**, which is formed by the union of the two vertebral arteries. This arterial circle lies just under the brain's center and sends branches to the cerebrum and other parts of the brain.

- The **superficial palmar arch** is formed by the union of the radial and ulnar arteries in the hand. It sends branches to the hand and the fingers **(see Fig. 14-5)**.
- The **mesenteric** arches are made up of communications between branches of the vessels that supply blood to the intestinal tract.
- One of several arterial arches in the foot is the **deep plantar arch**, formed by the union of the lateral plantar artery, which travels across the bases of the metatarsal bones, and the dorsalis pedis.

CHECKPOINTS 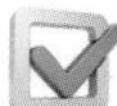

☐ **14-5** What are the subdivisions of the aorta, the largest artery?

☐ **14-6** What are the three branches of the aortic arch?

☐ **14-7** What areas are supplied by the brachiocephalic artery?

☐ **14-8** What is an anastomosis?

Systemic Veins

Whereas most arteries are located in protected and rather deep areas of the body, many of the principal systemic veins are found near the surface **(Fig. 14-7)**. The most important

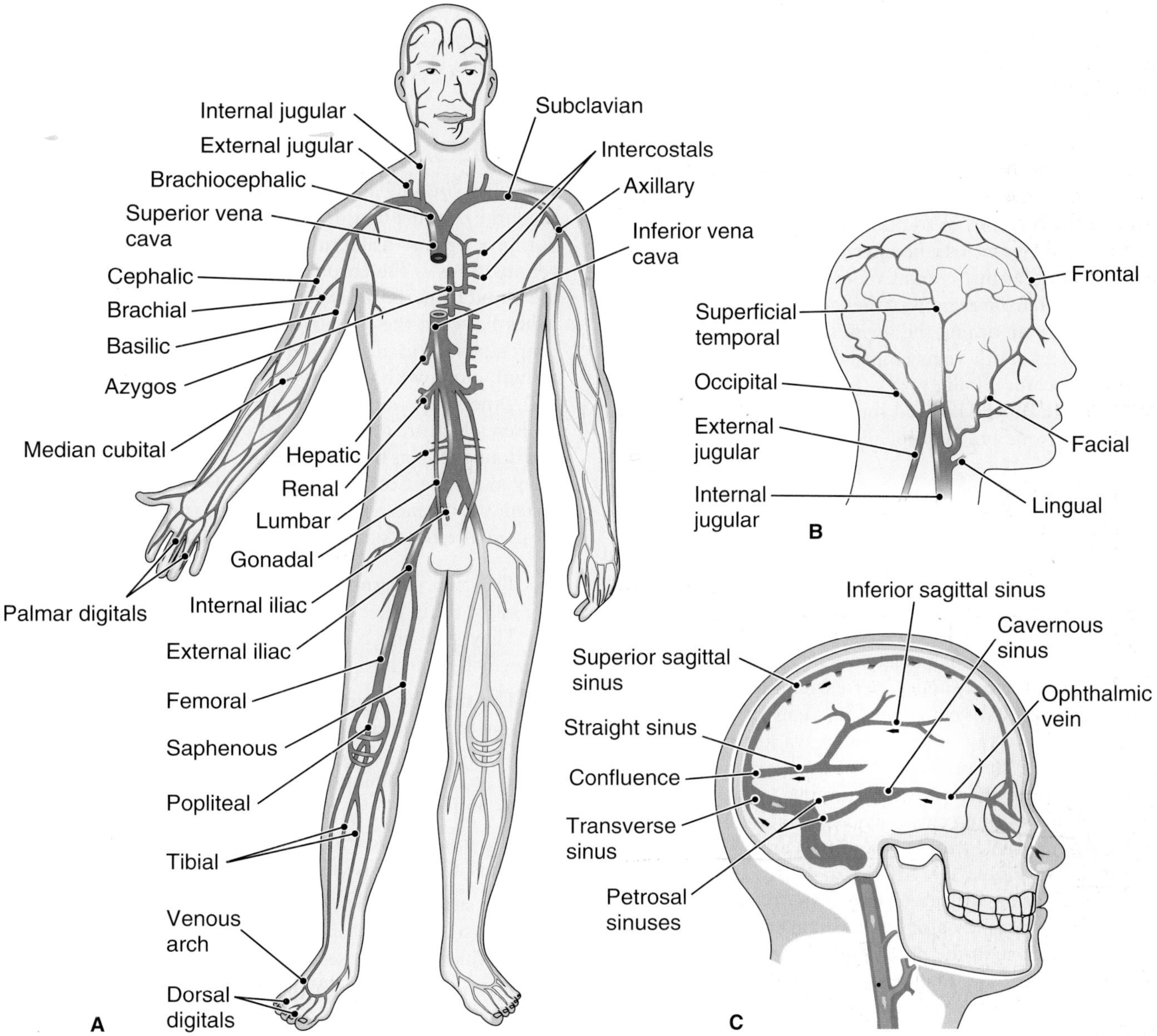

Figure 14-7 Principal systemic veins. A. Anterior view. **B.** Veins of the head and the neck, lateral view. **C.** Cranial venous sinuses, lateral view. ZOOMING IN How many brachiocephalic veins are there?

of the **superficial veins** are in the extremities, and include the following:

- The veins on the back of the hand and at the front of the elbow. Those at the elbow are often used for drawing blood for test purposes, as well as for intravenous injections. The largest of this venous group are the **cephalic** (seh-FAL-ik), the **basilic** (bah-SIL-ik), and the **median cubital** (KU-bih-tal) **veins.**
- The **saphenous** (sah-FE-nus) **veins** of the lower extremities, which are the body's longest veins. The great saphenous vein begins in the foot and extends up the medial side of the leg, the knee, and the thigh. It finally empties into the femoral vein near the groin.

The **deep veins** tend to parallel arteries and usually have the same names as the corresponding arteries **(see Fig. 14-7)**. Examples of these include the **femoral** and the **external** and **internal iliac** vessels of the lower body, and the **brachial, axillary,** and **subclavian** vessels of the upper extremities. (The femoral vein is where Reggie's problem originated in the case study.) Exceptions are found in the veins of the head and the neck. The two jugular (JUG-u-lar) veins on each side of the neck drain the areas supplied by the carotid arteries (*jugular* is from a Latin word meaning "neck"). The larger of the two veins, the **internal jugular,** receives blood from the large veins (cranial venous sinuses) that drain the head and also from regions of the face and neck. The smaller **external jugular** drains the areas supplied by the external carotid artery. Both veins empty directly into a subclavian vein. A **brachiocephalic vein** is formed on each side by the union of the subclavian and the jugular veins. (Remember, there is only *one* brachiocephalic artery.)

THE VENAE CAVAE AND THEIR TRIBUTARIES

Two large veins receive blood from the systemic vessels and empty directly into the heart's right atrium. The veins of the head, neck, upper extremities, and chest all drain into the **superior vena cava** (VE-nah KA-vah). This vessel is formed by the union of the right and left brachiocephalic veins, which drain the head, neck, and upper extremities. The unpaired **azygos** (AZ-ih-gos) **vein** drains the veins of the chest wall and empties into the superior vena cava just before the latter empties into the right atrium of the heart **(see Fig. 14-7)** (*azygous* is from a Greek word meaning "unpaired").

The **inferior vena cava,** which is much longer than the superior vena cava, returns blood from areas below the diaphragm. (See **Dissection Atlas Fig. A3-4.**) It begins in the lower abdomen with the union of the two common iliac veins. It then ascends along the abdomen's posterior wall, through a groove in the posterior part of the liver, through the diaphragm, and finally through the lower thorax to empty into the heart's right atrium.

The large veins below the diaphragm may be divided into two groups:

1. The right and left veins that drain paired parts and organs. They include the **external** and **internal iliac** veins from near the groin; four pairs of **lumbar veins** from the dorsal trunk and from the spinal cord; the **gonadal veins**—the **testicular veins** from the male testes and the **ovarian veins** from the female ovaries; the **renal veins** from the kidneys; and finally the large **hepatic veins** from the liver. For the most part, these vessels empty directly into the inferior vena cava. The left testicular in the male and the left ovarian in the female empty into the left renal vein, which carries this blood to the inferior vena cava; these veins thus constitute exceptions to the rule that the paired veins empty directly into the vena cava.
2. Unpaired veins that drain the spleen and parts of the digestive tract (stomach and intestine) empty into a vein called the **hepatic portal vein,** discussed shortly and shown in **Figure 14-8.** Unlike other lower veins, which empty into the inferior vena cava, the hepatic portal vein is part of a special system that enables blood to circulate through the liver before returning to the heart. This system, the hepatic portal system, will be described in more detail later.

VENOUS SINUSES

The word *sinus* means "space" or "hollow." A **venous sinus** is a large channel that drains blood low in oxygen, but does not have a vein's usual tubular structure. One example of a venous sinus is the **coronary sinus,** which receives most of the blood from the heart wall. (See **Fig. 13-6** in Chapter 13.) It lies between the left atrium and the left ventricle on the heart's posterior surface and empties directly into the right atrium, along with the two venae cavae.

Other important venous sinuses are the **cranial venous sinuses,** which are formed between the layers of the dura mater and drain the veins from throughout the brain **(see Fig. 14-7C)**. They also collect cerebrospinal fluid from the central nervous system (CNS) and return it to the bloodstream. The largest of the cranial venous sinuses are the following:

- The two **cavernous sinuses,** situated behind the eyeballs, drain the eyes' **ophthalmic** (of-THAL-mik) **veins.** They give rise to the **petrosal** (peh-TRO-sal) **sinuses,** which drain into the jugular veins.
- The **superior sagittal** (SAJ-ih-tal) **sinus** is a single long space located in the midline above the brain and in the fissure between the two cerebral hemispheres. It ends in an enlargement called the **confluence** (KON-flu-ens) **of sinuses.**
- The **inferior sagittal sinus** parallels the superior sagittal sinus and merges with the straight sinus.
- The **straight sinus** receives blood from the inferior sagittal sinus and a large cerebral vein and flows into the confluence of sinuses.
- The two **transverse sinuses,** also called the ***lateral sinuses***, begin posteriorly from the confluence of sinuses and then extend laterally. As each sinus extends around the skull's interior, it picks up additional blood. Nearly all of the blood leaving the brain eventually empties into one of the transverse sinuses. Each of these extends

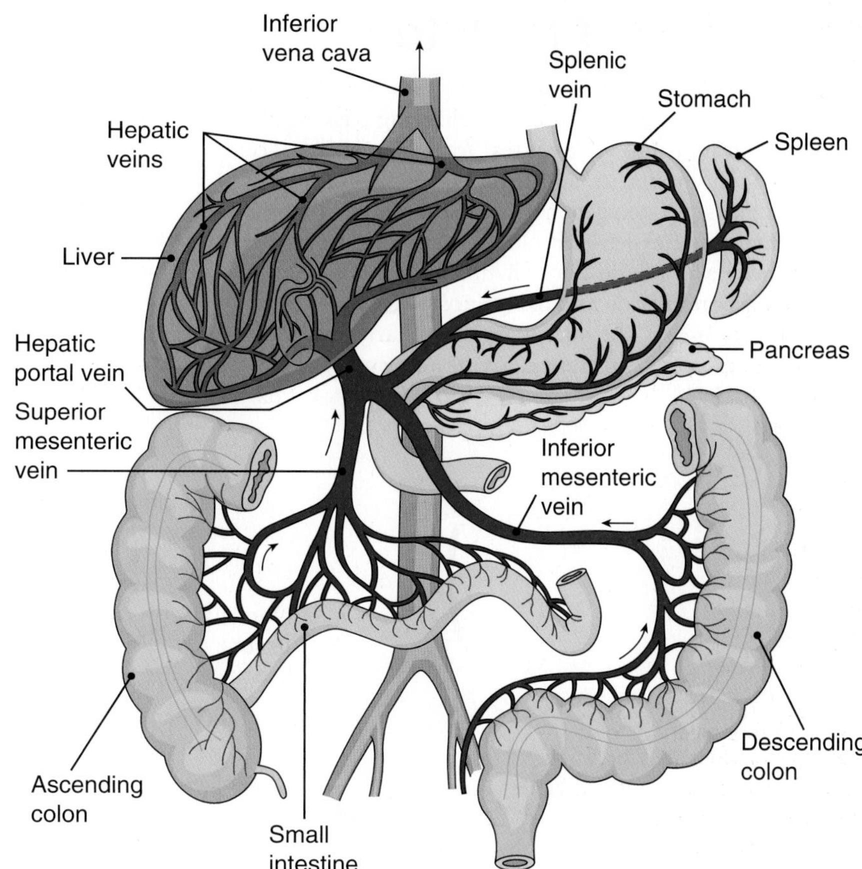

Figure 14-8 Hepatic portal system. KEY POINT Veins from the abdominal organs carry blood to the hepatic portal vein leading to the liver. Arrows show the direction of blood flow. ZOOMING IN What vessel do the hepatic veins drain into?

anteriorly to empty into an internal jugular vein, which then passes through a channel in the skull to continue downward in the neck.

THE HEPATIC PORTAL SYSTEM

Almost always, when blood leaves a capillary bed, it flows through venules and veins directly back to the heart. In a portal system, however, blood circulates through a second capillary bed, usually in a second organ, before it returns to the heart. A portal system is a kind of detour in the pathway of venous return that transports materials directly from one organ to another. Chapter 11 described the small local portal system that carries secretions from the hypothalamus to the pituitary gland. A much larger portal system is the **hepatic portal system**, which carries blood from the abdominal organs to the liver to be processed before it returns to the heart (Fig. 14-8).

The hepatic portal system includes the veins that drain blood from capillaries in the spleen, stomach, pancreas, and intestine. Instead of emptying their blood directly into the inferior vena cava, they deliver it through the hepatic portal vein to the liver. The portal vein's largest tributary is the **superior mesenteric vein**, which drains blood from the proximal portion of the intestine. It is joined by the **splenic vein** just under the liver. Other tributaries of the portal circulation are the **gastric**, **pancreatic**, and **inferior mesenteric veins.** As it enters the liver, the portal vein divides and subdivides into ever smaller branches.

Eventually, the portal blood flows into a vast network of sinuslike capillaries called **sinusoids** (SI-nus-oyds) (see Box 14-1). These enlarged capillary channels allow liver cells close contact with the blood coming from the abdominal organs. (Similar blood channels are found in the spleen and endocrine glands, including the thyroid and adrenals.) After leaving the sinusoids, blood is finally collected by the hepatic veins, which empty into the inferior vena cava.

The purpose of the hepatic portal system is to transport blood from the digestive organs and the spleen to the liver sinusoids, so that the liver cells can carry out their functions. For example, when food is digested, most of the end products are absorbed from the small intestine into the bloodstream and transported to the liver by the portal system. In the liver, these nutrients are processed, stored, and released as needed into the general circulation. The liver also breaks down alcohol, certain drugs, and various other toxins removed from the circulation.

CHECKPOINTS 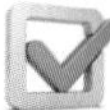

- 14-9 What is the difference between superficial and deep veins?
- 14-10 What two large veins drain the systemic blood vessels and empty into the right atrium?
- 14-11 What is a venous sinus?
- 14-12 The hepatic portal system takes blood from the abdominal organs to which organ?

Circulation Physiology

Circulating blood might be compared to a bus that travels around the city, picking up and delivering passengers at each stop on its route. Take gases, for example. As blood flows through capillaries surrounding the air sacs in the lungs, it picks up oxygen and unloads carbon dioxide. Later, when this oxygen-rich blood is pumped to capillaries in other parts of the body, it unloads the oxygen and picks up carbon dioxide and other substances generated by the cells (Fig. 14-9). The microscopic capillaries are of fundamental importance in these activities. It is only through the cells of these thin-walled vessels that the necessary exchanges can occur.

All living cells are immersed in a slightly salty liquid, the **interstitial** (in-ter-STISH-al) **fluid**, or *tissue fluid*. Looking again at Figure 14-9, one can see how this fluid serves as "middleman" between the capillary membrane and the neighboring cells. As water, oxygen, and other necessary cellular materials pass through the capillary walls, they enter the tissue fluid. Then, these substances make their way by diffusion to the cells. At the same time, carbon dioxide and other metabolic end products leave the cells and move in the opposite direction. These substances enter the

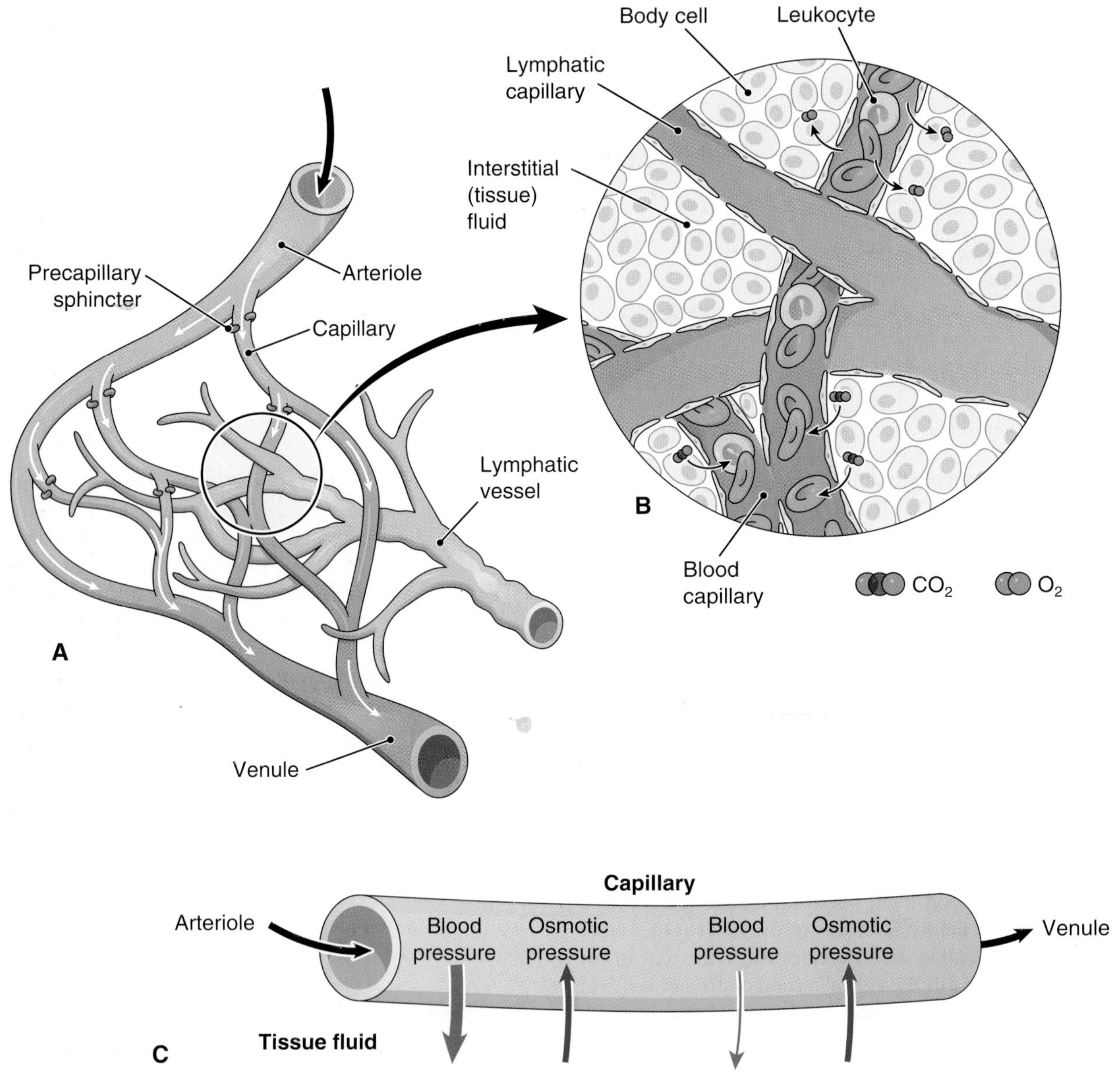

Figure 14-9 The role of capillaries. KEY POINT Capillaries are the point of exchanges between the bloodstream and the tissues. **A.** A capillary network. Note the lymphatic capillaries, which aid in tissue drainage. **B.** Materials, such as the gases oxygen and carbon dioxide, diffuse between the blood and the interstitial fluid. **C.** At the start of a capillary bed, blood pressure helps to push materials out of the blood. At the end of the capillary bed, osmotic pressure is the greater force and draws materials into the blood. The lymphatic system picks up excess water and proteins for return to the circulation.

capillaries and are carried away in the bloodstream for processing in other organs or elimination from the body.

CAPILLARY EXCHANGE

Diffusion is the main process by which substances move between the cells and the capillary blood. Recall that diffusion is the movement of a substance from an area where it is in higher concentration to an area where it is in lower concentration. Diffusion does not require transporters or cellular energy.

An additional force that moves materials from the blood into the tissues is the pressure of the blood as it flows through the capillaries **(see Fig. 14-9C)**. Blood pressure is the force that filters, or "pushes," water and dissolved materials out of the capillary into the tissue fluid. Fluid is drawn back into the capillary by osmotic pressure, the "pulling force" of substances dissolved and suspended in the blood. Osmotic pressure is maintained by plasma proteins (mainly albumin), which are too large in molecular size to go through the capillary wall. These processes result in the constant exchange of fluids across the capillary wall.

As blood enters the capillary bed, the force of its fluid pressure is greater than its opposing osmotic pressure. The tendency is for water and dissolved materials to move out of the capillaries and into the interstitial fluid. Water loss lowers blood pressure as blood flows through the capillaries. Thus, as blood leaves the capillary bed, the "pulling in" force of the blood osmotic pressure exceeds the "pushing out" force of the blood fluid pressure, and materials will tend to enter the capillaries.

The movement of blood through the capillaries is relatively slow, owing to the much larger cross-sectional area of the capillaries compared with that of the vessels from which they branch. This slow progress through the capillaries allows time for exchanges to occur.

Note that even when the capillary exchange process is most efficient, some water is left behind in the tissues. Also, some proteins escape from the capillaries into the tissues. The lymphatic system, discussed in Chapter 15, collects this extra fluid and protein and returns them to the circulation.

THE DYNAMICS OF BLOOD FLOW

Blood flow is carefully regulated to supply tissue needs without unnecessary burden on the heart. Some organs, such as the brain, liver, and kidneys, require large quantities of blood even at rest. The requirements of some tissues, such as the skeletal muscles and digestive organs, increase greatly during periods of activity. For example, the blood flow in muscle can increase up to 25 times during exercise. The volume of blood flowing to a particular organ can be regulated by changing the size of the blood vessels supplying that organ.

Vasomotor Changes An increase in a blood vessel's internal diameter is called **vasodilation**. This change allows for the delivery of more blood to an area. **Vasoconstriction** is a decrease in a blood vessel's internal diameter, causing a decrease in blood flow. These *vasomotor activities* result from the contraction or relaxation of smooth muscle in the walls of the blood vessels, mainly the arterioles. A **vasomotor** center in the medulla of the brain stem regulates vasomotor activities, sending its messages through the autonomic nervous system.

Blood flow into an individual capillary is regulated by a **precapillary sphincter** of smooth muscle that encircles the entrance to the capillary **(see Fig. 14-9)**. This sphincter widens to allow more blood to enter when tissues need more oxygen.

Blood's Return to the Heart Blood leaving the capillary networks returns in the venous system to the heart, and even picks up some speed along the way, despite factors that work against its return. Blood flows in a closed system and must continually move forward as the heart contracts. However, by the time blood arrives in the veins, little force remains from the heart's pumping action. Also, because the veins expand easily under pressure, blood tends to pool in the veins. Considerable amounts of blood are normally stored in these vessels. Finally, the force of gravity works against upward flow from regions below the heart. Several mechanisms help to overcome these forces and promote blood's return to the heart in the venous system. These are:

- **Contraction of skeletal muscles**. As skeletal muscles contract, they compress the veins and squeeze blood forward **(Fig. 14-10)**.
- **Valves in the veins**. They prevent back flow and keep blood flowing toward the heart.
- **Breathing**. Pressure changes in the abdominal and thoracic cavities during breathing also promote blood return in the venous system. During inhalation, the diaphragm flattens and puts pressure on the large abdominal veins. At the same time, chest expansion causes pressure to drop in the thorax. Together, these actions serve to both push and pull blood through the abdominal and thoracic cavities and return it to the heart.

As evidence of these effects, if a person stands completely motionless, especially on a hot day when the superficial vessels dilate, enough blood can accumulate in the lower extremities to cause fainting from insufficient oxygen to the brain.

CHECKPOINTS 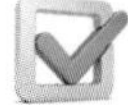

- 14-13 What force helps to push materials out of a capillary? What force helps to draw materials into a capillary?
- 14-14 Name the two types of vasomotor changes.
- 14-15 Where are vasomotor activities regulated?

THE PULSE

The ventricles regularly pump blood into the arteries about 70 to 80 times a minute. The force of ventricular contraction starts a wave of increased pressure that begins at the heart and travels along the arteries. This wave, called the

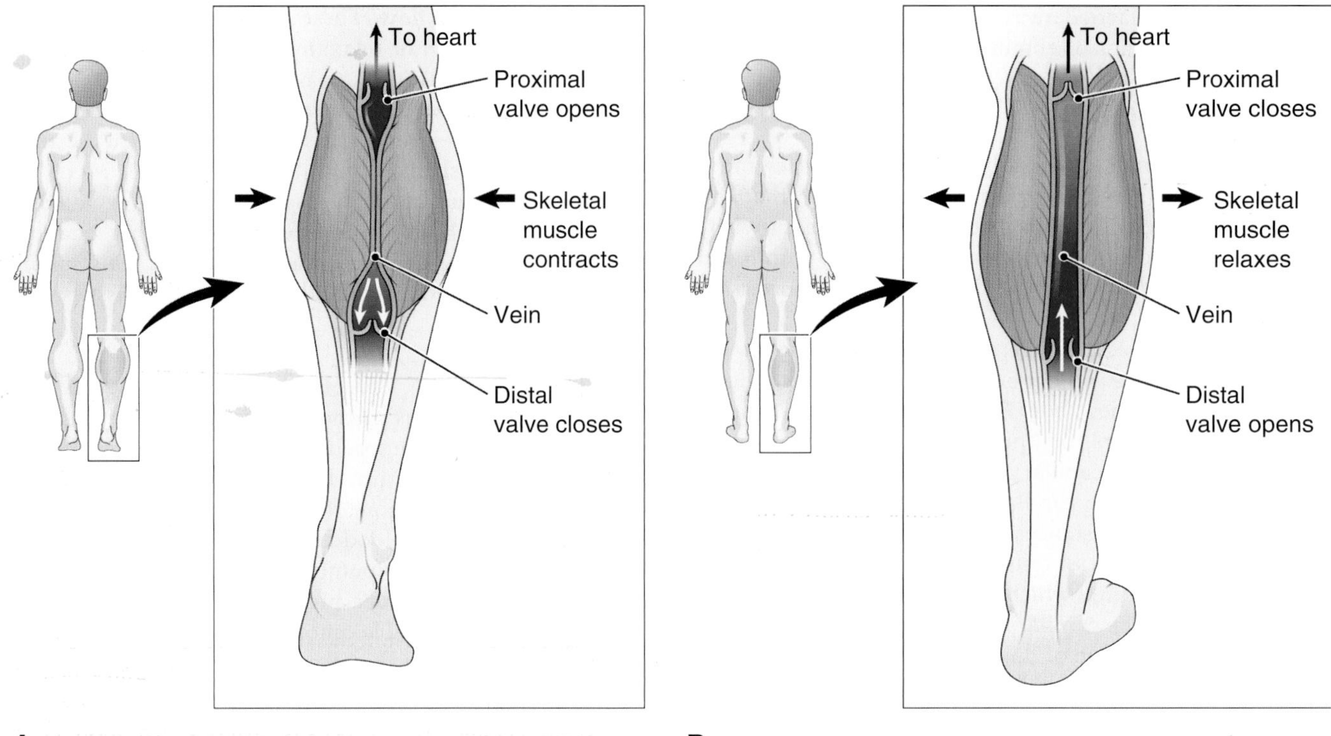

Figure 14-10 Blood return. KEY POINT Muscle contraction and valves keep blood flowing back toward the heart. **A.** Contracting skeletal muscle compresses the vein and drives blood forward, opening the proximal valve, while the distal valve closes to prevent backflow of blood. **B.** When the muscle relaxes again, the distal valve opens, and the proximal valve closes until blood moving in the vein forces it to open again. ZOOMING IN Which of the two valves shown is closer to the heart?

pulse, can be felt in any artery that is relatively close to the surface, particularly if the vessel can be pressed down against a bone. At the wrist, the radial artery passes over the bone on the forearm's thumb side, and the pulse is most commonly obtained here. Other vessels sometimes used for taking the pulse are the carotid artery in the neck and the dorsalis pedis on the top of the foot.

Normally, the pulse rate is the same as the heart rate, but if a heartbeat is abnormally weak, or if the artery is obstructed, the beat may not be detected as a pulse. In checking another person's pulse, it is important to use your second or third finger. If you use your thumb, you may be feeling your own pulse. When taking a pulse, it is important to gauge its strength as well as its regularity and rate.

Various factors may influence the pulse rate. We describe just a few here:

- The pulse is somewhat faster in small people than in large people, and usually is slightly faster in women than in men.
- In a newborn infant, the rate may be from 120 to 140 beats/min. As the child grows, the rate tends to become slower.
- Muscular activity influences the pulse rate. During sleep, the pulse may slow down to 60 beats/min, whereas during strenuous exercise, the rate may go up to well over 100 beats/min. For a person in good condition, the pulse does not go up as rapidly as it does in an inactive person, and it returns to a resting rate more quickly after exercise.
- Emotional disturbances may increase the pulse rate.
- Pulse rate increases with increased temperature, as in cases of infection.
- Excessive secretion of thyroid hormone may cause a rapid pulse.

BLOOD PRESSURE

Blood pressure is the force exerted by the blood against the walls of the vessels. This must be adjusted constantly to guarantee adequate blood flow to the tissues while preventing stress on the cardiovascular system.

Factors That Affect Blood Pressure As you will see from the next discussion, control of blood pressure is very complex and involves many systems. Some of the factors that affect blood pressure include:

Total Blood Volume This refers to the total amount of blood that is in the vascular system at a given time. Just as pressure will increase within a water bed as it fills, enabling you to adjust the firmness of your mattress, adding volume to the circulatory system increases blood pressure. The reverse is also true; loss of volume, as by hemorrhage for example, will lower blood pressure. The kidneys are important regulators of blood volume, as discussed in Chapter 19.

Cardiac Output As described in Chapter 13, the output of the heart, or cardiac output (CO), is the volume of blood pumped out of each ventricle in 1 minute. CO is the product of two factors:

- **Heart rate**, the number of times the heart beats each minute. The basic heart rate is set internally by the SA node but can be influenced by the autonomic nervous system, hormones, and other substances circulating in the blood, such as ions.
- **Stroke volume**, the volume of blood ejected from the ventricle with each beat. The sympathetic nervous system can stimulate more forceful heart contractions to increase blood ejection. Also, if more blood returns to the heart in the venous system, the increased blood volume stretches the heart muscle and promotes more forceful contractions. This response ensures that the heart will pump out as much blood as it receives and prevents pooling of blood in the ventricles.

Resistance to Blood Flow Resistance is opposition to blood flow due to friction generated as blood slides along the vessel walls. Because the effects of resistance are seen mostly in small arteries and arterioles that are at a distance from the heart and large vessels, this factor is often described as *peripheral resistance*. Resistance in the vessels is affected by the following factors:

- Blood vessel diameter: A narrow vessel offers more resistance to blood flow than a wider vessel, just as it is harder to draw fluid through a narrow straw than through a wide straw. Vasoconstriction increases resistance to flow and vasodilation lowers resistance. The medulla's vasomotor center, which controls a vessel's lumen diameter, responds mainly to sensory receptors in the large vessels. The carotid arteries and the aorta have **baroreceptors** (bar-o-re-SEP-torz) in their walls that respond to changes in pressure. When they are stretched by increased blood pressure, they transmit signals that result in vasodilation. At the same time, central controls slow the heart rate to reduce CO. With less stretching, the sympathetic nervous system causes the vessels to constrict and causes the heart rate to increase. Vasomotor activities are the most important determinant of peripheral resistance.
- Blood viscosity, or thickness: Just as a milkshake is harder to suck through a straw than milk is, increased blood viscosity will increase blood pressure. Under normal circumstances, blood viscosity remains within a constant range. However, loss of red cells, as in anemia, or loss of plasma proteins will decrease viscosity. Conversely, increased numbers of red blood cells, as in polycythemia, or a loss of plasma volume, as by dehydration, will increase viscosity. The hematocrit test described in Chapter 12 is one measure of blood viscosity; it measures the relative percentage of packed cells in whole blood.
- Blood vessel length: A longer vessel offers more resistance to blood flow than a shorter vessel. As blood vessel length is ordinarily constant, this is not a significant physiologic factor in peripheral resistance.

Blood Vessel Compliance and Elasticity

- The ease with which arteries expand to receive blood is termed their **compliance** (kom-PLI-ans). If vessels lose their capacity for expansion, as occurs with atherosclerosis, for example, they offer more resistance to blood flow. You have probably experienced this phenomenon if you have tried to blow up a firm, new balloon. More pressure is generated as you blow, and the balloon is a lot harder to inflate than a softer balloon, which expands more easily under pressure. Blood vessels lose compliance with aging, thus increasing resistance and blood pressure.
- The term **elasticity** (e-las-TIH-sih-te) describes the ability of blood vessels to return to their original size after being stretched. Think of an elasticized garment, a bathing suit for example. When new, its compliance (stretchability) is low, and it may be hard to get into, but it readily springs back to shape when removed. With time, its elasticity has decreased and its compliance has increased. It may be easier to put on, but it does not resume its original shape after wearing. Arteries stretch as they receive blood, near the heart for example, and then tend to recoil to their original size, putting pressure on the blood. This response helps to prevent wide fluctuations in blood pressure as the heart contracts and relaxes. Because arteries have more elastic tissue than veins, pressure is higher in the arterial system than in the venous system, and pressure drops continuously as blood travels away from the heart **(Fig. 14-11)**.

14

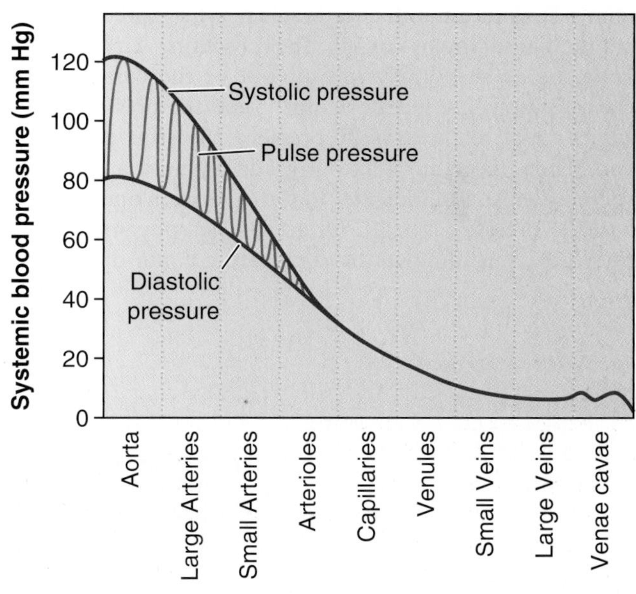

Figure 14-11 Blood pressure. KEY POINT Blood pressure declines as blood flows farther from the heart. Systolic pressure is the maximum pressure that develops in the arteries after heart muscle contraction; diastolic pressure is the lowest pressure in the arteries after relaxation of the heart. The difference between the two pressures (pulse pressure) declines as blood flows through the arteries. The small rises in the venae cavae represent the breathing pump that promotes venous return. ZOOMING IN In which vessels does the pulse pressure drop to zero?

Measurement of Blood Pressure The measurement and careful interpretation of blood pressure may prove a valuable guide in the care and evaluation of a person's health. Because blood pressure decreases as the blood flows from arteries into capillaries and finally into veins, healthcare providers ordinarily measure arterial pressure only, most commonly in the brachial artery of the arm. In taking blood pressure, two variables are measured:

- **Systolic pressure**, the maximum pressure that develops in the arteries after heart muscle contraction.
- **Diastolic pressure**, the lowest pressure measured in the arteries after relaxation of the heart muscle.

The wave of increased pressure that develops when the heart contracts represents the pulse, as previously described. The difference between the systolic and the diastolic pressures is called the *pulse pressure*. This value declines continuously as blood gets farther from the heart, dropping to zero by the time blood reaches the capillaries (see Fig. 14-11).

The instrument used to measure blood pressure is a **sphygmomanometer** (sfig-mo-mah-NOM-eh-ter) (Fig. 14-12), more simply called a blood pressure cuff or blood pressure apparatus. The sphygmomanometer is an inflatable cuff attached to a pressure gauge. Pressure is expressed in millimeters mercury (mm Hg), that is, the height to which the pressure can push a column of mercury in a tube. The examiner wraps the cuff around the patient's upper arm and inflates it with air until the brachial artery is compressed and the blood flow is cut off. Then, listening with a stethoscope, he or she slowly lets air out of the cuff until the first pulsations are heard. At this point, the pressure in the cuff is equal to the systolic pressure, and this pressure is read. Then, more air is let out gradually until a characteristic muffled sound indicates that the vessel is open and the diastolic pressure is read. Original-style sphygmomanometers display readings on a graduated column of mercury, but newer types display them on a dial. The newest devices measure blood pressure electronically: the examiner simply applies the cuff, which self-inflates and provides a digital reading. A typical normal systolic pressure is <120 mm Hg; a typical normal diastolic pressure is <80 mm Hg. Blood pressure is reported as systolic pressure first, then diastolic pressure, separated by a slash, such as 120/80. This reading would be reported verbally as "one twenty over eighty."

Considerable experience is required to ensure an accurate blood pressure reading. Often it is necessary to repeat measurements. Note also that blood pressure varies throughout the day and under different conditions, so a single reading does not give a complete picture. Some people typically have a higher reading in a doctor's office because of stress. People who experience such "white coat hypertension" may need to take their blood pressure at home while relaxed to get a more accurate reading. Box 14-2 explains how cardiac catheterization is used to measure blood pressure with high accuracy.

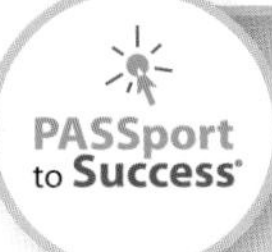

See the Student Resources on *thePoint* for career information on vascular technology. Vascular technologists collect information on the blood vessels and circulation to aid in diagnosis.

CHECKPOINTS

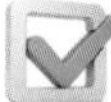

- 14-16 What is the definition of *pulse?*
- 14-17 What is the definition of blood pressure?
- 14-18 What is the most significant factor in determination of peripheral resistance?
- 14-19 What two components of blood pressure are measured?

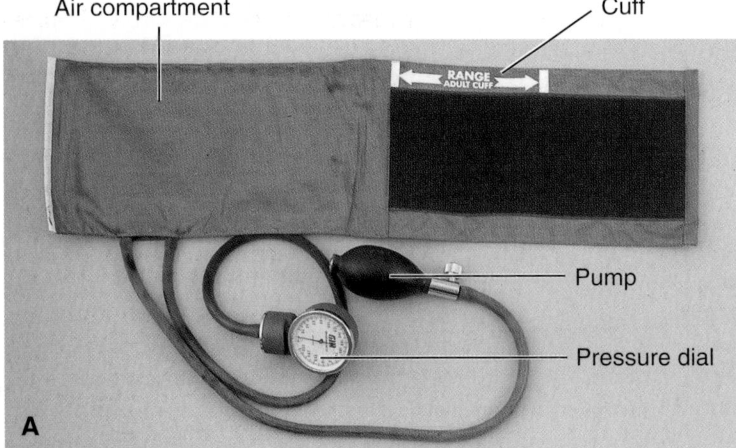

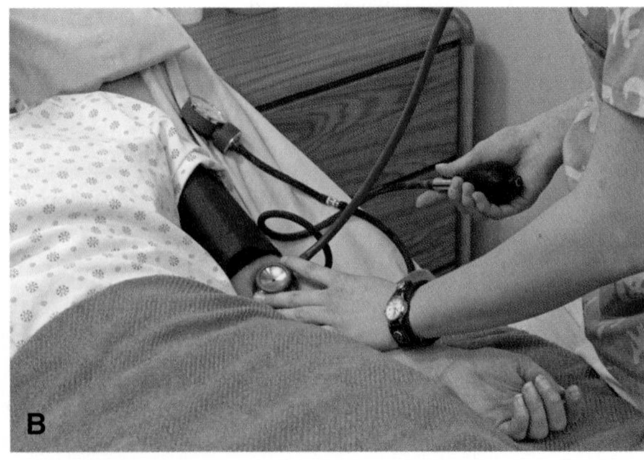

Figure 14-12 Measurement of blood pressure. A. A sphygmomanometer, or blood pressure cuff. **B.** Once the cuff is inflated, the examiner releases the pressure and listens for sounds in the vessels with a stethoscope. (A, Reprinted with permission from Bickley LS. *Bates' Guide to Physical Examination and History Taking*, 10th ed. Philadelphia, PA: Lippincott Williams & Wilkins, 2008; B, Reprinted with permission from Taylor C, Lillis C, LeMone P. *Fundamentals of Nursing*, 5th ed. Philadelphia, PA: Lippincott Williams & Wilkins, 2004.)

Box 14-2 *Clinical Perspectives*

Cardiac Catheterization: Measuring Blood Pressure from Within

Because arterial blood pressure decreases as blood flows farther away from the heart, measurement of blood pressure with a simple inflatable cuff around the arm is only a reflection of the pressure in the heart and pulmonary arteries. Precise measurement of pressure in these parts of the cardiovascular system is useful in diagnosing certain cardiac and pulmonary disorders.

More accurate readings can be obtained using a catheter (thin tube) inserted directly into the heart and large vessels. One type commonly used is the pulmonary artery catheter (also known as the Swan–Ganz catheter), which has an inflatable balloon at the tip. This device is threaded into the right side of the heart through a large vein. Typically, the right internal jugular vein is used because it is the shortest and most direct route to the heart, but the subclavian and femoral veins may be used instead. The catheter's position in the heart is confirmed by a chest x-ray and, when appropriately positioned, the atrial and ventricular blood pressures are recorded. As the catheter continues into the pulmonary artery, pressure in this vessel can be read. When the balloon is inflated, the catheter becomes wedged in a branch of the pulmonary artery, blocking blood flow. The reading obtained is called the **pulmonary capillary wedge pressure**. It gives information on pressure in the heart's left side and on resistance in the lungs. Combined with other tests, cardiac catheterization can be used to diagnose cardiac and pulmonary disorders such as shock, pericarditis, congenital heart disease, and heart failure.

A&P in Action Revisited

Reggie's Pulmonary Embolism

As soon as the blood clot broke free in Reggie's femoral vein, it began its journey to the heart. The clot (now called an embolus) traveled within the right femoral vein, which entered the abdominal cavity and widened, becoming the external iliac vein. The embolus flowed into the large right common iliac vein, mixing with pelvic blood from the internal iliac vein. Then, the embolus was carried toward the even larger inferior vena cava. As the embolus traveled superiorly toward the heart, it joined with blood from the kidneys and intestines. The inferior vena cava carried the embolus through the diaphragm into the thoracic cavity and into the right atrium of the heart. The embolus flowed past the tricuspid valve into the right ventricle, which contracted and propelled the embolus past the pulmonary valve and into the pulmonary trunk. The embolus entered the left pulmonary artery and then traveled through successively smaller arterial branches until finally it became wedged in one of the small arteries supplying blood to his left lung. Reggie had developed a pulmonary embolism!

Reggie felt a sharp crushing pain in his chest and woke with a start. He knew something was terribly wrong and pressed the panic button clipped to his hospital bed. Reggie's nurse rushed to his bedside and recognized that Reggie was in life-threatening danger. He received immediate treatment of tissue plasminogen activator (tPA) to dissolve the clots in his pulmonary artery and femoral vein and several doses of heparin to prevent more clots from forming. Reggie had survived his second medical emergency!

In this case, we followed an embolus as it traveled from Reggie's femoral vein to his pulmonary artery. Using the diagrams in this chapter, can you trace its pathway?

Chapter Wrap-Up

Summary Overview

A detailed chapter outline with space for note-taking is on *thePoint*. The figure below illustrates the main topics covered in this chapter.

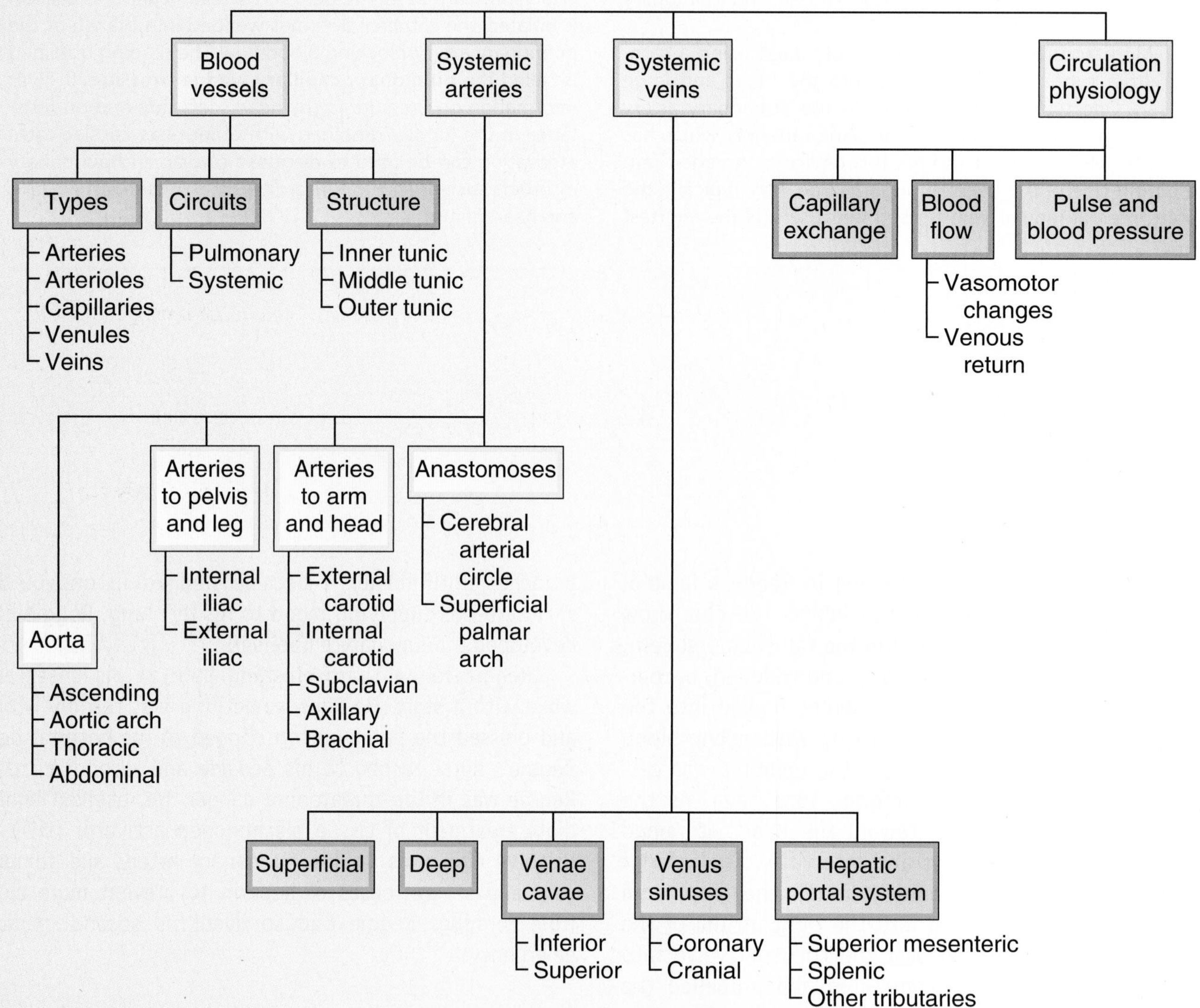

Key Terms

The terms listed below are emphasized in this chapter. Knowing them will help you organize and prioritize your learning. These and other boldface terms are defined in the Glossary with phonetic pronunciations.

aorta	compliance	sphygmomanometer	vein
arteriole	elasticity	valve	vena cava
artery	endothelium	vasoconstriction	venous sinus
baroreceptor	pulse	vasodilation	venule
capillary	sinusoid	vasomotor	

Word Anatomy

Scientific terms are built from standardized word parts (prefixes, roots, and suffixes). Learning the meanings of these parts can help you remember words and interpret unfamiliar terms.

WORD PART	MEANING	EXAMPLE
Systemic Arteries		
brachi/o	arm	The *brachiocephalic* artery supplies blood to the arm and head on the right side.
cephal/o	head	See preceding example.
clav/o	clavicle	The *subclavian* artery extends under the clavicle on each side.
cost/o	rib	The *intercostal* arteries are between the ribs.
celi/o	abdomen	The *celiac* trunk branches to supply blood to the abdominal organs.
gastr/o	stomach	The *gastric* artery goes to the stomach.
splen/o	spleen	The *splenic* artery goes to the spleen.
hepat/o	liver	The *hepatic* artery supplies blood to the liver.
enter/o	intestine	The *mesenteric* arteries supply blood to the intestines.
phren/o	diaphragm	The *phrenic* artery supplies blood to the diaphragm.
ped/o	foot	The dorsalis *pedis* artery supplies blood to the foot.
stoma	mouth	An *anastomosis* is a communication between two vessels.
Circulation Physiology		
bar/o	pressure	A *baroreceptor* responds to changes in pressure.
sphygm/o	pulse	A *sphygmomanometer* is used to measure blood pressure.
man/o	pressure	See preceding example.

Questions for Study and Review

BUILDING UNDERSTANDING

Fill in the Blanks

1. Capillaries receive blood from vessels called ______.
2. The specific part of the medulla oblongata that regulates blood flow is the ______.
3. The flow of blood into an individual capillary is regulated by a(n) ______.
4. Blood is delivered to the lungs by the _____ circuit.
5. The technical name for a blood pressure cuff is ______.

Matching > Match each numbered item with the most closely related lettered item.

___ 6. Supplies blood from the heart to the right arm and head
___ 7. Supplies blood from the heart to the kidneys
___ 8. Returns blood from the brain to the heart
___ 9. Returns blood from the small intestines to the heart
___ 10. Returns blood from the kidneys to the heart

a. jugular vein
b. superior mesenteric vein
c. brachiocephalic artery
d. renal artery
e. renal vein

Multiple Choice

___ 11. Which tissue makes up a blood vessel's inner tunic?
- a. smooth muscle
- b. epithelium
- c. connective tissue
- d. nervous tissue

___ 12. Which of the following vessels is the largest?
- a. aorta
- b. brachiocephalic trunk
- c. splenic artery
- d. superior mesenteric artery

___ 13. What is the main process of capillary exchange?
- a. endocytosis
- b. exocytosis
- c. osmosis
- d. diffusion

___ 14. Which vessel supplies oxygenated blood to the stomach, spleen, and liver?
- a. hepatic portal system
- b. superior mesenteric artery
- c. inferior mesenteric artery
- d. celiac trunk

___ 15. Which structure regulates vasomotor activities?
- a. medulla
- b. cerebellum
- c. cerebrum
- d. spinal cord

UNDERSTANDING CONCEPTS

16. Differentiate between the terms in each of the following pairs:
    - a. artery and vein
    - b. arteriole and venule
    - c. anastomosis and venous sinus
    - d. vasoconstriction and vasodilation
    - e. systolic and diastolic pressure
17. How does the structure of the blood vessels correlate with their function?
18. Trace a drop of blood from the left ventricle to the:
    - a. right side of the head and the neck
    - b. lateral surface of the left hand
    - c. right foot
    - d. liver
    - e. small intestine
19. Trace a drop of blood from capillaries in the wall of the small intestine to the right atrium. What is the purpose of going through the liver on this trip?
20. Describe three mechanisms that promote the return of blood to the heart in the venous system.
21. What physiological factors influence blood pressure?
22. Describe the blood vessels that contribute to the hepatic portal system.

CONCEPTUAL THINKING

23. Kidney disease usually results in the loss of protein from the blood into the urine. One common sign of kidney disease is edema. From your understanding of capillary exchange, explain why edema is often associated with kidney disease.

24. Cliff C., a 49-year-old self-described "couch potato," has high blood pressure. His doctor suspects that Cliff's lifestyle has contributed to atherosclerosis, a disease of the blood vessels characterized by a "narrowing of the arteries." How has this disorder contributed to Cliff's high blood pressure?

25. In Reggie's case, an embolus traveled from his femoral vein to his pulmonary artery. Describe the pathway the embolus would take if it traveled from his femoral vein to the middle cerebral artery supplying blood to his left frontal lobe. What deficits would you suspect to see from this brain stroke? (*Hint*: Refer to Chapter 9.)

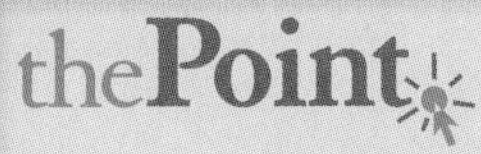

For more questions, see the learning activities on *thePoint*.

CHAPTER 15

The Lymphatic System and Immunity

A&P in Action

Mike's Second Case: Emergency Splenectomy

Alek, a fourth-year medical student, slumped into a chair in the lounge and closed his eyes. It was only a few hours into his shift, but he was already exhausted. Then, Alek's pager buzzed—*get to the operating room immediately*! Minutes later, he donned a sterile gown and gloves and entered the operating room, which buzzed with activity as the surgical team prepped the patient for emergency abdominal surgery. Alek listened carefully to the surgeon as he explained the case to the team. "Patient's name is Mike. He's 21 years old and was in a car accident about an hour ago. Paramedics noted significant bruising of the left upper quadrant, tachycardia, and hypotension." The surgeon glanced at the medical student and asked, "Alek, what does that suggest to you?"

Alek thought quickly and answered, "The location of the injury and cardiovascular problems suggest a ruptured spleen."

"That's exactly what the emergency team thought," replied the surgeon. "OK folks, let's open Mike up and see if Alek's right." Using a scalpel, the surgeon made a midsagittal incision through Mike's abdominal wall. Then, he made a transverse incision to open the left side of his abdominal cavity and suctioned out the blood that filled it. He located the purple-colored spleen in the left hypochondriac region and noted a large tear in the connective tissue capsule surrounding it. "You're right, Alek. We've got a ruptured spleen here, which we'll have to remove." The surgeon searched for the splenic artery supplying blood to the damaged organ and when he found it, tied it shut, and cut it. Then, he cut the ligaments that suspended the spleen between the stomach and transverse colon. Finally, he tied and cut the splenic vein and removed Mike's spleen. "OK," said the surgeon, "Let's close him up and get him to intensive care. Alek, good job today."

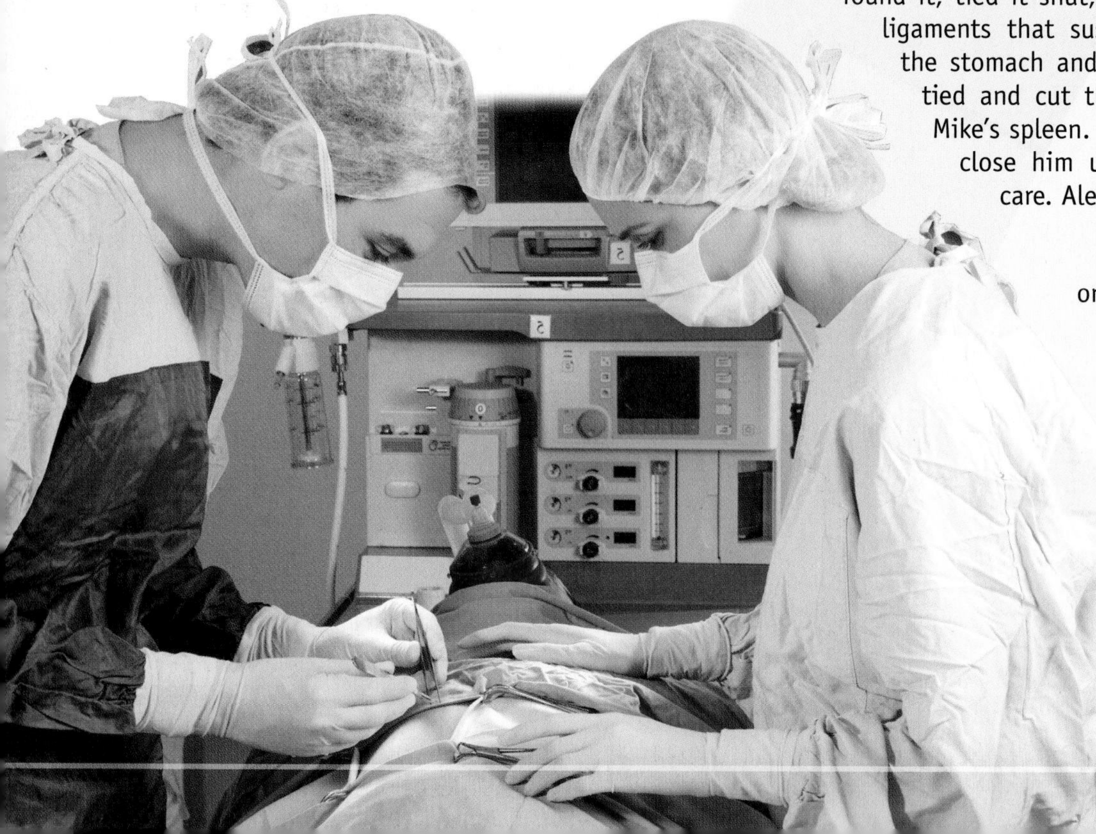

Mike's spleen, a lymphoid organ, was injured during a car accident and had to be removed. In this chapter, you will learn about the spleen and other organs that make up the lymphatic system. Later, we will check in on Mike and learn about splenectomy's long-term consequences.

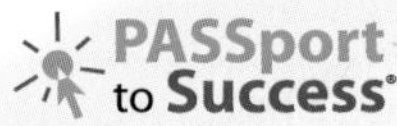

Ancillaries At-A-Glance

Visit *thePoint* to access the PASSport to Success and the following resources. For guidance in using these resources most effectively, see pp. ix–xviii.

Learning TOOLS

- Learning Style Self Assessment
- Live Advise Online Student Tutoring
- Tips for Effective Studying

Learning RESOURCES

- E-book: Chapter 15
- Web Figure: Chain of Events in Inflammation
- Web Chart: Lymphoid Tissue
- Animation: Acute Inflammation
- Animation: Immune Response
- Health Professions: Nurse Practitioner
- Health Professions: Clinical Massage Therapist
- Detailed Chapter Outline
- Answers to Questions for Study and Review
- Audio Pronunciation Glossary

Learning ACTIVITIES

- Pre-Quiz
- Visual Activities
- Kinesthetic Activities
- Auditory Activities

Learning Outcomes

After careful study of this chapter, you should be able to:

1. List the functions of the lymphatic system, ***p. 288***
2. Explain how lymphatic capillaries differ from blood capillaries, ***p. 289***
3. Name the two main lymphatic ducts and describe the area drained by each, ***p. 291***
4. List the major structures of the lymphatic system and give the locations and functions of each, ***p. 290***
5. Differentiate between nonspecific and specific body defenses and give examples of each, ***p. 295***
6. Briefly describe the inflammatory reaction, ***p. 296***
7. Define *antigen* and *antibody*, ***p. 298***
8. Compare and contrast T cells and B cells with respect to development and type of activity, ***p. 298***
9. Explain the role of antigen-presenting cells in specific immunity, ***p. 299***
10. Describe some protective effects of an antigen–antibody reaction, ***p. 301***
11. Differentiate between natural and artificial acquired immunity, ***p. 301***
12. Differentiate between active and passive immunity, ***p. 301***
13. Define the terms *vaccine* and *immune serum*, ***pp. 301, 303***
14. Describe the spleen's functions and the consequences of its removal, as described in the case study, ***pp. 286, 304***
15. Show how word parts are used to build words related to the lymphatic system (see Word Anatomy at the end of the chapter), ***p. 306***

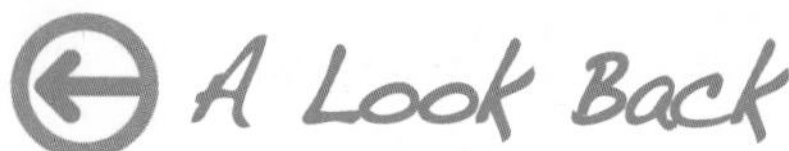

In Chapter 14 we learned that the blood leaves some fluid behind in the tissues as it travels through the capillary networks. The lymphatic system collects this fluid and returns it to the circulation. Lymph's return to the heart is governed by the same mechanisms that promote venous return of blood. The lymphatic system has other functions beside aiding in circulation, as we will see in this chapter.

The lymphatic system is a widespread system of tissues and vessels. Its organs are not grouped together but are scattered throughout the body, and it services almost all regions. Only bone marrow, cartilage, epithelium, and the central nervous system are not in direct communication with this system.

Functions of the Lymphatic System

The lymphatic system's functions are just as varied as its locations. These functions fall into three categories:

- **Fluid balance.** As blood circulates through the capillaries in the tissues, water and dissolved substances are constantly exchanged between the bloodstream and the interstitial (in-ter-STISH-al) fluids that bathe the cells. The volume of fluid that leaves the blood is not quite matched by the amount that returns to the blood, so there is always a slight excess of fluid left behind in the tissues. In addition, some proteins escape from the blood capillaries and are left behind. This fluid and protein would accumulate in the tissues if not for a second drainage pathway through lymphatic vessels (Fig. 15-1).

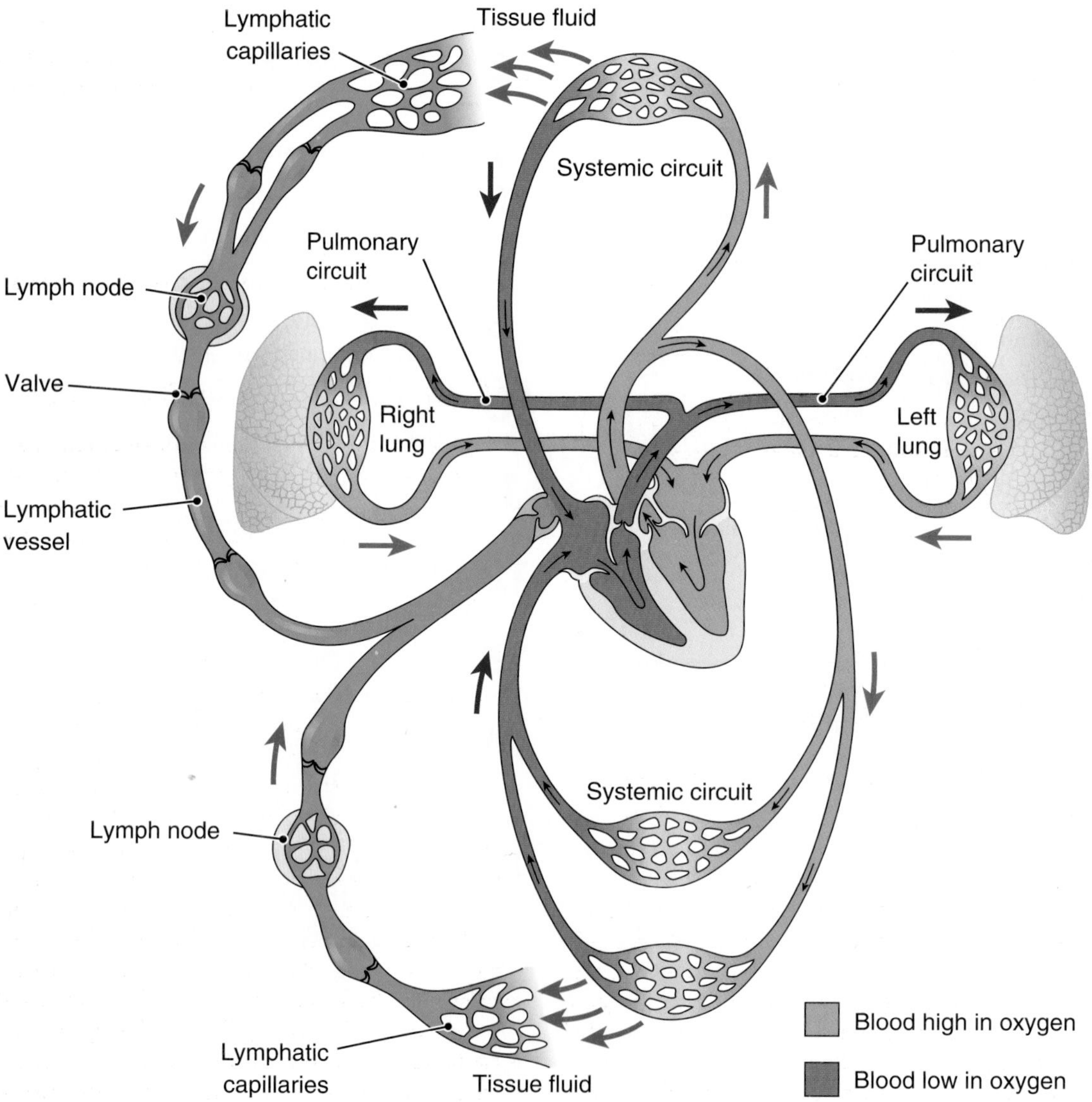

Figure 15-1 The lymphatic system in relation to the cardiovascular system. KEY POINT Lymphatic vessels pick up fluid in the tissues and return it to the blood in vessels near the heart. ZOOMING IN What type of blood vessel receives lymph collected from the body?

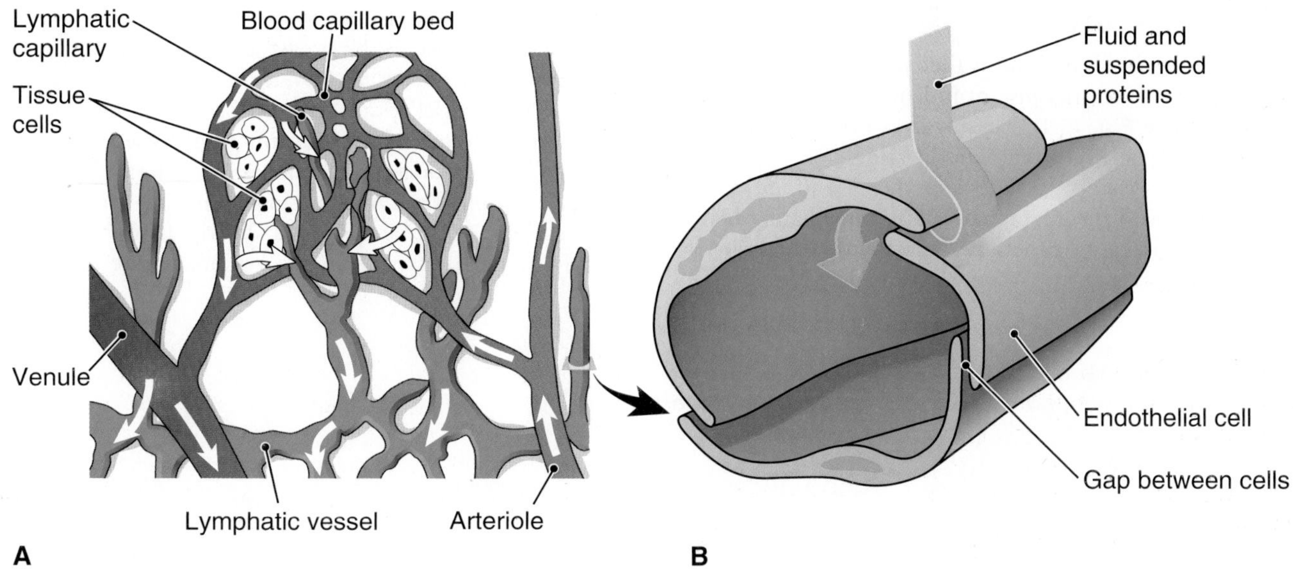

Figure 15-2 **Lymphatic drainage in the tissues.** KEY POINT Lymphatic capillaries pick up fluid and proteins from the tissues for return to the heart in lymphatic vessels. **A.** Blind-ended lymphatic capillaries in relation to blood capillaries. *Arrows* show the direction of flow. **B.** Structure of a lymphatic capillary. Fluid and proteins can enter the capillary with ease through gaps between the endothelial cells. Overlapping cells act as valves to prevent the material from leaving.

In addition to the blood-carrying capillaries, the tissues also contain microscopic lymphatic capillaries **(Fig. 15-2)**. These small vessels pick up excess fluid and protein from the tissues. They then drain into larger vessels, which eventually return these materials to the venous system near the heart.

The fluid that circulates in the lymphatic system is called **lymph** (limf), a clear fluid similar in composition to interstitial fluid. Although lymph is formed from the components of blood plasma, it differs from the plasma in that it has much less protein.

- **Protection.** The lymphatic system is an important component of the immune system, which fights infection. One group of white blood cells, the lymphocytes, can live and multiply in the lymphatic system, where they attack and destroy foreign organisms. Lymphoid tissue scattered throughout the body filters out pathogens, other foreign matter, tumor cells, and cellular debris found in body fluids.
- **Absorption of fats.** Following the chemical and mechanical breakdown of food in the digestive tract, most nutrients are absorbed into the blood through intestinal capillaries. Many digested fats, however, are too large to enter the blood capillaries and are instead absorbed into specialized lymphatic capillaries in the lining of the small intestine. Fats taken into these **lacteals** (LAK-te-als) are transported in lymphatic vessels until the lymph is added to the blood. More information on the lymphatic system's role in digestion is found in Chapter 17.

CHECKPOINT 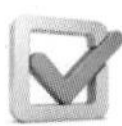

☐ 15-1 What are the three functions of the lymphatic system?

Lymphatic Circulation

Lymph travels through a network of small and large channels that are in some ways similar to the blood vessels. However, the system is not a complete circuit. It is a one-way system that begins in the tissues and ends when the lymph joins the blood **(see Fig. 15-1)**.

LYMPHATIC CAPILLARIES

The walls of the lymphatic capillaries resemble those of the blood capillaries in that they are made of one layer of flattened (squamous) epithelial cells. This thin layer, also called *endothelium*, allows for easy passage of soluble materials and water through the capillary wall **(see Fig. 15-2B)**. The gaps between the endothelial cells in the lymphatic capillaries are larger than those of the blood capillaries. The lymphatic capillaries are thus more permeable, allowing for easier entrance of relatively large protein molecules. The proteins do not move back out of the vessels because the endothelial cells overlap slightly, forming one-way valves to block their return.

Unlike the blood capillaries, the lymphatic capillaries arise blindly; that is, they are closed at one end and do not form a bridge between two larger vessels. Instead, one end simply lies within a lake of tissue fluid, and the other communicates with a larger lymphatic vessel that transports the lymph toward the heart **(see Fig. 15-2A)**.

LYMPHATIC VESSELS

The lymphatic vessels are thin-walled and delicate and have a beaded appearance because of indentations where valves are located **(see Fig. 15-1)**. These valves prevent back flow in the same way as do those found in veins.

Lymphatic vessels include superficial and deep sets **(Fig. 15-3)**. The surface lymphatics are immediately below the skin, often lying near the superficial veins. The deep vessels are usually larger and accompany the deep veins.

Lymphatic vessels are named according to location. For example, those in the breast are called mammary lymphatic vessels **(see Fig. 15-3D)**, those in the thigh are called femoral lymphatic vessels, and those in the leg are called tibial lymphatic vessels. At certain points, the vessels drain through **lymph nodes**, small masses of lymphatic tissue that filter the lymph. The nodes are in groups that serve a particular region, as will be described shortly. Lymphatic vessels carrying lymph away from the regional nodes eventually

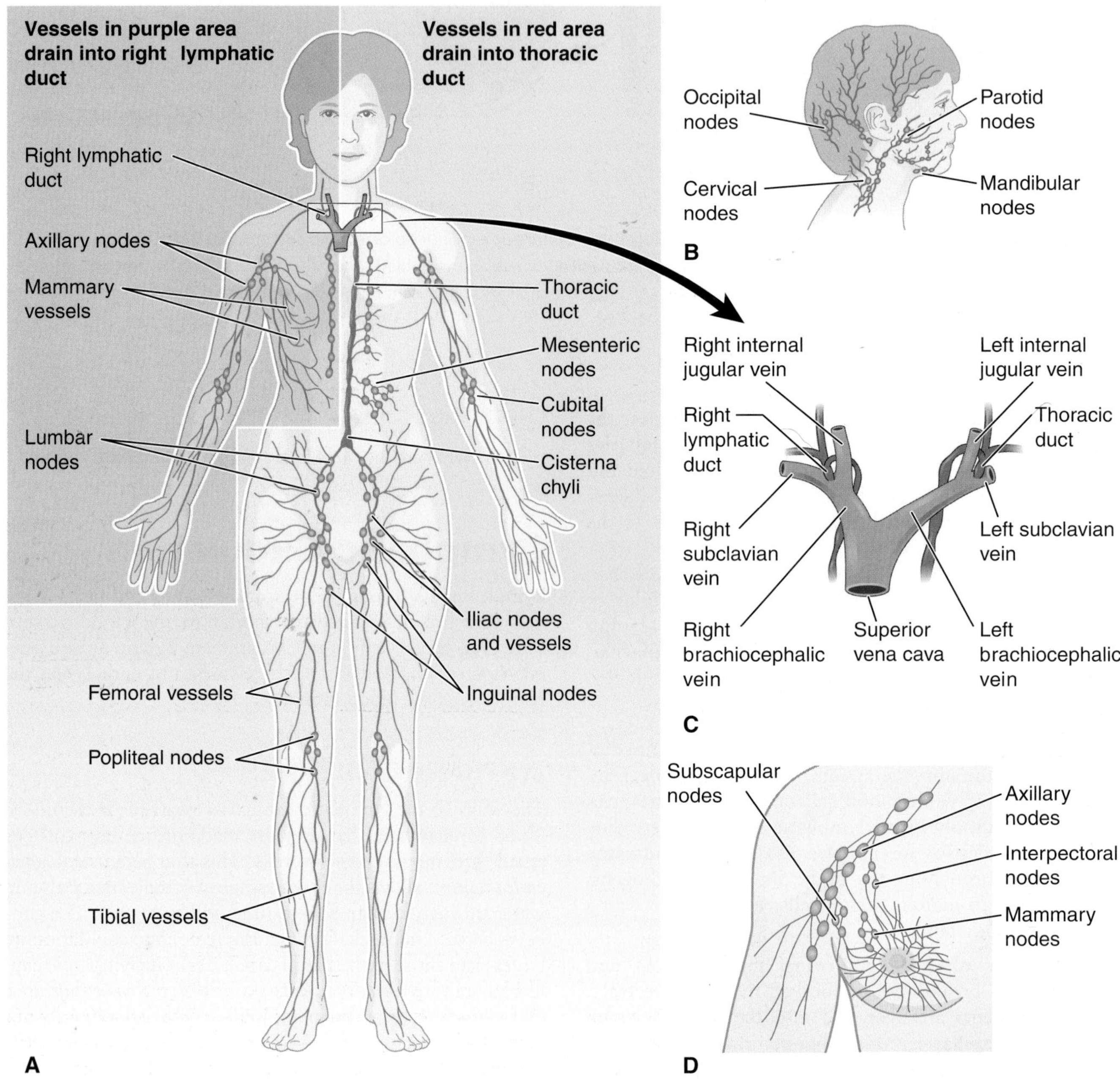

Figure 15-3 Vessels and nodes of the lymphatic system. KEY POINT Lymphatic vessels serve almost every area in the body. Lymph nodes are distributed along the path of the vessels. **A.** Lymph nodes and vessels, showing areas draining into the right lymphatic duct (*purple*) and the thoracic duct (*red*). **B.** Lymph nodes and vessels of the head. **C.** Drainage of right lymphatic duct and thoracic duct into subclavian veins. **D.** Lymph nodes and vessels of the mammary gland and surrounding areas. **ZOOMING IN** What are some nodes that receive lymph drainage from the breast?

drain into one of two terminal vessels, the right lymphatic duct or the thoracic duct, both of which empty into the bloodstream.

The Right Lymphatic Duct The **right lymphatic duct** is a short vessel, approximately 1.25 cm (1/2 in.) long, that receives only the lymph that comes from the body's superior right quadrant: the right side of the head, neck, and thorax, as well as the right upper extremity. The right lymphatic duct empties into the right subclavian vein near the heart (see Fig. 15-3C). Its opening into this vein is guarded by two pocket-like semilunar valves to prevent blood from entering the duct. The rest of the body is drained by the thoracic duct.

The Thoracic Duct The **thoracic duct**, or left lymphatic duct, is the larger of the two terminal vessels, measuring approximately 40 cm (16 in.) in length. As shown in Figure 15-3, the thoracic duct receives lymph from all parts of the body except those superior to the diaphragm on the right side. This duct begins in the posterior part of the abdominal cavity, inferior to the attachment of the diaphragm. The duct's first part is enlarged to form a cistern, or temporary storage pouch, called the **cisterna chyli** (sis-TER-nah KI-li). **Chyle** (kile) is the milky fluid that drains from the intestinal lacteals; it is formed by the combination of fat globules and lymph. Chyle passes through the intestinal lymphatic vessels and the lymph nodes of the mesentery (the membrane around the intestines), finally entering the cisterna chyli. In addition to chyle, all the lymph from below the diaphragm empties into the cisterna chyli, passing through the various clusters of lymph nodes. The thoracic duct then carries this lymph into the bloodstream.

The thoracic duct extends upward through the diaphragm and along the posterior thoracic wall into the base of the neck on the left side. Here, it receives the left jugular lymphatic vessels from the head and neck, the left subclavian vessels from the left upper extremity, and other lymphatic vessels from the thorax and its parts. In addition to the valves along the duct, there are two valves at its opening into the left subclavian vein to prevent the passage of blood into the duct.

MOVEMENT OF LYMPH

The segments of lymphatic vessels located between the valves contract rhythmically, propelling the lymph forward. The contraction rate is related to the fluid volume in the vessel—the more the fluid, the more rapid the contractions.

Lymph is also moved by the same mechanisms that promote venous return of blood to the heart. As skeletal muscles contract during movement, they compress the lymphatic vessels and drive lymph forward. Changes in pressures within the abdominal and thoracic cavities caused by breathing aid lymphatic movement during passage through these body cavities.

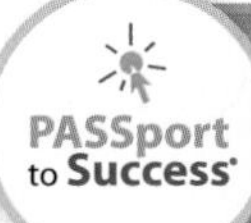

Massage therapy can improve lymphatic drainage and blood circulation as well as benefit muscles. See the Student Resources on *thePoint* for more information about this field.

CHECKPOINTS

☐ 15-2 What are the two differences between blood capillaries and lymphatic capillaries?

☐ 15-3 What are the two main lymphatic vessels?

Lymphoid Tissue

Lymphoid (LIM-foyd) **tissue** is distributed throughout the body and makes up the lymphatic system's specialized organs. The role of lymph nodes in lymphatic circulation has already been described. Here, we discuss the structure and function of lymph nodes and other lymphatic organs in greater detail.

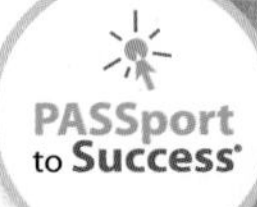

See the Student Resources on *thePoint* for a quick study chart on lymphoid tissue.

15

LYMPH NODES

The lymph nodes, as noted, are designed to filter the lymph as it travels through the lymphatic vessels (Fig. 15-4). They are also sites where lymphocytes of the immune system multiply and work to combat foreign organisms. The lymph nodes are small, rounded masses varying from pinhead size to as long as 2.5 cm (1 in.). Each has a fibrous connective tissue capsule from which partitions called *trabeculae* extend into the node's substance. At various points in the node's surface, afferent lymphatic vessels pierce the capsule to carry lymph toward open channels, or sinuses, in the node. An indented area, the *hilum* (HI-lum) is the exit point for efferent lymphatic vessels carrying lymph out of the node. At this location, other structures, including blood vessels and nerves, connect with the node. (*Hilum* is a general term for an indented region of an organ where vessels and nerves enter and leave).

A lymph node is divided into two regions: an outer cortex and an inner medulla. Each of these regions is subdivided into lymph-filled sinuses and cords of lymphatic tissue. The cortex contains pulplike *cortical nodules*, each of which has a *germinal center* where certain lymphocytes multiply. The medulla, has populations of immune cells, including lymphocytes and macrophages (phagocytes), along the *medullary sinuses*, which drain into the efferent lymphatic vessels.

Lymph nodes are seldom isolated. As a rule, they are grouped together in numbers varying from 2 or 3 to well over 100. Some of these groups are placed deeply,

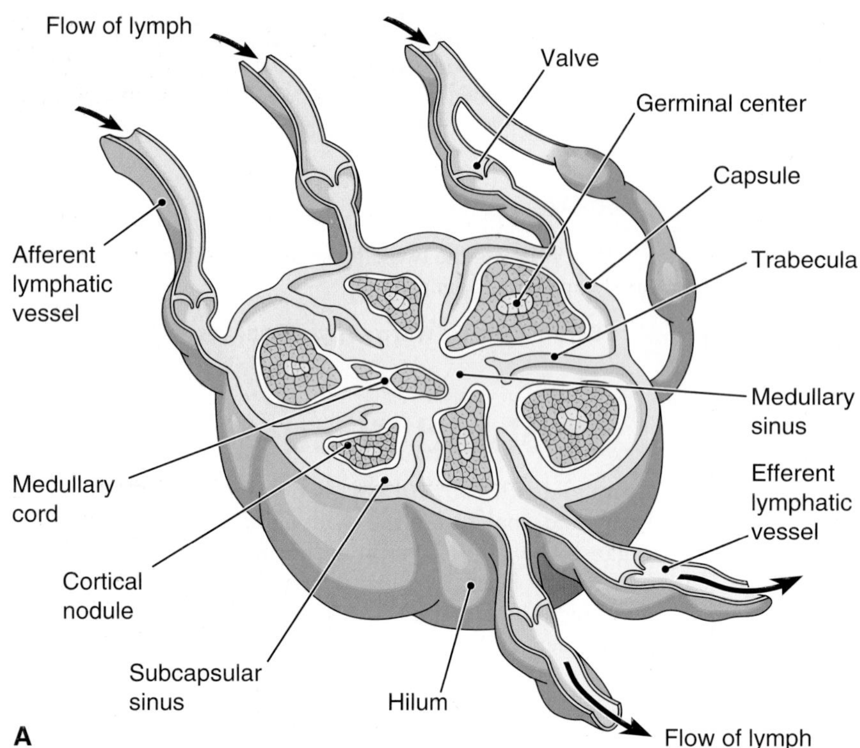

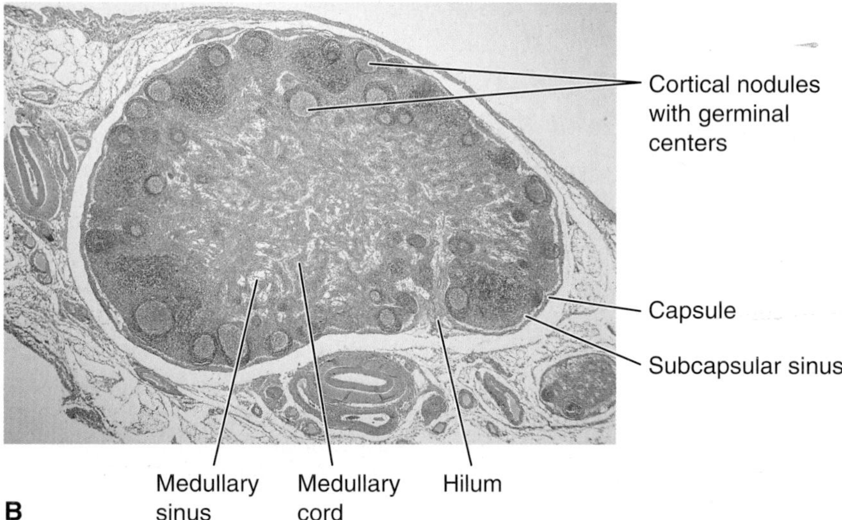

Figure 15-4 Lymph nodes. KEY POINT Lymph is filtered as it travels through a lymph node. Cells of the immune system also multiply in the nodes. **A.** Structure of a lymph node. Arrows indicate the flow of lymph. **B.** Section of a lymph node as seen under the microscope (low power). (B, Reprinted with permission from Cormack DH. *Essential Histology*, 2nd ed. Philadelphia, PA: Lippincott Williams & Wilkins, 2001.) ZOOMING IN What type of lymphatic vessel carries lymph into a node? What type of lymphatic vessel carries lymph out of a node?

whereas others are superficial. The main groups include the following:

- **Cervical nodes**, located in the neck in deep and superficial groups, drain various parts of the head and neck. They often become enlarged during upper respiratory infections.
- **Axillary nodes**, located in the axillae (armpits), may become enlarged after infections of the upper extremities and the breasts. Cancer cells from the breasts often metastasize (spread) to the axillary nodes, as noted in Box 15-1.
- **Tracheobronchial** (tra-ke-o-BRONG-ke-al) **nodes** are found near the trachea and around the larger bronchial tubes. In people who smoke, are exposed to smoke, or live in highly polluted areas, these nodes become filled with air-borne contaminants.
- **Mesenteric** (mes-en-TER-ik) **nodes** are found between the two layers of peritoneum that form the mesentery. There are some 100 to 150 of these nodes.
- **Inguinal nodes**, located in the groin region, receive lymph drainage from the lower extremities and from the external reproductive organs. When they become enlarged, they are often referred to as **buboes** (BU-bose), from which bubonic plague got its name.

Box 15-1 explains the role of lymph node biopsy in the treatment of cancer.

Box 15-1 *Hot Topics*

Sentinel Node Biopsy: Finding Cancer Before It Spreads

Ordinarily, the lymphatic system is one of the body's primary defenses against disease. In cancer, though, it can be a vehicle for the spread (metastasis) of disease. When cancer cells enter the lymphatic vessels, they are often trapped and killed within the lymph nodes by immune system cells. However, if the immune system is overwhelmed by cancer cells, some may escape the lymph nodes and travel to other parts of the body, where they may establish new tumors.

In breast cancer, the degree of invasion of nearby lymph nodes helps determine what treatments are required after surgical removal of the tumor. Until recently, a mastectomy often included the removal of nearby lymphatic vessels and nodes (a procedure called axillary lymph node dissection). Biopsy of the nodes determined whether or not they contained cancerous cells. If they did, radiation treatment or chemotherapy was required. In many women with early-stage breast cancer, however, the axillary nodes do not contain cancerous cells. In addition, about 20% of the women whose lymphatic vessels and nodes have been removed suffer impaired lymph flow, resulting in lymphedema, pain, disability, and an increased risk of infection.

Sentinel node biopsy is a diagnostic procedure that may minimize the need to perform axillary lymph node dissection, while still detecting metastasis. Surgeons use radioactive tracers to identify the first nodes that receive lymph from the area of a tumor. Biopsy of only these "sentinel nodes" reveals whether tumor cells are present, providing the earliest indication of metastasis. Research shows that sentinel lymph node biopsy is associated with less pain, fewer complications, and faster recovery than axillary lymph node dissection. However, clinical trials are ongoing to determine whether sentinel node biopsy is as successful as axillary dissection in finding cancer before it spreads.

THE SPLEEN

The **spleen** is an organ containing lymphoid tissue that filters blood. It is located in the superior left hypochondriac region of the abdomen, high up under the dome of the diaphragm, and normally is protected by the lower part of the rib cage **(Fig. 15-5)**. The spleen is a soft, purplish, and somewhat flattened organ, measuring approximately 12.5 to 16 cm (5 to 6 in.) long and 5 to 7.5 cm (2 to 3 in.) wide. The spleen's capsule, as well as its framework, is more elastic than that of the lymph nodes. It contains an involuntary muscle, which enables the splenic capsule to contract and also to withstand some swelling.

Not surprisingly, considering its role in blood filtration, the spleen has an unusually rich blood supply. The organ is filled with a soft pulp which not only cleanses the blood of impurities and cellular debris by filtration, but also harbors phagocytes and lymphocytes, which are active in immunity. The spleen is classified as part of the lymphatic system because it contains prominent masses of lymphoid tissue. However, it has wider functions than other lymphatic structures, including the following:

- Destroying old, worn-out red blood cells. The iron and other breakdown products of hemoglobin are then carried to the liver by the hepatic portal system to be reused or eliminated from the body.
- Producing red blood cells before birth
- Serving as a reservoir for blood, which can be returned to the bloodstream in case of hemorrhage or other emergency

Splenectomy (sple-NEK-to-me), or surgical removal of the spleen, is usually a well-tolerated procedure. Although

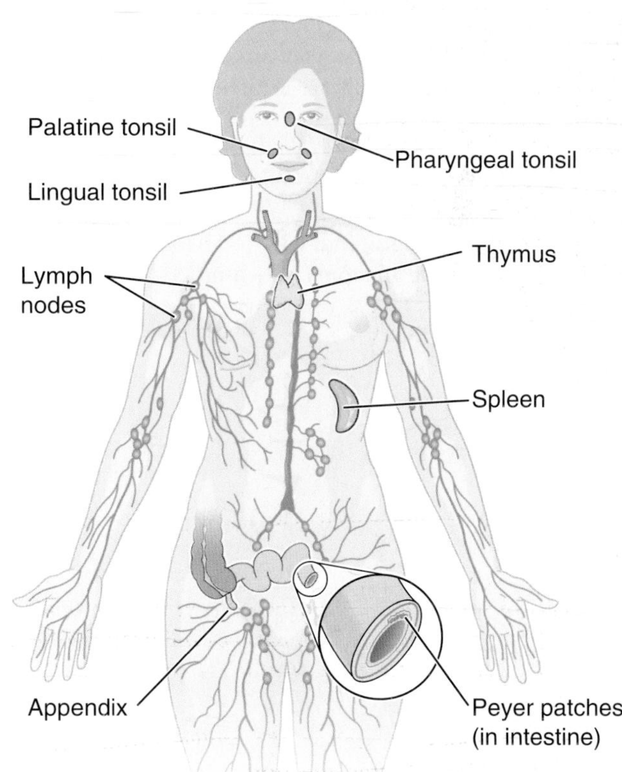

Figure 15-5 Location of lymphoid tissue. KEY POINT The lymphatic system is widespread and consists of vessels, nodes, organs, and other tissues.

15

the spleen is the body's largest lymphoid organ, other lymphoid tissues can take over its functions. There is evidence that splenectomy carries a risk of developing certain infections, especially in younger patients. Physicians might prescribe prophylactic antibiotics; educate patients about the risk; or perform a partial splenectomy if possible. In the case study, Mike's spleen was ruptured in a car accident and had to be removed. Physicians were alert to any complications that might follow his splenectomy.

THE THYMUS

The **thymus** (THI-mus), located in the superior thorax deep to the sternum, plays a role in immune system development during fetal life and infancy **(see Fig. 15-5)**. Certain lymphocytes, T cells, must mature in the thymus gland before they can perform their functions in the immune system. Removal of the thymus causes a generalized decrease in the production of T cells, as well as a decrease in the size of the spleen and of lymph nodes throughout the body.

The thymus is most active during early life. After puberty, the tissue undergoes changes; it shrinks in size and is gradually replaced by connective tissue and fat.

THE TONSILS

The **tonsils** are unencapsulated masses of lymphoid tissue located in the vicinity of the pharynx (throat) where they remove contaminants from materials that are inhaled or swallowed **(Fig. 15-6)**. The tonsils have deep grooves lined with lymphatic nodules. Lymphocytes attack pathogens trapped in these grooves. The tonsils are located in three areas:

- The **palatine** (PAL-ah-tine) **tonsils** are oval bodies located at each side of the soft palate. These are generally what is meant when one refers to "the tonsils."
- The single **pharyngeal** (fah-RIN-je-al) **tonsil** is commonly referred to as the **adenoid** (AD-eh-noyd) (a general term that means "gland-like"). It is located behind the nose on the posterior wall of the upper pharynx.
- The **lingual** (LING-gwal) **tonsils** are little mounds of lymphoid tissue at the posterior of the tongue.

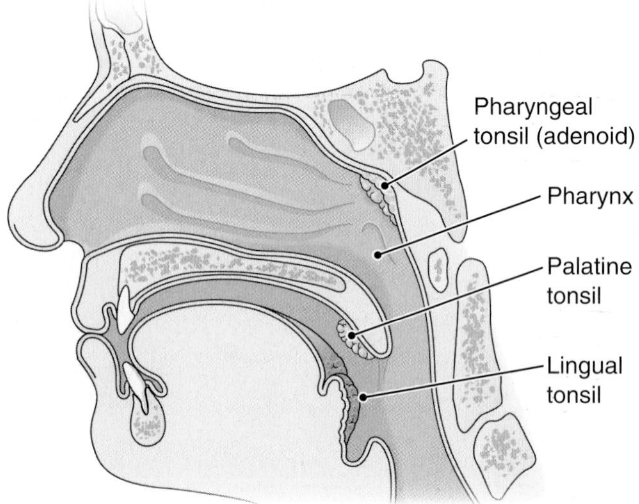

Figure 15-6 Location of the tonsils. KEY POINT All of the tonsils are in the vicinity of the pharynx (throat), where they filter impurities.

Any of these tonsils may become so loaded with bacteria that they become reservoirs for repeated infections and their removal is advisable. In children, a slight enlargement of any of them is not an indication for surgery, however, because all lymphoid tissue masses tend to be larger in childhood. A physician must determine whether these masses are abnormally enlarged, taking the patient's age into account, because the tonsils are important in immune function during early childhood. Surgery is considered if there is recurrent infection or if the enlarged tonsils make swallowing or breathing difficult. Their removal may also help children suffering from otitis media, because bacteria infecting the tonsils may travel to the middle ear.

OTHER LYMPHOID TISSUE

The **appendix** (ah-PEN-diks) is a fingerlike tube of lymphatic tissue, measuring approximately 8 cm (3 in.) long. It is attached, or "appended" to the first portion of the large intestine **(see Fig. 15-5)**. Like the tonsils, it seems to be noticed only when it becomes infected, causing appendicitis. However, the appendix may, like the tonsils, figure in the development of immunity.

In the mucous membranes lining portions of the digestive, respiratory, and urogenital tracts, there are areas of lymphatic tissue that help destroy foreign contaminants. By means of phagocytosis and production of antibodies, substances that counteract infectious agents, this **mucosal-associated lymphoid tissue**, or **MALT**, prevents microorganisms from invading deeper tissues.

Peyer (PI-er) **patches** are part of the MALT system. These clusters of lymphoid nodules are located in the mucous membranes lining the distal small intestine. Peyer patches, along with the tonsils and appendix, are included in the specific network known as GALT, or gut-associated lymphoid tissue. All of these lymphatic tissues associated with mucous membranes are now recognized as an important first barrier against invading microorganisms.

CHECKPOINTS 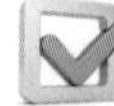

- ☐ 15-4 What is the function of the lymph nodes?
- ☐ 15-5 What is filtered by the spleen?
- ☐ 15-6 What kind of immune system cells develop in the thymus?
- ☐ 15-7 What is the general location of the tonsils?

The body is constantly exposed to harmful organisms such as bacteria and viruses. Fortunately, most of us survive contact with these invaders and even become more resistant to disease in the process. All of the defenses that protect us against disease constitute **immunity.** These defenses protect us against any harmful agent that enters the body, such as an infectious organism. They also protect against abnormal cells that arise within the body, such as tumor cells. Although immune defenses are critical to protection from cancer, this chapter will concentrate on immunity as it applies to invasion by infectious organisms. Some immune defenses are *nonspecific*; that is, they are effective against any harmful agent. Others are referred to as *specific*; that is, they act only against a certain agent and no others. Scientists use the term *immune system* to describe all the cells and tissues that protect us against foreign organisms or any cells different from our own normal cells.

Nonspecific Immunity

The features that protect the body against disease are usually considered successive "lines of defense," beginning with the relatively simple outer barriers and proceeding through progressively more complicated responses until the ultimate defense mechanism—specific immunity—is reached. Nonspecific defenses are inborn, or *innate*, that is, they are inherited along with all of a person's other characteristics. They include barriers and certain internal cellular and metabolic responses that protect against any foreign invaders or harmful substances.

THE FIRST LINE OF DEFENSE: BARRIERS

The first defense against invading organisms includes chemical and mechanical barriers, such as the following (Fig. 15-7):

- The skin serves as a mechanical barrier as long as it remains intact. A serious danger to burn victims, for example, is the risk of infection as a result of skin destruction.

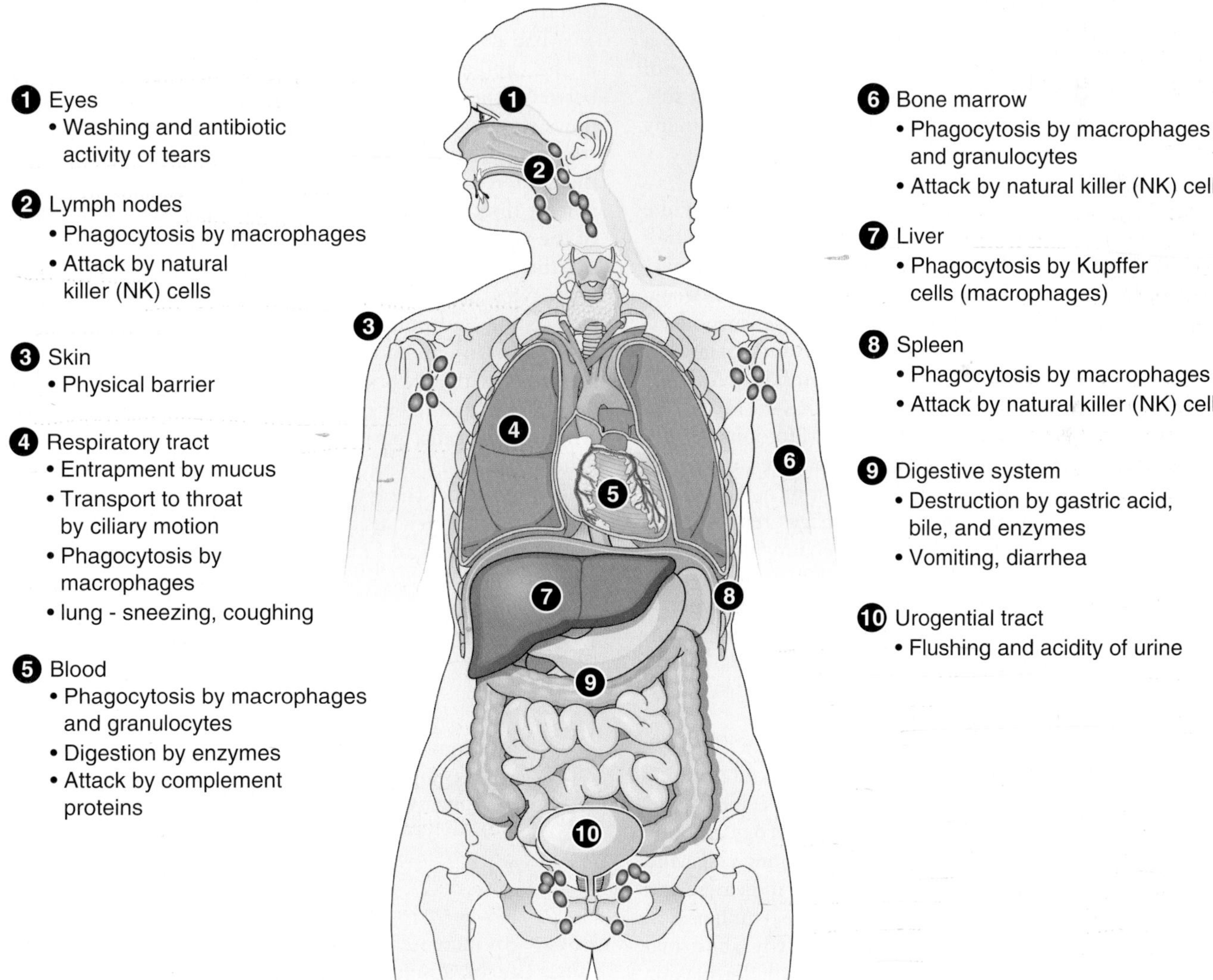

Figure 15-7 Nonspecific immunity. KEY POINT Various organs and systems contribute to our nonspecific (innate) defenses against foreign and abnormal antigens. The numbers show some sites of these activities. (Reprinted with permission from McConnell TH, *The Nature of Disease*, Philadelphia, PA: Lippincott Williams & Wilkins, 2007.)

15

- The mucous membranes that line the passageways leading into the body also act as barriers, trapping foreign material in their sticky secretions. The cilia in membranes in the upper respiratory tract help to sweep impurities out of the body.
- Body secretions, such as tears, perspiration, and saliva, wash away microorganisms and may contain acids, enzymes, or other chemicals that destroy invaders. Digestive juices destroy many ingested bacteria and their toxins (poisons).
- Certain reflexes aid in the removal of pathogens. Sneezing and coughing, for instance, tend to remove foreign matter, including microorganisms, from the upper respiratory tract. Vomiting and diarrhea are ways in which ingested toxins and bacteria may be expelled.

THE SECOND LINE OF DEFENSE: INTERNAL NONSPECIFIC RESPONSES

If an organism has overcome initial defenses, we have a number of internal activities that constitute a second line of defense **(see Fig. 15-7)**. Although we present them in a separate category, you will see later in this chapter that many participate in and promote specific immune responses.

Phagocytosis In the process of phagocytosis, white blood cells take in and destroy waste and foreign material. (See **Fig. 12-5** in Chapter 12.) Worn-out blood cells, bacteria, cancer cells, and other potentially harmful foreign substances are eliminated by phagocytosis. Neutrophils, a category of granular leukocytes, are important phagocytic white blood cells. (See **Table 12-2** in Chapter 12.) Another active phagocyte is the macrophage (MAK-ro-faj). (The name *macrophage* means "big eater.") Macrophages are large white blood cells derived from monocytes, a type of agranular leukocyte. Monocytes develop into macrophages upon entering the tissues. Some macrophages remain fixed in the tissues, for example, in the skin, liver, lungs, lymphoid tissue, bone marrow, and soft connective tissue throughout the body. In some organs, macrophages are given special names. For example, Kupffer (KOOP-fer) cells are macrophages located in the lining of the liver sinusoids (blood channels). In the lungs, where they ingest solid particles, macrophages are called *dust cells*.

Natural Killer Cells The natural killer (NK) cell is a type of lymphocyte different from those active in specific immunity, which are described later. NK cells can recognize body cells with abnormal membranes, such as tumor cells and cells infected with virus, and as their name indicates, can kill them on contact. NK cells are found in the lymph nodes, spleen, bone marrow, and blood. They destroy abnormal cells by secreting a protein that breaks down the plasma membrane, but the way in which they find their targets is not yet completely understood.

Inflammation **Inflammation** is a nonspecific defensive response to a tissue-damaging irritant. Any irritant can cause inflammation: friction, x-rays, fire, extreme temperatures, and wounds, as well as caustic chemicals and contact with allergens—all can be classified as irritants. Often, however, inflammation results from irritation caused by infection. With the entrance and multiplication of pathogens, a whole series of defensive processes begins. This inflammatory reaction is accompanied by four classic symptoms: heat, redness, swelling, and pain, as described below.

When tissues are injured, damaged cells release **histamine** (HIS-tah-mene) and other substances that cause the small blood vessels to dilate (widen) **(Fig. 15-8)**. They also release attractant substances that bring a variety of white blood cells to the area, including granulocytes, macrophages, and **mast cells**, which are similar to basophils but reside in the tissues. These cells also secrete vasodilators and other substances that promote and prolong the inflammatory response. Increased blood flow causes heat, redness, and swelling in the tissues. Some of these substances also irritate pain receptors.

The cellular secretions then cause the epithelial cells in the capillary walls to contract, thus widening the gaps between the cells and increasing permeability. As blood flows slowly through the vessels, granulocytes, mainly neutrophils, adhere to the vessel wall and then move through these altered walls into the tissue. Here, they can reach the irritant directly. Fluid from the blood plasma also leaks out of the vessels into the tissues and begins to clot, thus limiting the spread of infection to other areas. The mixture of leukocytes and fluid, the **inflammatory exudate**, contributes to swelling and puts pressure on nerve endings, adding to the pain of inflammation. Phagocytes are destroyed in large numbers as they work, and dead cells gradually accumulate in the area. The mixture of exudate, living and dead white blood cells, pathogens, and destroyed tissue cells is called "pus."

Meanwhile, the lymphatic vessels begin to drain fluid from the inflamed area and carry it toward the lymph nodes for filtration. The regional lymph nodes become enlarged and tender, a sign that they are performing their protective function by working overtime to produce phagocytic cells that "clean" the lymph flowing through them **(see Fig. 15-7)**.

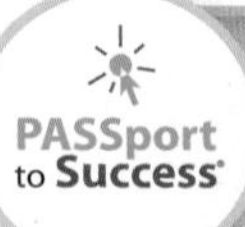

See the Student Resources on *thePoint* for a diagram summarizing the events in inflammation and for the *animation Acute* Inflammation.

Fever An increase in body temperature above the normal range can be a sign that body defenses are active. When phagocytes are exposed to infecting organisms, they release substances that raise body temperature. Fever boosts the immune system in several ways. It stimulates phagocytes, increases metabolism, and decreases certain disease organisms' ability to multiply.

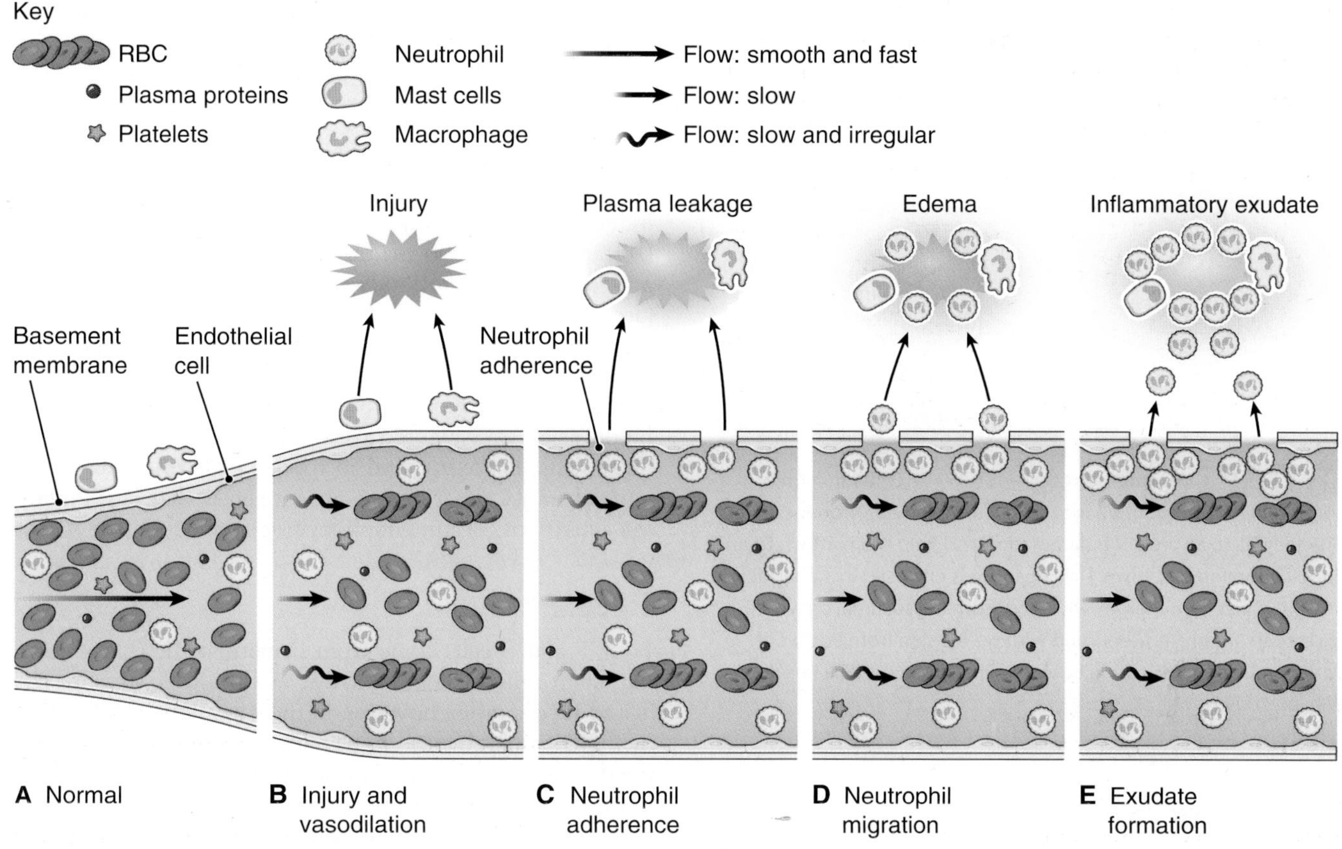

Figure 15-8 Inflammation. KEY POINT Acute inflammation involves components in blood and tissues. **A.** Normal capillary. **B** After injury, capillaries dilate and blood volume increases, but the flow rate slows and is irregular near the capillary wall. Tissue macrophages and mast cells migrate toward the injury. **C.** Injured endothelial cells become "sticky" and "leaky." Plasma leaks into the injury site. Granulocytes (mainly neutrophils) adhere to the endothelium. **D.** Plasma causes edema (swelling). Granulocytes migrate through the capillary wall. **E.** An inflammatory exudate forms from fluid and cells. (Reprinted with permission from McConnell TH, *The Nature of Disease*, Philadelphia, PA: Lippincott Williams & Wilkins, 2007.) ZOOMING IN What causes the heat, redness, swelling, and pain characteristic of inflammation?.

15

A common misperception is that fever is a dangerous symptom that should always be eliminated. Control of fever in itself does little to alter the course of an illness. Healthcare workers, however, should always be alert to fever development as a possible sign of a serious disorder and should recognize that an increased metabolic rate may have adverse effects on a weak patient's heart.

Interferon Certain cells infected with a virus release a substance that prevents nearby cells from producing more viruses. This substance was first found in cells infected with influenza virus, and it was called "interferon" because it "interferes" with multiplication and spread of the virus. Interferon is now known to be a group of substances. Each is abbreviated as IFN with a Greek letter, alpha (α), beta (β), or gamma (γ), to indicate different categories.

Pure interferons are now being produced by genetic engineering in microorganisms, making available adequate quantities for medical therapy. They are used to treat certain viral infections, such as hepatitis. Interferons are also of interest because they act nonspecifically on cells of the immune system. They have been used with varying success to boost the immune response in the treatment of malignancies, such as melanoma, leukemia, and Kaposi sarcoma, a cancer associated with AIDS. Interestingly, IFN-β is used to treat the autoimmune disorder multiple sclerosis (MS), because it stimulates cells that depress the immune response.

Complement The destruction of foreign cells sometimes requires the activity of a group of nonspecific proteins in the blood, together called **complement** (Fig. 15-9). Complement proteins are always present in the blood, but they must be activated by contact with foreign cell surfaces or by specific immune complexes (described shortly). Complement is so named because it complements (assists with) immune reactions. Some of complement's actions are to:

- Bind to foreign cells to help phagocytes recognize and engulf them
- Destroy cells by forming complexes that punch holes in plasma membranes
- Promote inflammation by increasing capillary permeability
- Attract phagocytes to an area of inflammation.

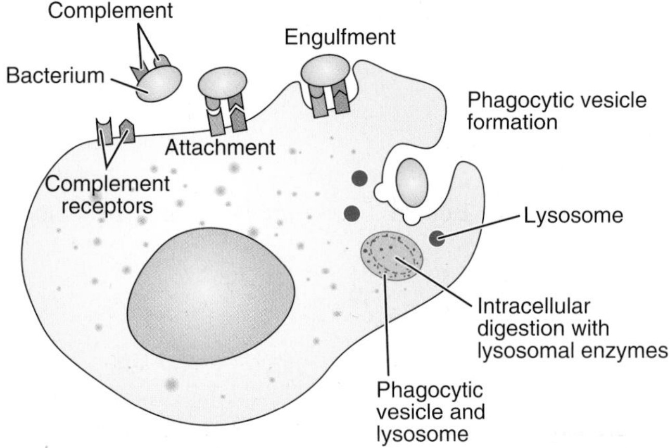

Figure 15-9 Complement. KEY POINT One function of complement is to aid in phagocytosis. Complement proteins attract phagocytes to an area of inflammation and help them attach to and engulf a foreign organism. The organism is enclosed in a phagocytic vesicle, which then merges with a lysosome. Lysosomal enzymes digest the organism. (Reprinted with permission from Porth CM, *Pathophysiology*, 7th ed. Philadelphia, PA: Lippincott Williams & Wilkins, 2005.)

CHECKPOINTS

- **15-8** What constitutes the first line of defense against the invasion of pathogens?
- **15-9** What are some factors in the second line of defense against infection?
- **15-10** What is complement?

Specific Immunity: The Final Line of Defense

Specific immunity to disease can be defined as an individual's power to resist or overcome the effects of a *particular* disease agent or its harmful products. In a broader sense, these defense mechanisms will recognize *any* foreign material and attempt to get rid of it, as occurs in tissue transplantation from one individual to another. Specific immunity is a selective process (i.e., immunity to one disease does not necessarily cause immunity to another). This selective characteristic is called **specificity** (spes-ih-FIS-ih-te).

Specific immunity is also termed **acquired immunity**, because it develops during a person's lifetime as he or she encounters various specific harmful agents. Another term used is *adaptive immunity*, because this response alters to provide protection against further challenges. If the following description of specific immunity seems complex, bear in mind that from infancy onward, your immune system is able to protect you from millions of foreign substances, even synthetic substances not found in nature. All the while, the system is kept in check, so that it does not usually overreact to produce allergies or mistakenly attack and damage your own body tissues.

ANTIGENS

Specific immunity is based on the body's ability to recognize a particular foreign substance. Any foreign substance that induces an immune response is called an **antigen** (AN-te-jen) **(Ag).** (The word is formed from *anti*body + *gen*, because an antigen generates antibody production.) Most antigens are large protein molecules, but carbohydrates and some lipids also may act as antigens. Normally, only nonself antigens stimulate an immune response. Such antigens can be found on the surfaces of pathogenic organisms, transfused blood cells, transplanted tissues, cancerous cells, and also on pollens, in toxins, and in foods. The critical feature of any substance described as an antigen is that it stimulates the activity of certain lymphocytes classified as T or B cells.

T CELLS

Both T and B cells come from hematopoietic (blood-forming) stem cells in bone marrow, as do all blood cells. The T and B cells differ, however, in their development and their method of action. Some of the immature stem cells migrate to the thymus and become T cells, which constitute about 80% of the lymphocytes in the circulating blood. While in the thymus, these T lymphocytes multiply and become capable of combining with specific foreign antigens, at which time they are described as *sensitized*. These thymus-derived cells produce an immunity that is said to be **cell-mediated immunity**.

There are several types of T cells, each with different functions. The different types and some of their functions are as follows:

- **Cytotoxic T cells** (T_c) destroy certain abnormal cells directly. They recognize cells infected with viruses or other intracellular pathogens, cancer cells, and foreign antigens present in transplanted tissue. They are able to form pores in the plasma membranes of these cells and insert enzymes that destroy the cell. They also produce substances that cause the cells to "self-destruct" by apoptosis.
- **Helper T cells** (T_h) are essential to the immune response through the release of substances known as **interleukins** (in-ter-LU-kinz) (IL). These substances stimulate the production of cytotoxic T cells as well as B cells and macrophages. (Interleukins are so named because they act between white blood cells). There are several subtypes of helper T cells, one of which is infected and destroyed by the AIDS virus (HIV). The HIV-targeted T cells have a special surface receptor (CD4) to which the virus attaches, as described later.
- **Regulatory T cells** (T_{reg}) suppress the immune response in order to prevent overactivity. These T cells may inhibit or destroy active lymphocytes.
- **Memory T cells** remember an antigen and start a rapid response if that antigen is contacted again.

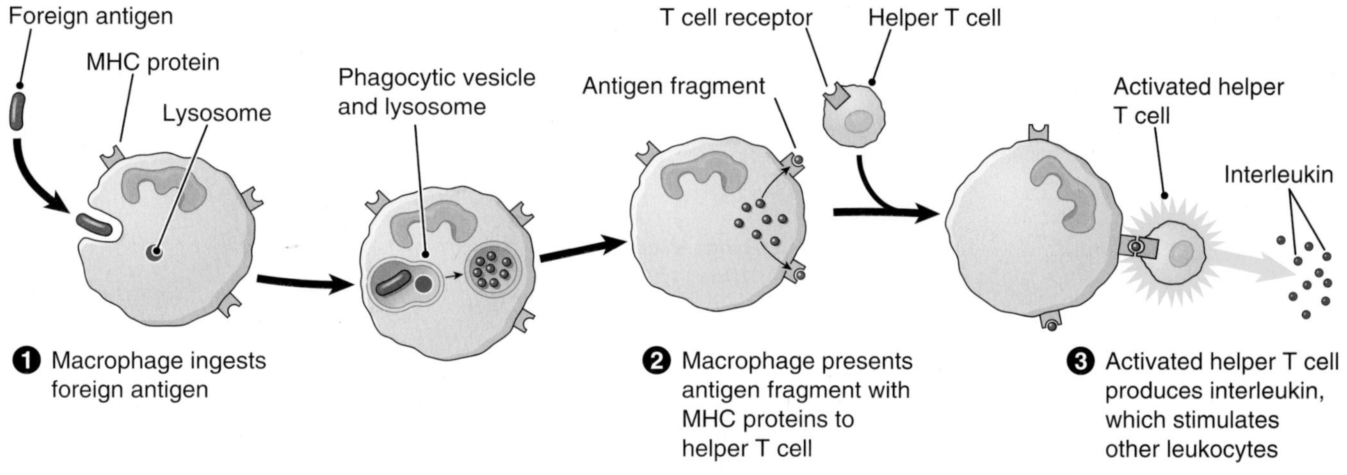

Figure 15-10 Activation of a helper T cell by a macrophage (antigen-presenting cell—APC). KEY POINT An antigen-presenting cell (APC) displays digested foreign antigen on its surface along with self major histocompatibility complex (MHC) antigen. A helper T cell is activated by contact with this complex and produces stimulatory interleukins. ZOOMING IN What is contained in the lysosome that joins the phagocytic vesicle?

The T cell portion of the immune system is generally responsible for defense against cancer cells, certain viruses, and other pathogens that grow within cells (intracellular parasites), as well as for the rejection of tissue transplanted from another person.

Antigen-Presenting Cells T cells cannot respond to foreign antigens directly. Instead, the antigen must be "presented" to them by an antigen-presenting cell (APC). The most important APCs are macrophages, which were discussed earlier, and *dendritic* cells large phagocytic cells with many fibrous processes. Like macrophages, dendritic cells are derived from monocytes. An APC acts as a processing center for foreign antigens. First, it ingests the foreign material, such as a disease organism, enclosing it in a vesicle. As is typical in phagocytosis, this vesicle then merges with a lysosome filled with digestive enzymes that break down the organism (Fig. 15-10). However, the APC then inserts fragments of the foreign antigen into its plasma membrane—in a sense, advertising them to helper T cells. They display the foreign antigen in combination with antigens that a T_h cell can recognize as belonging to the "self." Self-antigens are known as MHC (major histocompatibility complex) antigens because of their importance in cross-matching for tissue transplantation. They are also known as HLAs (human leukocyte antigens), because white blood cells are used in testing tissues for compatibility.

For a T_h cell to react with a foreign antigen, that antigen must be presented to the T_h cell along with the MHC proteins. A special receptor on the T_h cell must bind with both the MHC protein and the foreign antigen fragment (see Fig. 15-10). The activated T_h cell then produces ILs, which stimulate other leukocytes, such as B cells. There are many different types of ILs, and they participate at different points in the immune response. They are produced not only by leukocytes, but also by fibroblasts (cells in connective tissue that produce fibers) and by epithelial cells. Because ILs stimulate the cells active in immunity, they are used medically to boost the immune system.

CHECKPOINTS 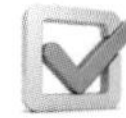

- 15-11 What is acquired immunity?
- 15-12 What is an antigen?
- 15-13 List four types of T cells.
- 15-14 What is the role of APCs in immunity?

B CELLS AND ANTIBODIES

B cells (B lymphocytes) are the second main class of lymphocytes active in immunity. Whereas T cells mature in the thymus, B cells mature in the red bone marrow before becoming active in the blood. B cells function in immunity by producing Y-shaped proteins called **antibodies (Ab)**, also known as **immunoglobulins (Ig)**, in response to a foreign antigen. (Globulins, in general, are a class of folded proteins described in Chapter 2. Another example of these proteins is hemoglobin.)

B cells have surface receptors that bind with a specific type of antigen (Fig. 15-11). Exposure to the antigen stimulates the cells to multiply rapidly and produce large numbers (clones) of **plasma cells.** These mature cells produce antibodies against the original antigen and release them into the blood, providing a form of immunity described as **humoral immunity** (the term *humoral* refers to body fluids). Humoral immunity is long term and generally protects against circulating antigens and bacteria that grow outside the cells (extracellular pathogens). All antibodies are contained in a portion of the blood plasma called the **gamma globulin** fraction.

The antibody that is produced in response to a specific antigen, such as a bacterial cell or a toxin, has a shape that

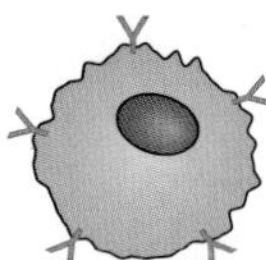

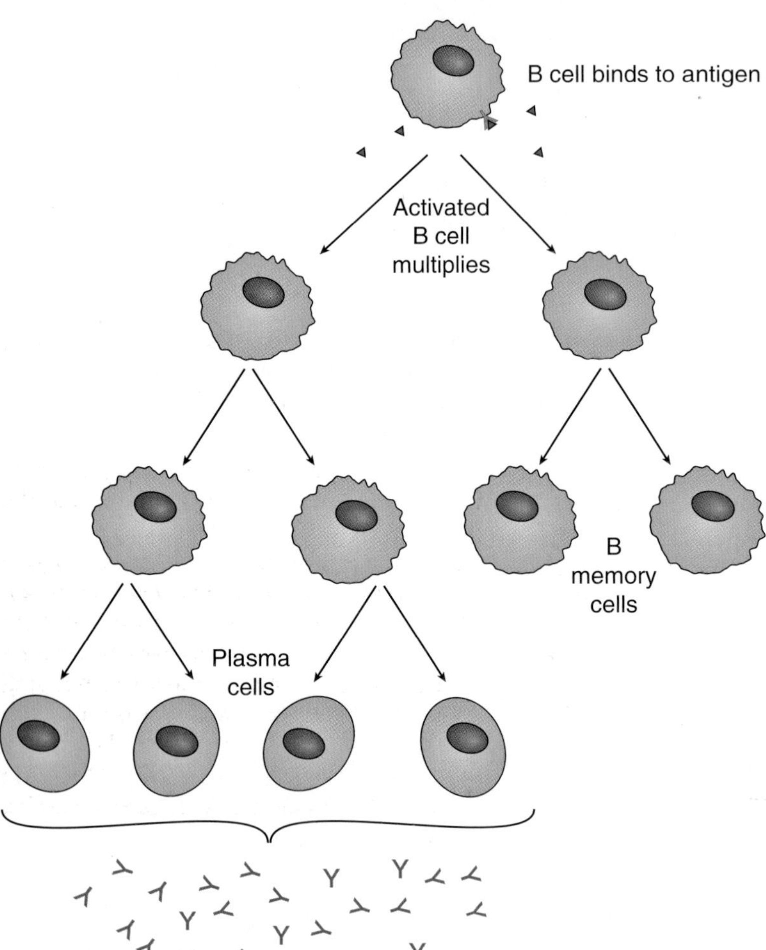

Figure 15-11 Activation of B cells. KEY POINT The B cell combines with a specific antigen. The cell divides to form plasma cells, which produce antibodies. Some of the cells develop into memory cells, which protect against reinfection. ZOOMING IN What two types of cells develop from activated B cells?

matches some part of that antigen, much in the same way that a key's shape matches the shape of its lock. The antibody can bind only to the antigen that caused its production. Antibodies do not destroy cells directly; rather, they assist in the immune response. For example, they prevent a pathogen's attachment to a host cell; help with phagocytosis; activate NK cells; and neutralize toxins. The antigen–antibody complex may activate the complement system, which helps in immunity, as previously described. These antigen–antibody interactions are illustrated and their protective effects are described in **Table 15-1**.

Notice in **Figure 15-11** that some of the activated B cells do not become plasma cells but, like certain T cells, become memory cells. These do not immediately produce antibodies. Instead, they circulate in the bloodstream and, upon repeated contact with an antigen, immediately begin dividing to produce many active plasma cells. Because of this "immunologic memory," one is usually immune to a childhood disease, such as chicken pox, after having it.

Figure 15-12 illustrates this secondary response. There are five different classes of antibodies distinguished by their locations and functions. The antibodies in this figure are designated as IgM (immunoglobulin M) and IgG (immunoglobulin G). IgM is the first type of antibody produced in an immune response, followed shortly by IgG. A second encounter with the antigen stimulates production of both types of antibodies, but has a much greater effect on IgG production. These and the other classes of immunoglobulins are described in **Box 15-2**.

CHECKPOINTS 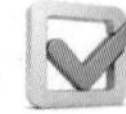

- [ ] **15-15** What is an antibody?
- [ ] **15-16** What type of cells produce antibodies?

Table 15-1 Antigen–Antibody Interactions and Their Effects

Interaction	Effects
Prevention of attachment	A pathogen coated with antibody is prevented from attaching to a cell.
Clumping of antigen	Antibodies can link antigens together, forming a cluster that phagocytes can ingest.
Neutralization of toxins	Antibodies bind to toxin molecules to prevent them from damaging cells.
Help with phagocytosis	Phagocytes can attach more easily to antigens that are coated with antibody.
Activation of complement	When complement attaches to antibody on a cell surface, a series of reactions begins that activates complement to destroy cells.
Activation of NK cells	NK cells respond to antibody adhering to a cell surface and attack the cell.

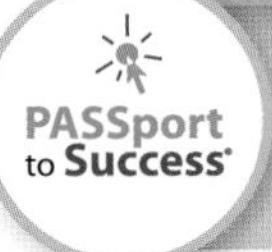

See the Student Resources on *thePoint* for the animation *Immune Response*.

NATURAL ACQUIRED IMMUNITY

As we have just seen, acquired immunity may develop naturally through contact with a specific disease organism. In this case, the infected person's T cells and antibodies act against the infecting agent or its toxins. The infection that triggers the immunity may be so mild as to cause no symptoms (is subclinical). Nevertheless, it stimulates the host's immune response. Moreover, each time a person is invaded by the disease organism, his or her cells will respond to the infection. Such immunity may last for years, and in some cases for life. Because the host is actively involved in generating protection, this type of immunity is described as *active*. Because the immunity is formed against harmful agents encountered in the normal course of life, it is called **natural active immunity** (Fig. 15-13).

Immunity also may be acquired naturally by the passage of antibodies from a mother to her fetus through the placenta. Because these antibodies come from an outside source, this type of immunity is called **natural passive immunity**. The antibodies obtained in this way do not last as long as actively produced antibodies, but they do help protect the infant for about 6 months, by which time the child's own immune system begins to function. Nursing an infant can lengthen this protective period because the mother's specific antibodies are present in her breast milk and colostrum (the first breast secretion). These are the only known examples of naturally acquired passive immunity.

Figure 15-12 Production of antibodies (Ab). KEY POINT Antibodies or immunoglobulins (Ig) are produced in response to a first encounter with a foreign antigen. A second exposure produces a greater response. Immunoglobulin M (IgM) and immunoglobulin G (IgG) are two of the five classes of antibodies.

ARTIFICIALLY ACQUIRED IMMUNITY

A person who has not been exposed to a particular antigen has no antibodies or T cells against that organism and may be defenseless against infection. Therefore, medical personnel may use artificial measures to establish immunity. As with naturally acquired immunity, artificially acquired immunity may be active or passive (see Fig. 15-13).

Artificial Active Immunity The administration of virulent pathogens to stimulate immunity obviously would be dangerous. Instead, laboratory workers treat the harmful agent to reduce its virulence before it is administered. In this way, the antibodies are produced without causing a serious illness. This protective process is known as immunization, or vaccination (vak-sin-A-shun), and the solution used is called a vaccine (vak-SENE). Ordinarily, the administration of a vaccine is a preventive measure designed to provide protection in anticipation of contact with a specific disease organism.

Originally, the word *vaccination* meant inoculation against smallpox. (The term even comes from the Latin word for *cow*, referring to cowpox, which was used to vaccinate against smallpox.) According to the World Health

Box 15-2 *A Closer Look*

Antibodies: A Protein Army That Fights Disease

Antibodies are proteins secreted by plasma cells (activated B cells) in response to specific antigens. They are all contained in a fraction of the blood plasma known as gamma globulin. Because the plasma contains other globulins as well, antibodies have become known as immunoglobulins (Ig). Immunologic studies have shown that there are several classes of immunoglobulins that vary in molecular size and in function (see below). Studies of these antibody fractions can be helpful in making a diagnosis. For example, high levels of IgM antibodies, because they are the first to be produced in an immune response, indicate a recent infection.

Class	Abundance	Characteristics and Function
IgG	75%	Found in the blood, lymph, and intestines Enhances phagocytosis, neutralizes toxins, and activates complement Crosses the placenta and confers passive immunity from mother to fetus
IgA	15%	Found in glandular secretions such as sweat, tears, saliva, mucus, and digestive juices Provides local protection in mucous membranes against bacteria and viruses Also found in breast milk, providing passive immunity to newborn
IgM	5%–10%	Found in the blood and lymph The first antibody to be secreted after infection Stimulates agglutination and activates complement
IgD	<1%	Located on the surface of B cells
IgE	<0.1%	Located on basophils and mast cells Active in allergic reactions and parasitic infections

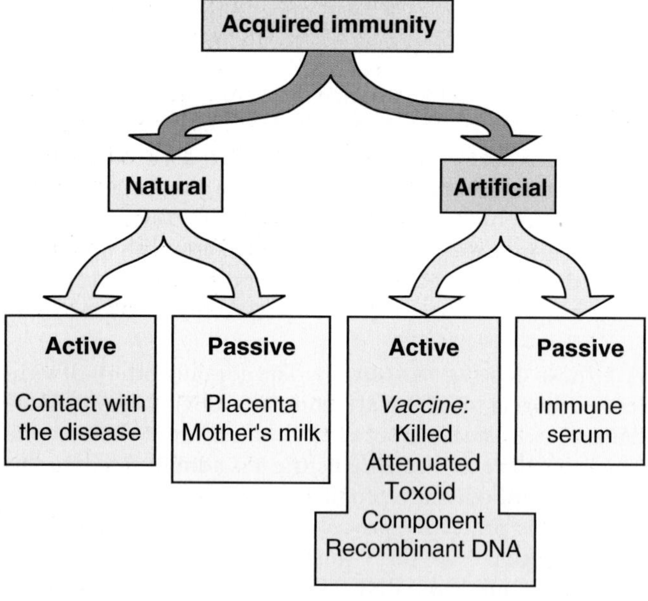

Figure 15-13 Specific immunity. KEY POINT Specific immunity, also called acquired or adaptive immunity, is a response to a particular antigen. Acquired immunity may develop naturally (as by contact with the disease) or by artificial means (as by vaccination). Both natural and artificial acquired immunity may be active (generated by the individual) or passive (provided from an outside source).

Organization, however, smallpox has now been eliminated as a result of widespread immunization programs. Mandatory vaccination against smallpox has been discontinued because the chance of adverse side effects from the vaccine is thought to be greater than the probability of contracting the disease.

All vaccines carry a small risk of adverse side effects and may be contraindicated in some cases. People who are immunosuppressed, for example, should not be given vaccines that contain live virus. Also, pregnant women should not receive live virus vaccine because the virus could cross the placenta and harm the fetus. In general, however, vaccines are extensively tested for safety and, for most people, their potential benefits far outweigh their risks.

Types of Vaccines Vaccines can be made with live organisms or with organisms killed by heat or chemicals. If live organisms are used, they must be nonvirulent for humans, such as the cowpox virus used for smallpox immunization, or they must be treated in the laboratory to weaken them as human pathogens. An organism weakened for use in vaccines is described as **attenuated**. Another type of vaccine is made from the toxin produced by a disease organism. The toxin is altered with heat or chemicals to reduce its harmfulness, but it can still function as an antigen to induce immunity. Such an altered toxin is called a **toxoid**.

Table 15-2 Childhood Immunizations (birth to 6 years)[a]

Vaccine	Disease(s)	Schedule
DTaP	Diphtheria, tetanus, pertussis (whooping cough)	2, 4, 6, and 15–18 mo; booster at 4–6 y Diphtheria and tetanus toxoid (Td) at 11–12 y
Hib	*Haemophilus influenza* type b (spinal meningitis)	2 and 4 mo or 2, 4, and 6 mo depending on type used
HAV	Hepatitis A virus	High risk children at 12–23 mo; second dose 6 mo later
HBV	Hepatitis B	Birth, 1–2 mo, 6–18 mo
Influenza	Influenza ("flu")	Yearly from 6 mo to 6 y
MMR	Measles, mumps, rubella	15 mo and 4–6 y
PCV	Pneumococcus (pneumonia, meningitis)	2, 4, 6, and 12–15 mo
Polio vaccine (IPV)	Poliomyelitis	2 and 4 mo, 6–18 mo, and 4–6 y
Rotavirus	Rotavirus gastroenteritis	2, 4, and 6 mo
Varicella	Chickenpox	12–15 mo and 4–6 y

[a]Recommended by the Advisory Committee on Immunization Practices (www.cdc.gov/vaccines/recs/acip), the American Academy of Pediatrics (www.aap.org), and the American Academy of Family Physicians (www.aafp.org). Information is also available through the National Immunization Program website (www.cdc.gov/vaccines).

The newest types of vaccines are produced from antigenic components of pathogens or by genetic engineering. By techniques of recombinant DNA, the genes for specific disease antigens are inserted into the genetic material of harmless organisms. The antigens produced by these organisms are extracted and purified and used for immunization. The hepatitis B vaccine is produced in this manner.

Boosters In many cases, an active immunity acquired by artificial (or even natural) means does not last a lifetime. Circulating antibodies can decline with time. To help maintain a high titer (level) of antibodies in the blood, repeated inoculations, called *booster shots*, are administered at intervals. The number of booster injections recommended varies with the disease and with an individual's environment or degree of exposure. On occasion, epidemics in high schools or colleges may prompt recommendations for specific boosters. Table 15-2 lists the vaccines currently recommended in the United States for childhood immunizations. The number and timing of doses varies with the different vaccines.

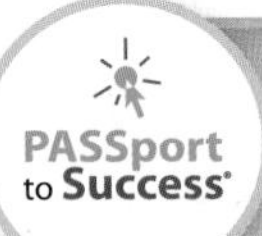

Nurse practitioners often prescribe and administer vaccines. See the Student Resources on *thePoint* to read about this career, and specifically about pediatric nurse practitioners.

Artificial Passive Immunity It takes several weeks to produce a naturally acquired active immunity and even longer to produce an artificial active immunity through the administration of a vaccine. Therefore, a person who receives a large dose of virulent organisms and has no established immunity to them is in great danger. To prevent illness, the person must quickly receive counteracting antibodies from an outside source. This is accomplished through the administration of an **immune serum**, or **antiserum**. The "ready-made" serum gives short-lived but effective protection against the organisms in the form of an artificially acquired passive immunity. Immune sera are used in emergencies, that is, in situations in which there is no time to wait until an active immunity has developed.

15

Preparation of Antisera Immune sera often are derived from animals, mainly horses. It has been found that the horse's tissues produce large quantities of antibodies in response to the injection of organisms or their toxins. After repeated injections, the horse is bled according to careful sterile technique; because of the animal's size, it is possible to remove large quantities of blood without causing injury. The blood is allowed to clot, and the serum is removed and packaged in sterile containers.

Injecting humans with serum derived from animals is not without its problems. The foreign proteins in animal sera may cause an often serious sensitivity reaction, called **serum sickness**. To avoid this problem, human antibody in the form of gamma globulin may be used.

CHECKPOINTS 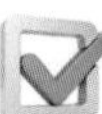

☐ **15-17** What is the difference between natural and artificial acquired immunity?

☐ **15-18** What is the difference between the active and passive forms of acquired immunity?

A&P in Action Revisited

Mike's Splenectomy

Mike lay in his hospital bed thinking about the past couple of days. After the surgery, his doctor had explained that removal of his spleen had been necessary because it had ruptured during the car accident. He was still coming to terms with what that meant. In fact, until today, he was not even sure what the spleen was!

Earlier in the morning, Mike's physician had come by to check in on him. During their conversation, Mike learned that the spleen is a bean-shaped purple organ about the size of a large bar of soap. It is normally located underneath the diaphragm in the upper left part of the abdomen. Given how little he knew about it, Mike was surprised to learn that one of the spleen's functions is to filter foreign substances from the blood and remove worn-out red blood cells. "You mean it's like an oil filter on a car?" asked Mike. "Sort of," replied the doctor. "But don't worry, other parts of your circulatory system will help clean your blood now."

Mike also learned that the spleen acts like a large lymph node, detecting and fighting disease-causing organisms. "So, now that my spleen is gone, am I going to be sick all the time?" asked Mike. "Well," answered his doctor, "as you recover, you'll need to take antibiotics to reduce the risk of infection. In the long term, if you have a fever or any sign of illness, come see me right away. In addition, make sure that you get your yearly flu vaccinations."

During this case, we saw that the spleen filters blood and protects the body from harmful organisms. Now that Mike is missing his spleen, he will need to keep his immune system healthy.

Chapter Wrap-Up

Summary Overview

A detailed chapter outline with space for note-taking is on *thePoint*. The figure below illustrates the main topics covered in this chapter.

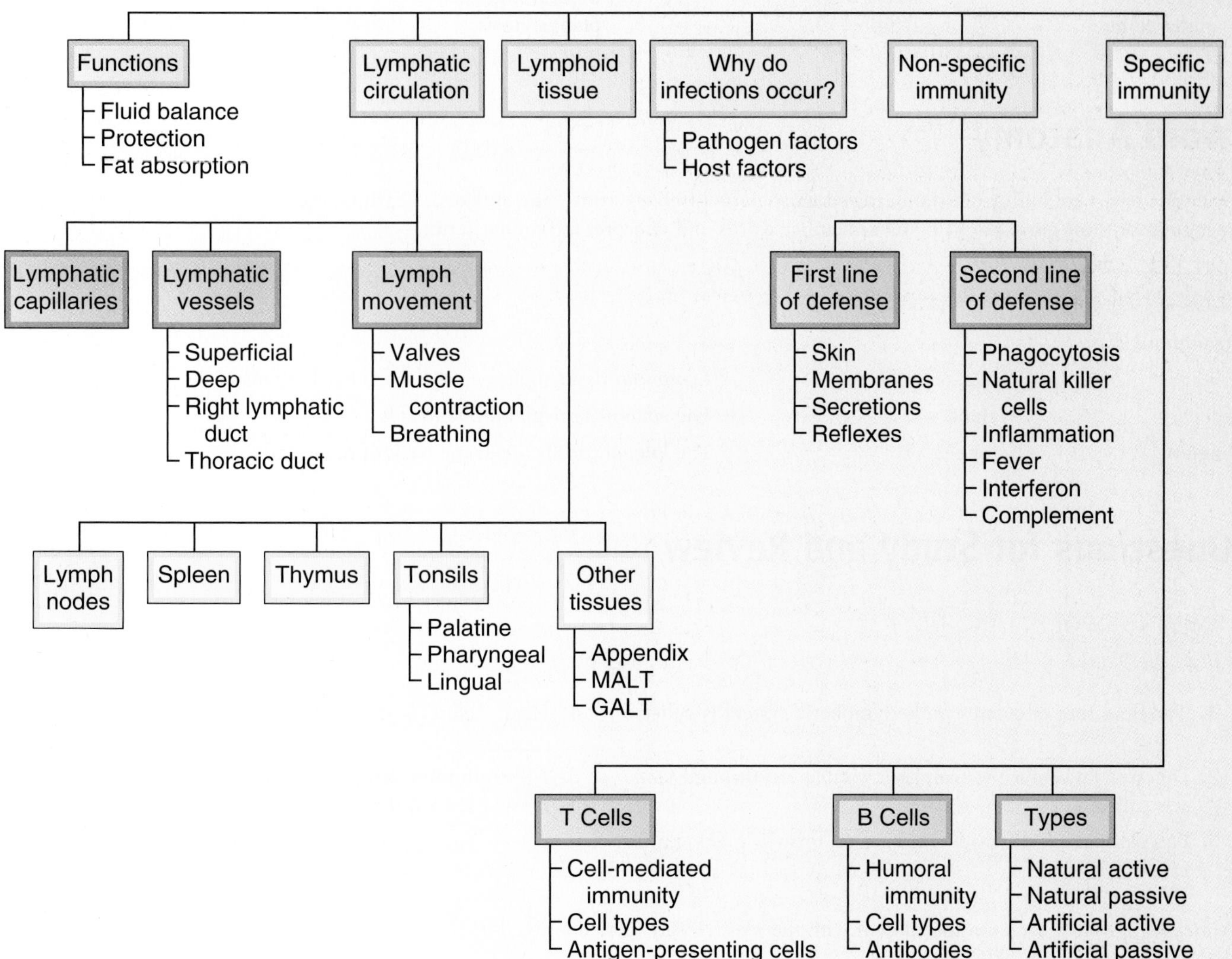

Key Terms

The terms listed below are emphasized in this chapter. Knowing them will help you organize and prioritize your learning. These and other boldface terms are defined in the Glossary with phonetic pronunciations.

adenoid
antibody
antigen
B cell
chyle
complement
gamma globulin
immunity
immunization
immunoglobulin
inflammation
interferon
interleukin
lymph
lymphatic duct
lymph node
lymphocyte
macrophage
mast cell
natural killer cell
phagocytosis
plasma cell
spleen
T cell
thymus
tonsil
vaccine

Word Anatomy

Scientific terms are built from standardized word parts (prefixes, roots, and suffixes). Learning the meanings of these parts can help you remember words and interpret unfamiliar terms.

WORD PART	MEANING	EXAMPLE
Lymphoid Tissue		
-oid	like, resembling	*Lymphoid* tissue makes up the specialized organs of the lymphatic system.
aden/o	gland	The *adenoids* are gland-like tonsils.
lingu/o	tongue	The *lingual* tonsils are at the back of the tongue.

Questions for Study and Review

BUILDING UNDERSTANDING

Fill in the Blanks

1. The fluid that circulates in the lymphatic system is called ______.
2. Digested fats enter the lymphatic circulation through vessels called______.
3. Fat globules and lymph combine to form a milky fluid called ______.
4. Heat, redness, swelling, and pain are classic signs of ______.
5. All antibodies are contained in a portion of the blood plasma termed the _____.

Matching > Match each numbered item with the most closely related lettered item.

___ **6.** Destroy foreign cells directly
___ **7.** Release interleukins, which stimulate other cells to join the immune response
___ **8.** Regulate the immune response to prevent overactivity
___ **9.** Tumor that occurs in lymphoid tissue
___ **10.** Manufacture antibodies when activated by antigens

a. regulatory T cells
b. memory T cells
c. cytotoxic T cells
d. B cells
e. helper T cells

Multiple Choice

___ **11.** Compared to plasma, lymph contains much less

a. fat
b. carbohydrate
c. protein
d. water

___ **12.** Which vessel returns lymph from the lower extremities to the cardiovascular system?

a. appendix
b. lacteal
c. right lymphatic duct
d. thoracic duct

___ **13.** Which of the following is part of the internal nonspecific response to infection?

a. tears
b. saliva
c. neutrophils
d. skin

___ **14.** Which of the following do damaged cells release?

a. interleukin
b. interferon
c. histamine
d. complement

___ **15.** Which cell matures in the thymus?

a. T cell
b. B cell
c. plasma cell
d. natural killer cell

UNDERSTANDING CONCEPTS

16. How does the structure of lymphatic capillaries correlate with their function? List some differences between lymphatic and blood capillaries.

17. Trace a globule of fat from a lacteal in the small intestine to the right atrium.

18. Describe the structure of a typical lymph node.

19. State the location of the spleen and list several of its functions.

20. What causes the symptoms of inflammation?

21. Differentiate between the terms in each of the following pairs:

a. interferon and interleukin
b. antibody and complement
c. nonspecific immunity and specific immunity
d. cell-mediated immunity and humoral immunity
e. active immunity and passive immunity
f. toxin and toxoid

22. Describe the events that must occur for a T cell to react with a foreign antigen. Once activated, what do the T cells do?

23. What role do antibodies play in immunity? How are they produced? How do they work?

24. Compare and contrast the four types of specific immunity.

CONCEPTUAL THINKING

25. Explain the absence of arteries in the lymphatic circulatory system.

26. In Mike's second case, he presented with hypotension and tachycardia due to a ruptured spleen. Explain how a ruptured spleen can cause these disorders.

27. In the case story, why was Mike treated with antibiotics and vaccinated for influenza following his splenectomy?

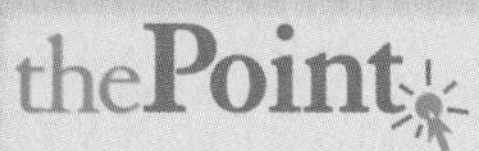

For more questions, see the learning activities on *thePoint*.

UNIT V

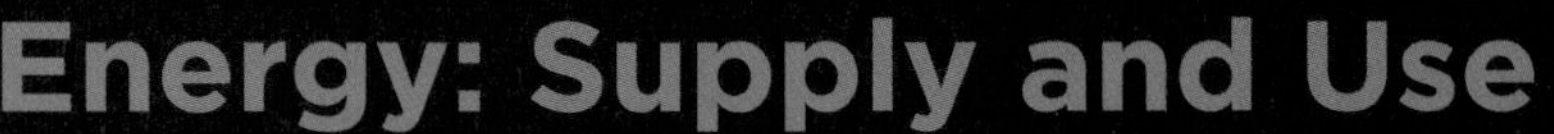

Energy: Supply and Use

The four chapters in this unit show how oxygen and nutrients are processed, taken up by the body fluids, and used by the cells to yield energy. This unit also describes how the stability of body functions (homeostasis) is maintained and how waste products are eliminated.

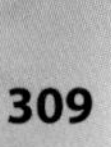

CHAPTER 16

The Respiratory System

A&P in Action

Emily's Case: Advances in Asthma Therapy

"Remind me to mention to Dr. Martinez that Emily still has that nagging cough," Nicole told her husband.

"I've been worried about that," he replied. "You know, I had asthma as a kid—I hope she doesn't. I could hardly do any sports without taking a couple puffs of my inhaler."

Later that week, Dr. Martinez listened carefully to 3-year-old Emily's lungs. He knew that the common symptoms of asthma—coughing, wheezing, and shortness of breath—were due to swelling of the airway tissues and spasm of the smooth muscle around them. "I don't hear any wheezing, but given the family history, we can't rule out asthma. In addition to the genetic component, asthma can have several environmental triggers such as respiratory infections, allergies, cold air, and exercise."

"Well," replied Nicole, "Emily did have a cold right before the coughing began. I haven't noticed any allergies, but now that I think about it, she did have a persistent cough last winter too. And, she is getting lots of exercise at preschool and dance class. If Emily does have asthma, will that limit her activities?"

"The asthma drugs we have now are much improved since your husband's youth. But first, we need to figure out what is causing Emily's cough. I'm going to order a chest x-ray to rule out infection. If Emily were a little bit older, we could measure her lung function with a spirometry test. For now, I'm going to ask you to monitor her for the next few weeks and see if anything exacerbates her symptoms. If she has asthma, we'll start daily treatment with a corticosteroid inhaler to control airway inflammation. Or, we could go with a long-term oral medication that prevents the lungs from producing leukotrienes, substances that cause constriction of smooth muscle in the airways. Emily will also need a short-term "rescue" inhaler in case of an acute attack."

Asthma is the most common chronic respiratory disease of childhood. In this chapter, we'll examine the respiratory system. Later in the chapter, we'll check in on Emily and learn about other medications used to treat asthma.

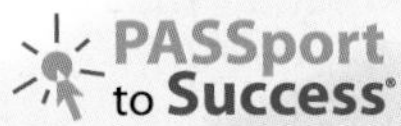

Ancillaries *At-A-Glance*

Visit *thePoint* to access the PASSport to Success and the following resources. For guidance in using these resources most effectively, see pp. ix–xviii.

Learning TOOLS

- Learning Style Self Assessment
- Live Advise Online Student Tutoring
- Tips for Effective Studying

Learning RESOURCES

- E-book: Chapter 16
- Web Figure: Principal muscles of breathing and lateral chest
- Animation: Pulmonary Ventilation
- Animation: Oxygen Transport
- Animation: Carbon Dioxide Exchange
- Health Professions: Respiratory Therapist
- Detailed Chapter Outline
- Answers to Questions for Study and Review
- Audio Pronunciation Glossary

Learning ACTIVITIES

- Pre-Quiz
- Visual Activities
- Kinesthetic Activities
- Auditory Activities

Learning Outcomes

After careful study of this chapter, you should be able to:

1. Define respiration and describe the four phases of respiration, ***p. 312***
2. Name and describe all the structures of the respiratory system, ***p. 313***
3. Explain the mechanism for pulmonary ventilation, ***p. 317***
4. Discuss the processes of internal and external gas exchange, ***p. 319***
5. List the ways in which oxygen and carbon dioxide are transported in the blood, ***p. 321***
6. Describe factors that control respiration, ***p. 322***
7. Discuss abnormal ventilation and give several examples of altered breathing patterns, ***p. 323***
8. Referring to the case study, discuss which parts of the respiratory system are affected by asthma, ***pp. 310, 326***
9. Show how word parts are used to build words related to respiration (see Word Anatomy at the end of the chapter), ***p. 328***

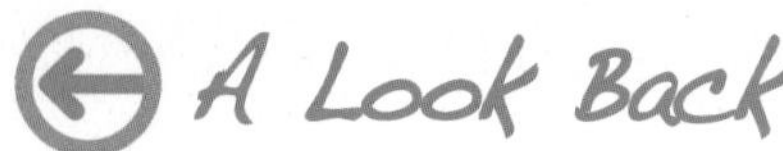

In Chapter 2, we talked about the properties of water that make it such a unique substance. Now we expand on the discussion to understand how water functions in respiration and gas exchange. The principles of diffusion, introduced in Chapter 3, apply to these exchanges. Finally, the ideas on compliance and elasticity, discussed in relation to the cardiovascular system, apply to respiratory physiology as well.

Phases of Respiration

Most people think of respiration simply as the process by which air moves into and out of the lungs—that is, *breathing*. By scientific definition, respiration is the process by which oxygen is obtained from the environment and delivered to the cells. Carbon dioxide is transported to the outside in a reverse pathway **(Fig. 16-1)**.

Respiration includes four phases:

- **Pulmonary ventilation,** which is the exchange of air between the atmosphere and the air sacs (alveoli) of the lungs. This is normally accomplished by the inhalation and exhalation of breathing.
- **External gas exchange,** which occurs in the lungs as oxygen (O_2) diffuses from the air sacs into the blood and carbon dioxide (CO_2) diffuses out of the blood to be eliminated.
- **Gas transport in the blood.** The circulating blood carries gases between the lungs and the tissues, supplying oxygen to the cells and bringing back carbon dioxide.

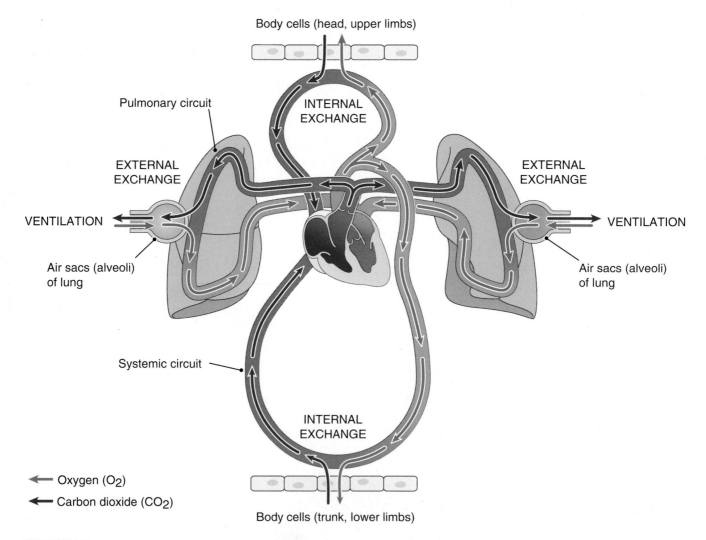

Figure 16-1 Overview of respiration. KEY POINT In ventilation, gases are moved into and out of the lungs. In external exchange, gases move between the air sacs (alveoli) of the lungs and the blood. In internal exchange, gases move between the blood and body cells. The circulation transports gases in the blood. ZOOMING IN From which side of the heart does blood leave to travel to the lungs? To which side does it return?

- **Internal gas exchange**, which occurs in the tissues as oxygen diffuses from the blood to the cells, whereas carbon dioxide travels from the cells into the blood.

The term *respiration* is also used to describe a related process that occurs at the cellular level. In cellular respiration, the cells take in oxygen and use it in the breakdown of nutrients. In this process, the cells release energy and carbon dioxide, a waste product of cellular respiration, as described in Chapter 18.

CHECKPOINT 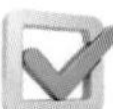

☐ 16-1 What are the four phases of respiration?

Structure of the Respiratory System

The respiratory system is a complex series of spaces and passageways that conduct air into and through the lungs (Fig. 16-2). These spaces include the nasal cavities; the pharynx, which is common to the digestive and respiratory systems; the voice box, or larynx; the windpipe, or trachea; and the lungs themselves, with their conducting tubes and air sacs. The entire system might be thought of as a pathway for gases between the atmosphere and the blood.

THE NASAL CAVITIES

Air enters the body through the openings in the nose called the **nostrils** or *nares* (NA-reze) (sing. naris). Immediately inside the nostrils, located between the roof of the mouth and the cranium, are the two spaces known as the **nasal cavities**. These two spaces are separated from each other by a partition, the **nasal septum**. The septum's superior portion is formed by a thin plate of the ethmoid bone that extends downward, and the inferior portion is formed by the vomer. (See Fig. 6-5A in Chapter 6.) An anterior extension of the septum is made of hyaline cartilage. The septum and the walls of the nasal cavity are covered with mucous membrane, consisting of stratified squamous (flat) epithelium, tissue that is resistant to wear.

On the lateral walls of each nasal cavity are three projections called the **conchae** (KONG-ke). (See Figs. 6-5A and 6-6 in Chapter 6.) The shell-like conchae greatly increase the surface area of the mucous membrane over which air travels on its way through the nasal cavities. This membrane contains many blood vessels that deliver heat and moisture. The membrane's cells secrete a large amount of fluid—up to

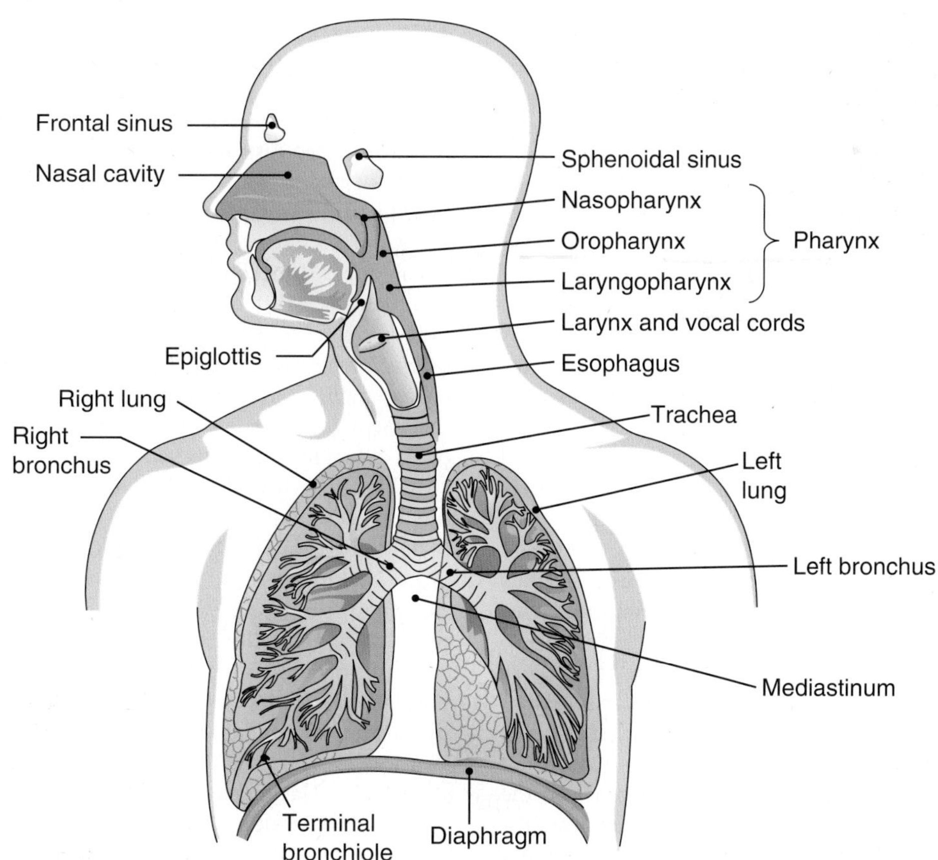

Figure 16-2 The respiratory system. KEY POINT The respiratory system consists of a series of airways that finally branch through the lungs. ZOOMING IN What organ is located in the medial depression of the left lung?

1 quart each day. The following changes occur as air comes in contact with the nasal lining:

- Foreign bodies, such as dust particles and pathogens, are filtered out by the hairs of the nostrils or caught in the surface mucus.
- Air is warmed by blood in the well-vascularized mucous membrane.
- Air is moistened by the liquid secretion.

To allow for these protective changes to occur, it is preferable to breathe through the nose rather than through the mouth.

As noted in Chapter 6, the paranasal sinuses are small cavities in the skull bones near the nose **(see Fig. 6-4)**. They are resonating chambers for the voice and lessen the skull's weight. These sinuses are lined with mucous membrane and communicate with the nasal cavities. They are highly susceptible to infection traveling from the nose and throat.

THE PHARYNX

The muscular **pharynx** (FAR-inks), or throat, carries air into the respiratory tract and carries foods and liquids into the digestive system **(see Fig. 16-2)**. The superior portion, located immediately behind the nasal cavity, is called the **nasopharynx** (na-zo-FAR-inks); the middle section, located posterior to the mouth, is called the **oropharynx** (o-ro-FAR-inks); and the most inferior portion is called the **laryngopharynx** (lah-rin-go-FAR-inks). This last section opens into the larynx toward the anterior and into the esophagus toward the posterior.

THE LARYNX

The **larynx** (LAR-inks), commonly called the *voice box* **(Fig. 16-3)**, is inferior to the pharynx and superior to the trachea. It has a framework of hyaline cartilage, one part of which is the *thyroid cartilage* that protrudes at the anterior of the neck. The projection formed by the thyroid cartilage is commonly called the *Adam's apple* because it is considerably larger in men than in women. The *cricoid* (KRI-koyd) *cartilage* forms a ring around the larynx below the thyroid cartilage. It is used as a landmark for medical procedures involving the trachea.

Folds of mucous membrane used in producing speech are located centrally in the superior larynx. These are the *vocal folds*, or **vocal cords (Fig. 16-4)**, which vibrate as air flows over them from the lungs. You can feel this vibration by placing your fingertips over the larynx at the center of your anterior throat and saying "Ah." Variations in the length and tension of the vocal cords and the distance between them regulate the pitch of sound. The amount of air forced over them regulates volume. A difference in the size of the larynx and the vocal cords is what accounts for the difference between adult male and female voices. In general, a man's larynx is larger than a woman's. His vocal cords are thicker and longer, so they vibrate more slowly, resulting in a lower range of pitch. Muscles of the pharynx,

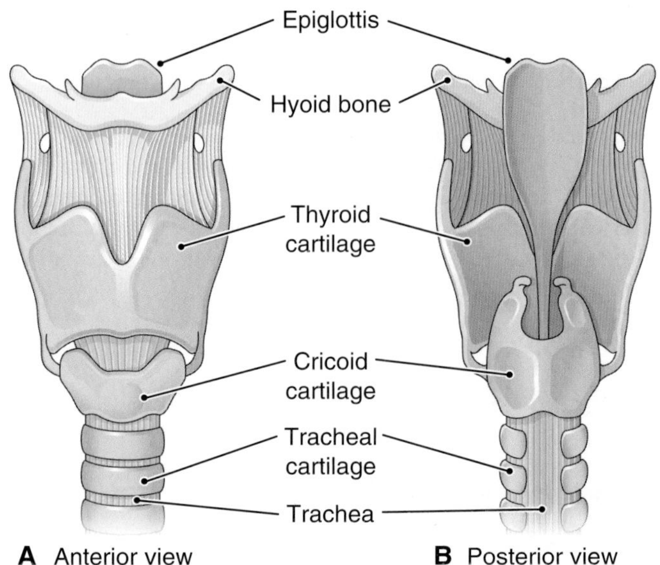

Figure 16-3 The larynx. KEY POINT The larynx is reinforced by hyaline cartilage, as is the trachea. The laryngeal cartilages include the epiglottis, thyroid cartilage, and cricoid cartilage.

tongue, lips, and face also are used to articulate words. The mouth, nasal cavities, paranasal sinuses, and the pharynx all serve as resonating chambers for speech, just as does the cabinet for an audio speaker. The space between the vocal cords is called the **glottis** (GLOT-is). This is somewhat open during normal breathing but widely open during forced breathing **(see Fig. 16-4)**.

Superior to the vocal cords are additional folds in the laryngeal mucous membrane. These are known as the *vestibular folds* **(see Fig. 16-4)**, sometimes called the "false vocal cords," because they do not contribute to speech production. Muscles in the larynx can bring these folds together to close off the glottis and help keep materials out of the respiratory tract during swallowing. They are also closed to help in holding one's breath against pressure in the thoracic cavity, as when straining to lift a heavy weight or to defecate.

The little leaf-shaped cartilage that covers the larynx during swallowing is called the **epiglottis** (ep-ih-GLOT-is). (The name means "above the glottis".) The glottis and epiglottis help keep food and liquids out of the remainder of the respiratory tract. As the larynx moves upward and forward during swallowing, the epiglottis moves downward, covering the opening into the larynx. You can feel the larynx move upward toward the epiglottis during this process by placing the pads of your fingers on your larynx as you swallow.

Despite laryngeal protections, it is possible to inhale or **aspirate** (AS-pih-rate) material into the respiratory tract. This might occur when someone is laughing or talking vigorously while eating, or an incapacitated individual inhales vomited gastric contents. Children can aspirate small objects or pieces of slippery food, such as hot dogs. Objects

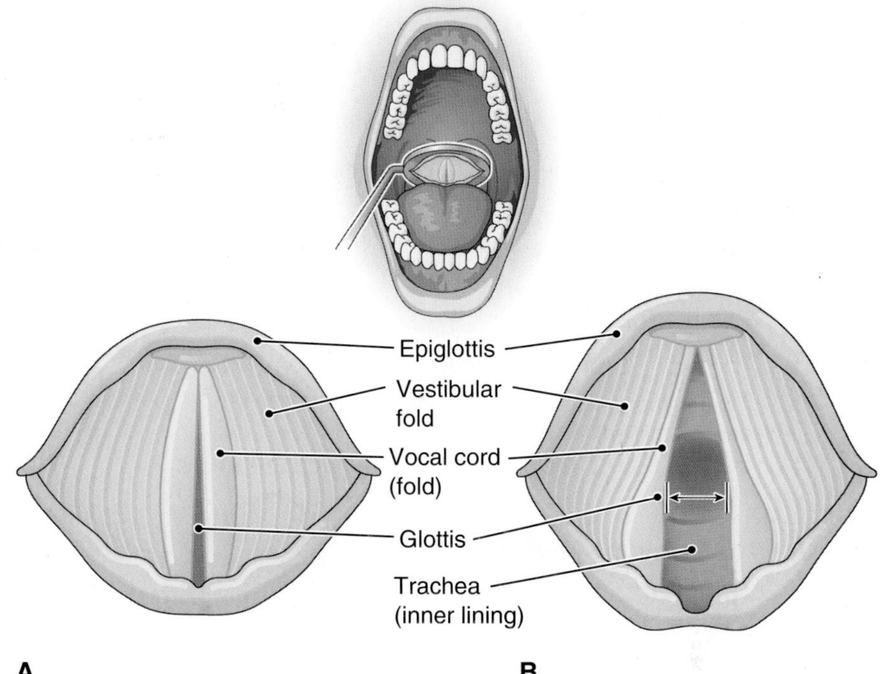

Figure 16-4 The vocal cords, superior view. KEY POINT The larynx contains the vocal cords, used in speech production. The glottis is the space between the vocal cords. The vestibular folds help close off the glottis when necessary. **A.** The glottis in closed position. **B.** The glottis in open position. ZOOMING IN What cartilage is named for its position above the glottis?

that enter the respiratory tract may cut off oxygen supply completely, resulting in suffocation, or become lodged in the respiratory passageways. If the object is not removed, infection and inflammation due to irritation are likely to result.

THE TRACHEA

The **trachea** (TRA-ke-ah), commonly called the *windpipe*, is a tube that extends from the inferior edge of the larynx to the upper part of the chest superior to the heart (see Fig. 16-2). The trachea's purpose is to conduct air between the larynx and the lungs.

A framework of separate cartilages reinforces the trachea and keeps it open. These cartilages, each shaped somewhat like a tiny horseshoe or the letter C, are found along the trachea's entire length (see Fig. 16-3). The open sections in the cartilages are lined up at their posterior so that the esophagus can expand into this region during swallowing.

CHECKPOINTS 

- 16-2 What happens to air as it passes over the nasal mucosa?
- 16-3 What are the three regions of the pharynx?
- 16-4 What are the scientific names for the throat, voice box, and windpipe?

THE BRONCHI

At its inferior end, the trachea divides into two mainstem, or primary, **bronchi** (BRONG-ki), which enter the lungs (Fig. 16-5). The right bronchus is considerably larger in diameter than the left and extends downward in a more vertical direction. Therefore, if a foreign body is inhaled, it is likely to enter the right lung. Each bronchus enters the lung at a notch or depression called the hilum (HI-lum). Blood vessels and nerves also connect with the lung here and, together with the bronchus, make up a region known as the *root* of the lung.

THE LINING OF THE AIR PASSAGEWAYS

The trachea, bronchi, and other conducting passageways of the respiratory tract are lined with a special type of epithelium (see Fig. 16-5B). Basically, it is simple columnar epithelium, but the cells are arranged in such a way that they appear stratified. The tissue is thus described as *pseudostratified*, meaning "falsely stratified." These epithelial cells secrete mucus to trap impurities and have cilia to create fluid movement within the conducting tubes. The cilia beat to drive impurities upward toward the throat, where they can be swallowed or eliminated by coughing, sneezing, or blowing the nose.

THE LUNGS

The **lungs** are the organs in which gas diffusion takes place through the extremely thin and delicate lung tissues. The two lungs are set side-by-side in the thoracic (chest) cavity (see Fig. 16-5A,C). Between them are the heart, the great blood vessels, and other organs of the mediastinum (the space and organs between the lungs). (See Fig. A3-5 in the Dissection Atlas for a photograph showing the lungs in relation to the heart and diaphragm.) On its medial side, the left lung has an indentation that accommodates the heart.

16

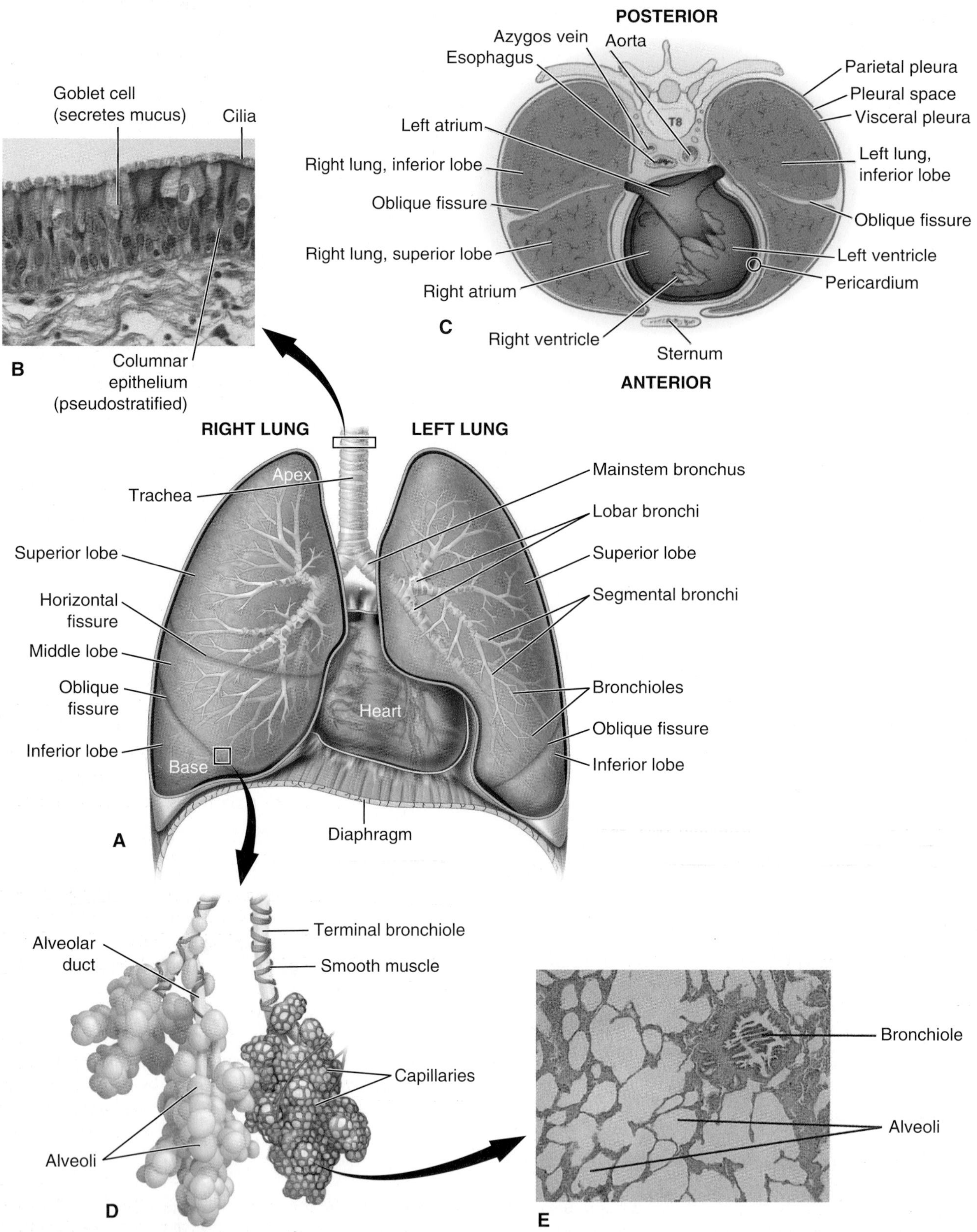

Figure 16-5 **The lungs.** KEY POINT The lungs are divided into lobes and segments that correspond to divisions of the bronchial tree. The histology of the respiratory tract differs in different regions. **A.** Position and structure of the lungs. **B.** Histology of the air passageways. **C.** Cross section of the thorax through the lungs, showing the visceral and parietal pleurae and the pleural space. **D.** Alveoli (air sacs). The left section of the diagram shows alveoli with capillaries removed. **E.** Histology of lung tissue (A and D, Reprinted with permission from McConnell TH, Hull KL. *Human Form Human Function*. Philadelphia, PA: Lippincott Williams & Wilkins, 2011; B, Reprinted with permission from Cormack DH. *Essential Histology*, 2nd ed. Philadelphia: Lippincott Williams & Wilkins, 2001; C, Reprinted with permission from Snell RS. *Clinical Anatomy*, 7th ed. Philadelphia, PA: Lippincott Williams & Wilkins, 2003; E, Courtesy of Dana Morse Bittus and BJ Cohen.)

Divisions of the Lungs The right lung is subdivided by a horizontal and an oblique fissure into three lobes (superior, middle, and inferior); the left lung is divided by a single oblique fissure into two lobes (superior and inferior). Each lobe is then further subdivided into segments and then lobules. These subdivisions correspond to subdivisions of the bronchi as they branch throughout the lungs.

Each mainstem bronchus enters the lung at the hilum and immediately subdivides. The right bronchus divides into three lobar, or secondary, bronchi, each of which enters one of the right lung's three lobes. The left bronchus gives rise to two lobar bronchi, which enter the left lung's two lobes. The bronchi subdivide again and again, becoming progressively smaller as they branch through lung tissue. The lobar bronchi become segmental bronchi as they branch into smaller segments of the lung. Because the bronchial subdivisions resemble the branches of a tree, they have been given the common name *bronchial tree*.

The Bronchioles The smallest of these conducting tubes are called **bronchioles** (BRONG-ke-oles). With branching, the histology of the tubes gradually changes. The bronchi contain small bits of cartilage, which give firmness to their walls and hold the passageways open so that air can pass in and out easily. As the bronchi become smaller, however, the cartilage decreases in amount. In the bronchioles, there is no cartilage at all; what remains is mostly smooth muscle, which is under the control of the autonomic (involuntary) nervous system. In Emily's asthma case study, it is spasms of this smooth muscle that constrict her airways and make breathing difficult.

The Alveoli At the end of the **terminal bronchioles**, the smallest subdivisions of the bronchial tree, there are clusters of tiny air sacs in which most gas exchange takes place. These sacs are the **alveoli** (al-VE-o-li) (sing. alveolus) **(see Fig. 16-5D)**. The wall of each alveolus is made of a single-cell layer of squamous epithelium. This thin wall provides easy passage for the gases entering and leaving the blood as the blood circulates through the millions of tiny capillaries covering the alveoli.

There are about 300 million alveoli in the human lungs. The resulting surface area in contact with gases approximates 60 m^2 (some sources say even more). This area is equivalent, as an example, to the floor surface of a classroom that measures about 24 by 24 ft. As with many other body systems, there is great functional reserve; we have about three times as much lung tissue as is minimally necessary to sustain life. Because of the many air spaces, the lung is light in weight; normally, a piece of lung tissue dropped into a glass of water will float. **Figure 16-5E** shows a microscopic view of lung tissue.

The pulmonary circuit brings blood to and from the lungs. In the lungs, blood passes through the capillaries around the alveoli, where gas exchange takes place.

The Lung Cavities and Pleura The lungs occupy a considerable portion of the thoracic cavity, which is separated from the abdominal cavity by the muscular partition known as the **diaphragm** (DI-ah-fram). A continuous doubled sac, the **pleura** (PLU-ra), covers each lung **(see Fig. 16-5C)**. The two layers of the pleura are named according to location. The portion that is attached to the chest wall is the parietal pleura, and the portion that is attached to the lung surface is the visceral pleura. Each closed sac completely surrounds the lung, except at the hilum, where the bronchus and blood vessels enter the lung.

Between the two layers of the pleura is the **pleural space**, containing a thin film of fluid that lubricates the membranes. The effect of this fluid is the same as between two flat pieces of glass joined by a film of water; that is, the surfaces slide easily on each other but strongly resist separation. Thus, the lungs are able to expand and contract effortlessly during breathing, but the pleural fluid keeps them from separating from the chest wall.

CHECKPOINTS 

- [ ] **16-5** What feature of the cells lining the respiratory passageways enables them to move impurities away from the lungs?
- [ ] **16-6** In what structures does gas exchange occur in the lung?
- [ ] **16-7** What is the name of the membrane that encloses the lung?

The Process of Respiration

Respiration involves ventilation of the lungs, exchange of gases, and their transport in the blood. Respiratory needs are met by central and peripheral controls of breathing.

PULMONARY VENTILATION

Ventilation is the movement of air into and out of the lungs, normally accomplished by breathing. There are two phases of ventilation: **inhalation**, which is the drawing of air into the lungs; and **exhalation**, or expiration, which is the expulsion of air from the lungs.

16

Inhalation In inhalation, the active phase of quiet breathing, respiratory muscles of the thorax and diaphragm contract to enlarge the thoracic cavity **(Fig. 16-6)**. During quiet breathing, the diaphragm's movement accounts for most of the increase in thoracic volume. The diaphragm is a strong, dome-shaped muscle attached to the body wall around the base of the rib cage. The diaphragm's contraction and flattening cause a piston-like downward motion that increases the chest's vertical dimension. Other muscles that participate in breathing are the external and internal intercostal muscles. These muscles run at different angles in two layers between the ribs. As the external intercostals contract for inhalation, they lift the rib cage upward and outward. Put the palms of your hands on either side of the rib cage to feel this action as you inhale. During forceful inhalation, the rib cage is moved further up and out by contraction of muscles in the neck and chest wall.

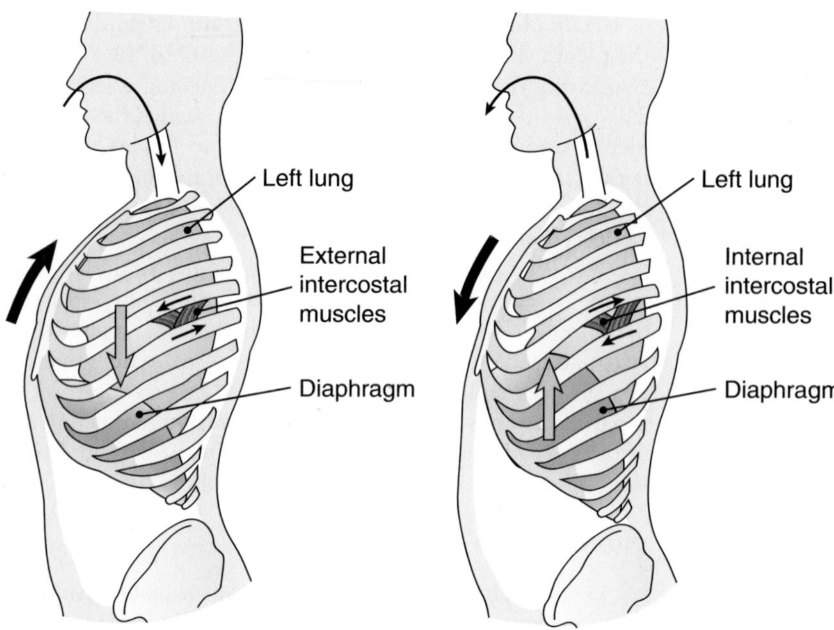

During inhalation the diaphragm presses the abdominal organs downward and forward.

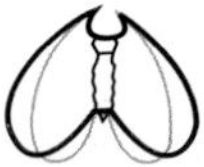

A. Action of rib cage in inhalation

During exhalation the diaphragm rises and recoils to the resting position.

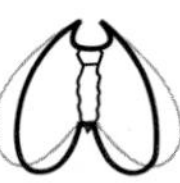

B. Action of rib cage in exhalation

Figure 16-6 Pulmonary ventilation. KEY POINT The diaphragm and intercostal muscles are involved in inhalation, the active phase of quiet breathing. These muscle relax in exhalation, the passive phase of quiet breathing. **A.** Inhalation. **B.** Exhalation. ZOOMING IN What muscles are located between the ribs?

As the thoracic cavity increases in size, gas pressure within the cavity decreases. This phenomenon follows a law in physics stating that when the volume of a given amount of gas increases, the pressure of the gas decreases. Conversely, when the volume decreases, the pressure increases. If you blow air into a tight balloon that does not expand very much, the gas particles are in close contact and will hit the wall of the balloon frequently, creating greater pressure **(Fig. 16-7)**. If you tap this balloon, it will spring back to its original shape. When you blow into a soft balloon that expands easily under pressure, the gas particles spread out into a larger volume and will not hit the balloon's wall as often. If you tap the balloon, your finger will make an indentation. Thus, pressure in the chest cavity drops as the thorax expands. When the pressure drops to slightly below the air pressure outside the lungs, air is drawn into the lungs, as by suction.

Air enters the respiratory passages and flows through the ever-dividing tubes of the bronchial tree. As the air travels this route, it moves more and more slowly through the many bronchial tubes until there is virtually no forward flow as it reaches the alveoli. The incoming air mixes with the residual air remaining in the respiratory passageways, so that the gases soon are evenly distributed. Each breath causes relatively little change in the gas composition of the alveoli, but normal continuous breathing ensures the presence of adequate oxygen and the removal of carbon dioxide.

As with expansion of blood vessels, discussed in Chapter 15, the ease with which one can expand the lungs and thorax in inhalation is called compliance. To understand some of the conditions that can affect lung compliance, we must look again at the properties of water, first introduced in Chapter 2. A thin film of water lines the alveoli. The moisture is necessary, because gases must go into solution before they can diffuse across the membrane in traveling between the air and capillary blood. Water has the property of high *surface tension* based on water molecules' attraction for each other as a result of hydrogen bonding **(see Box 2-1)**. You may have noticed that water will climb a short way up the inside of a narrow glass tube—the result of surface tension. A kind of "skin" forms at the surface of water that will support a light object or small insect, for example. Water's surface tension exerts an inward "pull" on the alveoli, causing them to resist expansion. To counteract this force, certain alveolar cells produce **surfactant** (sur-FAK-tant), a substance that reduces the surface tension of the fluids that line the alveoli. Surfactant is a mixture of lipoproteins that behaves much like a dish detergent, which reduces surface tension to aid in breaking down fats. Normal compliance of the lung tissue, aided by surfactant, allows the lungs to

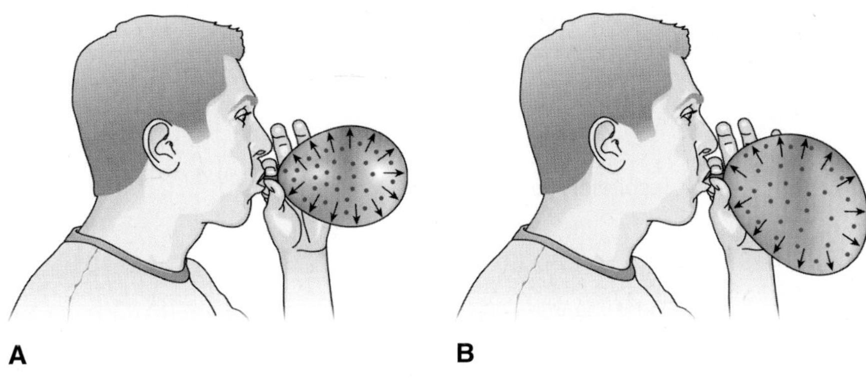

Figure 16-7 The relationship of gas pressure to volume. KEY POINT **A.** Inflation of a stiff balloon creates strong air pressure against the wall of the balloon. **B.** The same amount of air in a soft balloon spreads out into the available space, resulting in lower gas pressure. ZOOMING IN What happens to gas pressure as the volume of its container increases?

expand and fill adequately with air during inhalation. Compliance is decreased when the lungs resist expansion. Conditions that can decrease compliance include diseases that damage or scar lung tissue; fluid accumulation in the lungs; deficiency of surfactant; and interference with the action of breathing muscles.

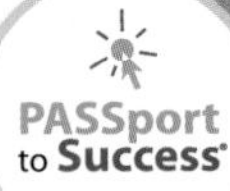

See the Student Resources on *thePoint* for illustrations of the breathing muscles and for the animation *Pulmonary Ventilation.*

Exhalation In exhalation, the passive phase of quiet breathing, the respiratory muscles relax, allowing the ribs and diaphragm to return to their original positions. The lung tissues are elastic and recoil to their original size during exhalation. Surface tension within the alveoli aids in this return to resting size. During forced exhalation, the internal intercostal muscles contract, pulling the bottom of the rib cage in and down. The muscles of the abdominal wall contract, pushing the abdominal viscera upward against the relaxed diaphragm. Even with maximum exhalation, however, you cannot expel all the air from your lungs. There is always a certain residual volume left to fill the airways and keep the lungs inflated.

Table 16-1 gives the definitions and average values for some of the breathing volumes and capacities that are important in evaluating respiratory function. A lung *capacity* is a sum of volumes. These same values are shown on a graph as they might appear on a tracing made by a **spirometer** (spi-ROM-eh-ter), an instrument for recording volumes of air inhaled and exhaled (Fig. 16-8). The tracing is a **spirogram** (SPI-ro-gram).

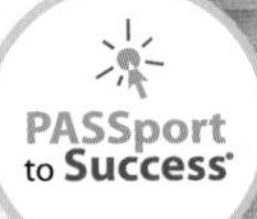

Respiratory therapists evaluate and treat breathing disorders. See the Student Resources on *thePoint* for a description of this career.

GAS EXCHANGE

External gas exchange is the movement of gases between the alveoli and the capillary blood in the lungs (Fig. 16-9). The barrier that separates alveolar air from the blood is composed of the alveolar wall and the capillary wall, both of which are extremely thin. This respiratory membrane is

16

Table 16-1 Lung Volumes and Capacities

Volume	Definition	Average Value (mL)
Tidal volume	The amount of air moved into or out of the lungs in quiet, relaxed breathing	500
Residual volume	The volume of air that remains in the lungs after maximum exhalation	1,200
Inspiratory reserve volume	The additional amount that can be breathed in by force after a normal inhalation	2,600
Expiratory reserve volume	The additional amount that can be breathed out by force after a normal exhalation	900
Vital capacity	The volume of air that can be expelled from the lungs by maximum exhalation after maximum inhalation	4,000
Functional residual capacity	The amount of air remaining in the lungs after normal exhalation	2,100
Total lung capacity	The total volume of air that can be contained in the lungs after maximum inhalation	5,200

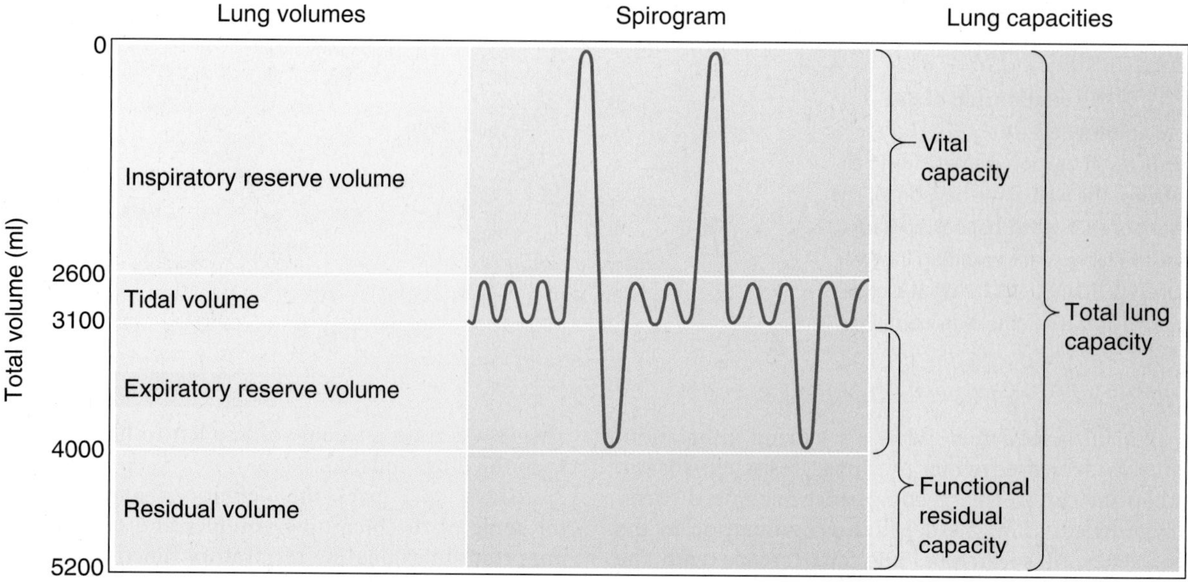

Figure 16-8 A spirogram. KEY POINT A spirogram is a tracing of lung volumes made with a spirometer, an instrument that measures volumes of air inhaled and exhaled. ZOOMING IN What lung volume cannot be measured with a spirometer? Which lung capacities cannot be measured with a spirometer?

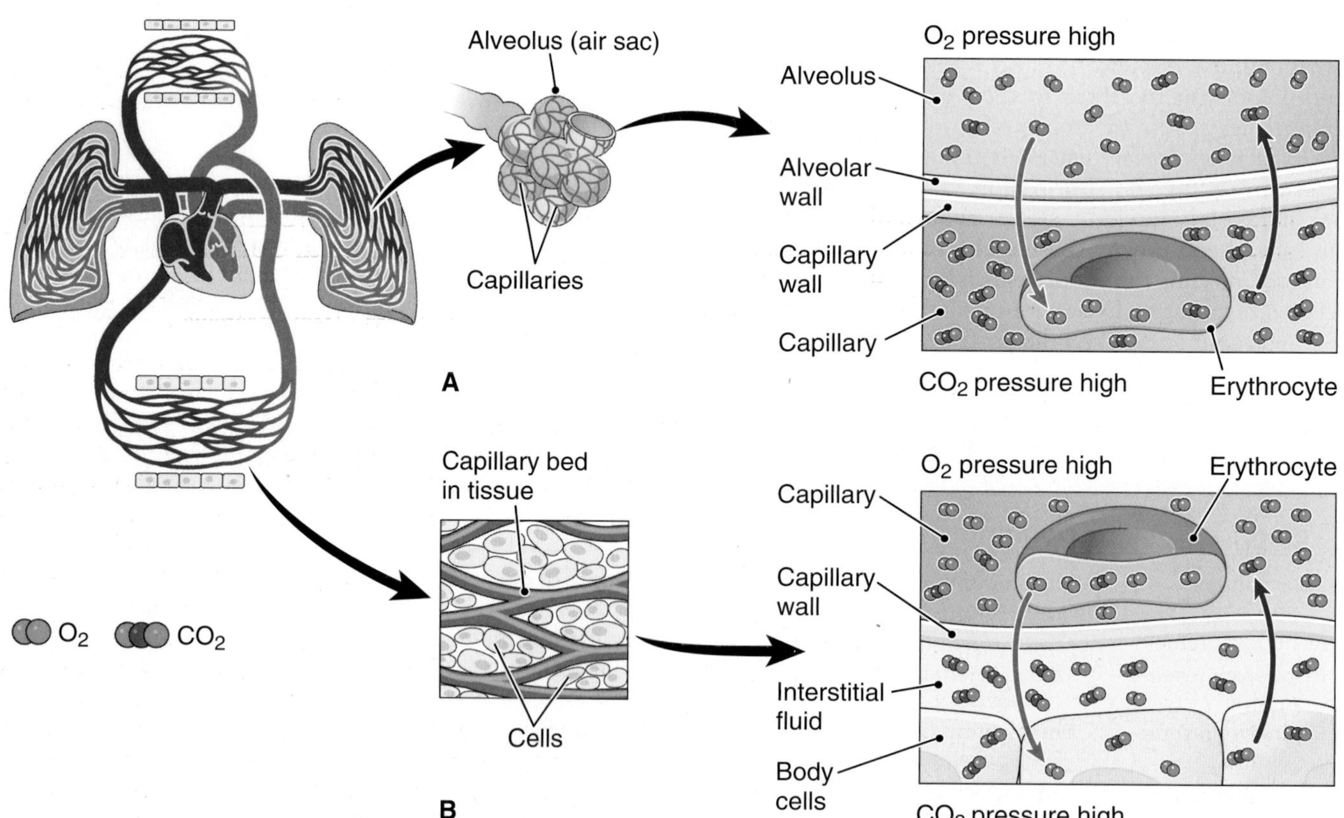

Figure 16-9 Gas exchange. KEY POINT Gas exchanges are based on relative partial pressures of oxygen and carbon dioxide on either side of a membrane. **A.** External exchange between the alveoli and the blood. Oxygen diffuses into the blood and carbon dioxide diffuses out, based on pressures of the two gases in the alveoli and in the blood. **B.** Internal exchange between the blood and the cells. Oxygen diffuses out of the blood and into tissues, while carbon dioxide diffuses from the cells into the blood.

not only very thin, but it is also moist. As previously noted, the moisture is important because the oxygen and carbon dioxide must go into solution before they can diffuse across the membrane.

The principle that governs gas exchange between the outside air and the tissues is the now familiar concept of diffusion. Recall that solutes diffuse down concentration gradients. Gases diffuse instead down individual *pressure gradients*, and the pressure of a gas is expressed in millimeters of mercury (mm Hg), as is blood pressure. If gases are in a mixture, the pressure of each individual gas in the mixture is called its **partial pressure**, symbolized with a P and a subscript of its formula. Thus, the partial pressures of oxygen and carbon dioxide are symbolized as Po_2 and Pco_2, respectively. Note that even though the gases are in a mixture, each diffuses independently of any other gas in that mixture.

The relative pressure of a gas on the two sides of a membrane determines the direction of diffusion **(see Fig. 16-9)**. The Po_2 in inspired air is higher than the Po_2 in the capillary blood of the lungs, because body cells have used oxygen in cellular respiration. In the lungs, therefore, oxygen will diffuse across the alveolar wall and into the capillaries. Because the cells generate carbon dioxide in cellular respiration, the Pco_2 in the pulmonary capillaries is higher than the Pco_2 in inspired air, and carbon dioxide diffuses out of the blood and into the alveoli.

In contrast, internal gas exchange takes place between the blood and the tissues, again based on the relative pressures of the two gases. The blood arriving in the tissues has been oxygenated in the lungs, and oxygen will pass into the oxygen-poor tissues. Carbon dioxide will diffuse out of the tissues and into the blood. Blood returning from the tissues and entering the lung capillaries through the pulmonary circuit is relatively low in oxygen and high in carbon dioxide. Again, the blood will pick up oxygen and give up carbon dioxide. After a return to the left side of the heart, it starts once more on its route through the systemic circuit.

TRANSPORT OF OXYGEN

A very small amount (1.5%) of the oxygen in the blood is carried in solution in the plasma. (Oxygen does dissolve in water, as shown by the fact that aquatic animals get their oxygen from water.) However, almost all (98.5%) of the oxygen that diffuses into the capillary blood in the lungs binds to hemoglobin in the red blood cells. If not for hemoglobin and its ability to hold oxygen in the blood, it would be impossible for the heart to supply enough oxygen to the tissues. The hemoglobin molecule is a large protein with four small iron-containing "heme" regions. Each heme portion can bind one molecule of oxygen.

Highly oxygenated blood (in systemic arteries and pulmonary veins) is 97% saturated with oxygen. That is, the total hemoglobin in the red cells is holding 97% of the maximum amount that it can hold. Blood low in oxygen (in systemic veins and pulmonary arteries) is usually about 70% saturated with oxygen. This 27% difference represents the oxygen that has been taken up by the cells. The terms *oxygenated* and *deoxygenated* are often used to describe blood that is high and low in oxygen, respectively. Note, however, that even blood that is described as deoxygenated still has a large reserve of oxygen. Even under conditions of high oxygen consumption, as in vigorous exercise, for example, the blood is never totally depleted of oxygen.

To enter the cells, oxygen must separate from hemoglobin. Normally, the bond between oxygen and hemoglobin is easily broken, and oxygen is released as blood travels into tissues where the oxygen pressure is relatively low. Cells are constantly using oxygen in cellular respiration and obtaining fresh supplies by diffusion from the blood. In addition, some conditions increase the rate of oxygen's release from hemoglobin. Increasing body temperature and increasing acidity, both generated by cellular activity, promote its release to the tissues.

The poisonous gas carbon monoxide (CO), at low partial pressure, binds with hemoglobin at the same molecular sites as does oxygen. However, it binds more tightly and displaces oxygen. Even a small amount of carbon monoxide causes a serious reduction in the blood's ability to carry oxygen.

For an interesting variation on normal gas transport, see **Box 16-1** on liquid ventilation.

TRANSPORT OF CARBON DIOXIDE

Carbon dioxide is produced continuously in the tissues as a byproduct of cellular respiration. It diffuses from the tissue cells into the blood and is transported to the lungs in three ways:

- About 10% is dissolved in the plasma and in the fluid within red blood cells. (Carbonated beverages are examples of water in which CO_2 is dissolved.)
- About 15% is combined with the protein portion of hemoglobin and with plasma proteins.
- About 75% is transported as an ion, known as a **bicarbonate** (bi-KAR-bon-ate) **ion**, which is formed when carbon dioxide undergoes a chemical change after it dissolves in blood fluids. It first combines with water to form **carbonic** (kar-BON-ik) **acid**, which then separates (ionizes) into hydrogen and bicarbonate ions.

16

The bicarbonate ion is formed slowly in the plasma but much more rapidly inside the red blood cells, where an enzyme called **carbonic anhydrase** (an-HI-drase) (CA) increases the reaction's speed. The bicarbonate formed in the red blood cells moves to the plasma and then is carried to the lungs. In the lungs, the process is reversed as bicarbonate reenters the red blood cells, joins with a hydrogen ion to form carbonic acid, and again under the effects of carbonic anhydrase, releases carbon dioxide and water. The carbon dioxide diffuses into the alveoli and is exhaled. For those with a background in chemistry, the equation for these reactions follows. The arrows going in both directions signify that the reactions are reversible. The upper arrows describe what happens as CO_2 enters the blood; the lower

Box 16-1 *Clinical Perspectives*

Liquid Ventilation: Breath in a Bottle

Researchers have been attempting for years to develop a fluid that could transport high concentrations of oxygen in the body. Such a fluid could substitute for blood in transfusions or be used to carry oxygen into the lungs. Early work on liquid ventilation climaxed in the mid-1960s when a pioneer in this field submerged a laboratory mouse in a beaker of fluid and the animal survived total immersion for more than 10 minutes. The fluid was a synthetic substance that could hold as much oxygen as does air.

A newer version of this fluid, a fluorine-containing chemical known as PFC, has been tested to ventilate the collapsed lungs of premature babies. In addition to delivering oxygen to the lung alveoli, it also removes carbon dioxide. The fluid is less damaging to delicate lung tissue than is air, which has to be pumped in under higher pressure. Others who might benefit from liquid ventilation include people whose lungs have been damaged by infection, inhaled toxins, asthma, emphysema, and lung cancer, but more clinical research is required. Scientists are also investigating whether liquid ventilation could be used to deliver drugs directly to lung tissue.

arrows indicate what happens as CO_2 is released from the blood to be exhaled from the lungs. CA represents the enzyme carbonic anhydrase.

$$CO_2 + H_2O \overset{CA}{\rightleftharpoons} H_2CO_3 \rightleftharpoons H^+ + HCO_3^-$$

carbon dioxide	water	carbonic acid	hydrogen ion	bicarbonate ion

Carbon dioxide is important in regulating the blood's pH (acid–base balance). As a bicarbonate ion is formed from carbon dioxide in the plasma, a hydrogen ion (H^+) is also produced. Therefore, the blood becomes more acidic as the amount of carbon dioxide in the blood increases. The exhalation of carbon dioxide shifts the blood's pH more toward the alkaline (basic) range. The bicarbonate ion is also an important buffer in the blood, acting chemically to help keep the pH of body fluids within a steady range of 7.35 to 7.45. Chapter 19 has more information on body fluids and the kidneys' role in regulating the composition of body fluids.

CHECKPOINTS 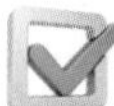

☐ **16-8** What are the two phases of quiet breathing? Which is active and which is passive?

☐ **16-9** What property of a gas determines its direction of diffusion across a membrane and in what units is this property expressed?

☐ **16-10** What substance in red blood cells holds almost all of the oxygen carried in the blood?

☐ **16-11** What is the main form in which carbon dioxide is carried in the blood?

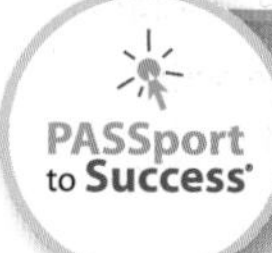

See the Student Resources on *thePoint* to view the animation *Oxygen Transport and Carbon Dioxide Exchange.*

REGULATION OF RESPIRATION

Regulation of respiration is a complex process that must keep pace with moment-to-moment changes in cellular oxygen requirements and carbon dioxide production. Centers in the central nervous system control the fundamental respiratory pattern. This pattern is modified by special receptors that detect changes in the blood's chemical composition. Other regulators of respiration are receptors in the airways, muscles, and joints.

Central Nervous Control Regulation of respiration depends primarily on a respiratory control center located partly in the medulla and partly in the pons of the brain stem. The control center's main part, located in the medulla, sets the basic pattern of respiration **(Fig. 16-10)**. This pattern can be modified by centers in the pons. These areas continuously regulate breathing, so that levels of oxygen, carbon dioxide, and acid are kept within normal limits.

From the respiratory center in the medulla, motor nerve fibers extend into the spinal cord. From the cervical (neck) part of the cord, these nerve fibers continue through the **phrenic** (FREN-ik) **nerve** (a branch of the vagus nerve) to the diaphragm and also to the intercostal muscles. The diaphragm and the other respiratory muscles are voluntary in the sense that they can be regulated consciously by messages from the higher brain centers, notably the cerebral cortex **(see Fig. 16-10A)**. It is possible for you to deliberately breathe more rapidly or more slowly or to hold your breath and not breathe at all for a while. In a short time, however, the respiratory center in the brain stem will override the voluntary desire to hold your breath, and breathing will resume. Most of the time, we breathe without thinking about it, and the respiratory center is in control.

Chemical Control Of vital importance in the control of respiration are **chemoreceptors** (ke-mo-re-SEP-tors) which, like the receptors for taste and smell, are sensitive to chemicals dissolved in body fluids (see Fig. 16-10B). The chemoreceptors that regulate respiration are located centrally (near the brain stem) and peripherally (in arteries).

The central chemoreceptors are on either side of the brain stem near the medullary respiratory center. These receptors respond to the CO_2 level in circulating blood, but the gas acts indirectly. CO_2 is capable of diffusing through the capillary blood–brain barrier. It dissolves in medullary interstitial fluid and separates into hydrogen ion and bicarbonate ion, as explained previously. It is the presence of hydrogen ion and its effect in lowering pH that actually stimulates the central chemoreceptors. The rise in blood CO_2 level, known as **hypercapnia** (hi-per-KAP-ne-ah), thus triggers ventilation.

The peripheral chemoreceptors that regulate respiration are found in structures called the *carotid* and *aortic bodies* (see Fig. 16-10B). The carotid bodies are located near the bifurcation (forking) of the common carotid arteries in the neck, whereas the aortic bodies are located in the aortic arch. These bodies contain sensory neurons that respond mainly to a decrease in oxygen supply. They are not usually involved in regulating breathing, because they do not act until oxygen drops to a very low level. Because there is usually an ample reserve of oxygen in the blood, carbon dioxide has the most immediate effect in regulating respiration at the level of the central chemoreceptors. When the carbon dioxide level increases, breathing must be increased to blow off the excess gas. Oxygen only becomes a controlling factor when its level falls considerably below normal, as in cases of lung disease or in high altitude environments where oxygen partial pressure is low.

Other Factors in Respiratory Control Illustrating the complexity of respiratory control, there are still additional factors that influence breathing (see Fig. 16-10B). Stimulation of pain receptors throughout the body can increase ventilation, acting through the brain's hypothalamus. Emotional responses can do the same. In the airways of the lungs, there are stretch receptors that stop inhalation to prevent overexpansion of the lungs. These are examples of mechanoreceptors, described in Chapter 10, that respond to changes in position. Finally, in muscles and joints, we have other mechanoreceptors that respond to movement and increase respiration as we move about. All these mechanoreceptors act through the medullary respiratory center.

ABNORMAL VENTILATION

In **hyperventilation** (hi-per-ven-tih-LA-shun), an increased amount of air enters the alveoli. This condition results from deep and rapid respiration that commonly occurs during anxiety attacks, or when a person is experiencing pain or other forms of stress. Hyperventilation causes an increase in the oxygen level and a decrease in the carbon dioxide level of the blood, a condition called **hypocapnia** (hi-po-KAP-ne-ah). Recall from the equation previously cited, that carbon dioxide determines blood pH by regulating hydrogen ion levels. In hyperventilation, the increased exhalation of carbon dioxide shifts the equation to the left, removing

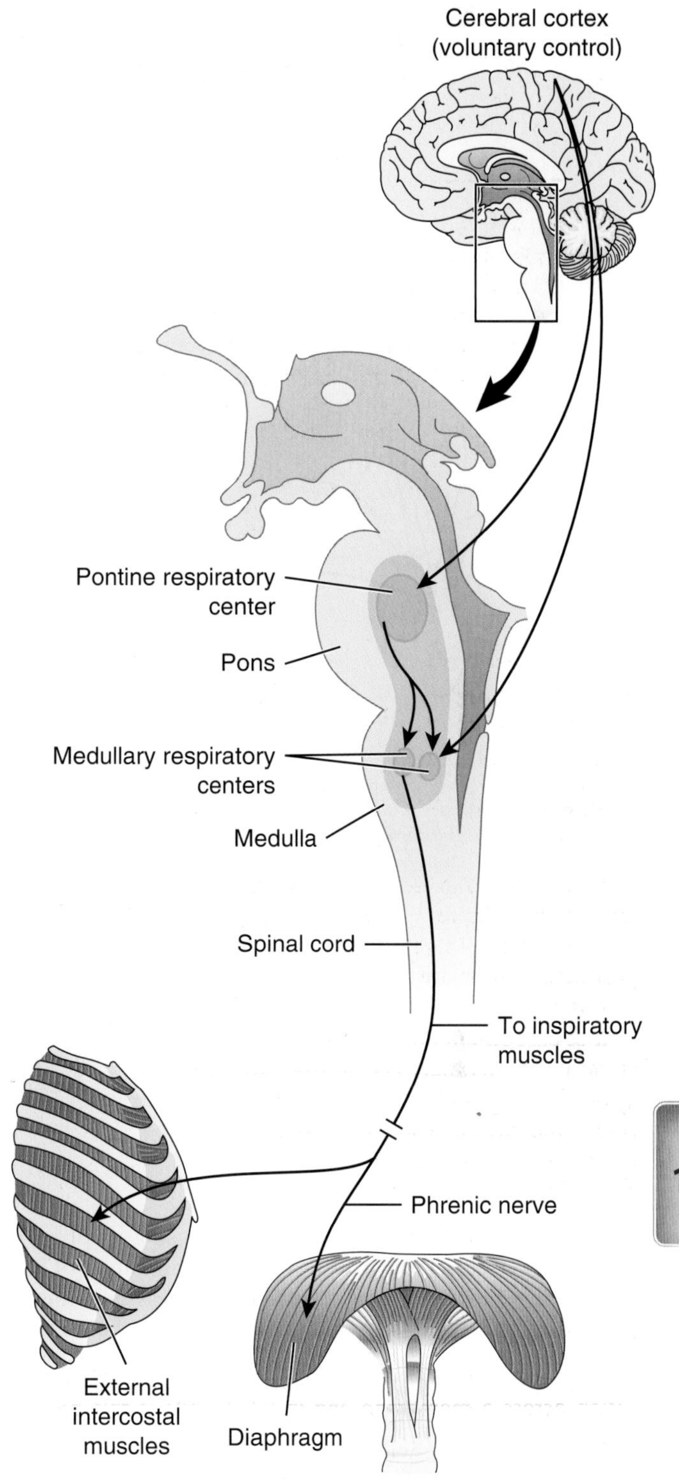

Figure 16-10 Regulation of respiration. KEY POINT Multiple factors control respiration to keep pace with need. **A.** Central nervous system control. Involuntary centers are located in the medulla and pons. They control contractions of the diaphragm and intercostal muscles through the vagus nerve (X). Voluntary control comes from the cerebral cortex. (Figure continues on next page.)

16

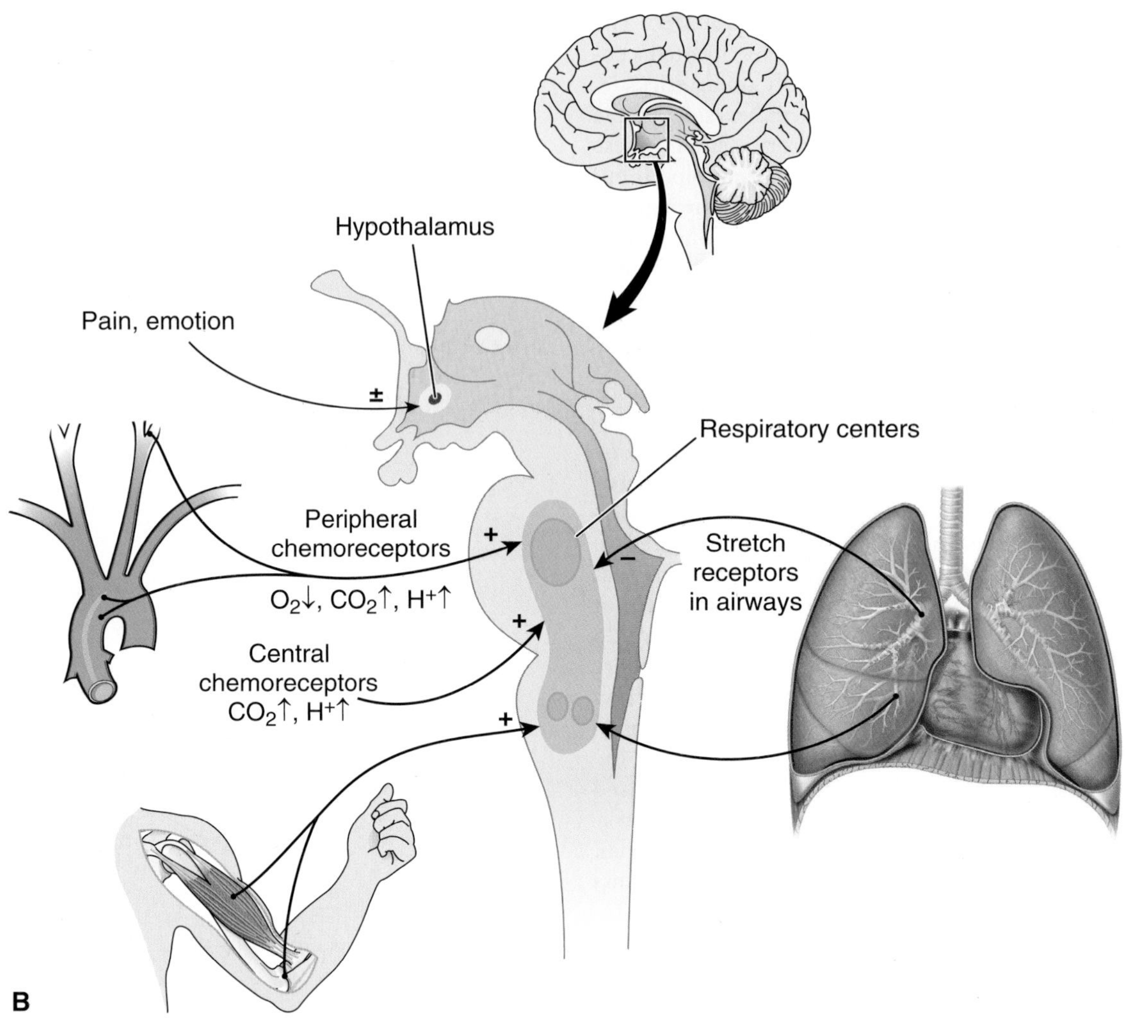

Figure 16-10 *(Continued)* **B.** Chemical and other factors that affect respiration. + indicates increased respiration; – indicates decreased respiration; ± means that response may vary with circumstances. For simplicity, the specific areas of the respiratory centers are not differentiated in this diagram.

acidic products from the blood and increasing its pH. This condition is referred to as *alkalosis*, excess alkalinity of body fluids. The change in pH results in dizziness and tingling sensations. Breathing may slow or even stop because the respiratory control center is not stimulated. Gradually, the carbon dioxide level returns to normal, and a regular breathing pattern is resumed. In extreme cases, a person may faint, and then breathing will involuntarily return to normal. In assisting a person who is hyperventilating, one should speak calmly, reassure him or her that the situation is not dangerous, and encourage even breathing using the diaphragm.

In **hypoventilation**, an insufficient amount of air enters the alveoli. The many possible causes of this condition include respiratory obstruction, lung disease, injury to the respiratory center, depression of the respiratory center, as by drugs, and chest deformity. Hypoventilation increases the blood's carbon dioxide concentration, shifting the equation cited previously to the right and decreasing the blood's pH. This condition is called *acidosis*, excess acidity of body fluids. The body responds to this condition by attempting to increase the rate and depth of respiration.

BREATHING PATTERNS

Normal breathing rates vary from 12 to 20 breaths per minute for adults. In children, rates may vary from 20 to 40 breaths per minute, depending on age and size. In infants, the respiratory rate may be more than 40 breaths per minute. Changes in respiratory rates are important in various disorders, and a healthcare provider should record them carefully. To determine the respiratory rate, the clinician counts the client's breathing for at least 30 seconds, usually by watching the chest rise and fall with each inhalation and exhalation. The count is then multiplied by 2 to obtain the rate in breaths per minute. It is best if the person does not realize that he or she is being observed because awareness of the measurement may cause a change in the breathing rate.

Box 16-2 *A Closer Look*

Adaptations to High Altitude: Living with Hypoxia

Our bodies work best at low altitudes where oxygen is plentiful. However, people are able to live at high altitudes where oxygen is scarce and can even survive climbing Mount Everest, the tallest peak on our planet, showing that the human body can adapt to both short-term and long-term hypoxic conditions. This adaptation process compensates for decreased atmospheric oxygen by increasing the efficiency of the respiratory and cardiovascular systems.

The body's immediate response to high altitude is to increase the rate of ventilation (hyperventilation) and raise the heart rate to increase cardiac output. Hyperventilation makes more oxygen available to the cells and increases blood pH (alkalosis), which boosts hemoglobin's capacity to bind oxygen. Over time, the body adapts in additional ways. Hypoxia stimulates the kidneys to secrete erythropoietin, prompting red bone marrow to manufacture more erythrocytes and hemoglobin. Also, capillaries proliferate, increasing blood flow to the tissues. Some people are unable to adapt to high altitudes, and for them, hypoxia and alkalosis lead to potentially fatal **altitude sickness**.

Successful adaptation to high altitude illustrates the principle of homeostasis and also helps to explain how the body adjusts to hypoxia associated with disorders such as chronic obstructive pulmonary disease.

Some Terms for Altered Breathing The following is a list of terms designating various respiratory abnormalities. These are symptoms, not diseases. Note that the word ending *-pnea* refers to breathing.

- **Hyperpnea** (hi-PERP-ne-ah) refers to an abnormal increase in the depth and rate of breathing.
- **Hypopnea** (hi-POP-ne-ah) is a decrease in the rate and depth of breathing.
- **Tachypnea** (tak-IP-ne-ah) is an excessive rate of breathing that may be normal, as in exercise.
- **Apnea** (AP-ne-ah) is a temporary cessation of breathing. Short periods of apnea occur normally during deep sleep. More severe sleep apnea can result from obstruction of the respiratory passageways or, less commonly, by failure in the central respiratory center.
- **Dyspnea** (disp-NE-ah) is a subjective feeling of difficult or labored breathing.
- **Orthopnea** (or-THOP-ne-ah) refers to a difficulty in breathing that is relieved by sitting in an upright position, either against two pillows in bed or in a chair.

Results of Inadequate Breathing Conditions that may result from decreased respiration include the following:

- **Cyanosis** (si-ah-NO-sis) is a bluish color of the skin and mucous membranes caused by an insufficient amount of oxygen in the blood.
- **Hypoxia** (hi-POK-se-ah) means a lower than normal oxygen level in the tissues. The term **anoxia** (ah-NOK-se-ah) is sometimes used instead, but is not as accurate because it means a total lack of oxygen.
- **Hypoxemia** (hi-pok-SE-me-ah) refers to a lower than normal oxygen partial pressure in arterial blood.

Box 16-2 offers information on adjusting to high altitudes and other hypoxic conditions.

CHECKPOINTS 

☐ 16-12 Where in the brain stem are the centers that set the basic pattern of respiration?

☐ 16-13 What is the name of the motor nerve that controls the diaphragm?

☐ 16-14 What gas is the main chemical controller of respiration?

16

Effects of Aging on the Respiratory Tract

With age, the tissues of the respiratory tract lose elasticity and become more rigid. Similar rigidity in the chest wall, combined with arthritis and loss of strength in the breathing muscles, results in an overall decrease in compliance and in lung capacity. However, there is a great deal of variation among individuals, and regular aerobic activity throughout adulthood (walking, running, swimming, etc.) can contribute significantly to maintaining respiratory function.

Reduction in protective mechanisms in the lungs, such as phagocytosis, leads to increased susceptibility to infection. The incidence of lung disease increases with age, but is hastened by cigarette smoking and by exposure to other environmental irritants.

A&P in Action Revisited

Emily's Asthma

It had been about a month since Emily's appointment with Dr. Martinez. During that time, her parents had monitored her breathing very carefully and had noticed patterns in her coughing bouts. "It does seem that Emily gets out of breath sooner than the other kids when she exercises," Emily's mother reported to Dr. Martinez during her follow-up appointment. "And now that the weather has cooled off, I do notice that she coughs more," continued Nicole.

"Let's take a listen to Emily's lungs," replied the doctor as he placed his stethoscope on the little girl's chest. "Yes," he continued, "I hear wheezing today, which suggests that Emily's airways are narrowed. Emily's chest x-ray came back negative for infection, but the radiologist did detect thickening of the bronchial walls. Based on these findings, your observations, and the family history, I think Emily has asthma."

Although Nicole had expected the doctor's diagnosis, it was still a shock to hear him say it. Seeing her look of alarm, Dr. Martinez continued, "Most kids with asthma lead very normal, active lives. The medications available today target asthma right at its source—inflammation. In fact, with proper treatment, many kids maintain near-normal pulmonary function. Let's start with an antiinflammatory in the form of a low-dose corticosteroid inhaler. If, after a few weeks, we don't see any improvement, I'll start Emily on an oral leukotriene modifier that she will take daily to control airway inflammation. I'm also going to prescribe another type of inhaler to use if Emily has a severe asthma episode. The inhaler contains a medication that relaxes the smooth muscle of her airways, giving her short-term relief of symptoms."

In this case, we learned that Emily's asthma was caused by airway inflammation. Medications that limit the inflammatory response in the respiratory passages can prevent the symptoms of asthma. For a review of the role of inflammation in normal body defense mechanisms, see Chapter 15.

Chapter Wrap-Up

Summary Overview

A detailed chapter outline with space for note-taking is on *thePoint*. The figure below illustrates the main topics covered in this chapter.

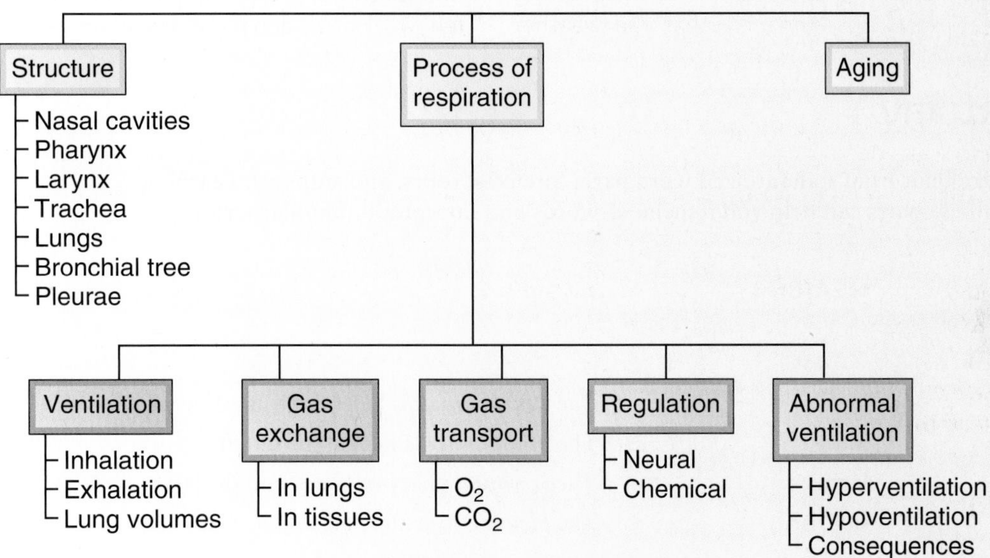

Key Terms

The terms listed below are emphasized in this chapter. Knowing them will help you organize and prioritize your learning. These and other boldface terms are defined in the Glossary with phonetic pronunciations.

alveolus (pl., alveoli)
bicarbonate ion
bronchiole
bronchus (pl., bronchi)
carbonic acid
carbonic anhydrase
chemoreceptor
compliance
diaphragm
epiglottis
hypercapnia
hypoxia
larynx
lung
pharynx
phrenic nerve
pleura
respiration
spirometer
surfactant
trachea
ventilation

Word Anatomy

Scientific terms are built from standardized word parts (prefixes, roots, and suffixes). Learning the meanings of these parts can help you remember words and interpret unfamiliar terms.

WORD PART	MEANING	EXAMPLE
Structure of the Respiratory System		
nas/o	nose	The *nasopharynx* is behind the nasal cavity.
or/o	mouth	The *oropharynx* is behind the mouth.
laryng/o	larynx	The *laryngeal* pharynx opens into the larynx.
pleur/o	side, rib	The *pleura* covers the lung and lines the chest wall (rib cage).
The Process of Respiration		
spir/o	breathing	A *spirometer* is an instrument used to record breathing volumes.
capn/o	carbon dioxide	*Hypercapnia* is a rise in the blood level of carbon dioxide.
-pnea	breathing	*Hypopnea* is a decrease in the rate and depth of breathing.
orth/o-	straight	*Orthopnea* can be relieved by sitting in an upright position.

Questions for Study and Review

BUILDING UNDERSTANDING

Fill in the Blanks

1. The exchange of air between the atmosphere and the lungs is called ______.
2. The space between the vocal cords is the ______.
3. The ease with which the lungs and thorax can be expanded is termed ______.
4. The diaphragm is innervated by the _____ nerve.
5. A lower than normal level of oxygen in the tissues is called ______.

Matching > Match each numbered item with the most closely related lettered item.

___ **6.** The amount of air remaining in the lungs after a normal exhalation

___ **7.** The amount of additional air that can be breathed out by force after a normal exhalation

___ **8.** The amount of air moved into or out of the lungs in quiet, relaxed breathing

___ **9.** The amount of air remaining in the lungs after maximum exhalation

___ **10.** The amount of air that can be expelled from the lungs by maximum exhalation after maximum inhalation

a. vital capacity
b. functional residual capacity
c. tidal volume
d. residual volume
e. expiratory reserve volume

Multiple Choice

___ **11.** Which bony projections increase nasal cavity surface area?

a. nares
b. septae
c. conchae
d. sinuses

___ **12.** Which structure contains the vocal cords?

a. pharynx
b. larynx
c. trachea
d. lungs

___ **13.** What covers the larynx during swallowing?

a. epiglottis
b. glottis
c. conchae
d. sinus

___ **14.** Which structure has the centers that regulate respiration?

a. cerebral cortex
b. diencephalon
c. brain stem
d. cerebellum

___ **15.** All of the following are true during forced expiration except

a. the diaphragm relaxes
b. the external intercostals contract
c. the abdominal muscles contract
d. the volume of the thoracic cavity decreases

UNDERSTANDING CONCEPTS

16. Differentiate between the terms in each pair:

a. internal and external gas exchange
b. pleura and diaphragm
c. inhalation and exhalation
d. spirometer and spirogram

17. Trace the path of air from the nostrils to the lung capillaries.

18. What is the function of the ciliated cells that line the respiratory passageways?

19. What is the relationship of gas pressure to volume? What happens to gas pressure in the lungs when the diaphragm contracts?

20. Compare and contrast oxygen and carbon dioxide transport in the blood.

21. Describe the direction in which oxygen and carbon dioxide diffuse during gas exchange. Why do the gases move in these directions?

22. Define hyperventilation and hypoventilation. What is the effect of each on blood CO_2 levels and blood pH?

23. What are chemoreceptors and how do they function to regulate breathing?

CONCEPTUAL THINKING

24. Jake, a sometimes exasperating 4-year-old, threatens his mother that he will hold his breath until "he dies." Should his mother be concerned that he might succeed?

25. Why is it important that airplane interiors are pressurized? If the cabin lost pressure, what physiological adaptations to respiration might occur in the passengers?

26. In Emily's case, an antiinflammatory medication was used to control her asthma symptoms. Explain how this drug works in the respiratory system.

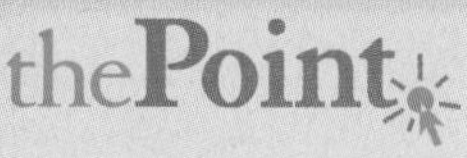

For more questions, see the learning activities on *thePoint*.

CHAPTER 17 The Digestive System

A&P in Action

Adam's Case: The Picture of Health

Adam was okay with everything his family doctor had described about his routine physical examination. "We'll draw some blood for testing," Dr. Michaels explained. "You didn't have anything to eat since last night, did you? We'll send your specimen to the lab to get information on your blood cells and blood chemistry, hemoglobin, lipoproteins, and such. You need to leave a urine sample to check for sugar, and then Annette will take your blood pressure and run an ECG. I'll be in to ask you some general questions and do some 'hands-on' examination, including, of course, a check on your prostate. And, Adam, since you are well past your 50th birthday, you need to stop stalling on getting that colonoscopy."

Sending in the stool sample later to test for signs of blood was not a problem for Adam, and he could live with the prostate exam, but he was not so happy about the colonoscopy! He had heard that the prep to clean out the colon was unpleasant. "You know," Adam protested, "I'm healthy and have no family history of colon cancer or polyps, so why do I need to do this?"

"Actually," replied Dr. Michaels, "most colorectal cancers appear in people with no symptoms and with no family history or genetic predisposition. In high-risk populations, we recommend testing even earlier and more frequently. There is a new 'virtual colonoscopy' procedure that uses computerized x-rays instead of an endoscope to generate detailed images of the colon, but for a baseline study, your proctologist might prefer the routine method. Besides, if we have to remove any polyps or other abnormal tissue, we'd have to resort to that anyway. When you're ready to leave the office, ask Jean at the front desk to set up an appointment for you."

As part of Adam's physical, the doctor examined many of Adam's organ systems, including his digestive system. Because of his age, the doctor recommended a closer inspection of Adam's colon. In this chapter, we will learn about the digestive tract and the accessory organs that contribute to digestion. We will also visit Adam again and find out how the colonoscopy went!

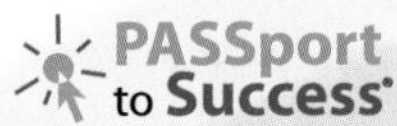

Ancillaries At-A-Glance

Visit *thePoint* to access the PASSport to Success and the following resources. For guidance in using these resources most effectively, see pp. ix–xviii.

Learning TOOLS

- Learning Style Self Assessment
- Live Advise Online Student Tutoring
- Tips for Effective Studying

Learning RESOURCES

- E-book: Chapter 17
- Animation: General Digestion
- Animation: Digestion of Carbohydrates
- Animation: Enzymes
- Animation: The Liver in Health and Disease
- Health Professions: Dental Hygienist
- Detailed Chapter Outline
- Answers to Questions for Study and Review
- Audio Pronunciation Glossary

Learning ACTIVITIES

- Pre-Quiz
- Visual Activities
- Kinesthetic Activities
- Auditory Activities

Learning Outcomes

After careful study of this chapter, you should be able to:

1. Name the three main functions of the digestive system, ***p. 334***
2. Describe the four layers of the digestive tract wall, ***p. 334***
3. Name and locate the two main layers and the subdivisions of the peritoneum, ***p. 335***
4. Name and locate the different types of teeth, ***p. 337***
5. Name and describe the functions of the digestive tract organs, ***p. 336***
6. Name and describe the functions of the accessory organs of digestion, ***p. 342***
7. Describe how bile travels into the digestive tract and functions in digestion, ***p. 344***
8. Explain the role of enzymes in digestion and give examples of these enzymes, ***p. 344***
9. Name the digestion products of fats, proteins, and carbohydrates, ***p. 344***
10. Define *absorption* and state how villi function in absorption, ***p. 346***
11. Explain the use of feedback in regulating digestion and give several examples, ***p. 346***
12. List several hormones involved in regulating digestion, ***p. 346***
13. Using the case study, describe the colonoscopy procedure and its role in diagnosing certain colon disorders, ***pp. 332, 348***
14. Show how word parts are used to build words related to digestion (see Word Anatomy at the end of the chapter), ***p. 350***

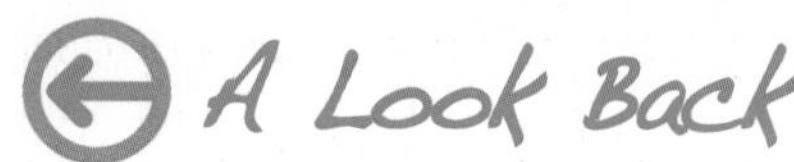

This chapter discusses some of the membranes and other tissue types introduced in Chapter 4. We also focus on the various organic substances and the activity of enzymes, described in Chapter 2.

General Structure and Function of the Digestive System

Every body cell needs a constant supply of nutrients. Cells use the energy contained in nutrients to do their work. In addition, they rearrange the nutrients' chemical building blocks to manufacture materials the body needs for metabolism, growth, and repair.

Food in its ingested form is too large to enter cells. It must first be broken down into particles small enough to pass through the cells' plasma membrane. This breakdown process is known as **digestion**. After digestion, the circulation must carry nutrients to the cells in every part of the body. The transfer of nutrients into the circulation is called **absorption**. Finally, undigested waste material must be eliminated. Digestion, absorption, and elimination are the three chief functions of the digestive system.

For our purposes, the digestive system may be divided into two groups of organs:

- The **digestive tract**, a continuous passageway beginning at the mouth, where food is taken in, and terminating at the anus, where the solid waste products of digestion are expelled from the body. The remainder of the digestive tract consists of the pharynx, esophagus, stomach, and small and large intestines, illustrated shortly.
- The **accessory organs**, which are necessary for the digestive process but are not a direct part of the digestive tract. They release substances into the digestive tract through ducts. These organs are the salivary glands, liver, gallbladder, and pancreas.

Before describing the individual organs of the digestive tract, we will pause to discuss the general structure of these organs. We will also describe the large membrane (peritoneum) that lines the abdominopelvic cavity, which contains most of the digestive organs.

THE WALL OF THE DIGESTIVE TRACT

Although modified for specific tasks in different organs, the wall of the digestive tract, from the esophagus to the anus, is similar in structure throughout (Fig. 17-1). The general

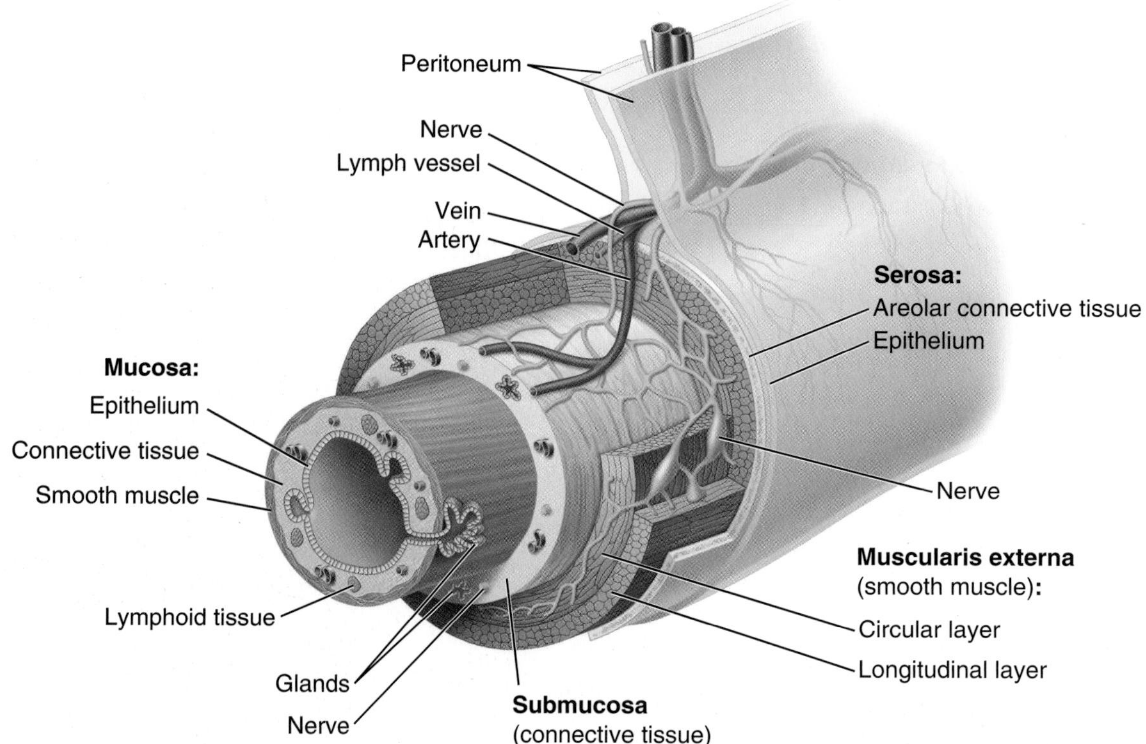

Figure 17-1 Wall of the digestive tract. KEY POINT The four layers are the mucosa, submucosa, muscularis externa (smooth muscle), and serosa. There is some variation in different organs. ZOOMING IN What type of tissue is between the submucosa and the serous membrane in the digestive tract wall? (Reprinted with permission from McConnell TH, Hull KL, *Human Form, Human Function*, Philadelphia, PA: Lippincott Williams & Wilkins, 2011.)

pattern consists of four layers, which are, from innermost to outermost:

1. Mucous membrane, or mucosa
2. Submucosa
3. Smooth muscle, the muscularis externa
4. Serous membrane, or serosa

First is the mucous membrane, or **mucosa**. From the mouth through the esophagus, and also in the anus, the mucosal epithelium consists of stratified squamous cells, which help to protect deeper tissues. Throughout the remainder of the digestive tract, the type of epithelium in the mucosa is simple columnar. Goblet cells within this epithelium secrete mucus to protect the system's lining. Beneath the epithelium is a layer of connective tissue followed by a very thin layer of smooth muscle. Many of the cells that secrete digestive juices are located in the mucosa. This layer also has lymphoid tissue associated with the immune system.

The layer of connective tissue beneath the mucosa is the **submucosa**, which contains blood vessels and some of the nerves that help regulate digestive activity. In the esophagus and small intestine, this layer also contains mucus-secreting glands.

The next layer, the **muscularis externa**, is composed of smooth muscle. Most of the digestive organs have two layers of smooth muscle: an inner layer of circular fibers, and an outer layer of longitudinal fibers. When a section of the circular muscle contracts, the organ's lumen narrows; when the longitudinal muscle contracts, a section of the wall shortens and the lumen becomes wider. These alternating muscular contractions create the wavelike movement, called **peristalsis** (per-ih-STAL-sis), that propels food through the digestive tract and mixes it with digestive juices. Nerves that control motility (movement) of the digestive organs are located in this smooth muscle layer.

The digestive organs in the abdominopelvic cavity have an outermost layer of serous membrane, or **serosa**, a thin, moist tissue composed of simple squamous epithelium and areolar (loose) connective tissue. This membrane forms the inner layer of the large serous membrane that extends throughout the abdominopelvic cavity, discussed next.

THE PERITONEUM

The **peritoneum** (per-ih-to-NE-um) is a thin, shiny serous membrane that lines the abdominopelvic cavity and also folds back to cover most of the organs contained within the cavity (Fig. 17-2). As noted in Chapter 4, the outer portion of this membrane, the layer that lines the cavity, is called the *parietal* (pah-RI-eh-tal) *peritoneum*; the layer that covers the organs is called the *visceral* (VIS-eh-ral) *peritoneum*. This slippery membrane allows the organs to slide over each other as they function. The peritoneum also carries blood

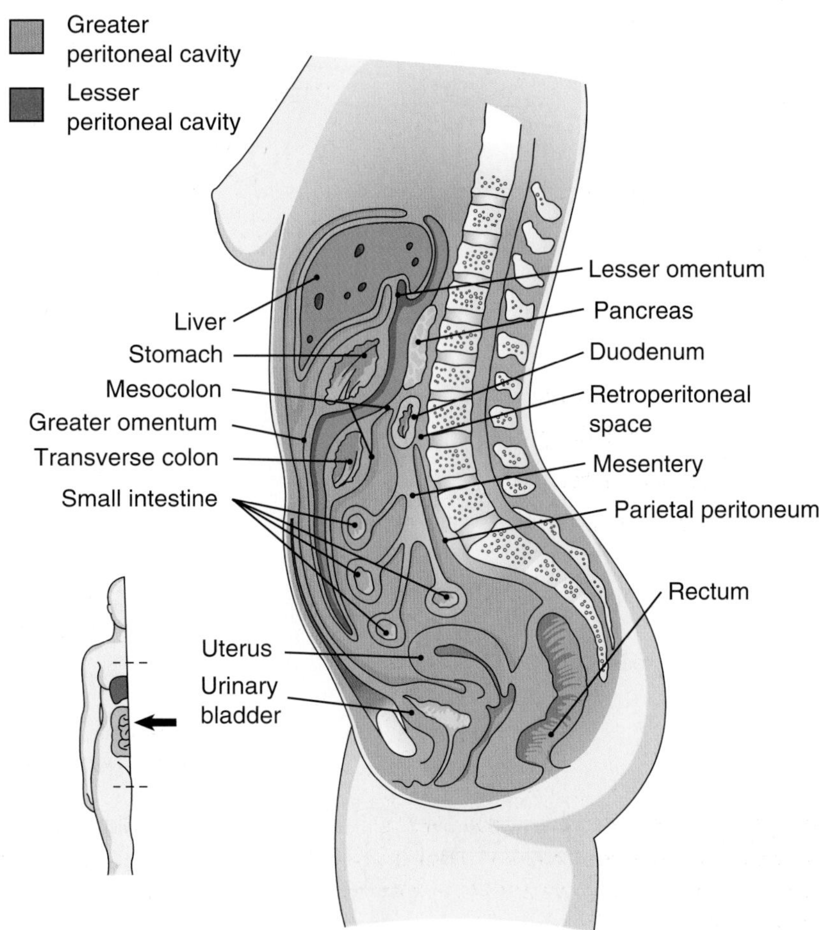

Figure 17-2 The abdominopelvic cavity and peritoneum. KEY POINT The parietal peritoneum lines the abdominopelvic cavity. Subdivisions of the visceral peritoneum fold over, supporting and separating individual organs. ZOOMING IN Which part of the peritoneum is around the small intestine?

vessels, lymphatic vessels, and nerves. In some places, it supports the organs and binds them to each other. The peritoneal cavity is the potential space between the membrane's two layers and contains serous fluid (peritoneal fluid). The *greater peritoneal cavity* is the main portion, located in the abdominal cavity and extending into the pelvic cavity (see Fig. 17-2). The *lesser peritoneal cavity* is formed by a smaller extension of these membranes dorsal to the stomach and liver to the posterior attachment of the diaphragm.

Subdivisions of the peritoneum around the various organs have special names. The mesentery (MES-en-ter-e) is a double-layered portion of the peritoneum shaped somewhat like a fan (see Fig. 17-2). The handle portion is attached to the posterior abdominal wall, and the expanded long edge is attached to the small intestine. Between the two membranous layers of the mesentery are the vessels and nerves that supply the intestine. The section of the peritoneum that extends from the colon to the posterior abdominal wall is the mesocolon (mes-o-KO-lon).

A large double layer of the peritoneum containing much fat hangs like an apron over the front of the intestine. This **greater omentum** (o-MEN-tum) extends from the lower border of the stomach into the pelvic cavity and then loops back up to the transverse colon. A smaller membrane, called the **lesser omentum**, extends between the stomach and the liver.

CHECKPOINTS 

- 17-1 Why does food have to be digested before cells can use it?
- 17-2 What are the typical four layers of the digestive tract wall?
- 17-3 What is the name of the large serous membrane that lines the abdominopelvic cavity and covers the organs it contains?

Organs of the Digestive Tract

As we study the organs of the digestive system, locate each in Figure 17-3. The digestive tract is a muscular tube extending through the body. It is composed of several parts: the

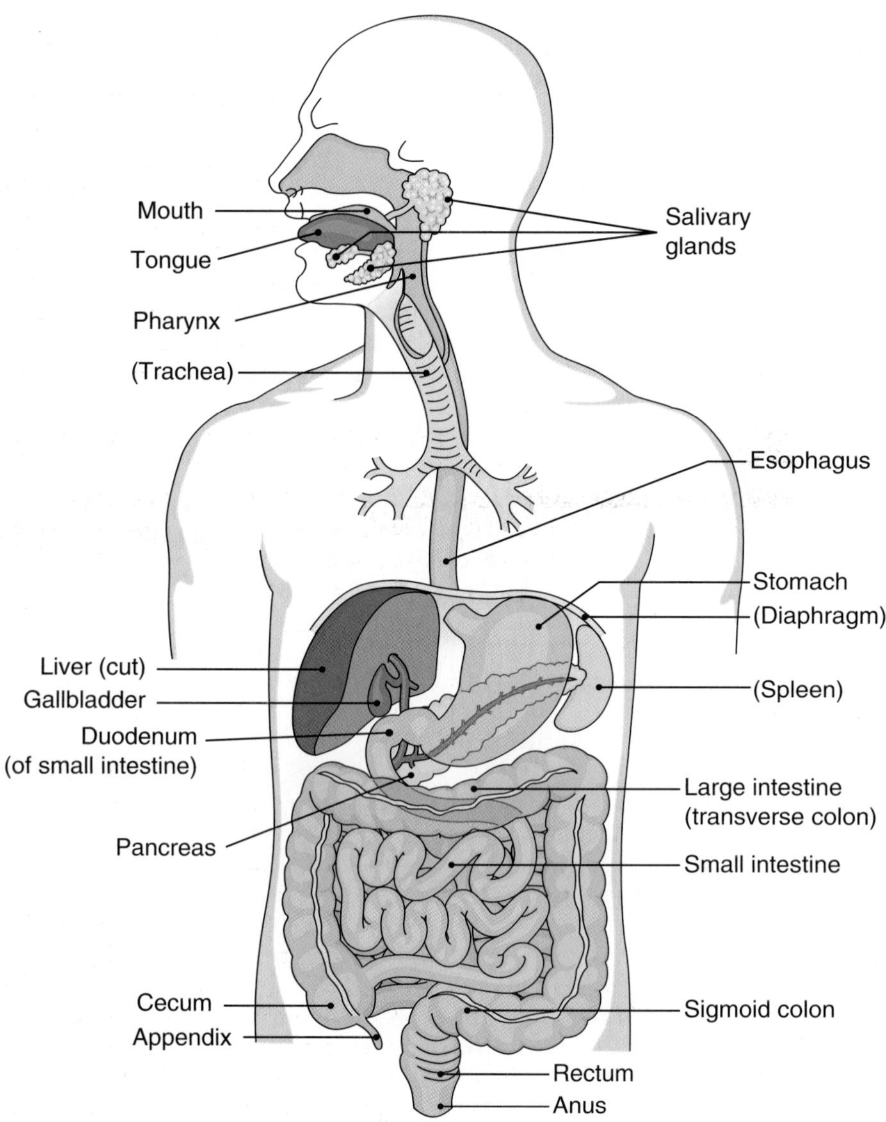

Figure 17-3 The digestive system. KEY POINT The digestive system extends from the mouth to the anus. Accessory organs secrete into the digestive tract. Nearby structures for orientation are shown in parentheses. ZOOMING IN Which accessory organs of digestion secrete into the mouth?

mouth, pharynx, esophagus, stomach, small intestine, and **large intestine.** The digestive tract is sometimes called the alimentary tract, from the word *aliment*, meaning "food." It is more commonly referred to as the **gastrointestinal (GI)** tract because of the major importance of the stomach and intestine in the digestive process.

The next section describes the structure and function of each digestive organ. These descriptions are followed by an overview of how the organs work together in digestion. See Dissection Atlas **Figure A3-7** for a photograph showing the abdominal digestive organs in place.

THE MOUTH

The mouth, also called the *oral cavity*, is where a substance begins its travels through the digestive tract **(Fig. 17-4)**. The mouth has the following digestive functions:

- It receives food, a process called **ingestion.**
- It breaks food into small portions. This is done mainly by the teeth in the process of chewing or **mastication** (mas-tih-KA-shun), but the tongue, cheeks, and lips are also used.
- It mixes the food with **saliva** (sah-LI-vah), which is produced by the salivary glands and secreted into the mouth. Saliva lubricates the food and has a digestive enzyme called *salivary amylase*, which begins starch digestion. The salivary glands will be described with the other accessory organs.
- It moves proper amounts of food toward the throat to be swallowed, a process called **deglutition** (deg-lu-TISH-un).

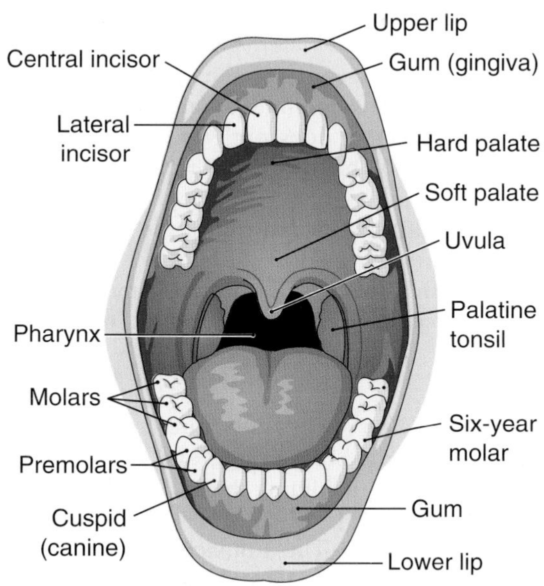

Figure 17-4 The mouth. KEY POINT Digestion begins in the mouth with enzymatic digestion of starch and mastication (chewing). The teeth and tonsils are visible in this view.

The **tongue** (TUNG), a muscular organ that projects into the mouth, aids in chewing and swallowing, and is one of the principal organs of speech. The tongue has a number of special surface receptors, called *taste buds*, which can differentiate taste sensations (e.g., bitter, sweet, sour, or salty) (see Chapter 10).

THE TEETH

The oral cavity also contains the teeth **(see Fig. 17-4)**. A child between 2 and 6 years of age has 20 teeth, known as the baby teeth or **deciduous** (de-SID-u-us) teeth. (The word deciduous means "falling off at a certain time," such as the leaves that fall off the trees in autumn.) A complete set of adult permanent teeth numbers 32. The cutting teeth, or **incisors** (in-SI-sors), occupy the anterior part of the oral cavity. The **cuspids** (KUS-pids), commonly called the *canines* (KA-nines) or *eyeteeth*, are lateral to the incisors. They are pointed teeth with deep roots that are used for more forceful gripping and tearing of food. The posterior **molars** (MO-lars) are the larger grinding teeth. There are two premolars and three molars. In an adult, each quadrant (quarter) of the mouth, moving from anterior to posterior, has two incisors, one cuspid, and five molars.

The first eight deciduous (baby) teeth to appear through the gums are the incisors. Later, the cuspids and molars appear. Usually, the 20 baby teeth all have appeared by the time a child has reached the age of 2 to 3 years. During the first 2 years, the permanent teeth develop within the upper jaw (maxilla) and lower jaw (mandible) from buds that are present at birth. The first permanent teeth to appear are the four 6-year molars, which come in before any baby teeth are lost. Because decay and infection of deciduous molars may spread to new, permanent teeth, deciduous teeth need proper care.

As a child grows, the jawbones grow, making space for additional teeth. After the 6-year molars have appeared, the baby incisors loosen and are replaced by permanent incisors. Next, the baby canines (cuspids) are replaced by permanent canines, and finally, the baby molars are replaced by the permanent bicuspids (premolars).

At this point, the larger jawbones are ready for the appearance of the 12-year, or second, permanent molar teeth. During or after the late teens, the third molars, or so-called *wisdom teeth*, may appear. In some cases, the jaw is not large enough for these teeth, or there are other abnormalities, so that the third molars may not erupt or may have to be removed. **Figure 17-5** shows the parts of a molar.

The main substance of the tooth is **dentin**, a calcified substance harder than bone. Within the tooth is a soft pulp containing blood vessels and nerves. The tooth's *crown* projects above the gum, the **gingiva** (JIN-jih-vah), and is covered with **enamel**, the hardest substance in the body. The *root* or roots of the tooth, located below the gum line in a bony socket, are covered with a rigid connective tissue (cementum) that helps to hold the tooth in place. A fibrous *periodontal ligament* joins the cementum

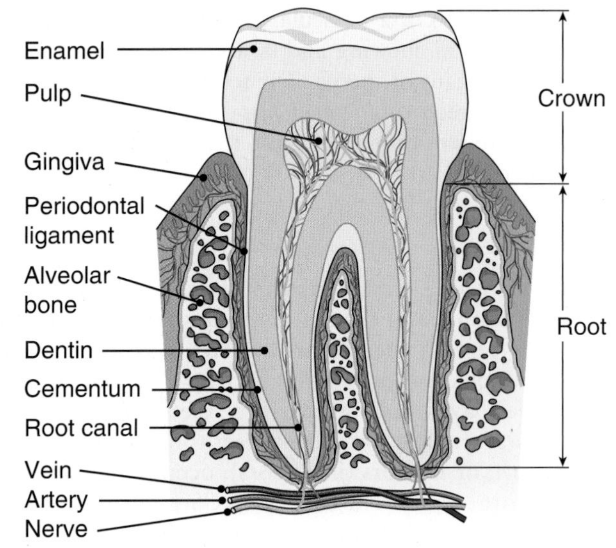

Figure 17-5 **A molar tooth.** KEY POINT The teeth grind food and break it apart. ZOOMING IN What is the common name for the gingiva?]

to the tooth socket. Each root has a canal containing extensions of the pulp.

THE PHARYNX

The pharynx (FAR-inks) is commonly referred to as the throat. It is a combined pathway for the respiratory and digestive systems, and was described in Chapter 16 (see Fig. 17-2). The oral part of the pharynx, the oropharynx, is visible when you look into an open mouth and depress the tongue. The palatine tonsils may be seen at either side of the oropharynx. The pharynx also extends upward to the nasal cavity, where it is referred to as the nasopharynx and downward to the larynx, where it is called the laryngopharynx. The **soft palate** is tissue that forms the posterior roof of the oral cavity. From it hangs a soft, fleshy, V-shaped mass called the **uvula** (U-vu-lah).

In swallowing, the tongue pushes a **bolus** (BO-lus) of food, a small portion of chewed food mixed with saliva, into the pharynx. Once the food reaches the pharynx, swallowing occurs rapidly by an involuntary reflex action. At the same time, the soft palate and uvula are raised to prevent food and liquid from entering the nasal cavity, and the tongue is raised to seal the back of the oral cavity. As described in Chapter 18, the entrance of the trachea is guarded during swallowing by the leaf-shaped cartilage, the epiglottis, which covers the opening of the larynx (see Fig. 16-3). The swallowed food is then moved into the esophagus.

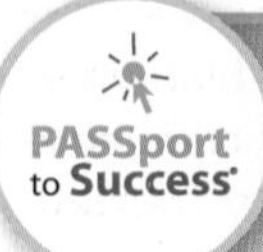

See the student resources on *thePoint* for information on dental hygienists and their role in maintaining the health of the teeth and gums.

THE ESOPHAGUS

The esophagus (eh-SOF-ah-gus) is a muscular tube about 25 cm (10 in.) long. Its musculature differs slightly from that of the other digestive organs because it has voluntary striated muscle in its upper portion, which gradually changes to smooth muscle along its length. In the esophagus, food is lubricated with mucus and moved by peristalsis into the stomach. No additional digestion occurs in the esophagus.

Before joining the stomach, the esophagus must pass through the diaphragm. It travels through an opening in the diaphragm called the **esophageal hiatus** (eh-sof-ah-JE-al hi-A-tus) (Fig. 17-6).

THE STOMACH

The stomach is an expanded J-shaped organ in the superior left region of the abdominal cavity (see Fig. 17-6). In addition to the two muscle layers already described, it has a third, inner oblique (angled) layer that aids in grinding food and mixing it with digestive juices. The left-facing arch of the stomach is the **greater curvature**, whereas the right surface forms the **lesser curvature**. The superior rounded portion under the left side of the diaphragm is the stomach's **fundus**. The region of the stomach leading into the small intestine is the **pylorus** (pi-LOR-us). The stomach's *body* is the largest part of the organ, located between the fundus and the pylorus.

Sphincters A sphincter (SFINK-ter) is a muscular ring that regulates the size of an opening. There are two sphincters that separate the stomach from the organs above and below.

Between the esophagus and the stomach is the **lower esophageal sphincter (LES)**. This muscle has also been called the *cardiac sphincter* because it separates the esophagus from the region of the stomach that is close to the heart. We are sometimes aware of the existence of this sphincter when it does not relax as it should, producing a feeling of being unable to swallow past that point.

Between the distal, or far, end of the stomach and the small intestine is the **pyloric** (pi-LOR-ik) **sphincter**. This sphincter and the stomach's pylorus, which leads to it, are important in regulating how rapidly food moves into the small intestine.

Functions of the Stomach The stomach serves as a storage pouch, digestive organ, and churn. When the stomach is empty, the lining forms many folds called rugae (RU-je) (see Fig. 17-6). These folds disappear as the stomach expands. (The stomach can stretch to hold one-half of a gallon of food and liquid.) Special cells in the stomach's lining secrete substances that mix together to form gastric juice (gastr/o is the word root for "stomach.") Some of the cells secrete a great amount of mucus to protect the organ's lining from digestive secretions.

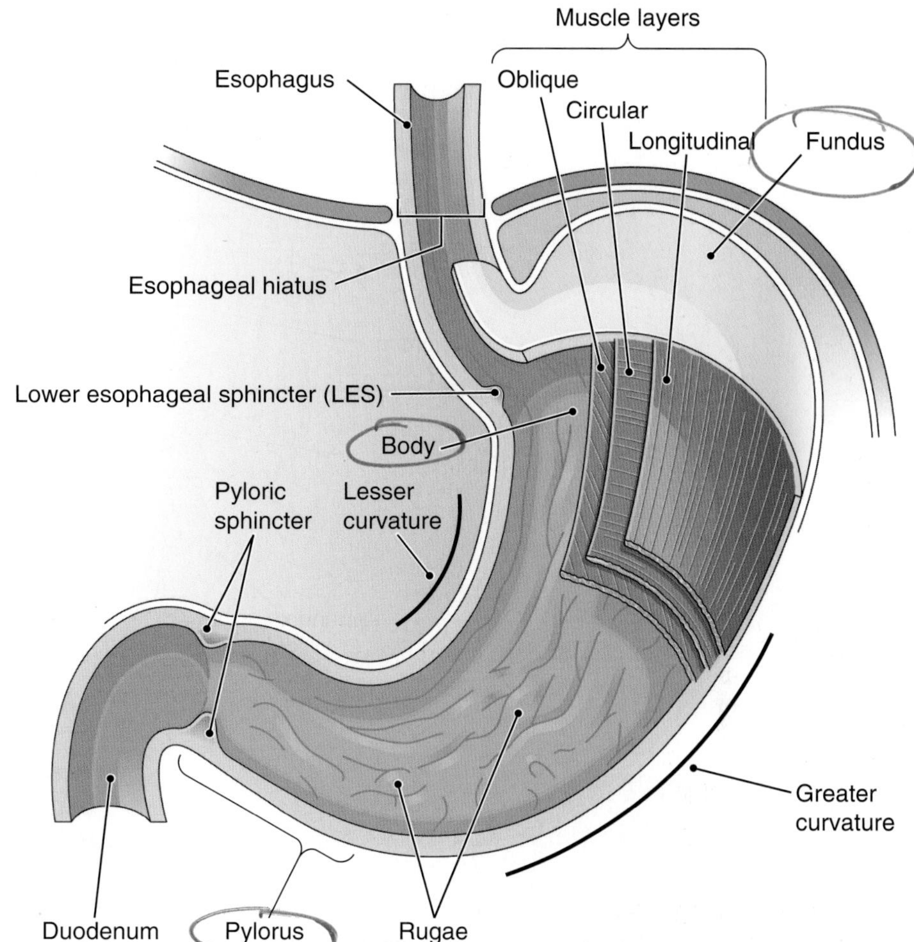

Figure 17-6 Longitudinal section of the stomach. KEY POINT The stomach's interior is shown, along with a portion of the esophagus and the duodenum. Sphincters regulate the organ's entrance and exit openings. ZOOMING IN Which additional muscle layer is in the wall of the stomach that is not found in the rest of the digestive tract?

Other cells produce the active components of the gastric juice, which are:

- Hydrochloric acid (HCl), a strong acid that unwinds proteins to prepare them for digestion and also destroys foreign organisms. HCl is produced in anticipation of eating and is produced in greater amounts when food enters the stomach.
- Pepsin, a protein-digesting enzyme. Pepsin is produced in an inactive form called *pepsinogen*, which is activated only when it contacts HCl.

Chyme (*kime*), from a Greek word meaning "juice," is the highly acidic, semiliquid mixture of gastric juice and food that leaves the stomach to enter the small intestine.

THE SMALL INTESTINE

The small intestine is the longest part of the digestive tract (Fig. 17-7). It is known as the small intestine because, although it is longer than the large intestine, it is smaller in diameter, with an average width of approximately 2.5 cm (1 in.). After death, when relaxed to its full length, the small intestine is approximately 6 m (20 ft) long. In life, the small intestine averages 3 m (10 ft) in length. The first 25 cm (10 in.) or so of the small intestine make up the **duodenum** (du-o-DE-num) (named for the Latin word for "twelve," based on its length of 12 finger widths). Beyond the duodenum are two more divisions: the **jejunum** (je-JU-num), which forms the next two-fifths of the small intestine, and the **ileum** (IL-e-um), which constitutes the remaining portion.

Functions of the Small Intestine The duodenal mucosa and submucosa contain glands that secrete large amounts of mucus to protect the small intestine from the strongly acidic chyme entering from the stomach. Mucosal cells of the small intestine also produce enzymes that digest proteins and carbohydrates. These enzymes are inserted into the cells' plasma membrane and act on nutrients that come in contact with the intestinal lining. In addition, digestive juices from the liver and pancreas enter the small intestine through a small opening in the duodenum. Most digestion takes place in the small intestine under the effects of these juices.

Minimal peristalsis occurs in the small intestine. This form of motility is too rapid to allow for effective digestion and absorption in the small intestine. A type of muscular activity termed **segmentation** operates here instead. In segmentation, the circular muscle in the organ's wall

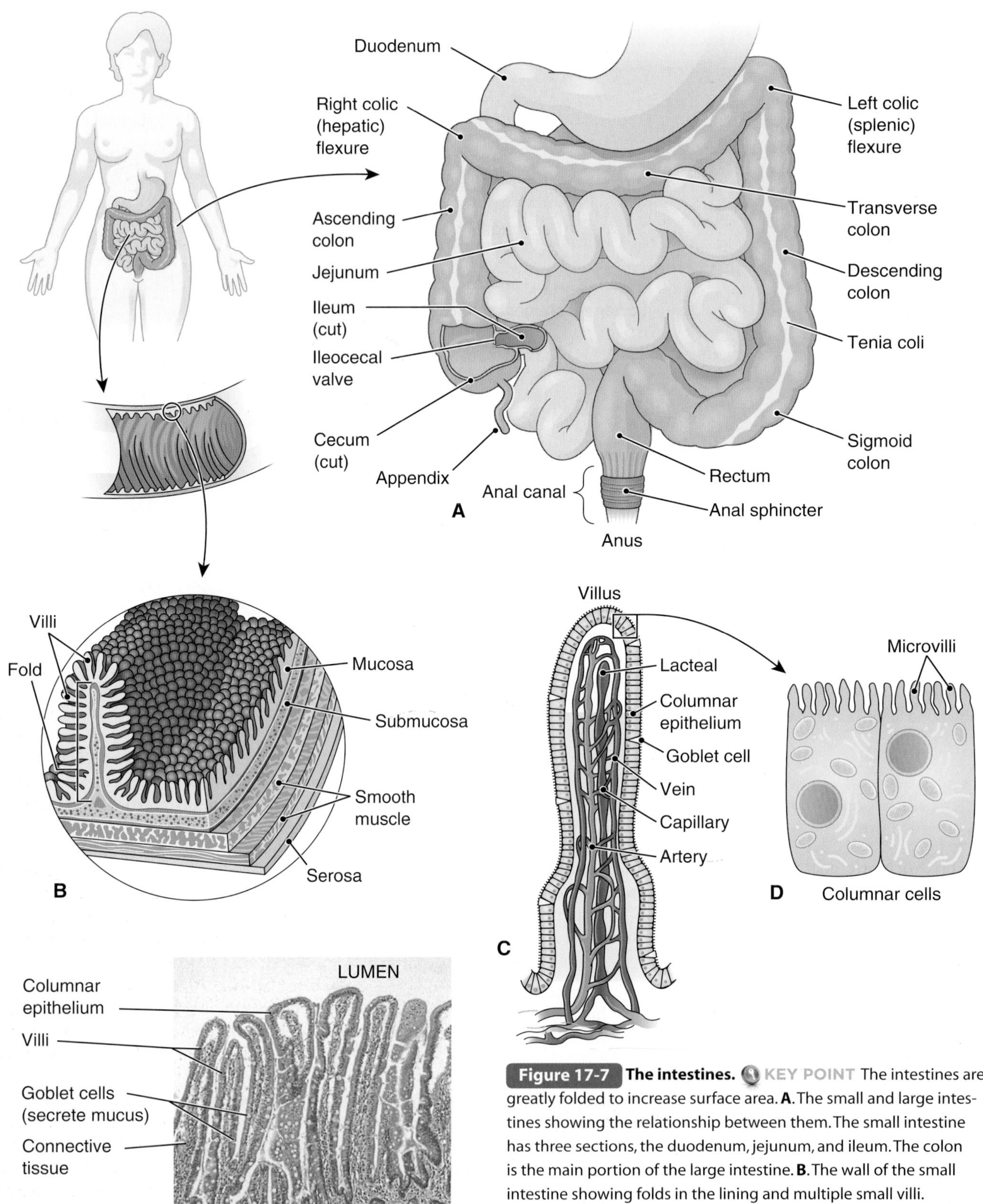

Figure 17-7 The intestines. KEY POINT The intestines are greatly folded to increase surface area. **A.** The small and large intestines showing the relationship between them. The small intestine has three sections, the duodenum, jejunum, and ileum. The colon is the main portion of the large intestine. **B.** The wall of the small intestine showing folds in the lining and multiple small villi. **C.** Drawing of a villus showing blood vessels, a lacteal of the lymphatic system and goblet cells that secret mucus. **D.** Columnar epithelial cells of the intestine with microvilli, folds of the plasma membrane. **E.** Micrograph of intestinal villi. (E Reprinted with permission from Cormack DH. *Essential Histology*, 2nd ed. Philadelphia, PA: Lippincott Williams & Wilkins, 2001.) ZOOMING IN Which portions of the small and large intestines join at the ileocecal valve?

Box 17-1 A Closer Look

The Folded Intestine: More Absorption with Less Length

Whenever materials pass from one system to another, they must travel through a cellular membrane. A major factor in how much transport can occur per unit of time is the total surface area of the membrane; the greater the surface area, the higher the rate of transport. The problem of packing a large amount of surface into a small space is solved in the body by folding the membranes. We do the same thing in everyday life. Imagine trying to store a bed sheet in the closet without folding it!

In the small intestine, where digested food must absorb into the bloodstream, there is folding of membranes down to the level of single cells.

- The 6 m long organ is coiled to fit into the abdominal cavity.
- The inner wall of the organ is thrown into circular folds called plicae circulares, which not only increase surface area, but aid in mixing.
- The mucosal villi project into the lumen, providing more surface area than a flat membrane would.
- The individual cells that line the small intestine have microvilli, tiny fingerlike folds of the plasma membrane that increase surface area tremendously.

Together, these structural features of the small intestine result in an absorptive surface area estimated to be about 250 m^2! Folding is present in other parts of the digestive system and in other areas of the body as well. Can you name other systems that show this folding pattern?

regularly contracts and relaxes in place, dividing the digestive contents and pushing portions back and forth. In this way, the material is thoroughly mixed with digestive juices and is placed in contact with the enzymes at the mucosal surface. Segmentation is regulated so that proximal segments contract before distal segments, slowly propelling the intestinal contents from the duodenum to the end of the ileum.

Most absorption of digested food, as well as water and electrolytes, also occurs through the walls of the small intestine. **Figure 17-7B** shows the wall and lining of the small intestine. Note that the lining, in addition to large circular folds, has millions of small extensions at the surface that aid in the absorption of nutrients, as described next.

Role of the Villi To increase the small intestine's surface area for absorption, the mucosa is formed into millions of tiny, fingerlike projections, or **villi** (VIL-li), which give the inner surface a velvety appearance. The epithelial cells of the villi also have small projecting folds of the plasma membrane known as **microvilli** **(see Fig. 17-7D)**. These extensions create a remarkable increase in the total surface area available for absorption in the small intestine.

Each villus contains blood vessels through which most digestion products are absorbed into the blood. Each one also contains a specialized lymphatic capillary called a **lacteal** (LAK-tele) through which fats are absorbed into the lymph. **Box 17-1** provides more information on the relationship of surface area to absorption.

THE LARGE INTESTINE

The large intestine is approximately 6.5 cm (2.5 in.) in diameter and approximately 1.5 m (5 ft) long **(see Fig. 17-7A)**. It is named for its wide diameter, rather than its length. The outer longitudinal muscle fibers in its wall form three separate surface bands. These bands, known as **teniae** (TEN-e-e) **coli,** draw up the organ's wall to give it its distinctive puckered appearance. (The name is also spelled *taeniae*; the singular is *tenia* or *taenia*).

Subdivisions of the Large Intestine The large intestine begins in the lower right region of the abdomen. The first part is a small pouch called the **cecum** (SE-kum). Between the ileum of the small intestine and the cecum is a sphincter, the **ileocecal** (il-e-o-SE-kal) **valve**, which prevents food from traveling backward into the small intestine. Attached to the cecum is a small, blind tube containing lymphoid tissue; its full name is **vermiform** (VER-mih-form) **appendix** (*vermiform* means "wormlike,") but usually just "appendix" is used.

The second portion, the **ascending colon**, extends superiorly along the right side of the abdomen toward the liver. It bends near the liver at the right colic (hepatic) flexure and extends across the abdomen as the **transverse colon.** It bends again sharply at the left colic (splenic) flexure and extends inferiorly on the left side of the abdomen into the pelvis, forming the **descending colon**. The distal colon bends backward into an S shape forming the **sigmoid colon** (named for the Greek letter *sigma*), which continues downward to empty into the **rectum**, a temporary storage area for indigestible or nonabsorbable food residue **(see Fig. 17-7A)**. The narrow terminal portion of the large intestine

Box 17-2 *Clinical Perspectives*

Endoscopy: A View From Within

Modern medicine has made great strides toward looking into the body without resorting to invasive surgery. An instrument that has made this possible in many cases is the **endoscope**, which is inserted into the body through an orifice or small incision and used to examine passageways, hollow organs, and body cavities. The first endoscopes were rigid lighted telescopes that could be inserted only a short distance into the body. Today, physicians are able to navigate the twists and turns of the digestive tract using long **fiberoptic endoscopes** composed of flexible bundles of glass or plastic that transmit light.

In the gastrointestinal tract, endoscopy can detect structural abnormalities, bleeding ulcers, inflammation, and tumors. In the case study, a colonoscopy was done to examine Adam's colon. In addition, endoscopes can be used to remove fluid samples or tissue specimens. Some surgery can even be done with an endoscope, such as polyp removal from the colon or expansion of a sphincter. Endoscopy can also be used to examine and operate on joints (arthroscopy), the bladder (cystoscopy), respiratory passages (bronchoscopy), and the abdominal cavity (laparoscopy).

Capsular endoscopy, a recent technological advance, has made examination of the gastrointestinal tract even easier. It uses a pill-sized camera that can be swallowed! As the camera moves through the digestive tract, it transmits video images to a data recorder worn on the patient's belt. Each camera is used only once; after about 24 hours, it is eliminated with the stool and flushed away.

is the **anal canal**, which leads to the outside of the body through an opening called the **anus** (A-nus). Visual examination of the colon is a part of Adam's physical examination in the case study. Box 17-2 provides more information about procedures such as the one Adam had.

Functions of the Large Intestine The large intestine secretes a great quantity of mucus, but no enzymes. Minimal digestion occurs in this organ, but some water is reabsorbed, and undigested food is stored, formed into solid waste material, called **feces** (FE-seze) or stool, and then eliminated.

At intervals, usually after meals, the involuntary muscles within the large intestine's walls propel solid waste toward the rectum. Stretching of the rectum stimulates smooth muscle contraction in the rectal wall. Aided by voluntary contractions of the diaphragm and the abdominal muscles, the feces are eliminated from the body in a process called **defecation** (def-e-KA-shun). An anal sphincter provides voluntary control over defecation (see Fig. 17-7A).

While food residue is stored in the large intestine, bacteria that normally live in the colon act on it to produce vitamin K and some of the B-complex vitamins.

CHECKPOINTS 

☐ 17-4 How many baby teeth are there and what is the scientific name for the baby teeth?

☐ 17-5 What type of food is digested in the stomach?

☐ 17-6 What are the three divisions of the small intestine?

☐ 17-7 How does the small intestine function in the digestive process?

☐ 17-8 What are the divisions of the large intestine?

☐ 17-9 What are the functions of the large intestine?

The Accessory Organs

The accessory organs release secretions through ducts into the digestive tract. Specifically, the salivary glands deliver their secretions into the mouth. The liver, gallbladder, and pancreas release secretions into the duodenum.

THE SALIVARY GLANDS

While food is in the mouth, it is mixed with **saliva** (sah-LI-vah), which moistens the food and facilitates mastication (chewing) and deglutition (swallowing). Saliva helps to keep the teeth and mouth clean. It also contains some antibodies and an enzyme (lysozyme) that help reduce bacterial growth.

This watery mixture contains mucus and an enzyme called **salivary amylase** (AM-ih-laze), which begins the digestive process by converting starch to sugar. Saliva is manufactured by three pairs of glands (Fig. 17-8):

- The **parotid** (pah-ROT-id) **glands**, the largest of the group, are located inferior and anterior to the ear.
- The **submandibular** (sub-man-DIB-u-lar) **glands**, also called *submaxillary* (sub-MAK-sih-ler-e) *glands*, are located near the body of the lower jaw.
- The **sublingual** (sub-LING-gwal) **glands** are under the tongue.

All these glands empty through ducts into the oral cavity.

THE LIVER

The **liver** (LIV-er), often referred to by the word root *hepat*, is the body's largest glandular organ (Fig. 17-9). It is located in the superior right portion of the abdominal cavity under the dome of the diaphragm. The lower edge of a normal-sized liver is level with the ribs' lower margin. The human

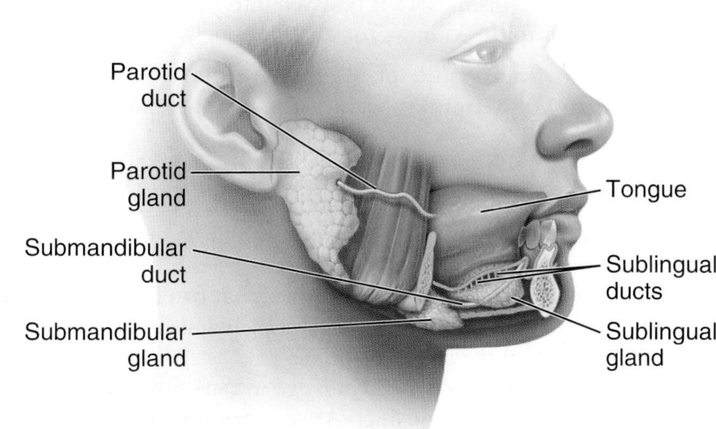

Figure 17-8 Salivary glands. KEY POINT Three groups of glands secret into the mouth through ducts. (Reprinted with permission from McConnell TH, Hull KL, *Human Form, Human Function*, Philadelphia, LWW, 2011.) ZOOMING IN Which salivary glands are directly below the tongue?

liver is the same reddish brown color as animal liver seen in the supermarket. It has a large right lobe and a smaller left lobe; the right lobe includes two inferior smaller lobes. The liver is supplied with blood through two vessels: the portal vein and the hepatic artery (the portal system and blood supply to the liver were described in Chapter 14). These vessels deliver about 1.5 quarts (1.6 L) of blood to the liver every minute. The hepatic artery carries blood high in oxygen, whereas the venous portal system carries blood that is low in oxygen and rich in digestive end products.

Functions of the Liver This most remarkable organ has many functions that affect digestion, metabolism, blood composition, and elimination of waste. Some of its major activities are:

- The manufacture of **bile**, a substance needed for the digestion of fats, discussed shortly.
- The storage of glucose (a simple sugar) in the form of glycogen, the animal equivalent of the starch found in plants. When the blood glucose level falls below normal, liver cells convert glycogen to glucose, which is released into the blood to restore a normal concentration.
- The modification of fats so that they can be used more efficiently by cells all over the body. The liver is also an important site for fat storage.
- The storage of some vitamins and iron.
- The formation of blood plasma proteins, such as albumin, globulins, and clotting factors.
- The destruction of old red blood cells and the recycling or elimination of their breakdown products. One byproduct, a pigment called **bilirubin** (BIL-ih-ru-bin), is eliminated in bile and gives the stool its characteristic dark color.

17

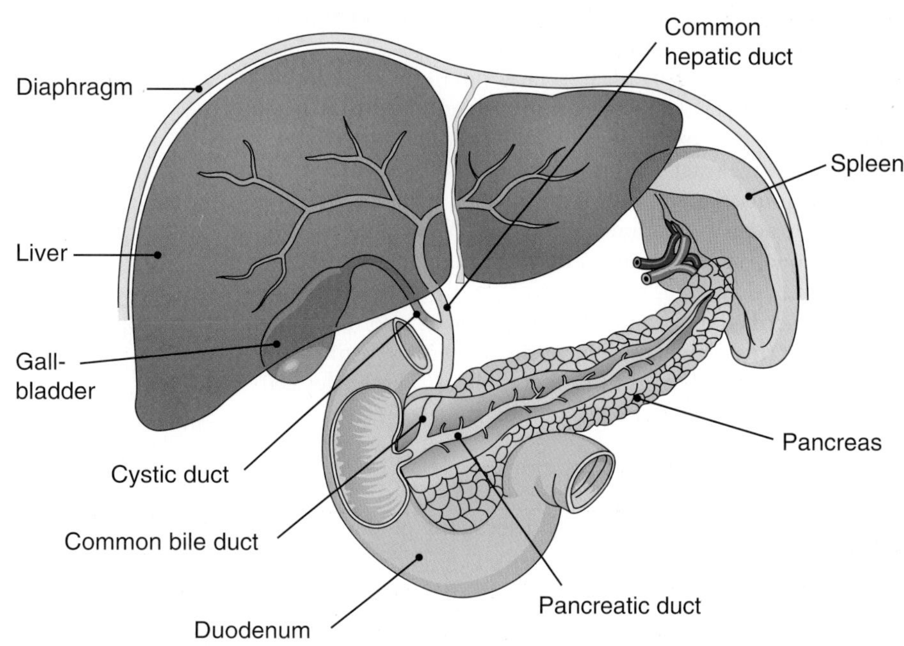

Figure 17-9 Accessory organs of digestion. KEY POINT The accessory organs secret digestive substances into the small intestine. ZOOMING IN Into which part of the intestine do these accessory organs secrete?

- The synthesis of **urea** (u-RE-ah), a waste product of protein metabolism. Urea is released into the blood and transported to the kidneys for elimination.
- The **detoxification** (de-tok-sih-fih-KA-shun) (removal of toxicity) of harmful substances, such as alcohol and certain drugs.

Bile The liver's main digestive function is the production of bile, a substance needed for the processing of fats. The salts contained in bile act like a detergent to **emulsify** fat; that is, to break up fat into small droplets that can be acted on more effectively by digestive enzymes. Bile also aids in fat absorption from the small intestine.

Bile leaves the lobes of the liver by two ducts that merge to form the **common hepatic duct**. After collecting bile from the gallbladder, this duct, now called the **common bile duct**, delivers bile into the duodenum. These and the other accessory ducts are shown in **Figure 17-9**.

THE GALLBLADDER

The **gallbladder** (GAWL-blad-er) is a muscular sac on the inferior surface of the liver that stores bile. Although the liver may manufacture bile continuously, the body needs it only a few times a day. Consequently, bile from the liver flows into the hepatic ducts and then up through the **cystic** (SIS-tik) **duct**, connected with the gallbladder **(see Fig. 17-9)**. When chyme enters the duodenum, the gallbladder contracts, squeezing bile through the cystic duct and into the common bile duct, leading to the duodenum.

THE PANCREAS

The **pancreas** (PAN-kre-as) is a long gland that extends from the duodenum to the spleen **(see Fig. 17-9)**. The pancreas produces enzymes that digest fats, proteins, carbohydrates, and nucleic acids. The protein-digesting enzymes are produced in inactive forms which must be converted to active forms in the small intestine by other enzymes.

The pancreas also releases large amounts of sodium bicarbonate ($NaHCO_3$), an alkaline (basic) fluid that neutralizes the acidic chyme in the small intestine, thus protecting the digestive tract's lining. These juices collect in a main duct that joins the common bile duct or empties into the duodenum near the common bile duct. Most people have an additional smaller pancreatic duct that opens into the duodenum.

As described in Chapter 11, the pancreas also functions as an endocrine gland, producing the hormones insulin and glucagon that regulate glucose metabolism. These islet cell secretions are released into the blood.

CHECKPOINTS 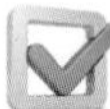

☐ **17-10** What are the names and locations of the salivary glands?

☐ **17-11** Which accessory organ secretes bile, and what is the function of bile in digestion?

☐ **17-12** What is the role of the gallbladder?

☐ **17-13** What accessory organ secretes sodium bicarbonate, and what is the function of this substance in digestion?

Enzymes and the Digestive Process

Although the individual organs of the digestive tract are specialized for digesting different types of food, the fundamental chemical process of digestion is the same for fats, proteins, and carbohydrates. In every case, this process requires enzymes. Recall from Chapter 2 **(see Fig. 2-11)** that enzymes are catalysts, substances that speed the rate of chemical reactions, but are not themselves changed or used up in the reaction.

Almost all enzymes are proteins, and they are highly specific in their actions. In digestion, an enzyme acts only in a certain type of reaction involving a certain type of nutrient molecule. For example, the carbohydrate-digesting enzyme amylase only splits starch into the disaccharide (double sugar) maltose. Another enzyme is required to split maltose into two molecules of the monosaccharide (simple sugar) glucose. Other enzymes split fats, or triglycerides, into their building blocks, glycerol, and fatty acids. Still others split proteins into smaller units called *peptides* and into their building blocks, amino acids (see Chapter 2).

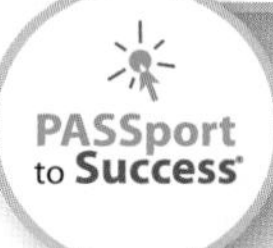

See the student resources on *thePoint* to review the animation on enzymes and view the animations *General Digestion* and *Digestion of Carbohydrates*.

THE ROLE OF WATER

Because water is added to nutrient molecules as they are split by enzymes, the process of digestion is referred to chemically as **hydrolysis** (hi-DROL-ih-sis), which means "splitting (lysis) by means of water (hydr/o)." In this chemical process, water's hydroxyl group (OH^-) is added to one fragment and the hydrogen ion (H^+) is added to the other, splitting the molecule. **Figure 17-10** shows the hydrolysis of a disaccharide into two monosaccharides. The building blocks of fats and proteins are separated in the same manner. Each hydrolysis reaction requires a specific enzyme and uses one molecule of water. About 7 L of water are secreted into the digestive tract each day, in addition to the nearly 2 L taken in with food and drink. You can now understand why so large an amount of water is needed. Water is not only used to produce digestive juices and to dilute food so that it can move more easily through the digestive tract, but is also used in the chemical process of digestion itself.

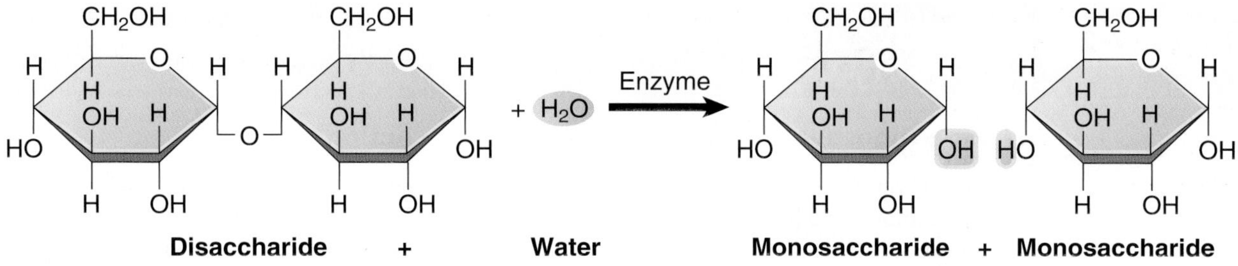

Figure 17-10 Hydrolysis. KEY POINT In digestion, water is added to compounds to split them into simpler building blocks. The figure shows the splitting of a disaccharide (double sugar) into two monosaccharides (simple sugars) by the addition of H^+ to one and OH^- to the other. The chemical bonds between the building blocks of fats and proteins are split in the same way. A specific enzyme is needed for every hydrolysis reaction.

DIGESTION, STEP-BY-STEP

Let us see what happens to a mass of food from the time it is taken into the mouth to the moment that it is ready to be absorbed (see Table 17-1).

In the mouth, the food is chewed and mixed with saliva, softening it so that it can be swallowed easily. Salivary amylase initiates the digestive process by changing some of the starches into maltose.

Digestion in the Stomach When the food reaches the stomach, it is acted on by gastric juice, with its hydrochloric acid (HCl) and enzymes. The hydrochloric acid has the important function of denaturing proteins, that is, unfolding them to prepare them for digestion. In addition, HCl activates the enzyme pepsin, which is secreted by gastric cells in an inactive form, as previously noted. Once activated by hydrochloric acid, pepsin works to digest protein; this enzyme is the first to digest nearly every type of protein in the diet. The stomach also secretes a fat-digesting enzyme (lipase), but it is of little importance in adults.

The food, gastric juice, and mucus (which is also secreted by cells of the gastric lining) are mixed to form chyme. This semiliquid substance is released gradually from the stomach through the pyloric sphincter into the small intestine for further digestion.

Digestion in the Small Intestine In the duodenum, the first part of the small intestine, chyme is mixed with the greenish-yellow bile delivered from the liver and the gallbladder through the common bile duct. Bile does not contain enzymes; instead, it contains bile salts that emulsify fats to allow the powerful secretions from the pancreas to act on them most efficiently.

Pancreatic juice contains a number of enzymes, including:

- **Lipase.** After bile divides fats into tiny particles, the pancreatic enzyme lipase digests almost all of them. In this process, the triglycerides, composed of glycerol and three fatty acids, are broken down into free fatty acids (two from each triglyceride) and monoglycerides (glycerol combined with one fatty acid). These breakdown products are more readily absorbable. If pancreatic lipase is absent, fats are expelled with the feces in undigested form.
- **Amylase.** This enzyme changes starch to maltose.
- **Trypsin** (TRIP-sin). This enzyme splits proteins into amino acids, which are small enough to be absorbed through the intestine.
- **Nucleases** (NU-kle-ases). These enzymes digest the nucleic acids DNA and RNA.

Table 17-1 Summary of Digestion

Organ	Activity	Nutrients Digested	Active Secretions
Mouth	Chews food and mixes it with saliva; forms it into bolus for swallowing	Starch	Salivary amylase
Esophagus	Moves food by peristalsis into stomach	—	—
Stomach	Stores food, churns food, and mixes it with digestive juices	Proteins	Hydrochloric acid, pepsin
Small intestine	Secretes enzymes, neutralizes acidity, receives secretions from pancreas and liver, absorbs nutrients and water into the blood or lymph	Fats, proteins, carbohydrates, nucleic acids	Intestinal enzymes, pancreatic enzymes, bile from liver
Large intestine	Reabsorbs some water; forms, stores, and eliminates stool	—	—

Table 17-2 Digestive Juices Produced by Digestive Tract Organs and Accessory Organs

Organ	Main Digestive Juices Produced	Action
Salivary glands	Salivary amylase	Begins starch digestion
Stomach	Hydrochloric acid (HCl)[a]	Breaks down proteins
	Pepsin	Begins protein digestion
Small intestine	Peptidases	Digest proteins to amino acids
	Lactase, maltase, sucrase	Digest disaccharides to monosaccharides
Pancreas	Sodium bicarbonate[a]	Neutralizes HCl
	Amylase	Digests starch
	Trypsin	Digests protein to amino acids
	Lipases	Digest fats to fatty acids and monoglycerides
	Nucleases	Digest nucleic acids
Liver	Bile salts[a]	Emulsify fats

[a]*Not enzymes.*

It is important to note that most digestion occurs in the small intestine under the action of pancreatic juice, which has the ability to break down all types of foods. When pancreatic juice is absent, serious digestive disturbances always occur.

The small intestine also produces a number of enzymes, including three that act on complex sugars to transform them into simpler, absorbable forms. These enzymes are **maltase, sucrase,** and **lactase,** which act on the disaccharides maltose, sucrose, and lactose, respectively.

Table 17-2 summarizes the main substances used in digestion. Note that, except for HCl, sodium bicarbonate, and bile salts, all the substances listed are enzymes.

CHECKPOINT 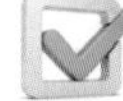

☐ 17-14 Which organ produces the most complete digestive secretions?

Absorption

The means by which digested nutrients reach the blood is known as **absorption.** Most absorption takes place through the villi in the mucosa of the small intestine (see Fig. 17-7D). Within each villus is an arteriole and a venule bridged with capillaries. Simple sugars, small proteins (peptides), amino acids, a few simple fatty acids, and most of the water in the digestive tract are absorbed into the blood through these capillaries. From here, they pass by way of the portal system to the liver, to be processed, stored, or released as needed.

ABSORPTION OF FATS

Most fats have an alternative method of reaching the blood. Instead of entering the blood capillaries, they are absorbed by the villi's more permeable lymphatic capillaries, the lacteals. The absorbed fat droplets give the lymph a milky appearance. The mixture of lymph and fat globules that drains from the small intestine after fat has been digested is called **chyle** (kile). Chyle merges with the lymphatic circulation and eventually enters the blood when the lymph drains into veins near the heart. The absorbed fats then move to the liver for further processing.

ABSORPTION OF VITAMINS AND MINERALS

Minerals and vitamins ingested with food are also absorbed from the small intestine. The minerals and some of the vitamins mix with water and are absorbed directly into the blood. Other vitamins are incorporated in fats and are absorbed along with the fats. Vitamin K and some B vitamins are produced by bacterial action in the colon and are absorbed from the large intestine.

CHECKPOINT 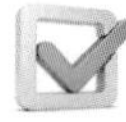

☐ 17-15 What is absorption?

Control of Digestion and Eating

As food moves through the digestive tract, its rate of movement and the activity of each organ it passes through must be carefully regulated. If food moves too slowly or digestive secretions are inadequate, the body will not get enough nourishment. If food moves too rapidly or excess secretions are produced, digestion and absorption may be incomplete or the digestive tract's lining may be damaged.

CONTROL OF DIGESTION

There are two types of control over digestion: nervous and hormonal. Both illustrate the principles of feedback control.

The nerves that control digestive activity are located in the submucosa and between the muscle layers of the organ walls (see Fig. 17-1). Instructions for action come from the autonomic (visceral) nervous system. In general, para-sympathetic

Table 17-3 Hormones Active in Digestion

Hormone	Source	Action
Gastrin	Stomach	Stimulates release of gastric juice
Gastric-inhibitory peptide (GIP)	Duodenum	Stimulates insulin release from pancreas when glucose enters duodenum; inhibits release of gastric juice
Secretin	Duodenum	Stimulates release of water and bicarbonate from pancreas; inhibits the stomach
Cholecystokinin (CCK)	Duodenum	Stimulates release of digestive enzymes from pancreas; stimulates release of bile from gallbladder; inhibits the stomach

stimulation increases activity, and sympathetic stimulation decreases activity. Excess sympathetic stimulation, as can be caused by stress, can slow food's movement through the digestive tract and inhibit mucus secretion, which is crucial to protecting the digestive tract's lining.

The digestive organs themselves produce the hormones involved in regulating digestion. The following is a discussion of some of these controls (Table 17-3).

The sight, smell, thought, taste, or feel of food in the mouth stimulates, through the nervous system, the secretion of saliva and the release of gastric juice. Once in the stomach, food stimulates the release into the blood of the hormone **gastrin**, which promotes stomach secretions and motility.

When chyme enters the duodenum, nerve impulses inhibit stomach motility, so that food will not move too rapidly into the small intestine. This action is a good example of negative feedback. At the same time, hormones released from the duodenum not only stimulate intestinal activity, but also feed back to the stomach to reduce its activity. **Gastric-inhibitory peptide (GIP)** is one such hormone. It acts on the stomach to inhibit the release of gastric juice. Its more important action is to stimulate insulin release from the pancreas when glucose enters the duodenum. (GIPs alternate name is *glucose-dependent insulinotropic peptide*, which stresses its role in glucose metabolism while keeping the same acronym). Another of these hormones, **secretin** (se-KRE-tin), stimulates the pancreas to release water and bicarbonate to dilute and neutralize chyme. **Cholecystokinin** (ko-le-sis-to-KI-nin) (**CCK**), stimulates the release of enzymes from the pancreas and causes the gallbladder to release bile.

CONTROL OF HUNGER AND APPETITE

Hunger is the desire for food, which can be satisfied by the ingestion of a filling meal. Hunger is regulated by hypothalamic centers that respond to nutrient levels in the blood. When these levels are low, the hypothalamus stimulates a sensation of hunger. Strong, mildly painful contractions of the empty stomach may stimulate a feeling of hunger. Messages received by the hypothalamus reduce hunger as food is chewed and swallowed and begins to fill the stomach. The short-term regulation of food intake works to keep the amount of food eaten within the limits of what the intestine can process. The long-term regulation of food intake maintains appropriate blood nutrient levels.

Appetite differs from hunger in that, although it is basically a desire for food, it often has no relationship to the need for food. Even after an adequate meal that has relieved hunger, a person may still have an appetite for additional food. A variety of factors, such as emotional state, cultural influences, habit, and memories of past food intake, can affect appetite. The regulation of appetite is not well understood. Despite day-to-day variations in food intake and physical activity, a healthy individual maintains a constant body weight and energy reserves of fat over long periods. With the discovery of the hormone leptin (from the Greek word *leptos*, meaning "thin,") researchers have been able to piece together one long-term mechanism for regulating weight. Leptin is produced by adipocytes in adipose tissue. When fat is stored because of excess food intake, the cells release more leptin. Centers in the hypothalamus respond to the hormone by decreasing food intake and increasing energy expenditure, resulting in weight loss. If this feedback mechanism is disrupted, obesity will result. Early hopes of using leptin to treat human obesity have dimmed, however, because obese people do not have a leptin deficiency. This system's failure in humans appears to be caused by the hypothalamus' inability to respond to leptin rather than our inability to make the hormone.

CHECKPOINTS 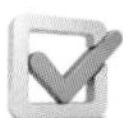

- ☐ 17-16 What are the two types of control over the digestive process?
- ☐ 17-17 What is the difference between hunger and appetite?

17

Effects of Aging on the Digestive System

With age, receptors for taste and smell deteriorate, leading to a loss of appetite and decreased enjoyment of food. A decrease in saliva and poor gag reflex make swallowing more difficult. Tooth loss or poorly fitting dentures may make chewing food more difficult.

Activity of the digestive organs decreases. These changes can be seen in poor absorption of certain vitamins and poor protein digestion. Slowing of peristalsis in the large intestine and increased consumption of easily chewed, refined foods contribute to the common occurrence of constipation.

The tissues of the digestive system require constant replacement. Slowing of this process contributes to a variety of digestive disorders, including gastritis, ulcers, and diverticulosis. As with many body systems, tumors and cancer occur more frequently with age.

A&P in Action Revisited

Adam's Colonoscopy

At his scheduled time, Adam reported to the hospital as an outpatient for his colonoscopy. He had stayed on a clear liquid diet for a day and done the required laxative prep to clear his colon. He met with Dr. Clarkson, a gastroenterologist (a physician who specializes in disorders of the gastrointestinal tract). Dr. Clarkson described the procedure. "We'll give you light sedation, and then use a flexible lighted endoscope with a camera to examine the entire colon. The procedure should take only about half an hour and has a very low risk. You have made arrangements for someone to go home with you, haven't you?" Adam said his brother was coming.

After the test, Dr. Clarkson reported that everything looked fine and that he would send the results to Dr. Michaels. "The good news, Adam, is that you have 10 years before you have to do this again. Maybe next time we'll be able to get our pictures with a small camera in a pill that you can swallow. That's already being tested. Scientists are also working on developing a screening test done by genetic study of cells sloughed off in the stool—and that won't require a prep."

Adam's case shows the importance of anatomic studies in the diagnosis and treatment of disease. Box 1-2 has general information on medical imaging, and various methods are mentioned in chapters and cases throughout this book. We will visit Adam again in Chapter 19 when he finds out that his prostate gland is affecting his urinary system.

Chapter Wrap-Up

Summary Overview

A detailed chapter outline with space for note-taking is on *thePoint*. The figure below illustrates the main topics covered in this chapter.

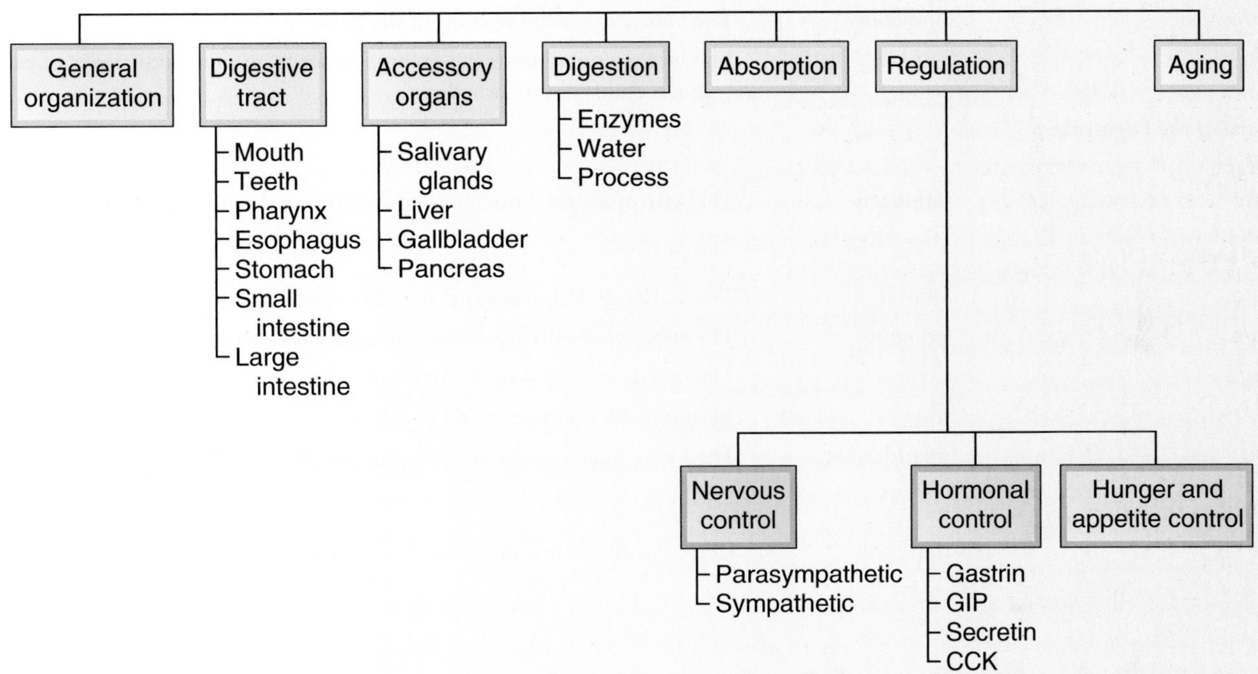

Key Terms

The terms listed below are emphasized in this chapter. Knowing them will help you organize and prioritize your learning. These and other bold face terms are defined in the Glossary with phonetic pronunciations.

absorption
bile
chyle
chyme
defecation
deglutition
digestion
duodenum
emulsify
esophagus
gallbladder
hydrolysis
ingestion
intestine
lacteal
liver
mastication
pancreas
peristalsis
peritoneum
saliva
sphincter
stomach
villi

Word Anatomy

Scientific terms are built from standardized word parts (prefixes, roots, and suffixes). Learning the meanings of these parts can help you remember words and interpret unfamiliar terms.

WORD PART	MEANING	EXAMPLE
General Structure and Function of the Digestive System		
ab-	away from	In *absorption*, digested materials are taken from the digestive tract into the circulation.
enter/o	intestine	The *mesentery* is the portion of the peritoneum around the intestine.
mes/o-	middle	The *mesocolon*, like the mesentery, comes from the middle layer of cells in the embryo, the mesoderm.
Organs of the Digestive Tract		
gastr/o	stomach	The *gastrointestinal* tract consists mainly of the stomach and intestine.
The Accessory Organs		
amyl/o	starch	The starch-digesting enzyme in saliva is salivary *amylase.*
lingu/o	tongue	The *sublingual* salivary glands are under the tongue.
hepat/o	liver	The *hepatic* portal system carries blood to the liver.
bil/i	bile	*Bilirubin* is a pigment found in bile.
cyst/o	bladder, sac	The *cystic* duct carries bile into and out of the gallbladder
Control of Digestion		
chole	bile, gall	*Cholecystokinin* is a hormone that activates the gallbladder (cholecyst/o).

Questions for Study and Review

BUILDING UNDERSTANDING

Fill in the Blanks

1. The wavelike movement of the digestive tract wall is called _____.

2. The small intestine is connected to the posterior abdominal wall by _____.

3. The liver can store glucose in the form of _____.

4. The parotid glands secrete _____.

5. Teeth are composed mainly of a hard calcified substance called _____.

Matching > Match each numbered item with the most closely related lettered item.

___ **6.** Digests starch
___ **7.** Begins protein digestion
___ **8.** Digests fats
___ **9.** Splits protein into amino acids
___ **10.** Emulsify fats

a. lipase
b. amylase
c. trypsin
d. pepsin
e. bile salts

Multiple Choice

___ **11.** The teeth break up food into small parts by a process called

a. absorption
b. deglutition
c. ingestion
d. mastication

___ **12.** Which organ secretes hydrochloric acid and pepsin?

a. salivary glands
b. stomach
c. pancreas
d. liver

___ **13.** What is the name for the double layer of peritoneum that extends from the lower border of the stomach and hangs over the intestine?

a. greater omentum
b. lesser omentum
c. mesentery
d. mesocolon

___ **14.** What is the soft, fleshy V-shaped mass of tissue that hangs from the soft palate called?

a. epiglottis
b. esophageal hiatus
c. uvula
d. gingiva

___ **15.** Which structure guards the entrance to the trachea during swallowing?

a. uvula
b. epiglottis
c. gingiva
d. bolus

UNDERSTANDING CONCEPTS

16. Differentiate between the terms in each of the following pairs:

a. digestion and absorption
b. parietal and visceral peritoneum
c. gastrin and gastric-inhibitory peptide
d. secretin and cholecystokinin

17. Name the four layers of the digestive tract. Which tissue makes up each layer? What is the function of each layer?

18. Describe the structure and function of the liver, pancreas, and gallbladder. How are the products of these organs delivered to the digestive tract?

19. Where does absorption occur in the digestive tract, and what structures are needed for absorption? Which types of nutrients are absorbed into the blood? Into the lymph?

20. How does the nervous system regulate digestion?

21. Name several hormones that regulate digestion.

CONCEPTUAL THINKING

22. Overuse of antacids can inhibit protein digestion. How?

23. Blockage of the common bile duct can cause autodigestion of the pancreas. Why?

24. In Adam's case, the proctologist described a colonoscopy done with a camera that is swallowed. Beginning in the mouth, trace the path the camera would take as it moves through the digestive tract toward the anus.

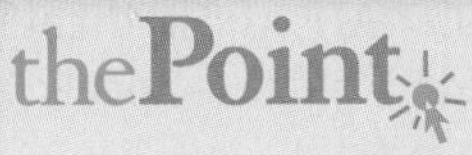

For more questions, see the learning activities on *thePoint*.

CHAPTER 18

Metabolism, Nutrition, and Body Temperature

A&P in Action

Becky's Second Case: Managing Her Metabolism

"Becky, are you sure you packed everything? Glucose monitor, insulin, needles..." asked Becky's mom as she loaded her daughter's knapsack and sleeping bag into the car. Becky rolled her eyes and said, "Yeah mom, I've got everything. Don't worry; I'll only be at camp for a week!"

Becky's mom sighed. She knew her daughter was right. Besides, *this* summer camp was for children with diabetes mellitus. Not only would she get to do all the fun things that kids normally do at camp, she would also be safe. After all, there was experienced medical staff on site and many of the camp counselors were diabetic themselves. Becky's mom knew that this was a great opportunity for her daughter to learn more about managing her condition and meet other kids with diabetes.

At camp, Becky was having a great time. Her cabin leader, Wanda, was really cool. Today, Wanda was going to teach them how to paddle a canoe! "OK girls," said Wanda, "before we head out to the dock, we need to check our blood glucose levels. Does anyone remember why?"

"Paddling a canoe takes a lot of effort and we have to make sure that we have energy for our muscles to do the work," answered Becky's bunkmate.

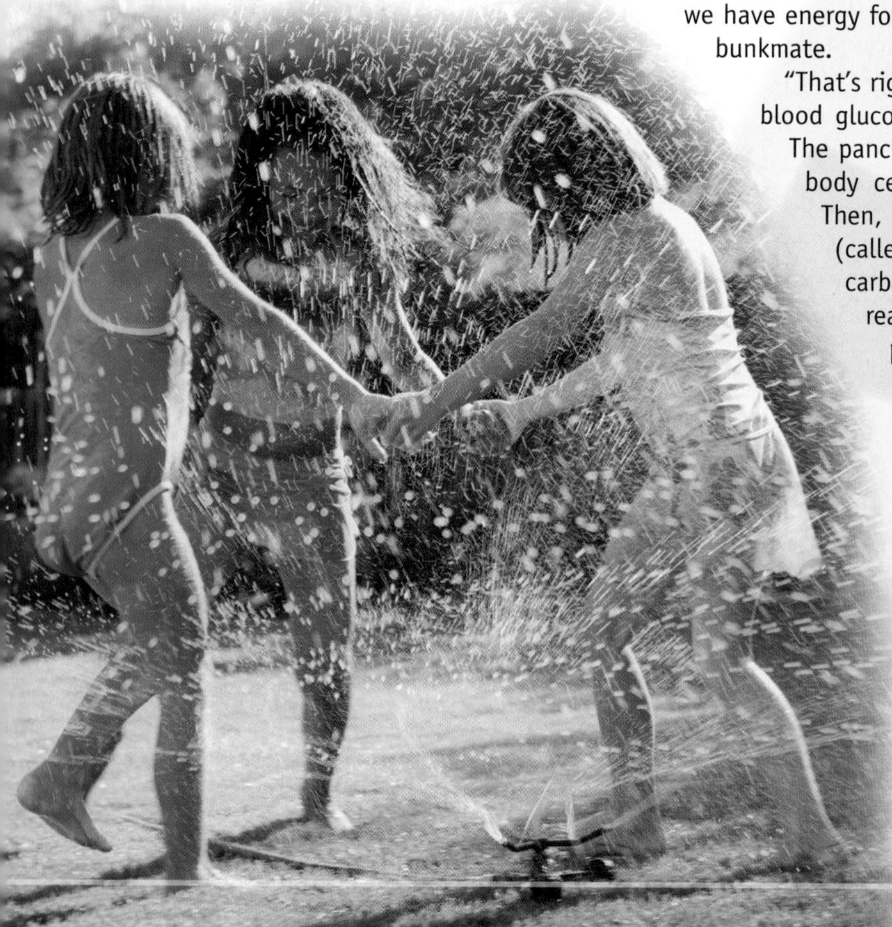

"That's right!" replied Wanda. She went on to explain that blood glucose is an important energy source for the body. The pancreas releases the hormone insulin, which signals body cells to absorb glucose from the blood stream. Then, the cells run a series of chemical reactions (called cellular respiration) that convert glucose into carbon dioxide and water. During these catabolic reactions, the cells manufacture adenosine triphosphate (ATP), which they use to run their cellular activities. People with type 1 diabetes mellitus do not make enough insulin, so their cells are not able to absorb glucose from the bloodstream and use it to make ATP. To ensure a constant supply of cellular ATP, these diabetics must monitor their blood glucose levels and inject themselves with insulin.

Diabetes mellitus is a disorder that affects glucose metabolism. In this chapter, we will learn more about metabolism as well as nutrition and body temperature regulation. Later in the chapter, we will revisit Becky and see what else she has learned at camp.

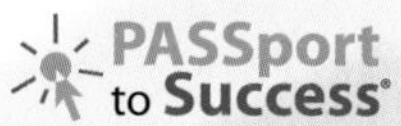

Ancillaries At-A-Glance

Visit *thePoint* to access the PASSport to Success and the following resources. For guidance in using these resources most effectively, see pp. ix–xviii.

Learning TOOLS

- Learning Style Self-Assessment
- Live Advise Online Student Tutoring
- Tips for Effective Studying

Learning RESOURCES

- E-book: Chapter 18
- Health Professions: Dietitian and Nutritionist
- Detailed Chapter Outline
- Answers to Questions for Study and Review
- Audio Pronunciation Glossary

Learning ACTIVITIES

- Pre-Quiz
- Visual Activities
- Kinesthetic Activities
- Auditory Activities

Learning Outcomes

After careful study of this chapter, you should be able to:

1. Differentiate between catabolism and anabolism, ***p. 354***
2. Differentiate between the anaerobic and aerobic phases of glucose catabolism and give the end products and the relative amount of energy released by each, ***p. 354***
3. Define *metabolic rate* and name several factors that affect the metabolic rate, ***p. 355***
4. Explain how carbohydrates, fats, and proteins are metabolized for energy, ***p. 355***
5. Compare the energy contents of fats, proteins, and carbohydrates, ***pp. 355, 356***
6. Define *essential amino acid*, ***p. 356***
7. Explain the roles of minerals and vitamins in nutrition and give examples of each, ***p. 357***
8. List the recommended percentages of carbohydrate, fat, and protein in the diet, ***p. 357***
9. Distinguish between simple and complex carbohydrates, giving examples of each, ***p. 358***
10. Compare saturated and unsaturated fats, ***p. 358***
11. Explain how heat is produced and lost in the body, ***p. 363***
12. Describe the role of the hypothalamus in regulating body temperature, ***p. 364***
13. Using the case study, suggest some dietary strategies for managing high blood glucose levels, ***pp. 352, 366***
14. Show how word parts are used to build words related to metabolism, nutrition, and body temperature (see Word Anatomy at the end of the chapter), ***p. 368***

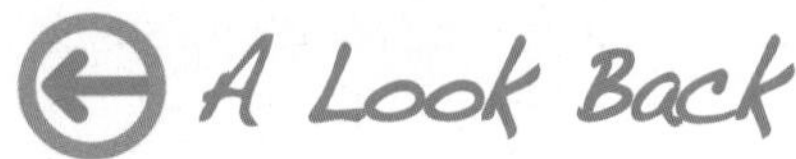

The concept of metabolism was introduced in Chapter 1 and applied to discussion of muscle function in Chapter 7. Nutritional studies also require knowledge of organic chemistry, introduced in Chapter 2 and further discussed in the previous chapter on digestion. Finally, maintenance of normal body temperature is an important factor in homeostasis.

Metabolism

Nutrients absorbed from the digestive tract are used for all the body's cellular activities, which together make up **metabolism.** In Chapter 1, we said that there are two types of metabolic activities (see Fig. 1-2):

- **Catabolism,** the breakdown of complex compounds into simpler components. Catabolism includes the digestion of food into small molecules and the release of energy from these molecules within the cell.
- **Anabolism,** the building of simple compounds into substances needed for cellular activities, growth and repair of tissues, and nutrient storage compounds.

Through the steps of catabolism and anabolism, there is a constant turnover of body materials as energy is consumed, cells function and grow, and waste products are generated.

CELLULAR RESPIRATION

Energy is released from nutrients in a series of reactions called **cellular respiration** (Fig. 18-1 and Table 18-1). In early studies on cellular respiration, scientists used glucose as the starting compound for the reactions. Glucose is a simple sugar that is a principal energy source for cells.

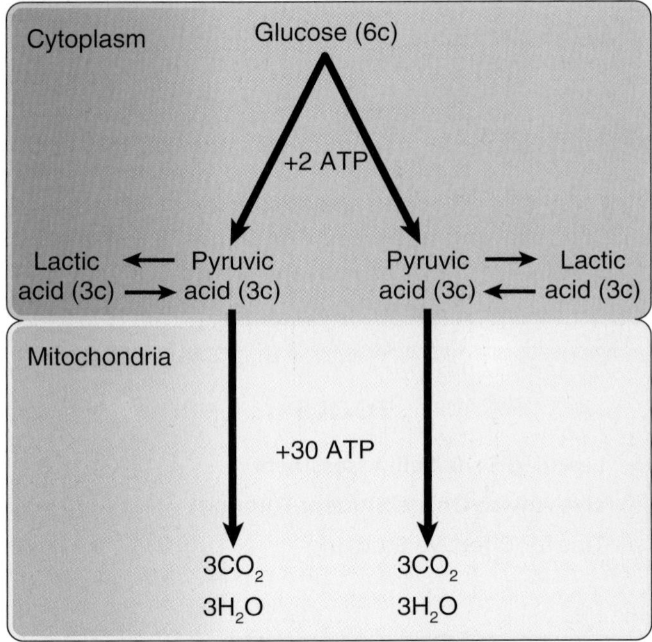

Figure 18-1 Cellular respiration. KEY POINT There are two stages of glucose catabolism, the first occurring without oxygen (anaerobic), followed by steps occurring with oxygen (aerobic). (The letter *c* represents a carbon atom, and the numbers show the number of carbon atoms in one molecule of the named substance.) In cellular respiration, glucose first yields two molecules of pyruvic acid. These initial steps occur in the cell's cytosol and do not require oxygen. The pyruvic acid is then fully catabolized in the mitochondria using oxygen. The final products of this phase are carbon dioxide and water and a large amount of adenosine triphosphate (ATP). Under anaerobic conditions, as during intense exercise, pyruvic acid is temporarily converted to lactic acid. When oxygen becomes available, the lactic acid is converted back to pyruvic acid for complete oxidation. ZOOMING IN What does pyruvic acid produce when it is metabolized anaerobically? What does it produce when metabolized completely using oxygen?

Anaerobic Glucose Catabolism The first steps in the breakdown of glucose do not require oxygen; that is, they are **anaerobic.** This phase of catabolism, known as **glycolysis** (gli-KOL-ih-sis), occurs in the cell's cytoplasm. It yields a small amount of energy, which is used to make ATP, the cell's energy compound. Each glucose molecule yields enough energy by this process to produce two molecules of ATP.

The anaerobic breakdown of glucose is incomplete and ends with formation of an organic product called **pyruvic** (pi-RU-vik) **acid.** This organic acid is further metabolized in the next phase of cellular respiration, which requires oxygen. In muscle cells that need to produce large amounts of ATP very rapidly, for example, at the start of exercise or during very intense exercise, pyruvic acid cannot be metabolized fast enough and accumulates in the cells. In this case,

Table 18-1 Summary of Cellular Respiration of Glucose

Phase	Location in Cell	End Product(s)	Energy Yield/Glucose
Anaerobic (glycolysis)	Cytoplasm	Pyruvic acid	2 adenosine triphosphate (ATP)
Aerobic	Mitochondria	Carbon dioxide and water	30 ATP

pyruvic acid is converted to a related compound called lactic acid. As lactic acid accumulates in the cells, it can spill over into the blood. Most physiologists do not believe that this lactic acid harms or inhibits the muscle cells in any way. It is simply converted back to pyruvic acid and fully metabolized either by other less active cells or by the cells that produced it when the later steps in metabolism catch up with the anaerobic yield.

Aerobic Glucose Catabolism To generate enough energy for survival, the body's cells must break pyruvic acid down more completely in the second phase of cellular respiration, which requires oxygen. These **aerobic** reactions occur within the cell's mitochondria. They result in transfer of most of the energy remaining in the nutrients to ATP. On average, cells are able to form about 30 molecules of ATP aerobically per glucose molecule. Statements on energy yields may differ slightly, because cells in different tissues vary in their metabolic pathways and in the amount of energy they use to power cellular respiration. In any case, this additional yield is quite an increase over anaerobic metabolism alone, generally resulting in a total of 32 molecules of ATP per glucose as compared to two.

During the aerobic steps of cellular respiration, the cells form carbon dioxide, which then must be transported to the lungs for elimination. In addition, water is formed by combining oxygen with the hydrogen that is removed from nutrient molecules. Because of the type of chemical reactions involved, and because oxygen is used in the final steps, cellular respiration is described as an **oxidation** of nutrients. Note that enzymes are required as catalysts in all these metabolic reactions. Many of the vitamins and minerals described later in this chapter are parts of these enzymes.

Although the oxidation of food is often compared to the burning of fuel, this comparison is inaccurate. Burning fuel results in a sudden and often wasteful release of energy in the form of heat and light. In contrast, metabolic oxidation occurs in small steps, and much of the energy released is stored as ATP for later use by the cells; some of the energy is released as heat, which is used to maintain body temperature, as discussed later in this chapter.

For those who know how to read chemical equations, the net balanced equation for cellular respiration, starting with glucose, is as follows:

$$\underset{\text{glucose}}{C_6H_{12}O_6} + \underset{\text{oxygen}}{6O_2} \rightarrow \underset{\text{carbon dioxide}}{6CO_2} + \underset{\text{water}}{6H_2O}$$

Metabolic Rate Metabolic rate refers to the rate at which energy is released from nutrients in the cells. It is affected by a person's size, body fat, sex, age, activity, and hormones, especially thyroid hormone (thyroxine). Metabolic rate is high in children and adolescents and decreases with age. **Basal metabolism** is the amount of energy needed to maintain life functions while the body is at rest. Thus, your *basal metabolic rate* (*BMR*) is the energy you expend each day simply to stay alive. Any activity you perform, even tapping a toe, increases your energy expenditure above your BMR.

The unit used to measure energy is the kilocalorie (kcal), which is the amount of heat needed to raise 1 kilogram of water 1°C. Nutrition information for the general public typically replaces the word *kilocalorie* with *Calorie (C)*. To estimate how many calories you need each day, taking into account your activity level, see **Box 18-1**.

NUTRIENT CATABOLISM

All three categories of nutrients can be oxidized for energy. All are broken down into their building blocks, which then can be converted to carbon dioxide and water with generation of ATP. But not all go through the complete steps of cellular respiration as previously described for glucose. They enter the process at different points in the pathway.

Carbohydrates As noted, glucose is a major source of energy for the body. Most of the carbohydrates in the diet are converted to glucose for further oxidation. Monosaccharides, such as fructose (fruit sugar), are converted directly to glucose. Starch, a polysaccharide, is split into its component glucose molecules, which are then metabolized. Some glucose reserves are stored in liver and muscle cells as glycogen (GLI-ko-jen), a complex carbohydrate built from glucose molecules. When glucose is needed for energy, glycogen is broken down to yield glucose. Muscle glycogen is used specifically in muscle tissue. The glucose from liver glycogen can be released into the bloodstream to power other cells. If we have more glucose in the blood than is needed for energy and glycogen storage, it is converted to fat and stored in adipose tissue and the liver.

Fats Although glucose was the starting compound used in early studies of catabolism, and glucose goes through the complete steps of cellular respiration, fatty acids are the other major energy source for cells. Fatty acids are broken into small fragments and then catabolized completely in mitochondria using oxygen. Most tissues can use fatty acids for energy. Brain tissue is one exception; it typically relies exclusively on glucose for its energy needs.

Ketone bodies are partially catabolized fatty acids produced in the liver. Under certain conditions that disrupt normal metabolism, these products may accumulate in the blood. For example, in uncontrolled diabetes mellitus, when fats are used for energy in place of unavailable glucose, and in cases of starvation or low carbohydrate intake, when the body metabolizes its stored fats, ketone bodies are produced in excess. Under these circumstances, the brain and other tissues can increase their use of these by-products. However, ketone bodies are acidic, and excesses disrupt the body's acid–base balance. We will say more about these changes in Chapter 19.

Fatty acids are a highly concentrated energy source and generate more ATP per molecule than does glucose. In fact, fat in the diet yields more than twice as much energy as do protein and carbohydrate (e.g., it is more "fattening"); fat yields 9 kcal of energy/g, whereas protein and carbohydrate each yields 4 kcal/g. Fat calories that are ingested in excess of need are also converted to fat and stored in adipose tissue.

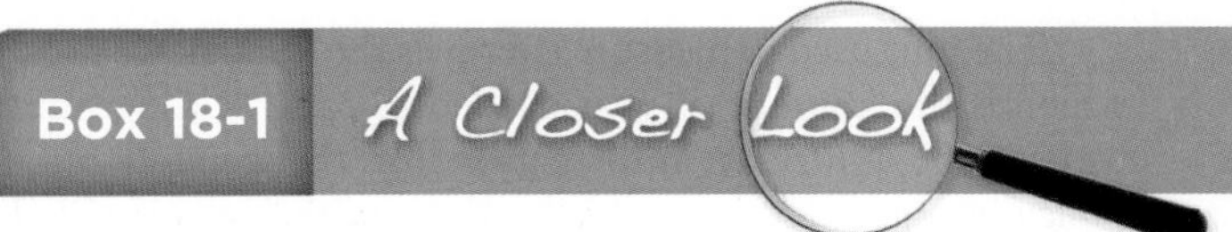

Calorie Counting: Estimating Daily Energy Needs

Have you ever wondered how many calories you need to eat each day in order to avoid gaining or losing weight? To answer that question, you first need to calculate your basal metabolic rate (BMR), and then estimate the calories you burn each day in physical activity. Adding those two numbers together should give you your daily calorie needs.

You can estimate your BMR with a simple formula. An average woman requires 0.9 kcal/kg/h, and a man, 1.0 kcal/kg/h. If you need to convert your body weight from pounds to kilograms (kg), divide your weight in pounds by 2.2. Next, multiply your body weight in kg by 0.9 if you are female, and by 1.0 if you are male. This gives you kcal burned per hour. Finally, multiply by 24 to find your BMR (the number of kcal you expend at rest per day).

For example, if you are female and weigh 132 lb, your equation would be as follows:

132 lb ÷ 2.2 lb/kg = 60 kg

0.9 kcal/kg/h × 60 kg = 54 kcal/h

54 kcal/h × 24 h/d = 1,296 kcal/d

Notice that, if you are male, you can skip step 2, since you'd simply be multiplying by 1.

To estimate your total energy needs for a day, you need to add to your BMR a percentage based on your current activity level ("couch potato" to serious athlete). These percentages are shown in the table that follows.

The equation to calculate total energy needs for a day is

BMR + (BMR × activity level)

Using the BMR from our previous example with different activity levels, the following equations apply:

At 25% activity:

1,296 kcal/d + (1,296 kcal/d × 25%) = 1,620 kcal/d

At 60% activity:

1,296 kcal/d + (1,296 kcal/d × 60%) = 2,073.6 kcal/d

As you can see, physical activity can help you maintain a healthful body weight. In this case, increased activity increased the individual's energy needs by more than 450 kcal per day!

Activity Level	Male	Female
Little activity ("couch potato")	25%–40%	25%–35%
Light activity (e.g., walking to and from class, but little or no intentional exercise)	50%–75%	40%–60%
Moderate activity (e.g., aerobics several times a week)	65%–80%	50%–70%
Heavy activity (serious athlete)	90%–120%	80%–100%

Proteins Before they are oxidized for energy, amino acids must have their nitrogen (amine) groups removed. This removal, called **deamination** (de-am-ih-NA-shun), occurs in the liver, where the nitrogen groups are then formed into urea by combination with carbon dioxide. The blood transports urea to the kidneys to be eliminated.

There are no specialized storage forms of proteins, as there are for carbohydrates (glycogen) and fats (adipose tissue). Protein consumed in excess of daily needs is not stored as protein, but is catabolized for energy or converted to fat. Conversely, when a person needs more proteins than are supplied in the diet, they must be obtained from body substance, such as muscle tissue or plasma proteins. Drawing on these resources becomes dangerous when needs are extreme. Fats and carbohydrates are described as "protein sparing," because they are used for energy before proteins are and thus spare proteins for the synthesis of necessary body components.

ANABOLISM

Instead of being oxidized for energy, nutrient molecules can be built anabolically into body materials. All of these synthesis reactions are catalyzed by enzymes.

Essential Amino Acids Eleven of the 20 amino acids needed to build proteins can be synthesized internally by metabolic reactions. These 11 amino acids are described as *nonessential* because they need not be taken in as food (Table 18-2). The remaining nine amino acids cannot be made metabolically and therefore must be taken in as part of the diet; these are the **essential amino acids.** Note that some nonessential amino acids may become essential under certain conditions, as during extreme physical stress, or in certain hereditary metabolic diseases.

Essential Fatty Acids There are two essential fatty acids, **linoleic** (lin-o-LE-ik) **acid** and **alpha-linolenic** (lin-o-LEN-ik) **acid,** which must be taken in as food. Linoleic acid is easily obtained through a healthful, balanced diet that includes plenty of vegetables and vegetable oils. In contrast, alpha-linolenic acid is found primarily in fatty fish and shellfish, dark green, leafy vegetables, and flaxseeds, soybeans, walnuts, and their oils. Thus, it is somewhat more difficult to obtain. We will say more about these fatty acids shortly when we discuss fats in a healthful diet.

Table 18-2 Amino acids

Nonessential Amino Acids[a]		Essential Amino Acids[b]	
Name	**Pronunciation**	**Name[c]**	**Pronunciation**
Alanine	AL-ah-nene	Histidine	HIS-tih-dene
Arginine	AR-jih-nene	Isoleucine	i-so-LU-sene
Asparagine	ah-SPAR-ah-jene	Leucine	LU-sene
Aspartic acid	ah-SPAR-tik AH-sid	Lysine	LI-sene
Cysteine	SIS-teh-ene	Methionine	meh-THI-o-nene
Glutamic acid	glu-TAM-ik AH-sid	Phenylalanine	fen-il-AL-ah-nene
Glutamine	GLU-tah-mene	Threonine	THRE-o-nene
Glycine	GLY-sene	Tryptophan	TRIP-to-fane
Proline	PRO-lene	Valine	VA-lene
Serine	SERE-ene		
Tyrosine	TI-ro-sene		

[a]*Nonessential amino acids can be synthesized by the body.*
[b]*Essential amino acids cannot be synthesized by the body; they must be taken in as part of the diet.*
[c]*If you are ever called upon to memorize the essential amino acids, the mnemonic (memory device) Pvt. T. M. Hill gives the first letter of each name.*

MINERALS AND VITAMINS

In addition to needing carbohydrates, fats, and proteins, the body requires minerals and vitamins.

Minerals are chemical elements needed for body structure, fluid balance, and such activities as muscle contraction, nerve impulse conduction, and blood clotting. Some minerals are components of vitamins. A list of the main minerals needed in a proper diet is given in Table 18-3. Some additional minerals not listed are also required for good health. Minerals needed in extremely small amounts are referred to as **trace elements**.

Vitamins are complex organic substances needed in very small quantities. Vitamins are parts of enzymes or other substances essential for metabolism, and vitamin deficiencies lead to a variety of nutritional diseases.

The water-soluble vitamins are the B vitamins and vitamin C. These are not stored and must be taken in regularly with food. The fat-soluble vitamins are A, D, E, and K. These vitamins are kept in reserve in fatty tissue. Excess intake of the fat-soluble vitamins can lead to toxicity. A list of vitamins is given in Table 18-4.

Certain substances are valuable in the diet as **antioxidants**. They defend against the harmful effects of reactive oxygen species (ROS), also described as *free radicals*, highly reactive and unstable molecules produced from oxygen in the normal course of metabolism (and also resulting from UV radiation, air pollution, and tobacco smoke). Free radicals contribute to aging and disease. Antioxidants react with ROS to stabilize them and minimize their harmful effects on cells. Vitamins C and E and beta-carotene, an orange pigment found in plants that is converted to vitamin A, are antioxidants. There are also many compounds found in plants (e.g., soybeans and tomatoes) that are antioxidants.

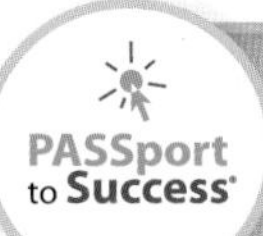

See the student resources on *thePoint* for information on dietitians and nutritionists, who study nutrition and metabolism and help people to plan healthful diets.

CHECKPOINTS

- 18-1 What are the two types of activities that make up metabolism?
- 18-2 What name is given to the series of cellular reactions that releases energy from nutrients?
- 18-3 What are the two main energy sources for cells?
- 18-4 What is meant when an amino acid or a fatty acid is described as essential?
- 18-5 What is the difference between vitamins and minerals?

Nutritional Guidelines

The relative amounts of carbohydrates, fats, and proteins that should be in the daily diet vary somewhat with the individual. Typical recommendations for the number of calories derived each day from the three types of food are as follows:

- Carbohydrate: 55% to 60%
- Fat: 30% or less
- Protein: 15% to 20%

It is important to realize that the type as well as the amount of each nutrient is a factor in good health. A weight loss

Table 18-3 Minerals

Mineral	Functions	Sources	Results of Deficiency
Calcium (Ca)	Formation of bones and teeth; blood clotting; nerve conduction; muscle contraction	Dairy products, eggs, green vegetables, legumes (peas and beans)	Rickets, tetany, osteoporosis
Phosphorus (P)	Formation of bones and teeth; found in ATP, nucleic acids	Meat, fish, poultry, egg yolk, dairy products	Osteoporosis, abnormal metabolism
Sodium (Na)	Fluid balance; nerve impulse conduction; muscle contraction	Most foods, especially processed foods, table salt	Weakness, cramps, diarrhea, dehydration dehydration
Potassium (K)	Fluid balance; nerve and muscle activity	Fruits, meats, seafood, milk, vegetables, grains	Muscular and neurologic disorders disorders
Chloride (Cl)	Fluid balance; hydrochloric acid in stomach	Meat, milk, eggs, processed food, table salt	Rarely occurs
Iron (Fe)	Oxygen carrier (hemoglobin, myoglobin)	Meat, eggs, fortified cereals, legumes, dried fruit	Anemia, dry skin, indigestion
Iodine (I)	Thyroid hormones	Seafood, iodized salt	Hypothyroidism, goiter
Magnesium (Mg)	Catalyst for enzyme reactions; carbohydrate metabolism	Green vegetables, grains, nuts, legumes	Spasticity, arrhythmia, vasodilation
Manganese (Mn)	Catalyst in actions of calcium and phosphorus; facilitator of many cellular processes	Many foods	Possible reproductive disorders
Copper (Cu)	Necessary for absorption and use of iron in formation of hemoglobin; part of some enzymes	Meat, water	Anemia
Chromium (Cr)	Works with insulin to regulate blood glucose levels	Meat, unrefined food, fats and oils	Inability to use glucose
Cobalt (Co)	Part of vitamin B_{12}	Animal products	Pernicious anemia
Zinc (Zn)	Promotes carbon dioxide transport and energy metabolism; found in enzymes	Meat, fish, poultry, grains, vegetables	Alopecia (baldness); possibly related to diabetes
Fluoride (F)	Prevents tooth decay	Fluoridated water, tea, seafood	Dental caries

diet should follow the same proportions as given above, but with a reduction in portion sizes.

CARBOHYDRATES

A healthful diet provides abundant complex carbohydrates, whereas simple sugars are kept to a minimum. Simple sugars are monosaccharides, such as glucose and fructose (fruit sugar), and disaccharides, such as sucrose (table sugar) and lactose (milk sugar). Simple sugars are a source of fast energy because they are metabolized rapidly. However, they boost pancreatic insulin output, and as a result, they cause blood glucose levels to rise and fall rapidly. It is healthier to maintain steady glucose levels, which normally range from approximately 85 to 125 mg/dL throughout the day.

The **glycemic effect** is a measure of how rapidly a particular food raises the blood glucose level and stimulates the release of insulin. The effect is generally low for whole grains, fruit, vegetables, legumes, and dairy products, and high for refined sugars and refined ("white") grains. Note, however, that the glycemic effect of a food also depends on when it is eaten during the day, and if or how it is combined with other foods.

Complex carbohydrates are polysaccharides. Examples are

- Starches, found in grains, legumes, and potatoes and other starchy vegetables
- Fibers, such as cellulose, pectins, and gums, which are the structural materials of plants

Fiber adds bulk to the stool and promotes elimination of toxins and waste. It also slows the digestion and absorption of carbohydrates, thus regulating the release of glucose. It helps in weight control by providing a sense of fullness and limiting caloric intake. Adequate fiber in the diet lowers cholesterol and helps to prevent diabetes, colon cancer, hemorrhoids, appendicitis, and diverticulitis. Foods high in fiber, such as whole grains, fruits, and vegetables, are also rich in vitamins and minerals (see Box 18-2). Becky, in the case study, has to learn about carbohydrates and other nutrients to help manage her diabetes.

FATS

Fats are subdivided into saturated and unsaturated forms based on their chemical structure. The fatty acids in

Table 18-4 Vitamins

Vitamins	Functions	Sources	Results of Deficiency
A (retinol)	Required for healthy epithelial tissue and for eye pigments; involved in reproduction and immunity	Orange fruits and vegetables, liver, eggs, dairy products, dark green vegetables	Night blindness, dry, scaly skin, decreased immunity
B_1 (thiamin)	Required for enzymes involved in oxidation of nutrients; nerve function	Pork, cereal, grains, meats, legumes, nuts	Beriberi, a disease of nerves
B_2 (riboflavin)	In enzymes required for oxidation of nutrients	Milk, eggs, liver, green leafy vegetables, grains	Skin and tongue disorders
B_3 (niacin, nicotinic acid)	Involved in oxidation of nutrients	Yeast, meat, liver, grains, legumes, nuts	Pellagra with dermatitis, diarrhea, mental disorders
B_6 (pyridoxine)	Amino acid and fatty acid metabolism; formation of niacin; manufacture of red blood cells	Meat, fish, poultry, fruit grains, legumes, vegetables	Anemia, irritability, convulsions, muscle twitching, skin disorders
Pantothenic acid	Essential for normal growth; energy metabolism	Yeast, liver, eggs, and many other foods	Sleep disturbances, digestive upset
B_{12} (cyanocobalamin)	Production of cells; maintenance of nerve cells; fatty acid and amino acid metabolism	Animal products	Pernicious anemia
Biotin (a B vitamin)	Involved in fat and glycogen formation, amino acid metabolism	Peanuts, liver, tomatoes, eggs, oatmeal, soy, and many other foods	Lack of coordination, dermatitis, fatigue
Folate (folic acid, a B vitamin)	Required for amino acid metabolism; DNA synthesis; maturation of red blood cells	Vegetables, liver, legumes, seeds	Anemia, digestive disorders, neural tube defects in the embryo
C (ascorbic acid)	Maintains healthy skin and mucous membranes, involved in synthesis of collagen; antioxidant	Citrus fruits, green vegetables, potatoes, orange fruits	Scurvy, poor wound healing, anemia, weak bones
D (calciferol)	Aids in absorption of calcium and phosphorus from intestinal tract	Fatty fish, liver, eggs, fortified milk, cereal	Rickets, bone deformities, osteoporosis
E (tocopherol)	Protects cell membranes; antioxidant	Seeds, green vegetables, nuts, grains, oils	Anemia, muscle and liver degeneration, pain
K	Synthesis of blood clotting factors; bone formation	Liver, cabbage, and leafy green vegetables	Hemorrhage, bacteria in digestive tract

18

Box 18-2 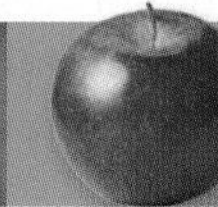 *Health Maintenance*

Dietary Fiber: Bulking Up

Dietary fiber is best known for its ability to improve bowel habits and promote weight loss. But fiber may also help to prevent diabetes, heart disease, and certain digestive disorders such as diverticulitis and gallstones.

Dietary fiber is an indigestible type of carbohydrate found in fruit, vegetables, and whole grains. The amount of fiber recommended for a 2,000-cal diet is 25 g/d, but most people in the United States tend to get only half this amount. One should eat fiber-rich foods throughout the day to meet the requirement. It is best to increase fiber in the diet gradually to avoid unpleasant symptoms, such as intestinal bloating and flatulence. If your diet lacks fiber, try adding the following foods over a period of several weeks:

- Whole grain breads, cereals, pasta, and brown rice. These add 1 to 3 more g of fiber per serving than the "white" product.
- Legumes, which include beans, peas, and lentils. These add 4 to 12 g of fiber per serving.
- Fruits and vegetables. Whole, raw, unpeeled versions contain the most fiber, and juices, the least. Apple juice has no fiber, whereas a whole apple has 3 g.
- Unprocessed bran. This can be sprinkled over almost any food: cereal, soups, and casseroles. One tablespoon adds 2 g of fiber. Be sure to take adequate fluids with bran.

saturated fats have more hydrogen atoms in their molecules because they have no double bonds between carbons atoms. In other words, their carbon atoms are fully "saturated" with hydrogen **(Fig. 18-2)**. Most saturated fats are from animal sources and are solid at room temperature, such as butter and lard. Also included in this group are the so-called tropical oils: coconut oil and palm oil.

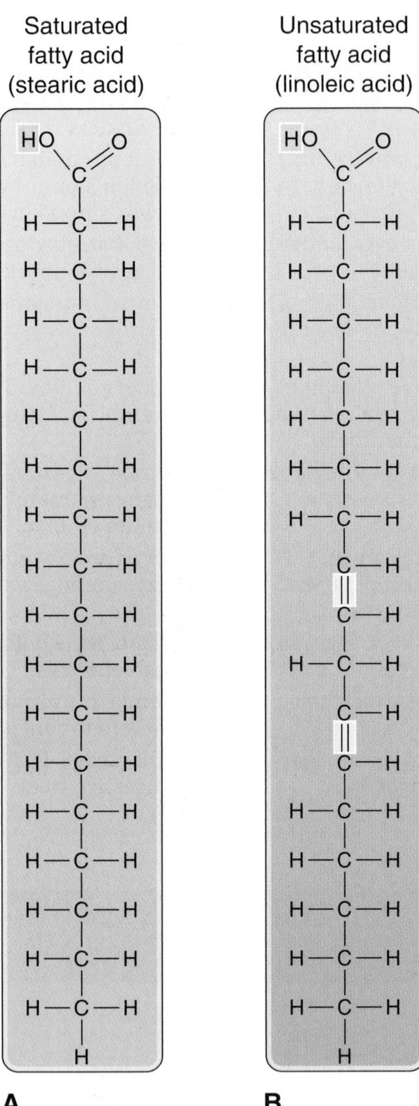

Figure 18-2 Saturated and unsaturated fats. KEY POINT Saturated and unsaturated fats differ in their bonding structure. **A.** Saturated fatty acids contain the maximum numbers of hydrogen atoms attached to carbons and no double bonds between carbon atoms. **B.** Unsaturated fatty acids have less than the maximum number of hydrogen atoms attached to carbons and one or more double bonds between carbon atoms (highlighted). The first carbon in the chain (**top**) is the alpha carbon; the last (**bottom**) is the omega carbon. The "omega" fatty acids are described according to how many carbons there are from the last double-bonded carbon in the chain to the omega carbon, such as omega-3, omega-6. Linoleic acid is an omega-6 fatty acid.

Unsaturated fats are derived from plants. They are liquid at room temperature and are generally referred to as oils, such as corn, peanut, olive, and canola oils. Their fatty acids have one or more double carbon bonds, which exclude hydrogen **(see Fig. 18-2)**. An unsaturated fatty acid is *monounsaturated* if it has a single double bond and polyunsaturated if it has more than one double bond. You may have heard or read about fatty acids described as "omega" acids with a number. This terminology refers to the position of the last double-bonded carbon in the chain with regard to the very last carbon, named the omega carbon for the last letter of the Greek alphabet. In the essential fatty acid linoleic acid, for example, the last double-bonded carbon is the sixth carbon from the omega carbon, so linoleic acid is an omega-6 fatty acid **(see Fig. 18-2B)**. The essential fatty acid alpha-linolenic acid is an omega-3 fatty acid. As to fat intake, a predominance of unsaturated fats in general, in addition to the previously mentioned essential fatty acids, contributes to a healthful diet.

Saturated fats should make up less than one-third of the fat in the diet (less than 10% of total calories). Diets high in saturated fats are associated with a higher than normal incidence of cancer, heart disease, and cardiovascular problems, although the relation between these factors is not fully understood.

Because most unsaturated fats are liquid and easily become rancid (spoil), commercial food manufacturers have used fats that are artificially saturated to extend shelf life and improve consistency of foods. These fats are listed on food labels as partially hydrogenated (HI-dro-jen-a-ted) vegetable oils and are found commonly in baked goods, processed peanut butter, vegetable shortening, and some solid margarines. Evidence shows that components of hydrogenated fats, known as *trans-fatty acids*, are more harmful than even natural saturated fats. They raise blood levels of LDL (the less healthful lipoproteins) and lower levels of HDLs (the healthful lipoproteins). Food manufacturers are responding to evidence that trans fats are harmful, and are making efforts to remove them from processed foods. Many countries now require labeling of trans fat content on food labels. In the United States., trans fat contents of 0.5 g or more per serving must be listed. Bear in mind, though, that restaurants still may be using trans fats in cooking, especially deep-frying.

PROTEINS

Because proteins, unlike carbohydrates and fats, are not stored in special reserves, protein foods should be taken in on a regular basis, with attention to obtaining the essential amino acids. Most animal proteins supply all of the essential amino acids and are described as complete proteins. Most plant proteins are lacking in one or more of the essential amino acids. People on strict vegetarian diets must learn to combine foods, such as legumes (e.g., beans and peas) with grains (e.g., rice, corn, or wheat), to obtain all the essential amino acids each day. **Figure 18-3** demonstrates the principles of combining two foods, legumes and grains, to supply essential amino acids that might be missing in one food

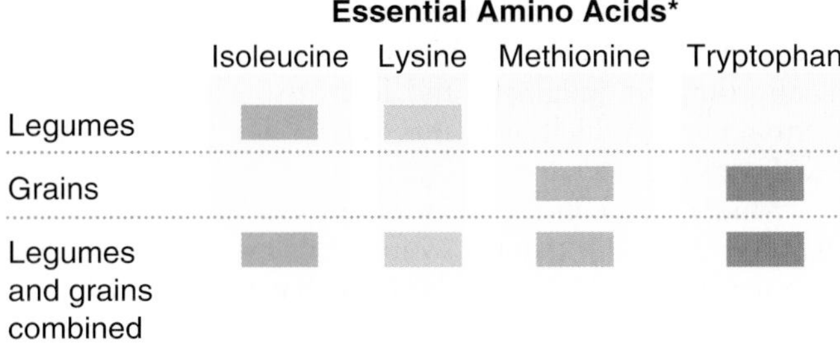

Essential Amino Acids*
Isoleucine
Lysine
Methionine
Tryptophan
Legumes
Grains
Legumes and grains combined
* There are 9 essential amino acids; the table includes 4 for the purposes of illustration.

Figure 18-3 Combining foods to obtain the essential amino acids. KEY POINT There are nine essential amino acids. If someone does not eat animal proteins, most of which supply all of the essential amino acids, foods must be combined to supply all the needed amino acids within the day. In this illustration, legumes and grains are combined to provide four of the nine essential amino acids.

or the other. Legumes are rich in isoleucine and lysine but poor in methionine and tryptophan, while grains are just the opposite. For illustration purposes, the table includes only the four missing essential amino acids (there are nine total). Traditional ethnic diets reflect these healthful combinations, for example, beans with corn or rice in Mexican dishes or chickpeas and lentils with wheat in Middle Eastern fare. Nuts and vegetables also provide plant proteins; thus, a peanut butter sandwich on whole grain bread or vegetables over rice are other complementary combinations.

MINERAL AND VITAMIN SUPPLEMENTS

The need for adding mineral and vitamin supplements to the diet is a subject of controversy. Some researchers maintain that adequate amounts of these substances can be obtained from a varied, healthful diet. Many commercial foods, including milk, cereal, and bread, are already fortified with minerals and vitamins. Others hold that pollution, depletion of the soils, and the storage, refining, and processing of foods make additional supplementation beneficial. Most agree, however, that children, elderly people, pregnant and lactating women, and teenagers, who often do not get enough of the proper foods, typically benefit from supplemental minerals and vitamins.

Some recent studies have concentrated on the need for vitamin D, which is produced when the skin is exposed to the UV radiation in sunlight. Dietary sources of vitamin D are fish, fish oils, and fortified foods, such as milk and cereal. People with dark skin living in Northern climates, those who do not go out in the sun or do so only with sunscreen, the elderly, and breast-fed babies who do not receive fortified formula are subject to deficiencies. Depending on age, diet, and life habits, people might need vitamin D supplements of up to 1000 IU per day.

When required, supplements should be selected by a physician or nutritionist to fit an individual's particular needs. Megavitamin dosages may cause unpleasant reactions and in some cases are hazardous. Fat-soluble vitamins have caused serious toxic effects when taken in excess of the established safe upper limit (UL).

USDA DIETARY GUIDELINES

The United States Department of Agriculture (USDA) has published dietary guidelines at regular intervals since 1916. The newest guidelines, My Plate **(Fig. 18-4)**, are updated and simplified to replace the Food Guide Pyramid in use since 1992. The plate in the new graphic is divided into four sections for fruits, grains, vegetables, and proteins in the relative proportion that each should make up in the diet. A fifth category, dairy, is represented by a cup, suggesting milk and milk products, such as cheeses and yogurt. Low-fat varieties are recommended, and for those who can't consume milk because of lactose intolerance or who choose not to consume milk, intakes of lactose-free products or other good sources of calcium are recommended. This mineral is also found in green vegetables and legumes.

A full description of the guidelines and much supplementary information can be found online at ChooseMyPlate.gov. Here you can click on each section of the plate to see what foods are in each group. The protein section specifies a nutrient category rather than a type of food. Foods high in proteins are meat, poultry, seafood, and eggs, but proteins are also found in plant products, such as seeds, nuts, legumes, and grains. The guidelines accommodate individual variation. So, on the Web site, you can get a personalized estimate of what and how much you should eat based on your height, weight, age, sex, and

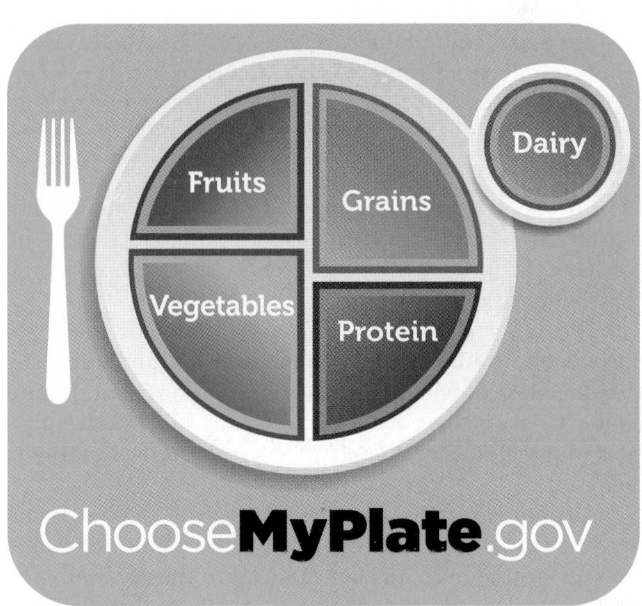

Figure 18-4 USDA dietary guidelines. The plate shows the recommended proportion of each food category in the diet. (MyPlate, U.S. Department of Agriculture/Center for Nutrition Policy and Promotion, www.choosemyplate.gov.)

level of physical activity. You can also assess your diet and plan healthy menus.

The guidelines stress

- Moderation. A single serving or portion is smaller than most people think.
- Variety in the diet. Foods in all the groups are needed each day for good health.
- Eating fruits and vegetables. Most people need more of these in their diets.
- Choice of unrefined foods, such as whole grains, and unprocessed foods. At least one-half the grains in the diet should be whole grains.
- Drinking water instead of sugary beverages
- The importance of exercise for good health

The plate graphic does not include oils, solid fats, or sugars. Although oils in moderation are important for health, solid fats and added sugars (SoFAS) are described as "empty calories" that provide calories but little nutrition. These are "extras" that you can eat within your recommended daily energy limit after you meet your nutritional needs. Of course, you could also select additional foods from among the recommended nutrient-rich groups to satisfy your energy needs. Limiting salt intake, especially in processed foods and restaurant fare, is also important.

The dietary guidelines are updated regularly. Issues always under consideration include weight control and giving attention to special groups, such as children, older adults, and pregnant or breast-feeding women. Any guidelines also should accommodate people with special needs or dietary preferences, such as people with gluten allergies, those who are lactose intolerant, strict vegetarians (vegans) who eat no animal products, and vegetarians who eat dairy products and eggs (lacto-ovo vegetarians).

ALCOHOL

Alcohol yields energy in the amount of 7 kcal/g, but it is not considered a nutrient because it does not yield useful end products. In fact, alcohol interferes with metabolism and contributes to a variety of disorders.

The body can metabolize about one-half ounce of pure alcohol (ethanol) per hour. This amount translates into one glass of wine, one can of beer, or one shot of hard liquor. Consumed at a more rapid rate, alcohol accumulates in the bloodstream and affects many cells, notably in the brain.

Alcohol is rapidly absorbed through the stomach and small intestine and is detoxified by the liver. When delivered in excess to the liver, alcohol can lead to the accumulation of fat as well as inflammation and scarring of liver tissue. It can eventually cause cirrhosis (*sih-RO-sis*), which involves irreversible changes in liver structure. Alcohol metabolism ties up enzymes needed for oxidation of nutrients and also results in by-products that acidify body fluids. Other effects of alcoholism include obesity, malnutrition, cancer, ulcers, and fetal alcohol syndrome. Health professionals advise pregnant women not to drink any alcohol. In addition, alcohol impairs judgment and leads to increased involvement in motor vehicle accidents, drownings, falls, and other accidental injuries.

Moderate alcohol consumption is defined as no more than one drink per day for women and two drinks per day for men. Current research suggests that moderate alcohol consumption is compatible with good health and may even have a beneficial effect on the cardiovascular system.

CHECKPOINTS 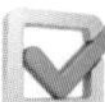

- [ ] **18-6** What is the normal range of blood glucose?
- [ ] **18-7** What are typical recommendations for the relative amounts of carbohydrates, fats, and proteins in the diet?
- [ ] **18-8** What is the difference between saturated and unsaturated fats?
- [ ] **18-9** What are some adverse effects of excess alcohol consumption?

WEIGHT CONTROL

Body mass index (BMI) is a measurement used to evaluate body size. It is based on the ratio of weight to height (**Fig. 18-5**). BMI is calculated by dividing weight in kilograms by height in meters squared. (For those not accustomed to using the metric system, an alternate method is to divide weight in pounds by the square of height in inches and multiply by 703.) A healthy range for this measurement is 18.5 to 24.9.

BMI does not take into account the relative amount of muscle and fat in the body. For example, a

Calculation of body mass index (BMI)

Formula:

$$\text{BMI} = \frac{\text{Weight (kg)}}{\text{Height (m)}^2}$$

Conversion:

Kilograms = pounds ÷ 2.2

Meters = inches ÷ 39.4

Example:

A woman who is 5′4″ tall and weighs 134 pounds has a BMI of 23.5.

Weight: 134 pounds ÷ 2.2 = 61 kg

Height: 164 inches ÷ 39.4 = 1.6 m; $(1.6)^2 = 2.6$

$$\text{BMI} = \frac{61 \text{ kg}}{2.6 \text{ m}} = 23.5$$

Figure 18-5 Calculation of body mass index (BMI). KEY POINT BMI is a measurement used to evaluate body size based on the ratio of weight to height. ZOOMING IN What is the BMI of a male 5′10″ in height who weighs 170 pounds? (Round off to one decimal place.)

bodybuilder might be healthy with a higher than typical BMI because muscle has a higher density than fat. Researchers have also noted that people of different ethnicities commonly have different levels of body fat at the same BMI. Finally, BMI does not give a fair indication of overweight or obesity in people over age 65 or in children.

Overweight and Obesity Overweight is defined as a BMI of 25 to 30, and obesity as a BMI greater than 30. Although the prevalence of overweight among Americans has fluctuated between 31 and 34% since national surveys began in 1960, it is common knowledge that obesity has increased in these decades. In 1962, the US obesity rate was below 14%. In 2008, 33% of Americans were obese.

The causes of obesity are complex, involving social, economic, genetic, psychological, and metabolic factors. Obesity shortens the life span and is associated with cardiovascular disease, diabetes, some cancers, and other diseases. Unfortunately, obesity rates have also increased among American children. Some researchers hold that obesity has a closer correlation to chronic disease than poverty, smoking, or drinking alcohol.

Scientists are studying the nervous and hormonal controls over weight, but so far they have not found any effective and safe drugs for weight control. For most people, a varied diet eaten in moderation and regular exercise are the surest ways to avoid obesity. At least 30 minutes of moderate to vigorous exercise every day is recommended for health and weight maintenance. At least 60 minutes a day is recommended for weight loss.

UNDERWEIGHT

A BMI of less than 18.5 is defined as underweight. People who are underweight can have as much difficulty gaining weight as others have losing it. The problem of underweight may result from rapid growth, eating disorders, allergies, illness, or psychological factors. It is associated with low reserves of energy, reproductive disturbances, and nutritional deficiencies. To gain weight, people have to increase their intake of calories, but they should also engage in regular exercise to add muscle tissue and not just fat.

Nutrition and Aging

With age, a person may find it difficult to maintain a balanced diet. Often, the elderly lose interest in buying and preparing food or are unable to do so. Because metabolism generally slows, and less food is required to meet energy needs, nutritional deficiencies may develop. With age, the ability to synthesize vitamin D declines and the kidneys are less able to convert it to its active form. Older adults may need supplements of vitamin D as well as calcium to prevent loss of bone density. The senses of smell and taste become less acute with age, diminishing appetite. Medications may interfere with appetite and with the absorption and use of specific nutrients.

It is important for older people to seek out foods that are "nutrient dense," that is, foods that have a high proportion of nutrients in comparison with the number of calories they provide. Exercise helps to boost appetite and maintain muscle tissue, which is more active metabolically.

Body Temperature

Heat is an important by-product of the many chemical activities constantly occurring in body tissues. At the same time, heat is always being lost through a variety of outlets. Under normal conditions, a number of regulatory devices keep body temperature constant within quite narrow limits. Maintenance of a constant temperature despite both internal and external influences is one phase of homeostasis, the tendency of all body processes to maintain a normal state despite forces that tend to alter them.

HEAT PRODUCTION AND HEAT LOSS

Heat is a by-product of the cellular oxidations that generate energy. The amount of heat produced by a given organ varies with the kind of tissue and its activity. While at rest, muscles may produce as little as 25% of total body heat, but when muscles contract, heat production is greatly multiplied, owing to their increased metabolic rate. Under basal conditions (at rest), the liver and other abdominal organs produce about 50% of total body heat. The brain produces only 15% of body heat at rest, and an increase in nervous tissue activity produces little increase in heat production. High heat-generating tissues do not become much warmer than others because the circulating blood distributes the heat fairly evenly.

Factors Affecting Heat Production The rate at which heat is produced is affected by a number of factors, including exercise, hormone production, food intake, and age. Hormones, such as thyroxine from the thyroid gland and epinephrine (adrenaline) from the adrenal medulla, increase heat production.

The intake of food is also accompanied by increased heat production. The nutrients that enter the blood after digestion are available for increased cellular metabolism. In addition, the glands and muscles of the digestive system generate heat as they set to work. These responses do not account for all the increase, however, nor do they account for the much greater increase in metabolism after a meal containing a large amount of protein.

Mechanisms of Heat Loss Although 15% to 20% of heat loss occurs through the respiratory system and with urine and feces, more than 80% of heat loss occurs through the skin. Networks of blood vessels in the skin's dermis (deeper part) can bring considerable quantities of blood

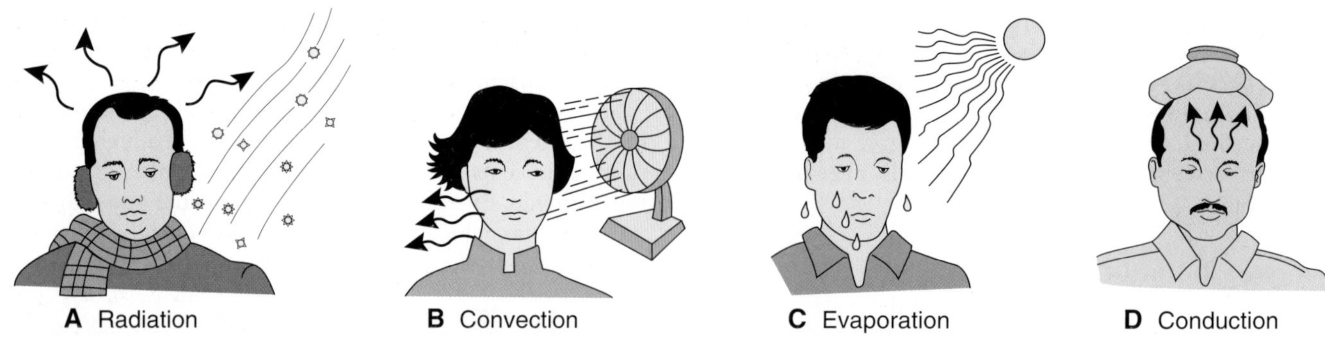

Figure 18-6 Mechanisms of heat loss. KEY POINT There are four processes that promote heat loss of body heat to the environment. **A.** Radiation—Heat travels away as heat waves or rays. **B.** Convection—Heat transfer is promoted by movement of a cooler medium. **C.** Evaporation—Heat is used to change a liquid (such as sweat) to a vapor. **D.** Conduction—Heat is transferred to a cooler object. (Reprinted with permission from Taylor C, et al. *Fundamentals of Nursing*, 5th ed. Philadelphia, PA: Lippincott Williams & Wilkins, 2005.) ZOOMING IN What will happen in **(B)** if the fan speed is increased? What will happen in **(C)** as environmental humidity increases?

near the surface, so that heat can be dissipated to the outside. This release can occur in several ways (Fig. 18-6):

- In **radiation**, heat travels from its source as heat waves or rays. Radiation does not require contact between the heat source and the heat receiver.
- In **convection,** heat transfer is promoted by movement of a cooler contacting medium. For example, if the air around the skin is put in motion, as by an electric fan, the layer of heated air next to the body is constantly carried away and replaced with cooler air. Another example of convection is the transfer of heat from muscle tissue to circulating blood.
- In **evaporation**, heat is lost in the process of changing a liquid to the vapor state. Heat from the skin is used to evaporate sweat from the skin's surface, just as heat applied to a pot of water will be used to convert the water to steam.
- In **conduction**, a warm object transfers heat energy to a cooler object. For example, heat can be transferred from the skin directly to an ice pack.

To illustrate evaporation, rub some alcohol on your skin; it evaporates rapidly, using so much heat that your skin feels cold. Perspiration does the same thing, although not as quickly. The rate of heat loss through evaporation depends on the humidity of the surrounding air. When humidity exceeds 60% or so, perspiration does not evaporate as readily, making one feel very uncomfortable unless some other means of heat loss is available, such as convection caused by a fan.

Prevention of Heat Loss Factors that play a part in heat loss through the skin include the volume of tissue compared with the amount of skin surface. A child loses heat more rapidly than does an adult. Such parts as fingers and toes are affected most by exposure to cold because they have a great amount of skin compared with total tissue volume.

If the surrounding air temperature is lower than that of the body, excessive heat loss is prevented by both natural and artificial means. Clothing checks heat loss by trapping insulating air in both its material and its layers. An effective natural insulation against cold is the layer of fat under the skin. The degree of insulation depends on the thickness of the subcutaneous layer. Even when skin temperature is low, this fatty tissue prevents the deeper tissues from losing much heat. On the average, this layer is slightly thicker in females than in males.

TEMPERATURE REGULATION

Body temperature remains almost constant despite wide variations in the rate of heat production or loss, because of internal temperature-regulating mechanisms.

The Role of the Hypothalamus Many body areas take part in heat regulation, but the most important center is the hypothalamus, the area of the brain located just above the pituitary gland. Regulation is based on the temperature of the blood circulating through the brain and also on input from temperature receptors in the skin.

If these two factors indicate that too much heat is being lost, impulses are sent quickly from the hypothalamus to the sympathetic branch of the autonomic (involuntary) nervous system, which in turn causes constriction of the skin's blood vessels to reduce heat loss. Other impulses are sent to the muscles to cause shivering, a rhythmic contraction that results in increased heat production. Furthermore, epinephrine output may be increased if necessary. Epinephrine increases cellular metabolism for a short period, and this in turn increases heat production.

If there is danger of overheating, the hypothalamus stimulates the sweat glands to increase their activity. Impulses from the hypothalamus also cause cutaneous blood vessels to dilate, so that increased blood flow will promote heat loss. The hypothalamus may also induce muscle relaxation to minimize heat production.

Muscles are especially important in temperature regulation because variations in the activity of these large tissue masses can readily increase or decrease heat generation. Because muscles form roughly one-third of the body, either an involuntary or an intentional increase in their activity can produce enough heat to offset a considerable decrease in the environmental temperature.

Age Factors Very young and very old people are limited in their ability to regulate body temperature when exposed to environmental extremes. A newborn infant's body temperature decreases if the infant is exposed to a cool environment for a long period. Elderly people are also not able to produce enough heat to maintain body temperature in a cool environment.

With regard to overheating in these age groups, heat loss mechanisms are not fully developed in the newborn. The elderly do not lose as much heat from their skin as do younger people. Both groups should be protected from extreme temperatures.

Normal Body Temperature The normal temperature range obtained by either a mercury or an electronic thermometer may extend from 36.2°C to 37.6°C (97°F to 100°F). Body temperature varies with the time of day. Usually, it is lowest in the early morning because the muscles have been relaxed and no food has been taken in for several hours. Body temperature tends to be higher in the late afternoon and evening because of physical activity and food consumption.

Normal temperature also varies in different parts of the body. Skin temperature obtained in the axilla (armpit) is lower than mouth temperature, and mouth temperature is a degree or so lower than rectal temperature. It is believed that, if it were possible to place a thermometer inside the liver, it would register a degree or more higher than rectal temperature. The temperature within a muscle might be even higher during activity.

Although the Fahrenheit scale is used in the United States, in most parts of the world, temperature is measured with the **Celsius** (SEL-se-us) thermometer. On this scale, the ice point is at 0° and the normal boiling point of water is at 100°, the interval between these two points being divided into 100 equal units. The Celsius scale is also called the **centigrade scale** (think of 100 cents in a dollar).

Fever Fever (FE-ver) is a condition in which the body temperature is higher than normal. An individual with a fever is described as febrile (FEB-ril). Usually, the presence of fever is due to an infection, but there can be many other causes, such as malignancies, brain injuries, toxic reactions, reactions to vaccines, and diseases involving the central nervous system (CNS). Sometimes, emotional upsets can bring on a fever. Whatever the cause, the effect is to reset the body's thermostat in the hypothalamus.

Curiously enough, fever is usually preceded by a chill—that is, a violent attack of shivering and a sensation of cold that blankets and heating pads seem unable to relieve. As a result of these reactions, heat is generated and stored and, when the chill subsides, the body temperature is elevated.

The old adage that a fever should be starved is completely wrong. During a fever, there is an increase in metabolism that is usually proportional to the fever's intensity. The body uses available sugars and fats, and there is an increase in the use of protein. During the first week or so of a fever, there is definite evidence of protein destruction, so a high-calorie diet with plenty of protein is recommended.

When a fever ends, sometimes the return of temperature to normal occurs very rapidly. This sudden drop in temperature is called the **crisis**, and it is usually accompanied by symptoms indicating rapid heat loss: profuse perspiration, muscular relaxation, and dilation of blood vessels in the skin. A gradual drop in temperature, in contrast, is known as **lysis**. A drug that reduces fever is described as **antipyretic** (an-ti-pi-RET-ik).

The mechanism of fever production is not completely understood, but we might think of the hypothalamus as a thermostat that during fever is set higher than normal. This change in the heat-regulating mechanism often follows the introduction of a foreign protein or the entrance into the bloodstream of bacteria or their toxins. Substances that produce fever are called **pyrogens** (PI-ro-jens).

Up to a point, fever may be beneficial because it steps up phagocytosis (the process by which white blood cells destroy bacteria and other foreign material), inhibits the growth of certain organisms, and increases cellular metabolism, which may help recovery from disease.

CHECKPOINTS 

- ☐ **18-10** What are some factors that affect heat production in the body?
- ☐ **18-11** What part of the brain is responsible for regulating body temperature?
- ☐ **18-12** What is normal body temperature?

A&P in Action Revisited

Becky Learns to Manage Her Diabetes

"Hi Mom!" Becky shouted into the camp phone. "No, everything's fine... Actually, I'm calling because I knew you were probably worried! I'm having an awesome time. I've gone canoeing, hiking, and swimming every day. At night, we've been sitting around the campfire telling ghost stories... Yeah, I've made some new friends too—everyone's really great. Wanda, my cabin leader, is so cool. She has diabetes too and she knows a lot about it. We did this neat experiment the other day where we tested our blood glucose levels before and after going on a hike. Did you know that glucose levels drop after exercise because the body uses glucose to make ATP? ... And at lunch today we learned that foods are made up of carbohydrates, fats, and proteins. Did you know that glucose is a carbohydrate? And that some foods can raise your blood sugar really fast. Wanda called it the 'glycemic effect' or something like that. Anyways, that's why it's better to eat brown bread and fruit instead of white bread and candy. We also learned about saturated and unsaturated fats. Tell Dad that when I get home he and I need to talk. If he keeps eating all those fatty foods he likes, he's going to get heart disease!"

In this case, we saw that diabetes mellitus is an endocrine disorder that prevents cells from metabolizing glucose. To review the endocrine system, see Chapter 11.

Chapter Wrap-Up

Summary Overview

A detailed chapter outline with space for note-taking is on *thePoint*. The figure below illustrates the main topics covered in this chapter.

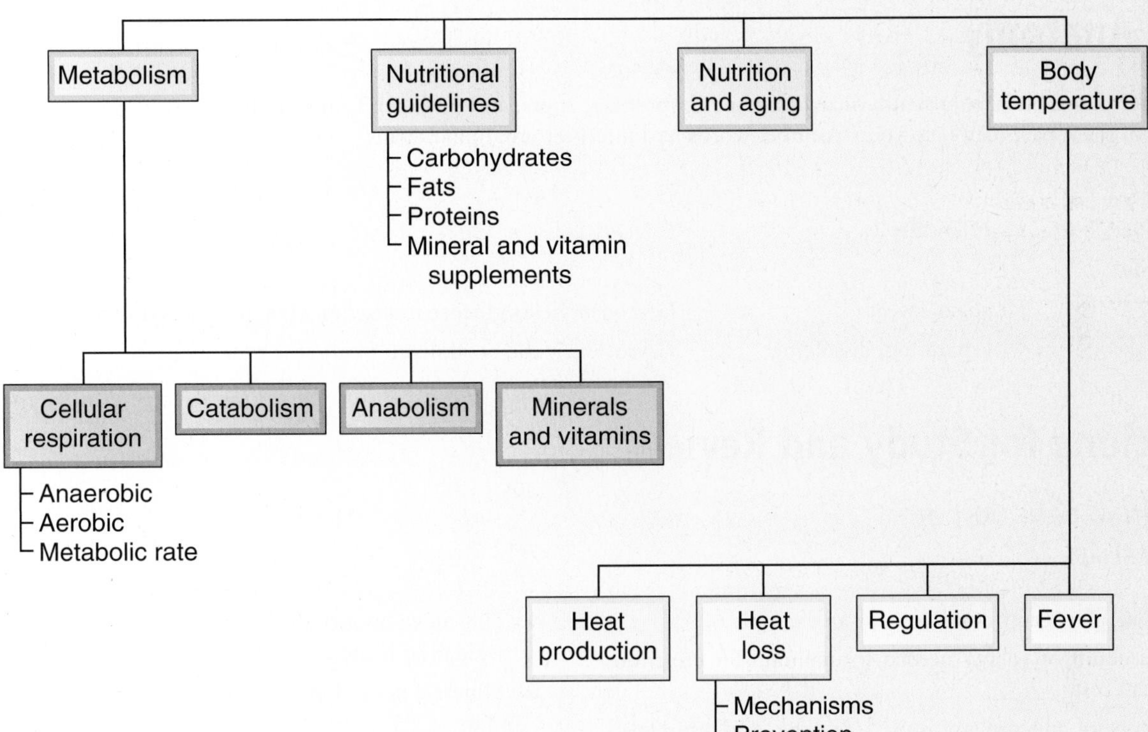

Key Terms

The terms listed below are emphasized in this chapter. Knowing them will help you organize and prioritize your learning. These and other boldface terms are defined in the Glossary with phonetic pronunciations.

anabolism
basal metabolism
catabolism
cellular respiration
glucose
glycogen
glycolysis
hypothalamus
kilocalorie
metabolic rate
mineral
oxidation
vitamin

Word Anatomy

Scientific terms are built from standardized word parts (prefixes, roots, and suffixes). Learning the meanings of these parts can help you remember words and interpret unfamiliar terms.

WORD PART	MEANING	EXAMPLE
Metabolism		
glyc/o	sugar, sweet	*Glycogen* yields glucose molecules when it breaks down.
-lysis	separating, dissolving	*Glycolysis* is the breakdown of glucose for energy.

Questions for Study and Review

BUILDING UNDERSTANDING

Fill in the Blanks

1. Building glycogen from glucose is an example of _____.

2. The amount of energy needed to maintain life functions while at rest is _____.

3. Reserves of glucose are stored in liver and muscle as _____.

4. The most important area of the brain for temperature regulation is the _____.

5. Minerals needed in extremely small amounts are referred to as _____.

Matching > Match each numbered item with the most closely related lettered item:

___ **6.** Major energy source for the body

___ **7.** Chemical element required for normal body function

___ **8.** Complex organic substance required for normal body function

___ **9.** Energy storage molecule with only single bonds between carbon atoms

___**10.** Energy storage molecule with one or more double bonds between carbon atoms

a. saturated fat

b. vitamin

c. mineral

d. unsaturated fat

e. glucose

Multiple Choice

___ **11.** By what method is nitrogen removed during amino acid catabolism?

a. oxidation
b. the glycemic effect
c. lysis
d. deamination

___ **12.** Which of the following would have the lowest glycemic effect?

a. glucose
b. sucrose
c. lactose
d. starch

___ **13.** Which organ catabolizes alcohol?

a. small intestine
b. liver
c. pancreas
d. spleen

___ **14.** What are amino acids that cannot be made by metabolism called?

a. essential
b. nonessential
c. antioxidants
d. reactive oxygen species

UNDERSTANDING CONCEPTS

15. In what part of the cell does anaerobic respiration occur and what are its end products? In what part of the cell does aerobic respiration occur? What are its end products?

16. About how many kilocalories are released from a tablespoon of butter (14 g)? a tablespoon of sugar (12 g)? a tablespoon of egg white (15 g)?

17. If you eat 2,000 kcal a day, how many kilocalories should come from carbohydrates? from fats? from protein?

18. How is heat produced in the body? What structures produce the most heat during increased activity?

19. Emily's body temperature increased from 36.2°C to 36.5°C and then decreased to 36.2°C. Describe the feedback mechanism regulating Emily's body temperature.

20. Differentiate between the terms in the following pairs:

a. conduction and convection
b. radiation and evaporation
c. antioxidants and reactive oxygen species
d. catabolism and anabolism

CONCEPTUAL THINKING

21. The oxidation of glucose to form ATP is often compared to the burning of fuel. Why is this analogy inaccurate?

22. In the case study, Becky learned about the glycemic effect. In order to prevent hyperglycemia (high blood sugar), which foods should Becky avoid or eat in moderation?

23. It is a hot summer day and you are trying to keep cool by sitting in front of a fan, but you are still sweating profusely. Describe the two mechanisms of heat loss that you are employing.

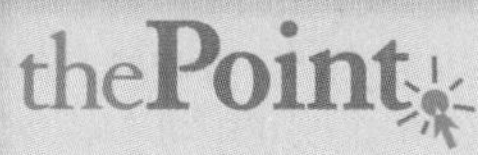

For more questions, see the learning activities on *thePoint*.

CHAPTER 19

The Urinary System and Body Fluids

A&P in Action

Adam's Second Case: Urinary Blockade

Adam rolled out of bed and glanced at the clock as he rushed to the bathroom. *Jeez, it's only been a couple of hours since the last time I had to pee, he thought. Hopefully this time it won't take as long*. Sure enough, Adam had difficulty voiding. Even once he was able to get started, he only managed to produce a small volume of urine. Lately, this was happening more and more frequently. At first, he chalked it up to getting older, but now he wondered if he had some sort of bladder or kidney infection. As he climbed back into bed, Adam decided that he would make an appointment with his family doctor.

"So let me get this straight," said Dr. Michaels. "Over the last several weeks, you've experienced increased frequency and urgency of urination, even at night (nocturia). While urinating, you've had hesitation in starting, decreased volume, and diminished force of the stream. And even after urination, you still feel that your urinary bladder is not completely empty." Based on Adam's symptoms, Dr. Michaels suspected that Adam's prostate gland (a male reproductive organ) was causing problems for his urinary system. The prostate gland lies immediately inferior to the urinary bladder, where it surrounds the first part of the urethra. If the gland becomes enlarged, it can obstruct the urethra and prevent the urinary bladder from emptying completely. At 55 years old, Adam was in the right age range for this condition.

Dr. Michaels' suspicions were confirmed by the digital rectal exam. Adam's prostate was large and rubbery. The doctor carefully palpated the prostate's surface with his finger—he could not detect any nodules on its smooth surface. "Adam, my initial diagnosis is that you have benign prostatic hypertrophy—your prostate has grown larger and is preventing urine from passing out of your urinary bladder. Your prostate's surface is smooth though, which suggests that the growth is not cancerous, but we'll have to get that ruled out. I'm going to order some blood tests and urinalyses, as well as refer you to a urologist."

Adam's prostate is causing problems for his urinary system. In this chapter, we will examine the anatomy and physiology of the urinary system. Later, we will learn how Adam's disorder is resolved.

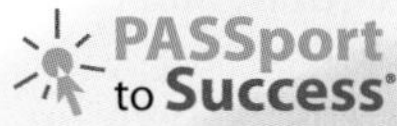

Ancillaries At-A-Glance

Visit *thePoint* to access the PASSport to Success and the following resources. For guidance in using these resources most effectively, see pp. ix–xviii.

Learning TOOLS

- Learning Style Self-Assessment
- Live Advise Online Student Tutoring
- Tips for Effective Studying

Learning RESOURCES

- E-book: Chapter 19
- Web Chart: Kidney Regulation of Blood Pressure
- Web Chart: The Role of Hormones in Electrolyte Balance
- Animation: Renal Function
- Health Professions: Hemodialysis Technician
- Detailed Chapter Outline
- Answers to Questions for Study and Review
- Audio Pronunciation Glossary

Learning ACTIVITIES

- Pre-Quiz
- Visual Activities
- Kinesthetic Activities
- Auditory Activities

Learning Outcomes

After careful study of this chapter, you should be able to:

1. Describe the organs of the urinary system and give the functions of each, ***pp. 372***
2. List the systems that eliminate waste and name the substances eliminated by each, ***p. 373***
3. List the activities of the kidneys in maintaining homeostasis, ***p. 373***
4. Trace the path of a drop of blood as it flows through the kidney, ***p. 373***
5. Describe a nephron, ***p. 373***
6. Name the four processes involved in urine formation and describe the action of each, ***p. 374***
7. Identify hormones involved in urine formation and cite the function of each, ***p. 377***
8. Describe the components and functions of the juxtaglomerular (JG) apparatus, ***p. 378***
9. Describe the process of micturition, ***p. 380***
10. Name three normal constituents of urine, ***p. 381***
11. Compare intracellular and extracellular fluids, ***p. 382***
12. List four types of extracellular fluids, ***p. 382***
13. Name the systems that are involved in water balance, ***p. 383***
14. Explain how thirst is regulated, ***p. 383***
15. Define *electrolytes* and describe some of their functions, ***p. 383***
16. Describe the role of hormones in electrolyte balance, ***p. 385***
17. Describe three methods for regulating the pH of body fluids, ***p. 385***
18. Referring to the case study, describe how urethral blockage can affect kidney function, ***pp. 370, 386***
19. Show how word parts are used to build words related to the urinary system and body fluids (see Word Anatomy at the end of the chapter), ***p. 388***

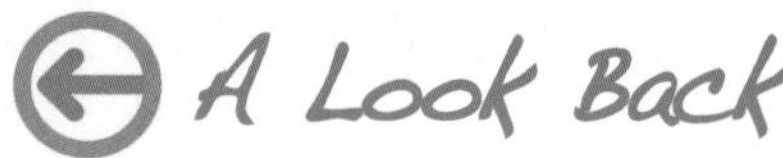

The importance of body fluid volume and composition has been stressed throughout previous chapters, beginning with the discussion of water in Chapter 2. Most of the water lost in a day is through the urine produced by the kidneys. The kidneys not only help regulate total fluid volume, but also the electrolyte and acid-base balance of body fluids. This chapter concludes with a discussion of the electrolytes important in all of metabolism and their relative distribution in intracellular and extracellular fluids.

Systems Involved in Excretion

The urinary system is also called the *excretory system* because one of its main functions is **excretion**, removal and elimination of unwanted substances from the blood. The urinary system has many other functions as well, including regulation of the volume, acid–base balance (pH), and electrolyte composition of body fluids.

The main parts of the urinary system, shown in Figure 19-1, are as follows:

- Two kidneys. These organs extract wastes from the blood, balance body fluids, and form urine.
- Two **ureters** (U-re-ters). These tubes conduct urine from the kidneys to the urinary bladder.
- A single **urinary bladder**. This reservoir receives and stores the urine brought to it by the two ureters.
- A single urethra (u-RE-thrah). This tube conducts urine from the bladder to the outside of the body for elimination.

Although the focus of this chapter is the urinary system, some other systems are mentioned here as well, because they also function in excretion and in maintaining fluid

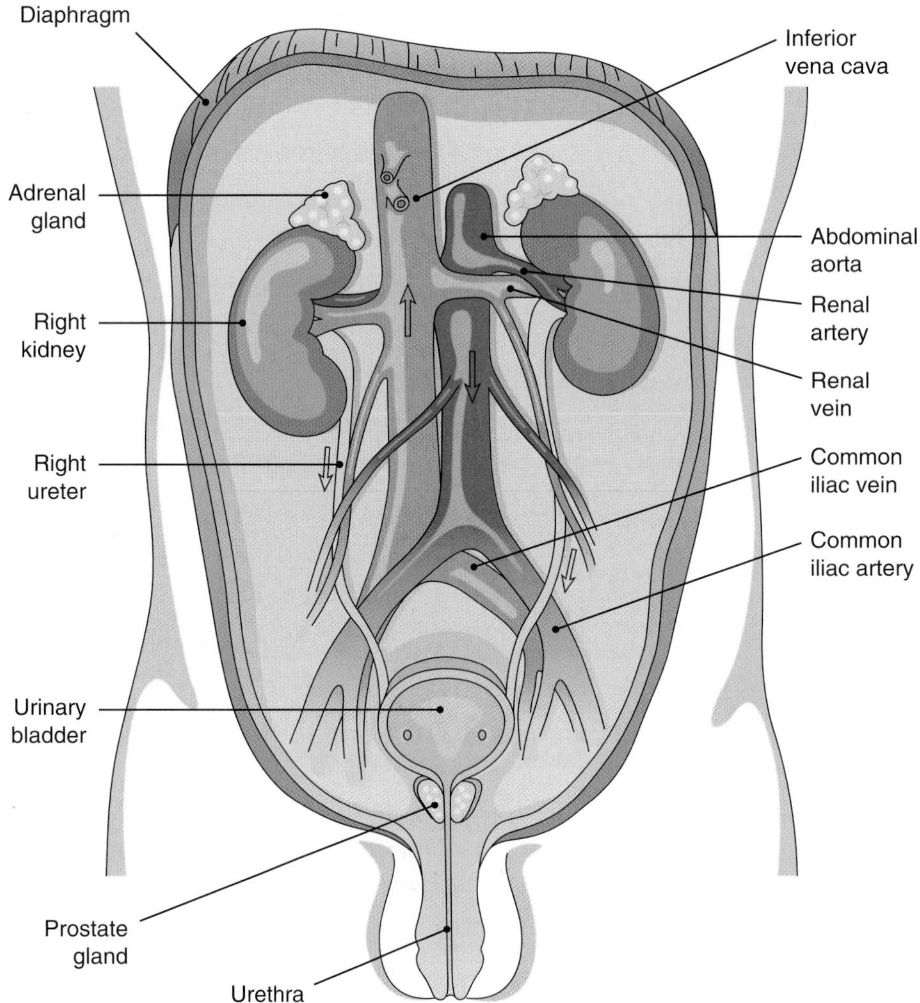

Figure 19-1 Male urinary system. The urinary system along with nearby blood vessels and the adrenal glands are shown. **ZOOMING IN** What vessel supplies blood to the renal artery? What vessel receives blood from the renal vein?

homeostasis. These systems and some of the substances they eliminate are the following:

- The **digestive system** eliminates water, some salts, and bile, in addition to digestive residue, all of which are contained in the feces. The liver is important in eliminating the products of red blood cell destruction and in breaking down certain drugs and toxins.
- The **respiratory system** eliminates carbon dioxide and water. The latter appears as vapor, as can be demonstrated by breathing on a windowpane or a mirror, where the water condenses.
- The skin, or **integumentary system**, excretes water, salts, and very small quantities of nitrogenous wastes. These all appear in perspiration, although water also evaporates continuously from the skin without our being conscious of it.

CHECKPOINTS 

- 19-1 What are the organs of the urinary system?
- 19-2 What are some systems other than the urinary system that eliminate waste?

The Kidneys

The kidneys interact with other systems as prime regulators of homeostasis. After a brief overview of the kidney's many activities, we will describe its structure and specific roles in urine formation and regulation of blood pressure.

KIDNEY ACTIVITIES

The kidneys are involved in the following processes:

- Excretion of unwanted substances, such as cellular metabolic waste, excess salts, and toxins. One product of amino acid metabolism is nitrogen-containing waste material, chiefly **urea** (u-RE-ah). After synthesis in the liver, urea is transported in the blood to the kidneys for elimination. The kidneys have a specialized mechanism for the elimination of urea and other nitrogenous (ni-TROJ-en-us) wastes.
- Water balance. Although the amount of water gained and lost in a day can vary tremendously, the kidneys can adapt to these variations by altering urine output so that the volume of body water remains remarkably stable from day to day.
- Acid–base balance of body fluids. Acids are constantly being produced by cellular metabolism. Certain foods can yield acids or bases, and people may also ingest antacids, such as bicarbonate. However, if the body is to function normally, the pH of body fluids must remain in the range of 7.35 to 7.45.
- Blood pressure regulation. The kidneys depend on blood pressure to filter the blood. If blood pressure falls, potentially limiting filtration, specialized kidney cells release renin. This enzyme activates a blood protein, angiotensin, that causes blood vessels to constrict, thus raising blood pressure. Angiotensin has additional effects as described later in the chapter.
- Regulation of red blood cell production. When the kidneys do not get enough oxygen, they produce the hormone **erythropoietin** (eh-rith-ro-POY-eh-tin) (**EPO**), which stimulates red cell production in the bone marrow.

KIDNEY STRUCTURE

The kidneys lie against the back muscles in the upper abdomen at about the level of the last thoracic and first three lumbar vertebrae. The right kidney is slightly lower than the left to accommodate the liver. **(see Fig. 19-1)** Each kidney is firmly enclosed in a membranous **renal capsule** made of fibrous connective tissue **(Fig. 19-2)**. In addition, there is a protective layer of fat called the *adipose capsule* around the organ. An outermost layer of fascia (connective tissue) anchors the kidney to the peritoneum and abdominal wall. The kidneys, as well as the ureters, lie posterior to the peritoneum (see Chapter 19). Thus, they are not in the peritoneal cavity but rather in an area known as the **retroperitoneal** (ret-ro-per-ih-to-NE-al) **space**. See **Figure A3-8** in Appendix 3 for a dissection photograph showing the kidneys and renal vessels in place.

Blood Supply The kidney's blood supply is illustrated in **Figure 19-2**. Blood is brought to the kidney by a short branch of the abdominal aorta called the **renal artery**.

After entering the kidney, the renal artery subdivides into smaller and smaller branches, which eventually make contact with the kidney's functional units, the **nephrons** (NEF-ronz). Blood leaves the kidney by vessels that finally merge to form the **renal vein**, which carries blood into the inferior vena cava for return to the heart.

19

Organization The kidney is a somewhat flattened organ approximately 10 cm (4 in.) long, 5 cm (2 in.) wide, and 2.5 cm (1 in.) thick **(see Fig. 19-2)**. On the medial border, there is a notch called the **hilum**, where the renal artery, the renal vein, and the ureter connect with the kidney. The lateral border is convex (curved outward), giving the entire organ a bean-shaped appearance.

The kidney is divided into two regions: the renal cortex and the renal medulla **(see Fig. 19-2)**. The **renal cortex** is the kidney's outer portion. The internal **renal medulla** contains tubes in which urine is formed and collected. These tubes form a number of cone-shaped structures called **renal pyramids.** The tips of the pyramids point toward the **renal pelvis**, a funnel-shaped basin that forms the upper end of the ureter. Cuplike extensions of the renal pelvis surround the tips of the pyramids and collect urine; these extensions are called **calyces** (KA-lih-seze; singular, **calyx**, KA-liks). The urine that collects in the pelvis then passes down the ureters to the bladder.

The Nephron As is the case with most organs, the kidney's most fascinating aspect is too small to be seen with the naked

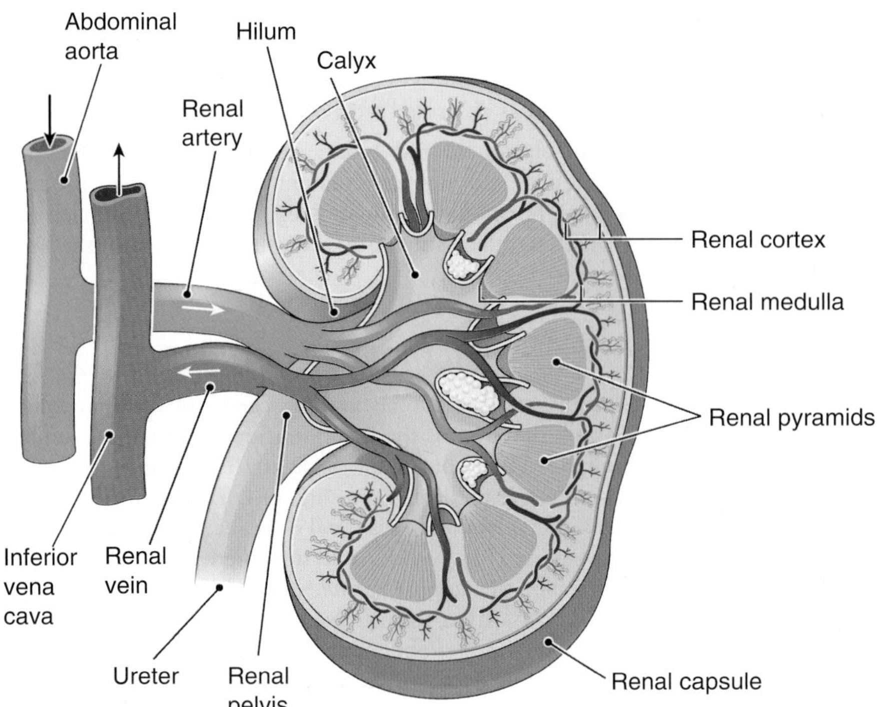

Figure 19-2 Kidney structure and the renal blood supply. KEY POINT A longitudinal section through the kidney shows its internal structure. The renal artery branches to all regions of the kidney. Venous drainage combines to flow into the renal vein. ZOOMING IN What is the outer region of the kidney called? What is the inner region of the kidney called?

eye. This basic unit, which actually does the kidney's work, is the **nephron** (Fig. 19-3). Each nephron begins with a hollow, cup-shaped bulb known as the **glomerular** (glo-MER-u-lar) **capsule** or *Bowman capsule*. This structure gets its name from the cluster of capillaries it contains, which is called the **glomerulus** (a word that comes from the Latin meaning "ball of yarn.") This combined unit of the glomerulus with its glomerular capsule is the nephron's filtering device. The remainder of the nephron is essentially a tiny coiled tube, the **renal tubule**, which consists of several parts. The coiled portion leading from the glomerular capsule is called the **proximal tubule,** also known as the *proximal convoluted* (KON-vo-lu-ted) *tubule* (PCT), to describe its twisted form. The renal tubule then uncoils to form a hairpin-shaped segment called the **nephron loop**, or *loop of Henle*. The first part of the loop, which carries fluid toward the medulla, is the **descending limb** (see Fig. 19-3). The part that continues from the loop's turn and carries fluid away from the medulla, is the **ascending limb.** Continuing from the ascending limb, the tubule coils once again into the **distal tubule**, or *distal convoluted tubule* (**DCT**), so called because it is farther along the tubule from the glomerular capsule than is the proximal tubule. Each renal tubule empties into a collecting duct, which then continues through the medulla toward the renal pelvis.

Each kidney contains about one million nephrons; if all these coiled tubes were separated, straightened out, and laid end to end, they would span some 120 km (75 mi.)! Figure 19-4 is a microscopic view of kidney tissue showing several glomeruli, each surrounded by a glomerular capsule. This figure also shows sections through renal tubules.

A small blood vessel, the **afferent arteriole**, supplies the glomerulus with blood; another small vessel, called the **efferent arteriole**, carries blood from the glomerulus. When blood leaves the glomerulus, it does not head immediately back toward the heart. Instead, it flows into a capillary network that surrounds the renal tubule. These **peritubular capillaries** are named for their location.

In most cases, the glomerulus, glomerular capsule, and the proximal and distal tubules of the nephron are within the renal cortex. The nephron loop and collecting duct extend into the medulla (see Fig. 19-3).

CHECKPOINTS 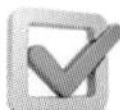

☐ 19-3 The kidneys are located in the retroperitoneal space. Where is this space?

☐ 19-4 What vessel supplies blood to the kidney and what vessel drains blood from the kidney?

☐ 19-5 What are the outer and inner regions of the kidney called?

☐ 19-6 What is the functional unit of the kidney called?

☐ 19-7 What name is given to the coil of capillaries in the glomerular (Bowman) capsule?

FORMATION OF URINE

The following explanation of urine formation describes a complex process, involving many back-and-forth exchanges between the bloodstream and the kidney tubules. As fluid filtered from the blood travels slowly through the nephron's twists and turns, there is ample time for exchanges to take place. These processes together allow the kidney to "fine tune" body fluids as they adjust the urine's composition.

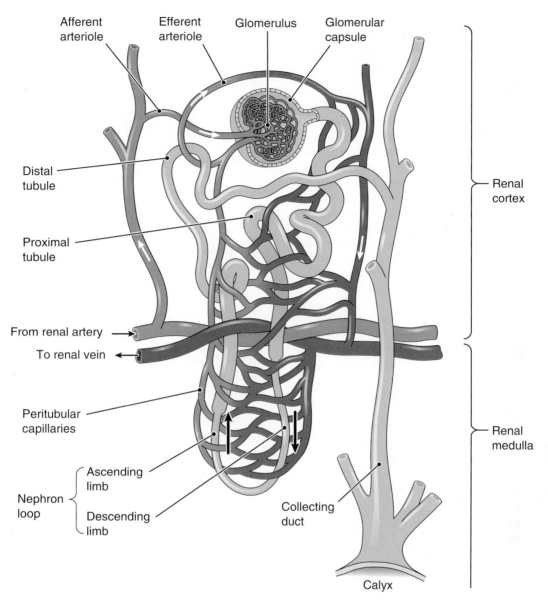

Figure 19-3 A nephron and its blood supply. KEY POINT The nephron regulates the proportions of urinary water, waste, and other materials according to the body's constantly changing needs. Materials that enter the nephron can be returned to the blood through the surrounding capillaries. ZOOMING IN Which of the two convoluted tubules arises closer to the glomerular capsule? Following along the length of the nephron, which convoluted tubule is farther away from the glomerular capsule?

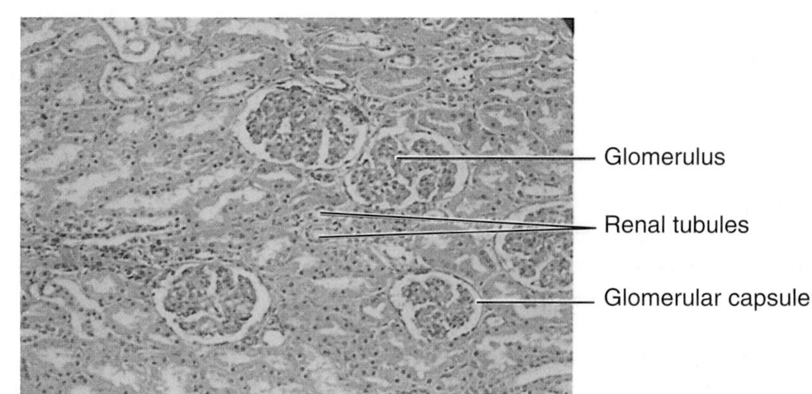

Figure 19-4 Microscopic view of the kidney. KEY POINT The glomeruli and glomerular capsules are visible along with cross sections of the renal tubules. (Courtesy of Dana Morse Bittus and BJ Cohen.)

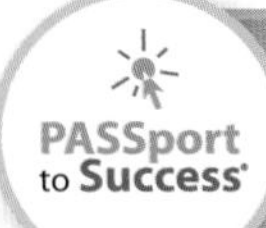

See the student resources on *thePoint* for the animation *Renal Function,* which shows the process of urine formation in action.

Glomerular Filtration The process of urine formation begins with the glomerulus in the glomerular capsule. The walls of the glomerular capillaries are sieve-like and permit the free flow of water and soluble materials through them. Like other capillary walls, however, they are impermeable (im-PER-me-abl) to blood cells and large protein molecules, and these components remain in the blood **(Fig. 19-5).**

Because the diameter of the afferent arteriole is slightly larger than that of the efferent arteriole **(see Fig. 19-5),** blood can enter the glomerulus more easily than it can leave. Thus, blood pressure in the glomerulus is about three to four times higher than that in other capillaries. To understand this effect, think of placing your thumb over the end of a garden hose as water comes through. As you make the diameter of the opening smaller, water is forced out under higher pressure. As a result of increased fluid (hydrostatic) pressure in the glomerulus, materials are constantly being pushed out of the blood and into the nephron's glomerular capsule. As described in Chapter 3, the movement of water and dissolved materials through a membrane under pressure is called *filtration*. This movement of materials under pressure from the blood into the capsule is therefore known as **glomerular filtration.**

The fluid that enters the glomerular capsule, called the **glomerular filtrate,** begins its journey along the renal tubule. In addition to water and the normal soluble substances in the blood, other substances, such as vitamins and drugs, also may be filtered and become part of the glomerular filtrate.

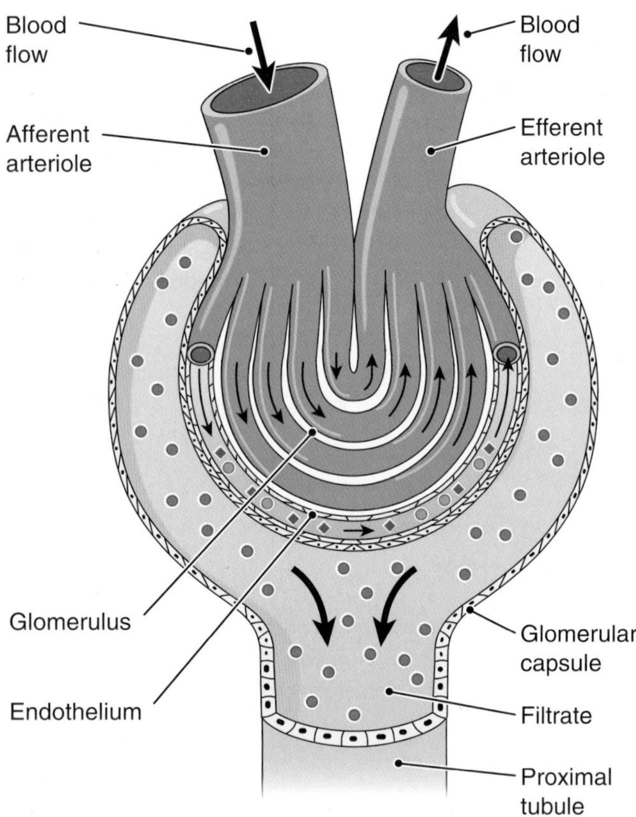

Figure 19-5 Glomerular filtration: the first step in urine formation. KEY POINT Blood pressure inside the glomerulus forces water and dissolved substances into the glomerular capsule. Blood cells and proteins remain behind in the blood. The smaller diameter of the efferent arteriole as compared with that of the afferent arteriole maintains high hydrostatic (fluid) pressure. In this simple illustration, only one capillary is cut away, but filtration occurs through all the vessels, and the glomerular capillaries are actually in a cluster, as shown in other figures.

Tubular Reabsorption The kidneys form about 160 to 180 L of filtrate each day. However, only 1 to 1.5 L of urine are eliminated daily. Clearly, most of the water that enters the nephron is not excreted with the urine, but rather, is returned to the circulation. In addition to water, many other substances the body needs, such as nutrients and ions, pass into the nephron as part of the filtrate, and these also must be returned. Therefore, the process of filtration that occurs in the glomerular capsule is followed by a process of **tubular reabsorption.** As the filtrate travels through the renal tubule, water and other needed substances leave the tubule and enter the surrounding tissue fluid, the interstitial fluid (IF). They move by several processes previously described in Chapter 3, including:

- Diffusion. The movement of substances from an area of higher concentration to an area of lower concentration (following the concentration gradient).
- Osmosis. Diffusion of water through a semipermeable membrane.
- Active transport. Movement of materials through the plasma membrane against the concentration gradient using energy and transporters.

Several hormones, including aldosterone and atrial natriuretic peptide (ANP), affect tubular reabsorption **(Table 19-1).**

The substances that leave the nephron and enter the IF then enter the peritubular capillaries and return to the circulation. In contrast, most of the urea and other nitrogenous waste materials are kept within the tubule to be eliminated with the urine.

Tubular Secretion Before the filtrate leaves the body as urine, the kidney makes final adjustments in composition by means of **tubular secretion.** In this process, some substances are actively moved from the blood into the nephron. Potassium ions are moved into the urine in this manner.

Table 19-1 Substances that Affect Renal Function

Substance	Source	Action
Aldosterone (al-DOS-ter-one)	Hormone released from the adrenal cortex when blood pressure falls or blood potassium levels are too high	Promotes reabsorption of sodium and water in the kidney to conserve water and increase blood pressure
Atrial natriuretic peptide (na-tre-u-RET-ik) (ANP)	Atrial myocardial cells; released when blood pressure is too high	Causes kidney to excrete sodium and water to decrease blood volume and blood pressure
Antidiuretic hormone (an-te-di-u-RET-ik) (ADH)	Made in the hypothalamus and released from the posterior pituitary; released when blood becomes too concentrated or blood pressure falls	Promotes water reabsorption from the distal tubule and collecting duct to concentrate the urine and conserve water
Renin (RE-nin)	Enzyme produced by renal cells when blood pressure falls	Activates angiotensin in the blood
Angiotensin (an-je-o-TEN-sin)	Protein in the blood that is activated by renin	Causes constriction of blood vessels to raise blood pressure; increases fluid volume by stimulating thirst and promoting release of aldosterone and ADH

Importantly, the kidneys regulate the acid–base (pH) balance of body fluids by the active secretion of hydrogen ions. Some drugs, such as penicillin, also are actively secreted into the nephron for elimination.

Concentration of the Urine The amount of water that is eliminated with the urine is regulated by a complex mechanism within the nephron. This process is called the **countercurrent mechanism** because it involves fluid traveling in opposite directions within the ascending and descending limbs of the nephron loop. The countercurrent mechanism is illustrated in Figure 19-6. Its essentials are as follows.

As the filtrate passes through the nephron loop, electrolytes, especially sodium, are actively pumped out by the

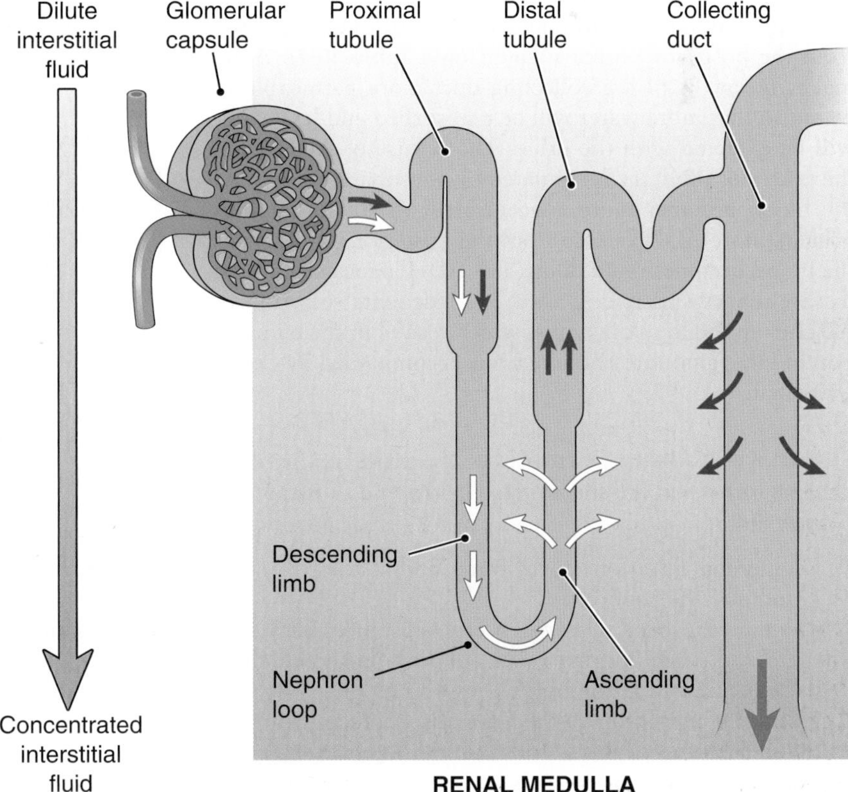

Figure 19-6 Concentration of urine by the countercurrent mechanism. KEY POINT Urine concentration is regulated by means of intricate exchanges of water and electrolytes, mainly sodium, in the nephron loop, distal tubule, and collecting duct. The intensity of color shows the increasing concentration of the interstitial fluid moving from the cortex to the medulla. As urine flows through the collecting ducts, water is drawn out by the hypertonic interstitial fluid, thus concentrating the urine. ADH increases the permeability of the collecting duct, allowing more water to leave the urine.

19

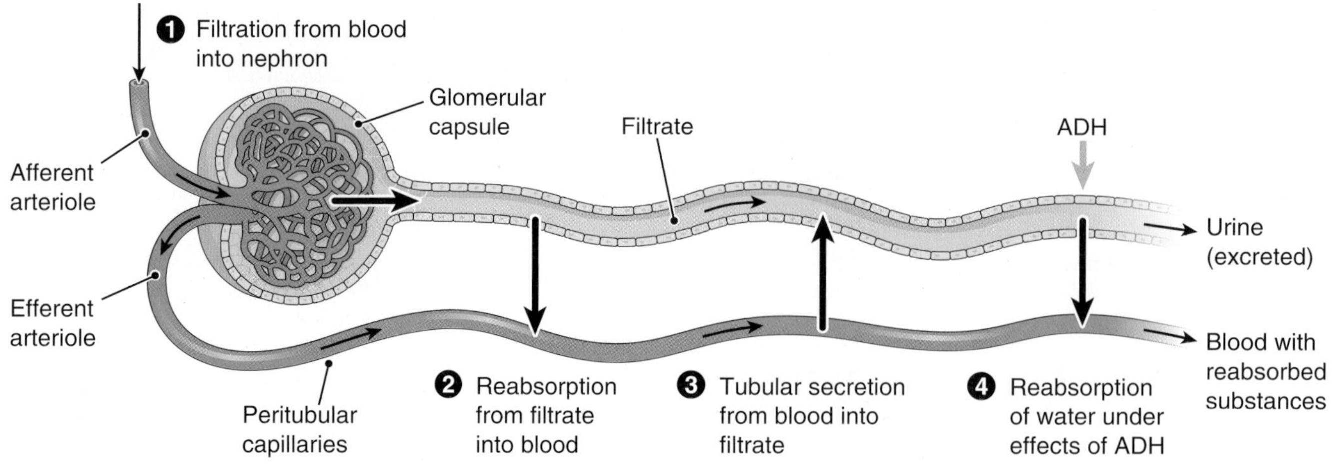

Figure 19-7 **Summary of urine formation in a nephron.** KEY POINT Four processes involved in urine formation are shown. ZOOMING IN What vessels absorb materials that leave the nephron?

nephron's cells, resulting in an increased concentration of the IF deep within the medulla. Because the ascending limb of the loop is not very permeable to water, the filtrate at this point becomes increasingly dilute **(see Fig. 19-6)**. As this dilute filtrate passes through the more permeable collecting duct, the concentrated fluids around the nephron draw water out to be returned to the blood. (Remember, according to the laws of osmosis, water follows salt.) In this manner, the urine becomes more concentrated as it leaves the nephron and its volume is reduced.

Water reabsorption from the collecting duct is influenced by **antidiuretic hormone** (**ADH**), a hormone released from the posterior pituitary gland **(see Table 19-1)**. ADH makes the walls of the collecting duct more permeable to water, so that more water will be reabsorbed and less water will be excreted with the urine. The release of ADH from the posterior pituitary is regulated by a feedback system. As the blood becomes more concentrated, the hypothalamus triggers more ADH release from the posterior pituitary; as the blood becomes more dilute, less ADH is released. In the disease diabetes insipidus, there is inadequate secretion of ADH from the hypothalamus, which results in the elimination of large amounts of dilute urine accompanied by excessive thirst.

Summary of Urine Formation The processes involved in urine formation are summarized below and illustrated in **Figure 19-7**.

1. Glomerular filtration moves water and solutes from the blood into the nephron.
2. Tubular reabsorption moves useful substances back into the blood while keeping waste products in the nephron to be eliminated in the urine.
3. Tubular secretion moves additional substances from the blood into the nephron for elimination. Movement of hydrogen ions is one means by which the pH of body fluids is balanced.
4. The countercurrent mechanism concentrates the urine and reduces the volume excreted. The pituitary hormone ADH allows more water to be reabsorbed from the nephron.

CONTROL OF BLOOD PRESSURE

The kidneys have an internal mechanism for maintaining adequate filtration pressure. A specialized portion of the nephron, the **juxtaglomerular (JG) apparatus**, is involved in this control. The JG apparatus includes cells in the distal tubule, which carries urine from the nephron into the collecting duct, and cells in the afferent arteriole, which carries blood into the glomerulus. As seen in **Figure 19-8**, the first portion of the distal tubule curves backward toward the glomerulus to pass between the afferent and efferent arterioles (*juxtaglomerular* means "near the glomerulus.") At the point where the distal tubule makes contact with the afferent arteriole, there are specialized cells in each that together make up the JG apparatus.

Receptors in the distal tubule respond to low sodium content in the filtrate leaving the nephron. Note that low sodium in the filtrate correlates with low volume. When stimulated, these receptors trigger cells in the afferent arteriole to secrete the enzyme **renin** (RE-nin) **(see Table 19-1)**. This enzyme initiates the process that activates angiotensin, a protein that elevates blood pressure by several mechanisms. It promotes the release of aldosterone and ADH and stimulates thirst, raising blood pressure by increasing blood volume. It also causes vasoconstriction and stimulates heart activity through the sympathetic nervous system. **Box 19-1** has more details on these events and their clinical applications.

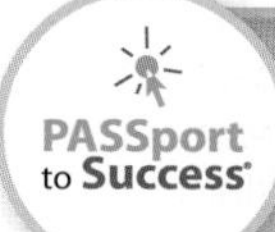

See the student resources on *thePoint* for a flow chart summarizing kidney regulation of blood pressure.

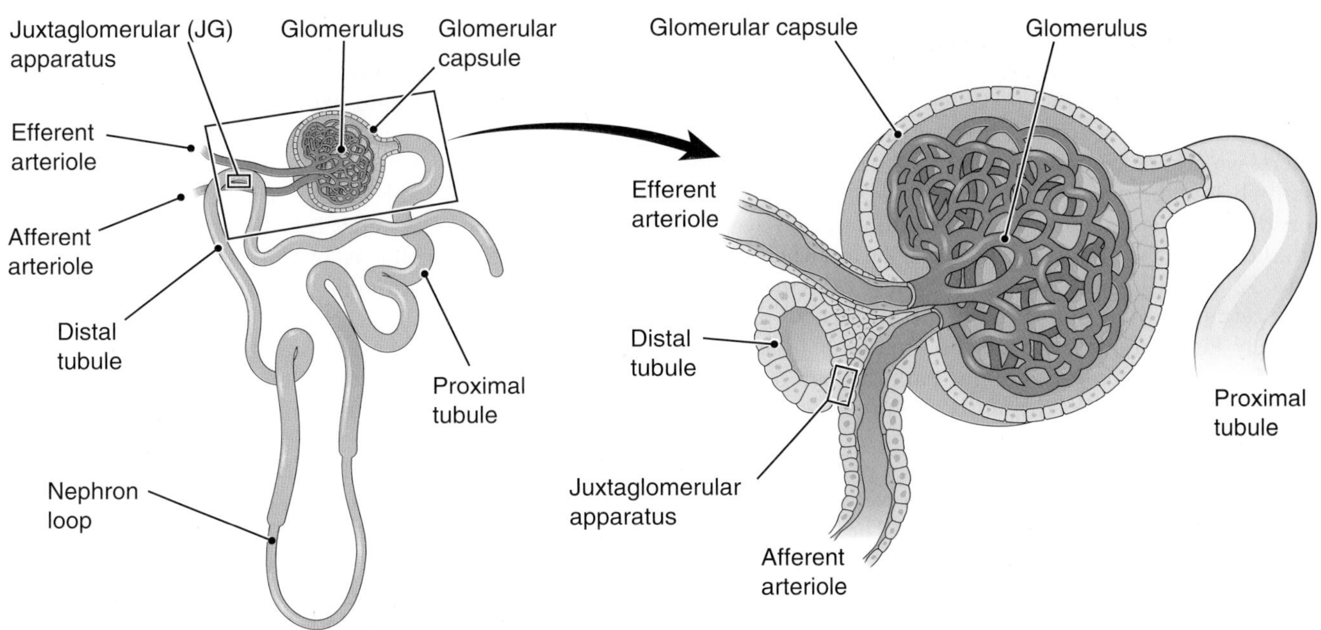

Figure 19-8 **The juxtaglomerular (JG) apparatus.** KEY POINT Note how the distal tubule contacts the afferent arteriole (right). Cells in these two structures make up the JG apparatus, which releases renin to raise blood pressure.

CHECKPOINTS 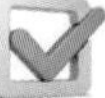

☐ 19-8 What is glomerular filtration?

☐ 19-9 What are the four processes involved in the formation of urine?

☐ 19-10 What substance is produced by the JG apparatus and under what conditions is it produced?

Elimination of Urine

Urine is excreted from the kidneys into the two ureters, which transport urine to the bladder. It is then stored until eliminated from the body via the urethra. Let us take a closer look at each of these organs.

Box 19-1 *A Closer Look*

The Renin-Angiotensin Pathway: The Renal Route to Blood Pressure Control

In addition to forming urine, the kidneys play an integral role in regulating blood pressure. When blood pressure drops, cells of the juxtaglomerular (JG) apparatus secrete the enzyme renin into the blood. Renin acts on another blood protein, **angiotensinogen**, which is manufactured by the liver. Renin converts angiotensinogen into **angiotensin I** by cleaving off some amino acids from the end of the protein. Angiotensin I is then converted into **angiotensin II** by yet another enzyme called angiotensin-converting enzyme (ACE), which is manufactured by capillary endothelium, especially in the lungs. Angiotensin II increases blood pressure in four ways:

1. It increases cardiac output and stimulates vasoconstriction.
2. It stimulates the release of aldosterone, a hormone that acts on the nephron's distal tubule to increase sodium reabsorption, and secondarily, water reabsorption.
3. It stimulates the release of antidiuretic hormone (ADH), which acts directly on the distal tubules and collecting ducts to increase water reabsorption.
4. It stimulates thirst centers in the hypothalamus, resulting in increased fluid consumption.

The combined effects of angiotensin II produce a dramatic increase in blood pressure. In fact, angiotensin II is estimated to be four to eight times more powerful than norepinephrine, another potent stimulator of hypertension, and thus is a good target for blood pressure-controlling drugs. One class of drugs used to treat hypertension is the **ACE inhibitors**, which control blood pressure by blocking the production of angiotensin II.

THE URETERS

Each of the two ureters is a long, slender, muscular tube that extends from the kidney down to and through the inferior portion of the urinary bladder **(see Fig. 19-1)**. The ureters, which are located posterior to the peritoneum and distally below the peritoneum, are entirely extraperitoneal (outside the peritoneum). Their length naturally varies with the size of the individual; they may be anywhere from 25 to 32 cm (10 to 13 in.) long. Nearly 2.5 cm (1 in.) of the terminal distal ureter enters the bladder by passing obliquely (at an angle) through the inferior bladder wall **(Fig. 19-9)**. Because of this oblique path through the wall, a full bladder compresses the ureter and prevents the backflow of urine.

The ureteral wall includes a lining of epithelial cells, a relatively thick layer of involuntary muscle, and finally, an outer coat of fibrous connective tissue. The epithelium is the transitional type, which flattens from a cuboidal shape as the tube stretches. This same type of epithelium lines the renal pelvis, the bladder, and the proximal portion of the urethra. The ureteral muscles are capable of the same rhythmic contraction (peristalsis) that occurs in the digestive system. Urine is moved along the ureter from the kidneys to the bladder by gravity and by peristalsis at frequent intervals.

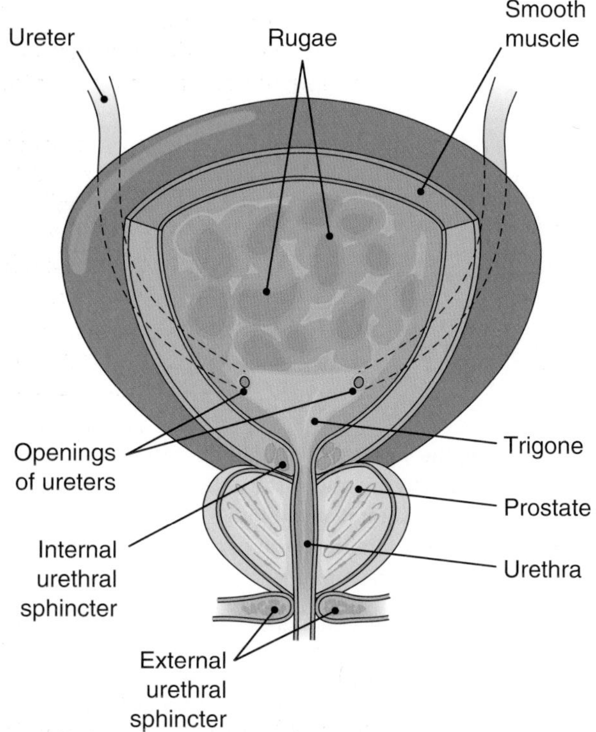

Figure 19-9 The male urinary bladder. KEY POINT The interior of the bladder is folded into rugae. Internal and external sphincters regulate urination. The trigone is a triangular region in the floor of the bladder marked by the openings of the ureters and the urethra. ZOOMING IN What gland does the urethra pass through in the male?

THE URINARY BLADDER

When it is empty, the urinary bladder **(see Fig. 19-9)** is located below the parietal peritoneum and posterior to the pubic symphysis. When filled, it pushes the peritoneum upward and may extend well into the abdominal cavity proper. The urinary bladder is a temporary reservoir for urine, just as the gallbladder is a storage sac for bile.

The bladder wall has many layers. It is lined with mucous membrane containing transitional epithelium. The bladder's lining, like that of the stomach, is thrown into folds called *rugae* when the organ is empty. Beneath the mucosa is a layer of connective tissue, followed by a three-layered coat of involuntary smooth muscle that can stretch considerably. Finally, there is an incomplete coat of peritoneum that covers only the bladder's superior portion.

When the bladder is empty, the muscular wall becomes thick, and the entire organ feels firm. As the bladder fills, the muscular wall becomes thinner, and the organ may increase from a length of 5 cm (2 in.) up to as much as 12.5 cm (5 in.) or even more. A moderately full bladder holds about 470 mL (1 pint) of urine.

The **trigone** (TRI-gone) is a triangular-shaped region in the floor of the bladder. It is marked by the openings of the two ureters and the urethra **(see Fig. 19-9)**. As the bladder fills with urine, it expands upward, leaving the trigone at the base stationary. This stability prevents stretching of the ureteral openings and the possible backflow of urine into the ureters.

THE URETHRA

The **urethra** is the tube that extends from the bladder to the outside **(see Fig. 19-1)** and is the means by which the bladder is emptied. The urethra differs in males and females; in the male, it is part of both the reproductive system and the urinary system, and it is much longer than is the female urethra.

The male urethra is approximately 20 cm (8 in.) in length. Proximally, it passes through the prostate gland, where it is joined by two ducts carrying male reproductive cells (spermatozoa) from the testes and glandular secretions. From here, it leads to the outside through the **penis** (PE-nis), the male organ of copulation. The male urethra serves the dual purpose of draining the bladder and conveying semen with spermatozoa.

The urethra in the female is a thin-walled tube about 4 cm (1.5 in.) long. It is posterior to the pubic symphysis and is embedded in the muscle of the anterior vaginal wall. The external opening, called the **urinary meatus** (me-A-tus), is located just anterior to the vaginal opening between the labia minora. The female urethra drains the bladder only and is entirely separate from the reproductive system.

URINATION

The process of expelling (voiding) urine from the bladder is called **urination** or *micturition* (mik-tu-RISH-un). This process is controlled both voluntarily and involuntarily with the aid of two muscular rings (sphincters) that surround the urethra **(see Fig. 19-9)**. Near the bladder's outlet is an involuntary **internal urethral sphincter** formed by a continuation of the bladder's smooth muscle. Below this muscle is a voluntary **external urethral sphincter** formed by the muscles of the pelvic floor. By learning to control the voluntary sphincter, one can gain control over the bladder's emptying.

As the bladder fills with urine, stretch receptors in its wall send impulses to a center in the lower part of the spinal cord. Motor impulses from this center stimulate contraction of the bladder wall, forcing urine outward as both the internal and external sphincters are made to relax. In the infant, this emptying occurs automatically as a simple reflex. Early in life, a child learns to control urination from higher centers in the brain until an appropriate time, a process known as *toilet training*. The impulse to urinate will override conscious controls if the bladder becomes too full.

The bladder can be emptied voluntarily by relaxing the muscles of the pelvic floor and increasing the pressure in the abdomen. The resulting increased pressure in the bladder triggers the spinal reflex that leads to urination.

THE URINE

Urine is a yellowish liquid that is approximately 95% water and 5% dissolved solids and gases. The pH of freshly collected urine averages 6.0, with a range of 4.5 to 8.0. Diet may cause considerable variation in pH as well as color and odor. For example, some people's urine takes on an unusual odor when they eat asparagus.

The amount of dissolved substances in urine is indicated by its **specific gravity**. The specific gravity of pure water, used as a standard, is 1.000. Because of the dissolved materials it contains, urine has a specific gravity that normally varies from 1.002 (very dilute urine) to 1.040 (very concentrated urine). When the kidneys are diseased, they lose the ability to concentrate urine, and the specific gravity no longer varies as it does when the kidneys function normally.

Normal Constituents of Urine Some of the dissolved substances normally found in the urine are the following:

- **Nitrogenous waste products**, including the following:
  - urea, formed from amine groups released in protein catabolism
  - uric acid from the breakdown of purines, which are found in some foods and nucleic acids
  - creatinine (kre-AT-ih-nin), a breakdown product of muscle creatine
- **Electrolytes**, including sodium chloride (as in common table salt) and different kinds of sulfates and phosphates. Electrolytes are excreted in appropriate amounts to keep their blood concentration constant.
- **Pigment**, Urochrome, a yellow substance derived from the breakdown of hemoglobin, is the main pigment in urine. Small amount of bilirubin and other bile pigments are also found in normal urine. Beets and other dark foods can add color, as can B vitamins, vitamin C and food dyes. Also certain drugs can cause color to appear in the urine.

CHECKPOINTS

- ☐ **19-11** What is the name of the tube that carries urine from the kidney to the bladder?
- ☐ **19-12** What openings form the bladder's trigone?
- ☐ **19-13** What is the name of the tube that carries urine from the bladder to the outside?
- ☐ **19-14** What are some normal constituents of urine?

The Effects of Aging on the Urinary System

Even without renal disease, aging causes the kidneys to lose some of their ability to concentrate urine. With aging, progressively more water is needed to excrete the same amount of waste. Older people find it necessary to drink more water than young people, and they eliminate larger amounts of urine (polyuria), even at night (nocturia).

Beginning at about 40 years of age, there is a decrease in the number and size of the nephrons. Often, more than half of them are lost before the age of 80 years. There may be an increase in blood urea nitrogen (BUN) without serious symptoms. Elderly people are more susceptible than young people to urinary system infections. Childbearing may cause damage to the pelvic floor musculature, resulting in urinary tract problems in later years.

Enlargement of the prostate, common in older men, may cause obstruction and back pressure in the ureters and kidneys **(see Fig. 19-1)**. If this condition is untreated, it will cause permanent damage to the kidneys. Adam, in the case study, is confronted with this problem. Changes with age, including decreased bladder capacity and decreased muscle tone in the bladder and urinary sphincters, may predispose to incontinence. However, most elderly people (60% in nursing homes, and up to 85% living independently) have no incontinence.

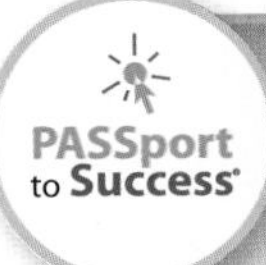

See the student resources on *thePoint* for information about a career as a hemodialysis technician who treats patients who have defective kidney function.

Body Fluids

Water is important to living cells as a solvent, a transport medium, and a participant in metabolic reactions. The force of water in the vessels helps to maintain blood pressure, which is important for maintaining blood flow and capillary exchange. The normal proportion of body water varies from 50% to 70% of a person's weight. It is highest in the young and in thin, muscular individuals. As the amount of fat increases, the percentage of water in the body decreases, because adipose tissue holds

19

very little water compared with muscle tissue. In infants, water makes up 75% of the total body mass. That's why infants are in greater danger from dehydration than adults.

REGULATION OF BODY FLUIDS

Various electrolytes (salts), nutrients, gases, waste, and special substances, such as enzymes and hormones, are dissolved or suspended in body water. The composition of body fluids is an important factor in homeostasis. Whenever the volume or chemical makeup of these fluids deviates even slightly from normal, disease results. The constancy of body fluids is maintained in the following ways:

- The thirst mechanism helps maintain a constant fluid volume by adjusting water intake.
- Kidney activity helps keep water volume and electrolytes constant by adjusting urine output.
- Hormones control thirst and kidney activity.
- Buffers, respiration, and kidney function regulate body fluid pH (acidity and alkalinity).

The maintenance of proper fluid balance involves many of the principles discussed in earlier chapters, such as pH and buffers; the effects of respiration on pH; tonicity of solutions; and forces influencing capillary exchange. Some of these chapters are referenced in the following sections.

FLUID COMPARTMENTS

Although body fluids have much in common no matter where they are located, there are some important differences between fluid inside and outside cells. Accordingly, fluids are grouped into two main compartments (Fig. 19-10):

- **Intracellular fluid** (ICF) is contained within the cells. About two-thirds to three-fourths of all body fluids are in this category.
- **Extracellular fluid** (ECF) includes all body fluids outside of cells. In this group are the following:
    - **Interstitial** (in-ter-STISH-al) **fluid**, or more simply, tissue fluid. This fluid is located in the spaces between the cells in tissues throughout the body. It is estimated that tissue fluid constitutes about 15% of body weight.
    - **Blood plasma**, which constitutes about 4% of body weight.
    - **Lymph**, the fluid that drains from the tissues into the lymphatic system. This is about 1% of body weight.
    - **Fluid in special compartments**, such as cerebrospinal fluid, the aqueous and vitreous humors of the eye, serous fluid, and synovial fluid. Together, these make up about 1% to 3% of total body fluids.

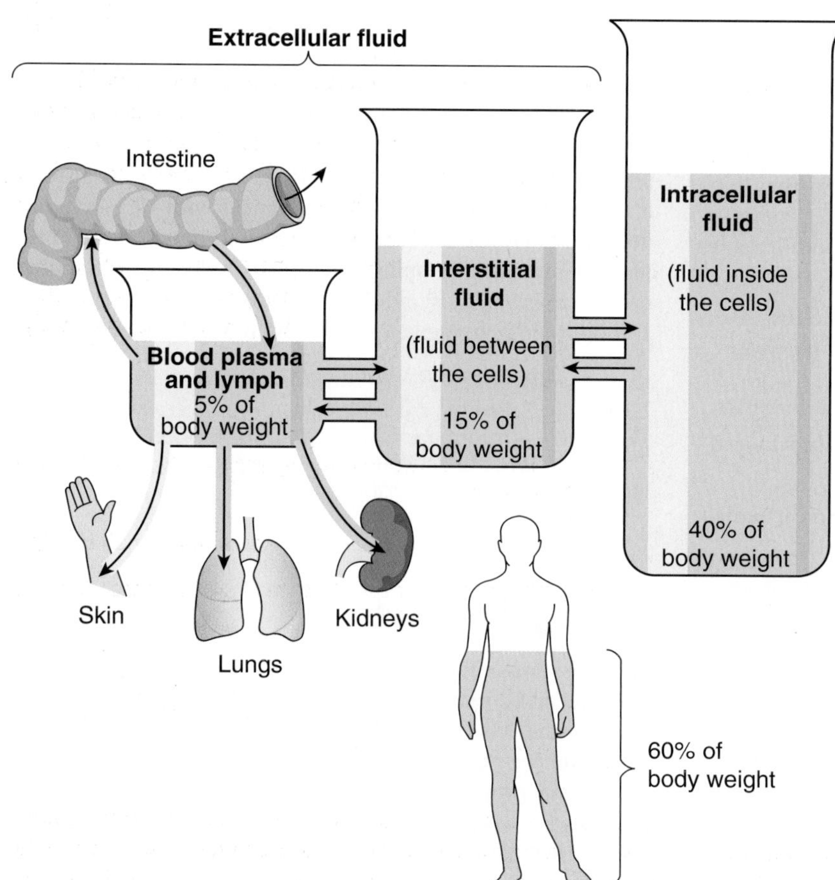

Figure 19-10 Main fluid compartments showing relative percentage by weight of body fluid. KEY POINT Fluid percentages vary but total about 60% of body weight. Fluids are constantly exchanged among compartments, and each day fluids are lost and replaced. ZOOMING IN What are some avenues through which water is lost?

Fluids are not locked into one compartment. There is a constant interchange between compartments as fluids are transferred between blood and interstitial fluid and between interstitial fluid and intracellular fluid (see Fig. 19-10). Also, fluids are lost and replaced on a daily basis.

WATER BALANCE

In a healthy person, the quantity of water gained in a day is approximately equal to the quantity lost (output) (Fig. 19-11). The quantity of water consumed in a day (intake) varies considerably among individuals, and is typically increased in hot weather; however, the average adult in a comfortable environment takes in about 2,300 mL of water (about 2½ quarts) daily. About two-thirds of this quantity comes from drinking water and other beverages; about one-third comes from foods, such as fruits, vegetables, and soups. About 200 mL of water is produced each day as a by-product of cellular respiration. This water, described as *metabolic water*, brings the total average gain to 2,500 mL each day.

The same volume of water is constantly being lost from the body by the following routes:

- The **kidneys** excrete the largest quantity of water lost each day. About 1 to 1.5 L of water are eliminated daily in the urine.
- The **skin**. Although sebum and keratin help prevent dehydration, water is constantly evaporating from the skin's surface. Larger amounts of water are lost from the skin as sweat when it is necessary to cool the body.
- The **lungs** expel water along with carbon dioxide.
- The **intestinal tract** eliminates water along with the feces.

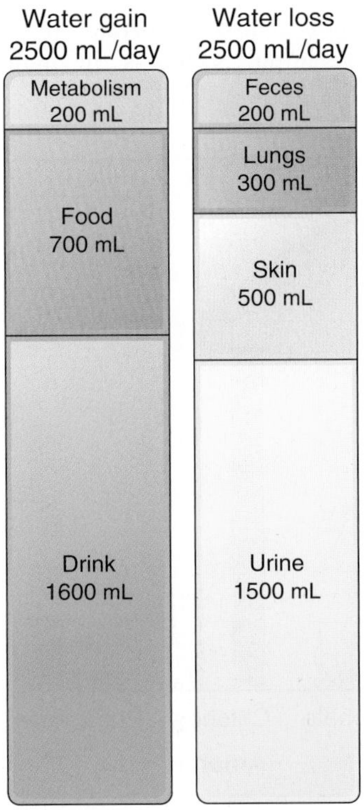

In many disorders, it is important for the health care team to know whether a patient's intake and output are equal; in such a case, a 24-hour intake–output record is kept. The intake record includes *all* the liquid the patient has taken in. This means fluids administered intravenously as well as those consumed by mouth. The health care provider must account for water, other beverages, and liquid foods, such as soup and ice cream. The output record includes the quantity of urine excreted in the same 24-hour period as well as an estimation of fluid losses due to fever, vomiting, diarrhea, bleeding, wound discharge, or other causes.

Water gain 2500 mL/day
Metabolism 200 mL
Food 700 mL
Drink 1600 mL

Water loss 2500 mL/day
Feces 200 mL
Lungs 300 mL
Skin 500 mL
Urine 1500 mL

Figure 19-11 Daily gain and loss of water. KEY POINT In a healthy person, water gained in a day is approximately equal to the quantity lost. ZOOMING IN In what way is the most water lost in a day?

SENSE OF THIRST

As you can see by studying Figure 19-11, it is essential to take in enough fluid each day to replace physiologic losses. Our thirst mechanism prompts us to drink water. The control center for the sense of thirst is located in the brain's hypothalamus. This center plays a major role in the regulation of total fluid volume. A decrease in fluid volume or an increase in the concentration of body fluids stimulates the thirst center, causing a person to drink water or other fluids containing large amounts of water. Dryness of the mouth also causes a sensation of thirst. Excessive thirst, such as that caused by excessive urine loss in cases of diabetes, is called **polydipsia** (pol-e-DIP-se-ah). (See Box 19-2 on receptors involved in water balance.)

The thirst center should stimulate enough drinking to balance fluids, but this is not always the case. During vigorous exercise, especially in hot weather, the body can dehydrate rapidly, and people may not drink enough to replace needed fluids. In addition, if plain water is consumed, the dilution of body fluids may depress the thirst center. Athletes who are exercising very strenuously may need to drink beverages with some carbohydrates for energy and also some electrolytes to keep fluids in balance. Margaret, in the case study, will have to be careful about maintaining her fluid balance.

CHECKPOINTS 

☐ 19-15 What are the two main compartments into which body fluids are grouped?

☐ 19-16 What are the four routes for water loss from the body?

☐ 19-17 Where is the control center for the sense of thirst located?

Electrolytes and Their Functions

Electrolytes are important constituents of body fluids. These compounds separate into positively and negatively charged ions in solution. Positively charged ions are

Box 19-2 A Closer Look

Osmoreceptors: Thinking about Thirst

Osmoreceptors are specialized neurons that help to maintain water balance by detecting changes in the concentration of extracellular fluid (ECF). They are located in the hypothalamus of the brain in an area adjacent to the third ventricle, where they monitor the osmotic pressure (concentration) of the circulating blood plasma.

Osmoreceptors respond primarily to small increases in sodium, the most common cation in ECF. As the blood becomes more concentrated, sodium draws water out of the cells, initiating nerve impulses. Traveling to different regions of the hypothalamus, these impulses may have two different but related effects:

- They stimulate the hypothalamus to produce antidiuretic hormone (ADH), which is then released from the posterior pituitary. ADH travels to the kidneys and causes these organs to conserve water.
- They stimulate the thirst center of the hypothalamus, causing increased consumption of water. Almost as soon as water consumption begins, however, the sensation of thirst disappears. Receptors in the throat and stomach send inhibitory signals to the thirst center, preventing overconsumption of water and allowing time for ADH to affect the kidneys.

Both of these mechanisms serve to dilute the blood and other body fluids. Both are needed to maintain optimal water balance. If either fails, a person soon becomes dehydrated.

called **cations;** negatively charged ions are called **anions.** Electrolytes are so named because they conduct an electric current in solution.

MAJOR IONS

A few of the most important cations and anions are reviewed next. **Figure 19-12** shows the distribution of common electrolytes in the different fluid compartments.

- Cations (positive ions):
  - > **Sodium** is chiefly responsible for maintaining osmotic balance and body fluid volume. It is the main positive ion in extracellular fluids. Sodium is required for nerve impulse conduction and is important in maintaining acid–base balance.
  - > **Potassium** is also important in the transmission of nerve impulses and is the major positive ion

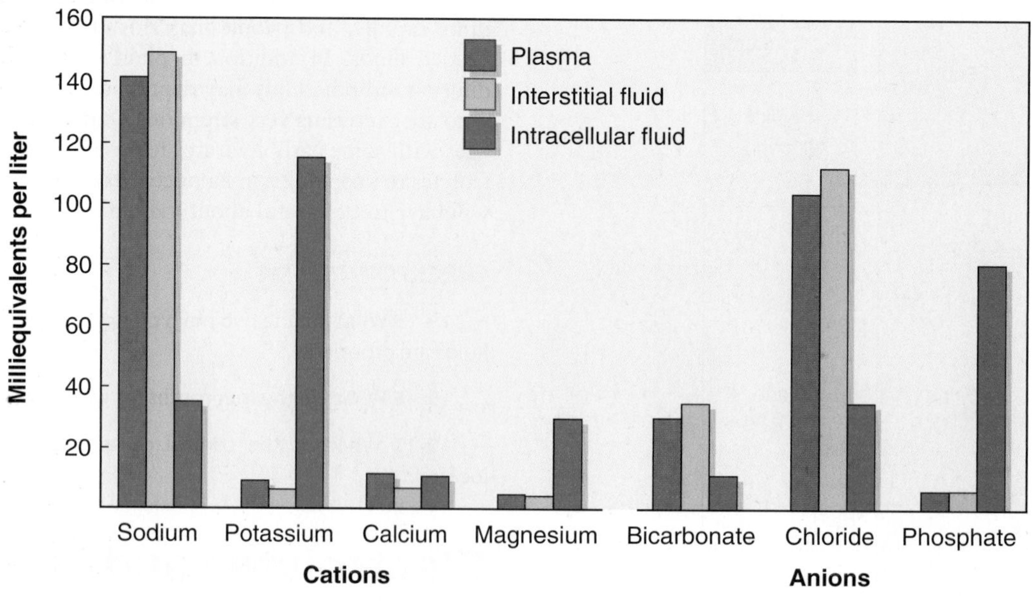

Figure 19-12 Distribution of some major ions in intracellular and extracellular fluids. KEY POINT Ion distribution varies in the different fluid compartments. Plasma and interstitial fluid are extracellular fluids. Ions are measured in milliequivalents (mEq), a unit based on atomic weight and valence. ZOOMING IN What ions are highest in extracellular fluids? In intracellular fluids? (Reprinted with permission from Taylor CR, Lillis C. *Fundamentals of Nursing*, 6th ed. Philadelphia, PA: Lippincott Williams & Wilkins, 2008.)

in ICF. Potassium is involved in enzymatic activities, and it helps regulate the chemical reactions by which carbohydrate is converted to energy and amino acids are converted to protein.

  - **Calcium** is required for bone formation, muscle contraction, nerve impulse transmission, and blood clotting.
  - **Magnesium** is necessary for muscle contraction and for the action of some enzymes.

- Anions (negative ions):
  - **Bicarbonate** is an important buffer in body fluids.
  - **Chloride** is essential for the formation of hydrochloric acid in the stomach. It also helps to regulate fluid balance and pH. It is the most abundant anion in extracellular fluids.
  - **Phosphate** is essential in carbohydrate metabolism, bone formation, and acid–base balance. Phosphates are found in plasma membranes, nucleic acids (DNA and RNA), and ATP.

ELECTROLYTE BALANCE

The body must keep electrolytes in the proper concentration in both intracellular and extracellular fluids. The maintenance of water and electrolyte balance is one of the most difficult problems for health providers in caring for patients. Although some electrolytes are lost in the feces and through the skin as sweat, the job of balancing electrolytes is left mainly to the kidneys.

Several hormones are involved in balancing electrolytes (see Chapter 11). Aldosterone, produced by the adrenal cortex, promotes the reabsorption of sodium (and thus, water) and the elimination of potassium. In Addison disease, in which the adrenal cortex does not produce enough aldosterone, there is a loss of sodium and water and an excess of potassium.

When the blood concentration of sodium rises above the normal range, the pituitary secretes more antidiuretic hormone (ADH). This hormone increases water reabsorption in the kidney to dilute the excess sodium.

The most recently discovered hormone active in electrolyte regulation comes from the heart. Atrial natriuretic peptide (ANP) is secreted by specialized atrial myocardial cells when blood pressure rises too high. ANP causes the kidneys to excrete sodium and water, thus decreasing blood volume and lowering blood pressure. The name comes from *natrium*, the Latin name for sodium, and the adjective for *uresis*, which refers to urination.

Parathyroid hormone increases blood calcium levels by causing the bones to release calcium and the kidneys to reabsorb calcium. Vitamin D (the hormone calcitriol), once it is activated in the liver and kidneys, increases intestinal absorption of calcium.

CHECKPOINTS 

☐ 19-18 What is the main cation in extracellular fluid? In intracellular fluid?

☐ 19-19 What is the main anion in extracellular fluid?

☐ 19-20 What are some mechanisms for regulating electrolytes in body fluids?

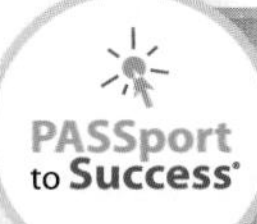

See the student resources on *thePoint* for a summary chart of hormones and electrolyte balance.

Acid–Base Balance

The pH scale is a measure of how acidic or basic (alkaline) a solution is. As described in Chapter 2, the pH scale measures the hydrogen ion (H^+) concentration in a solution. Body fluids are slightly alkaline, with a pH range of 7.35 to 7.45. These fluids must be kept within a narrow pH range, or damage, even death, will result. A shift in either direction by three-tenths of a point on the pH scale, to 7.0 or 7.7, is fatal.

REGULATION OF pH

The body constantly produces acids in the course of metabolism. Catabolism of fats yields fatty acids and ketones; anaerobic metabolism during intense exercise generates hydrogen ions; carbon dioxide dissolves in the blood and yields carbonic acid (see Chapter 16). Conversely, a few abnormal conditions may cause alkaline shifts in pH. Several systems act together to counteract these changes and maintain acid–base balance:

- **Buffer systems**. Buffers are substances that prevent sharp changes in hydrogen ion (H^+) concentration and thus maintain a relatively constant pH. Buffers work by accepting or releasing these ions as needed to keep the pH steady. The main buffer systems in the body are bicarbonate buffers, phosphate buffers, and proteins, such as hemoglobin in red blood cells and plasma proteins.
- **Respiration**. The role of respiration in controlling pH was described in Chapter 16. Recall that carbon dioxide release from the lungs makes the blood more alkaline by reducing the amount of carbonic acid formed. In contrast, carbon dioxide retention makes the blood more acidic. Respiratory rate can adjust pH for short-term regulation.
- **Kidney function**. The kidneys regulate pH by reabsorbing or eliminating hydrogen ions as needed. The kidneys are responsible for long-term pH regulation. The activity of the kidneys was described earlier in this chapter.

CHECKPOINTS 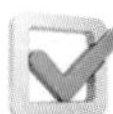

☐ 19-21 What are three mechanisms for maintaining the acid–base balance of body fluids?

A&P in Action Revisited

Adam Has Prostate Surgery to Prevent Kidney Damage

The urologist inserted the cystoscope into Adam's urethra, carefully guiding it toward the urinary bladder. When he examined the bladder's mucous membrane lining, he did not see any urinary stones or tumors of the rugae. He did note that the neck of Adam's urinary bladder was occluded by his enlarged prostate. This observation fitted with the results of the pyelogram (a special radiograph of the urinary system) he had ordered for Adam a week earlier. The x-ray images indicated a blockage in the neck of the urinary bladder, which prevented urine from exiting. The back pressure of the urine was causing distention of the ureters (hydroureter) and kidneys (hydronephrosis). The doctor removed the cystoscope and reported his findings to his patient. "Adam, Dr. Michaels' diagnosis was correct. The blockage in your urinary system is due to enlargement of your prostate gland. If we don't treat this now, your kidneys are at risk of severe damage and renal failure. I suggest we do a procedure called a *transurethral prostatectomy* to remove the prostatic overgrowth and reestablish urine flow."

A few days later, Adam was back at the hospital for his surgery. The urologist inserted an instrument called a resectoscope into Adam's urethra. With the electrical loop at the end of the instrument, he removed pieces of the prostate and cauterized blood vessels to control bleeding. By the end of the surgery, the urologist had resected enough of the prostate to restore normal urine flow. It would take Adam a few weeks to recover, but soon he would be back to normal.

During this case, we saw that enlargement of the prostate gland can seriously affect urinary system function. To learn more about the prostate gland and other organs of the male reproductive system, see Chapter 20.

Chapter Wrap-Up

Summary Overview

A detailed chapter outline with space for note-taking is on *thePoint*. The figure below illustrates the main topics covered in this chapter.

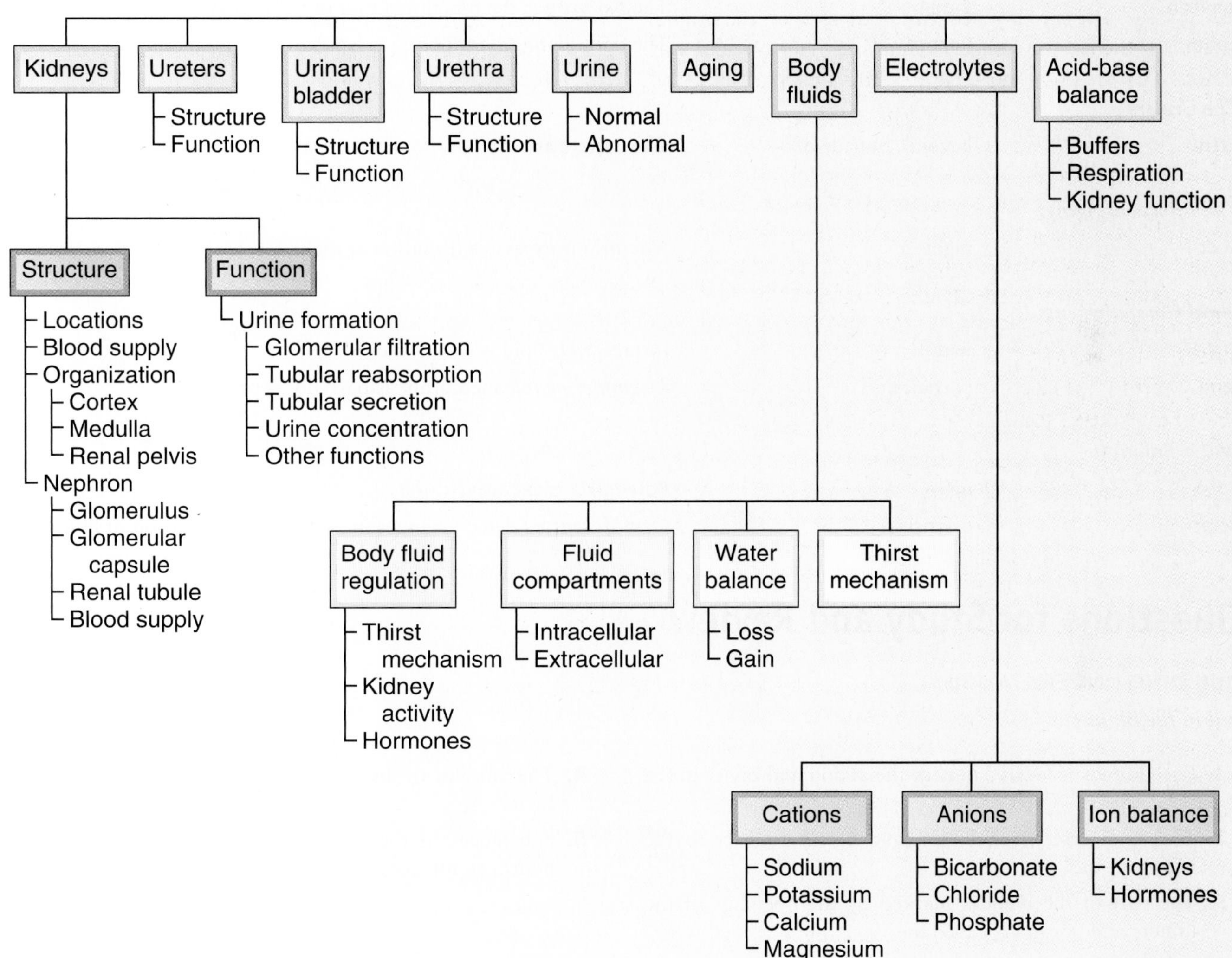

Key Terms

The terms listed below are emphasized in this chapter. Knowing them will help you organize and prioritize your learning. These and other boldface terms are defined in the Glossary with phonetic pronunciations.

angiotensin
anion
antidiuretic hormone (ADH)
buffer
calculi
cation
erythropoietin
excretion
extracellular
glomerular filtrate
glomerulus
interstitial
intracellular
kidney
micturition
nephron
pH
reabsorption
renin
urea
ureter
urethra
urinalysis
urinary bladder
urine

Word Anatomy

Scientific terms are built from standardized word parts (prefixes, roots, and suffixes). Learning the meanings of these parts can help you remember words and interpret unfamiliar terms.

WORD PART	MEANING	EXAMPLE
The Kidneys		
retro-	backward, behind	The *retroperitoneal* space is posterior to the peritoneal cavity.
ren/o	kidney	The *renal* artery carries blood to the kidney.
nephr/o	kidney	The *nephron* is the functional unit of the kidney.
juxta-	next to	The *juxtaglomerular* apparatus is next to the glomerulus.
The Ureters		
extra-	beyond, outside of	The ureters are *extraperitoneal.*
The Effects of Aging		
noct/i	night	*Nocturia* is excessive urination at night.
Fluid Compartments		
intra-	within	*Intracellular* fluid is within a cell.
semi-	partial, half	A *semipermeable* membrane is partially permeable.
Water Balance		
poly-	many	*Polydipsia* is excessive thirst.
osmo-	osmosis	*Osmoreceptors* detect changes in osmotic concentration of fluids.

Questions for Study and Review

BUILDING UNDERSTANDING

Fill in the Blanks

1. Each kidney is located outside the abdominal cavity in the _____ space.
2. The renal artery, renal vein, and ureter connect to the kidney at the _____.
3. The part of the bladder marked by the openings of the ureters and urethra is called the _____.
4. The amount of dissolved substances in urine is indicated by its _____.
5. Substances in the blood that prevent sharp changes in hydrogen ion concentration are called _____.

Matching > Match each numbered item with the most closely related lettered item.

_____ **6.** Produced by the kidney in response to low blood pressure

_____ **7.** Stimulates vasoconstriction

_____ **8.** Produced by the kidney in response to hypoxia

_____ **9.** Stimulates kidneys to produce concentrated urine

_____ **10.** Produced by the liver during protein catabolism

a. urea

b. erythropoietin

c. antidiuretic hormone

d. renin

e. angiotensin

Multiple Choice

___ **11.** What is the functional unit of the renal system?

a. renal capsule
b. kidney
c. nephron
d. juxtaglomerular apparatus

___ **12.** Where is the nephron loop located?

a. cortex
b. medulla
c. pelvis
d. calyx

___ **13.** How does fluid move out of the glomerulus?

a. filtration
b. diffusion
c. osmosis
d. active transport

___ **14.** Voluntary control of which structure is responsible for the ability to delay urination?

a. trigone
b. internal urethral sphincter
c. external urethral sphincter
d. urinary meatus

___ **15.** What is the fluid located in the spaces between cells called?

a. cytoplasm
b. plasma
c. interstitial fluid
d. lymph

UNDERSTANDING CONCEPTS

16. List four organ systems active in excretion. What are the products eliminated by each?

17. Compare and contrast the following terms:

a. glomerular capsule and glomerulus
b. afferent and efferent arteriole
c. proximal and distal tubule
d. ureter and urethra

18. Trace the pathway of a urea molecule from the afferent arteriole to the urinary meatus.

19. Describe the four processes involved in the formation of urine.

20. Compare the male urethra and female urethra in structure and function.

21. List some of the dissolved substances normally found in urine.

22. Explain the role of the hypothalamus in water balance.

23. How do the respiratory and renal systems regulate pH?

CONCEPTUAL THINKING

24. A class of antihypertensive drugs called loop diuretics prevents sodium reabsorption in the nephron loop. How could a drug like this lower blood pressure?

25. In Adam's second case study, enlargement of the prostate gland led to hydronephrosis. What effect might this have on glomerular filtration?

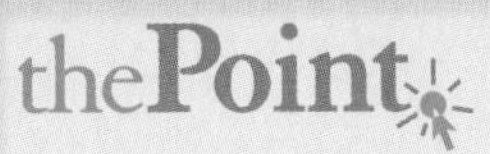

For more questions, see the learning activities on *thePoint*.

UNIT VI

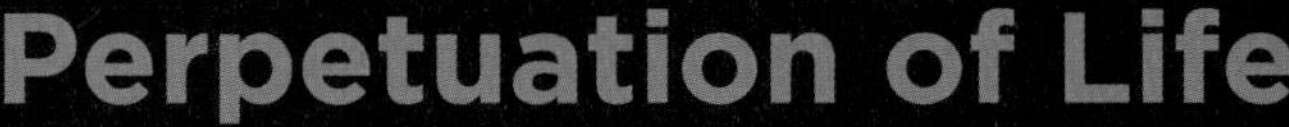

Perpetuation of Life

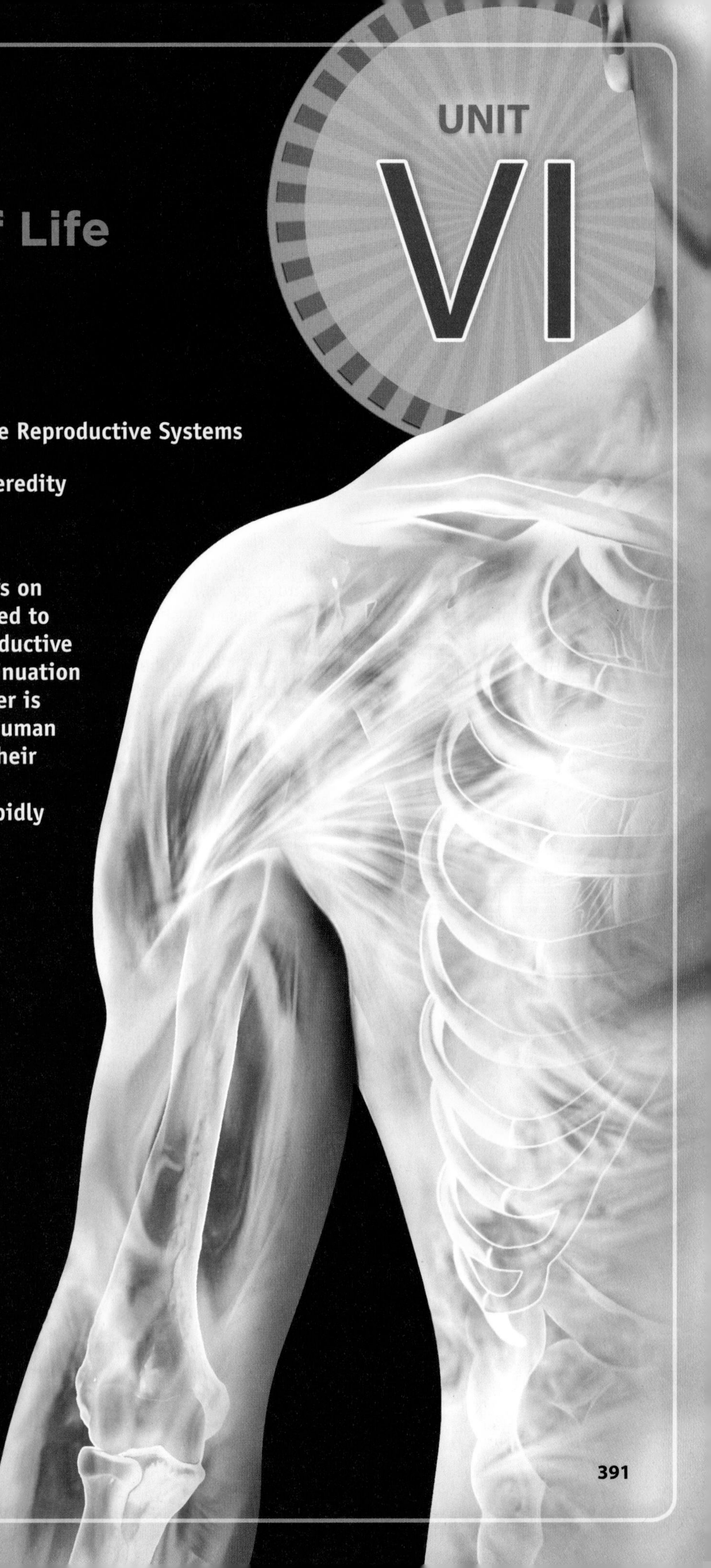

The final unit includes two chapters on the structures and functions related to reproduction and heredity. The reproductive system is not necessary for the continuation of the life of the individual but rather is needed for the continuation of the human species. The reproductive cells and their genes have been studied intensively during recent years as part of the rapidly advancing science of genetics.

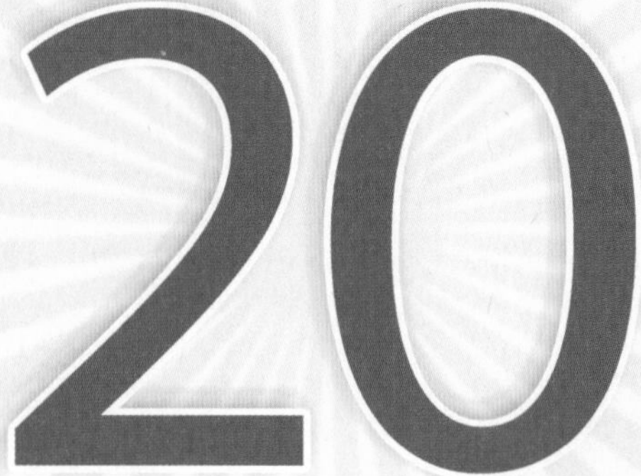

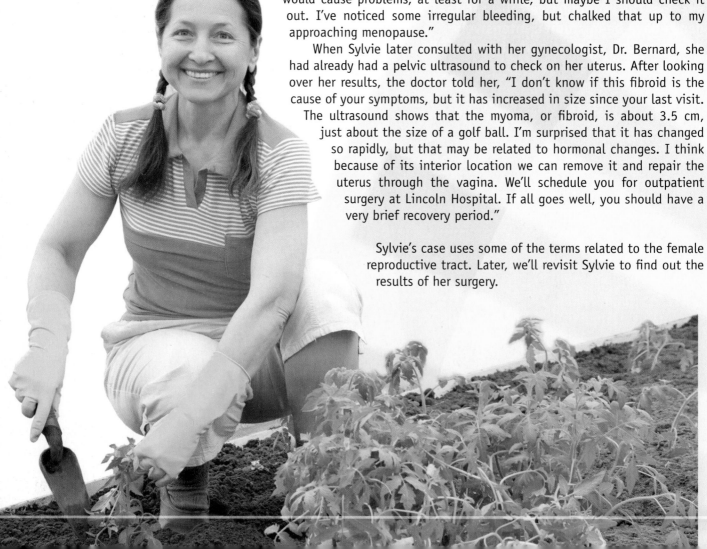

CHAPTER 20

The Male and Female Reproductive Systems

A&P in Action

Sylvie's Case: Removal of a Benign Uterine Tumor

"Ooh," Sylvie complained to her husband as she came into the house from gardening. "I know it's unusually hot this summer, but I'm having a hard time gardening this year for some reason. I feel a pull in my hip and groin and some discomfort in my belly. Maybe I've pulled a muscle; I should make an appointment for a massage and maybe talk to the trainers at the gym about getting some exercises to stretch out my hip muscles." "Maybe you should make an appointment with your gynecologist," Jon suggested. "Remember when you went for your annual exam he said he wanted to watch something?" "Right," Sylvie replied, "he said something about a small, benign tumor in my uterus. A fibroid, I think he called it. He didn't think it would cause problems, at least for a while, but maybe I should check it out. I've noticed some irregular bleeding, but chalked that up to my approaching menopause."

When Sylvie later consulted with her gynecologist, Dr. Bernard, she had already had a pelvic ultrasound to check on her uterus. After looking over her results, the doctor told her, "I don't know if this fibroid is the cause of your symptoms, but it has increased in size since your last visit. The ultrasound shows that the myoma, or fibroid, is about 3.5 cm, just about the size of a golf ball. I'm surprised that it has changed so rapidly, but that may be related to hormonal changes. I think because of its interior location we can remove it and repair the uterus through the vagina. We'll schedule you for outpatient surgery at Lincoln Hospital. If all goes well, you should have a very brief recovery period."

Sylvie's case uses some of the terms related to the female reproductive tract. Later, we'll revisit Sylvie to find out the results of her surgery.

PASSport to Success

Ancillaries At-A-Glance

Visit *thePoint* to access the PASSport to Success and the following resources. For guidance in using these resources most effectively, see pp. ix–xviii.

Learning TOOLS

- Learning Style Self-Assessment
- Live Advise Online Student Tutoring
- Tips for Effective Studying

Learning RESOURCES

- E-book: Chapter 20
- Web Chart: Reproductive Hormones
- Animation: Ovulation and Fertilization
- Health Professions: Physician Assistant
- Detailed Chapter Outline
- Answers to Questions for Study and Review
- Audio Pronunciation Glossary

Learning ACTIVITIES

- Pre-Quiz
- Visual Activities
- Kinesthetic Activities
- Auditory Activities

Learning Outcomes

After careful study of this chapter, you should be able to:

1 Identify the male and female gametes and state the purpose of meiosis, ***p. 394***

2 Name the gonads and accessory organs of the male reproductive system and cite the function of each, ***p. 394***

3 Describe the composition and function of semen, ***p. 397***

4 Draw and label a spermatozoon, ***p. 396***

5 Identify the two hormones that regulate the production and development of the male gametes, ***p. 398***

6 Name the gonads and accessory organs of the female reproductive system and cite the function of each, ***p. 399***

7 List in the correct order the hormones produced during the menstrual cycle and cite the source of each, ***p. 402***

8 Describe the changes that occur during and after menopause, ***p. 403***

9 Cite the main methods of birth control in use, ***p. 403***

10 Referring to the case study, discuss some procedures used to diagnose and treat uterine disorders, ***pp. 392, 407***

11 Show how word parts are used to build words related to the reproductive systems (see Word Anatomy at the end of the chapter), ***p. 409***

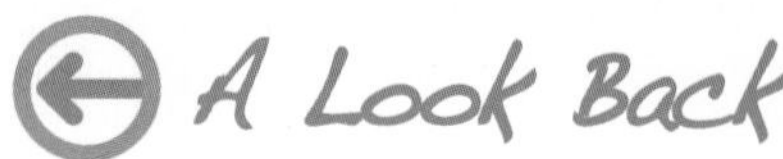

In this chapter we return once again to the concept of negative feedback in describing how this mechanism controls reproductive activities in males and females. We also provide more details on the production and action of the sex hormones, first introduced in Chapter 11.

The chapters in this unit deal with what is certainly one of the most interesting and mysterious attributes of life: the ability to reproduce. The simplest forms of life, one-celled organisms, usually need no partner to reproduce; they simply divide by themselves. This form of reproduction is known as **asexual** (nonsexual) reproduction.

In most animals, however, reproduction is **sexual**, meaning that there are two kinds of individuals, males and females, each of which has specialized cells designed specifically for the perpetuation of the species. These specialized sex cells are known as **gametes** (GAM-etes), or *germ cells*. In the male, they are called **spermatozoa** (sper-mah-to-ZO-ah; sing., spermatozoon) or simply sperm cells; in the female, they are called **ova** (O-vah; sing., ovum), or eggs.

Gametes are characterized by having half as many chromosomes as are found in any other body cell. During their formation, they go through a special process of cell division, called **meiosis** (mi-O-sis), which halves the number of chromosomes (see Fig. 21-1). In humans, meiosis reduces the chromosome number in a cell from 46 to 23. The role of meiosis in reproduction is explained in more detail in Chapter 21.

The male and female reproductive systems each include two groups of organs, primary and accessory:

- The primary organs are the **gonads** (GO-nads), or sex glands; they produce the gametes and manufacture hormones. The male gonad is the testis and the female gonad is the ovary, as explained shortly.
- The **accessory organs** include a series of ducts that transport the gametes as well as various exocrine glands.

The Male Reproductive System

The gonads and accessory organs of the male reproductive system are shown in Figure 20-1. (See Figure A3-9 in the Dissection Atlas for a photograph of the male reproductive system.)

THE TESTES

The male gonads, the paired **testes** (TES-teze; sing., testis), are located outside of the body proper, suspended between the thighs in a sac called the **scrotum** (SKRO-tum). The testes are oval organs measuring approximately 4.0 cm (1.5 in.) in length and approximately 2.5 cm (1 in.) in each of the other two dimensions. During embryonic life, each testis develops from tissue near the kidney.

A month or two before birth, the testis normally descends (moves downward) through the **inguinal** (ING-gwih-nal) **canal** in the abdominal wall into the scrotum (Fig. 20-2). There, the testis is suspended by a **spermatic cord** that extends through the inguinal canal (see Fig. 20-1). This cord contains blood vessels, lymphatic vessels, nerves, and the tube (ductus deferens) that transports spermatozoa away from the testis. The gland must descend completely if it is to function normally; to produce spermatozoa, the testis must be kept at the temperature of the scrotum, which is several degrees lower than that of the abdominal cavity.

Internal Structure Most of the specialized tissue of the testis consists of tiny coiled **seminiferous** (seh-mih-NIF-er-us) **tubules** (see Fig. 20-1B). Primitive cells in the walls of these tubules develop into mature spermatozoa, aided by neighboring cells called **sustentacular** (sus-ten-TAK-u-lar) (Sertoli) **cells**. These so-called "nurse cells" nourish and protect the developing spermatozoa. They also secrete a protein that binds testosterone in the seminiferous tubules.

Specialized **interstitial** (in-ter-STISH-al) **cells** that secrete the male sex hormone **testosterone** (tes-TOS-teh-rone) are located between the seminiferous tubules. An older name for these cells is *Leydig* (LI-dig) *cells*. Figure 20-3 is a microscopic view of the testis in cross section, showing the seminiferous tubules, interstitial cells, and developing spermatozoa.

Testosterone From the testis, testosterone diffuses into surrounding fluids and is then absorbed into the bloodstream. This hormone has three functions:

- Development and maintenance of the reproductive structures
- Development of spermatozoa
- Development of **secondary sex characteristics**, traits that characterize males and females but are not directly concerned with reproduction. In males, these traits include a deeper voice, broader shoulders, narrower hips, a greater percentage of muscle tissue, and more body hair than are found in females.

The Spermatozoa Spermatozoa are tiny individual cells illustrated in Figure 20-4. They are so small that at least 200 million are contained in the average ejaculation (release of semen). After puberty, sperm cells are manufactured continuously in the testes' seminiferous tubules.

The spermatozoon has an oval head that is mostly a nucleus containing chromosomes. The **acrosome** (AK-ro-some), which covers the head like a cap, contains enzymes that help the sperm cell to penetrate the ovum.

Whiplike movements of the tail (flagellum) propel the sperm through the female reproductive tract to the ovum. The cell's middle region (midpiece) contains many mitochondria that provide energy for movement.

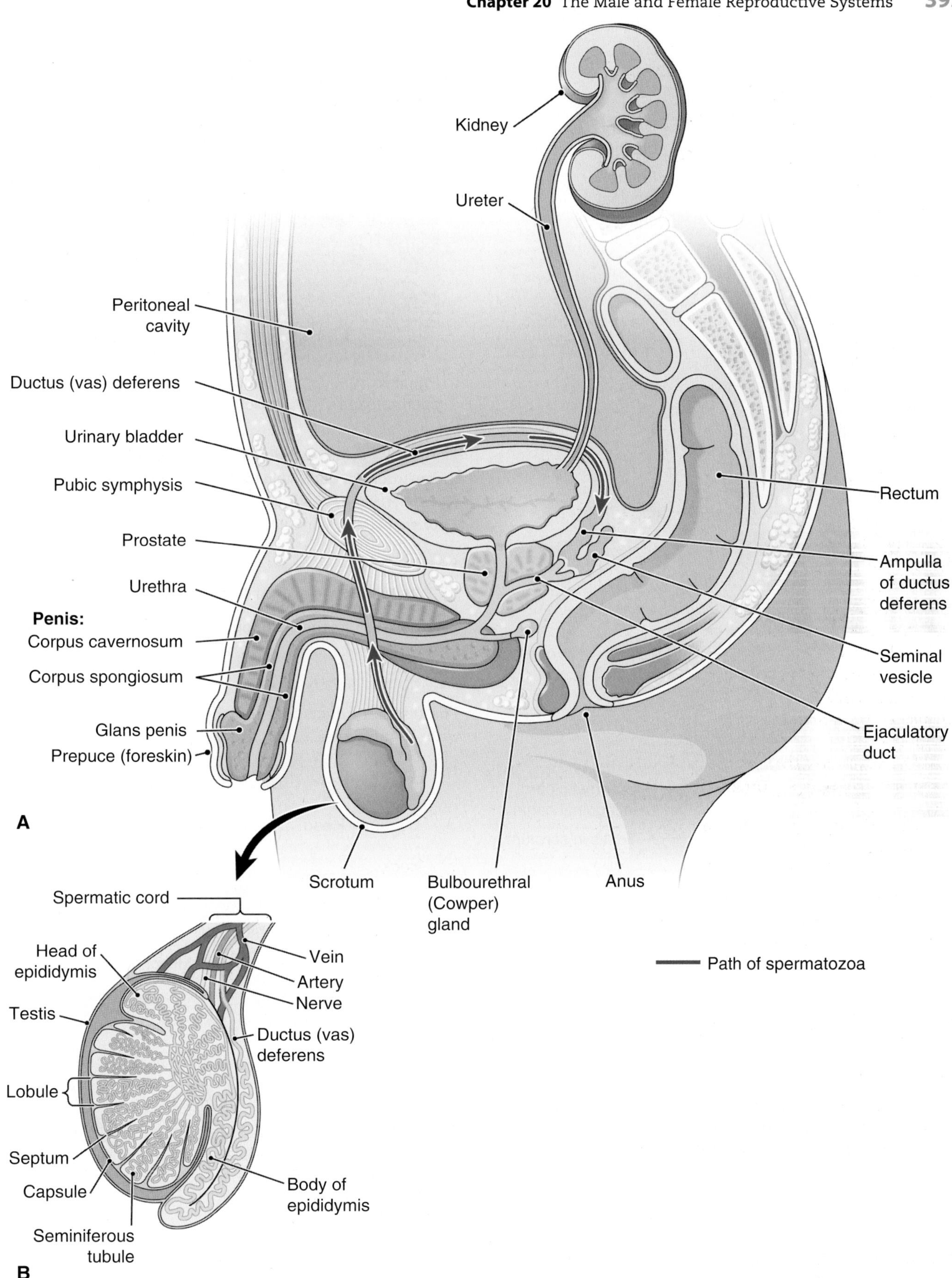

Figure 20-1 **Male reproductive system. A.** The internal and external portions of the male reproductive system are shown along with the urinary system. **B.** Structure of the testis also showing the epididymis and spermatic cord. ZOOMING IN What four glands empty secretions into the urethra? What duct receives secretions from the epididymis?

20

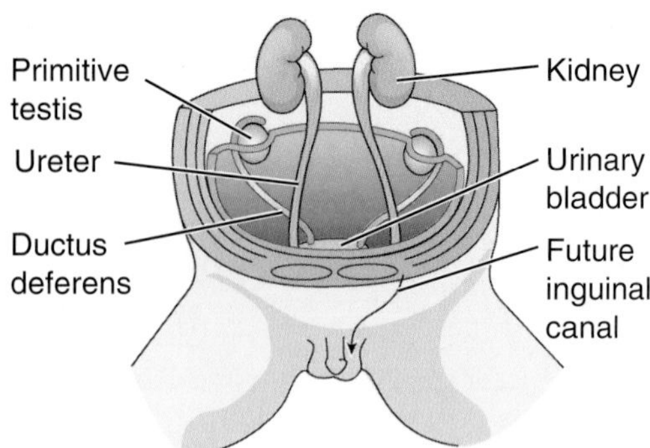

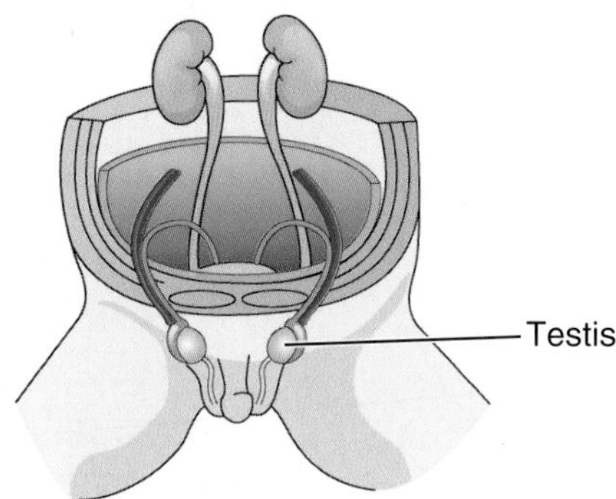

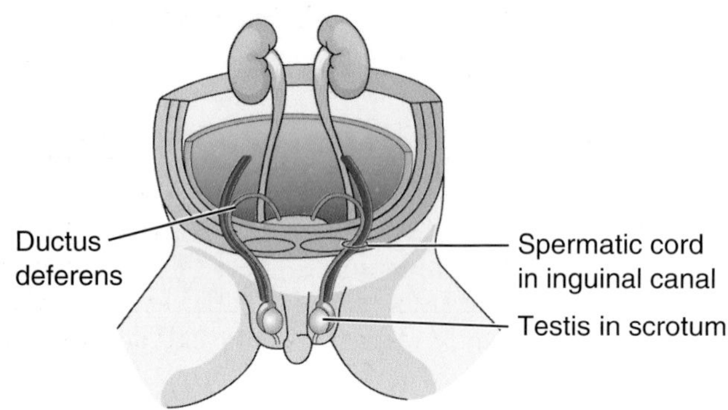

Figure 20-2 **Descent of the testes.** KEY POINT During fetal development the testis moves down the inguinal canal into the scrotum. Drawings show formation of the inguinal canals and descent of the testes at three different times during fetal development. **A.** At 7 weeks, the testis is in the dorsal abdominal wall. **B.** At 7 months, the testis is passing through the inguinal canal. **C.** At 9 months, the testis is in the scrotum, suspended by the spermatic cord. (Reprinted with permission from Cohen BJ. *Medical Terminology*, 6th ed. Philadelphia, PA: Lippincott Williams & Wilkins, 2011.)

CHECKPOINTS 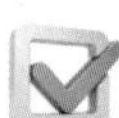

☐ 20-1 What is the process of cell division that halves the chromosome number in a cell to produce a gamete?

☐ 20-2 What is the male gamete called?

☐ 20-3 What is the male gonad?

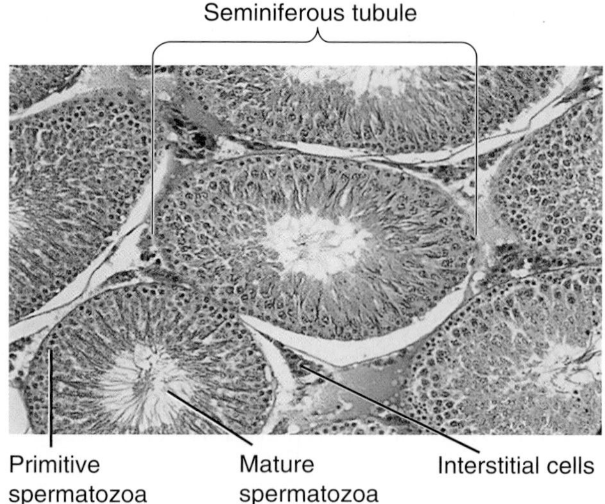

Figure 20-3 **Microscopic view of the testis.** KEY POINT Spermatozoa develop within the testis' seminiferous tubules. ZOOMING IN Where are the interstitial cells located? (Courtesy of Dana Morse Bittus and BJ Cohen.)

☐ 20-4 What is the main male sex hormone?

☐ 20-5 What are the main subdivisions of a spermatozoon?

ACCESSORY ORGANS

The system of ducts that transports the spermatozoa begins with tubules inside the testis itself. From these tubules,

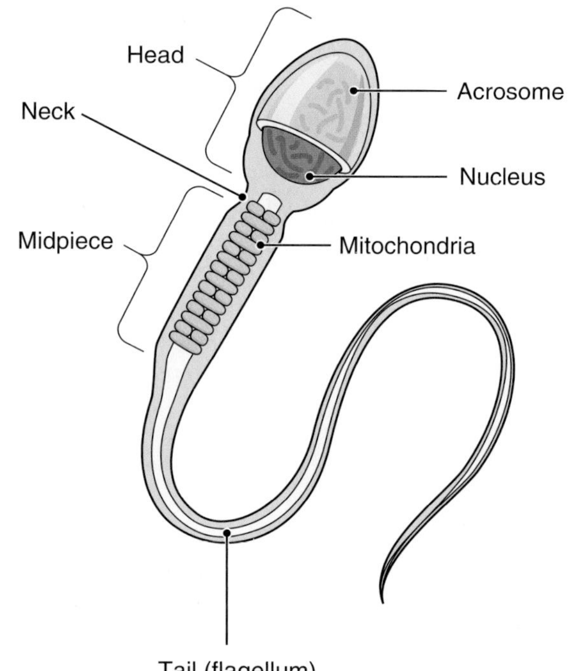

Figure 20-4 **Human spermatozoon.** The diagram shows major structural features of the male gamete. ZOOMING IN What organelles provide energy for sperm cell motility?

the cells collect in a greatly coiled tube called the **epididymis** (ep-ih-DID-ih-mis), which is 6 m (20 ft) long and is located on the surface of the testis inside the scrotal sac **(see Fig. 20-1)**. While they are temporarily stored in the epididymis, the sperm cells mature and become motile, able to move or "swim" by themselves.

The epididymis finally extends upward as the **ductus deferens** (DEF-er-enz), also called the *vas deferens*. This tube, contained in the spermatic cord, continues through the inguinal canal into the abdominal cavity. Here, it separates from the remainder of the spermatic cord and curves behind the urinary bladder. The ductus deferens then joins with the duct of the **seminal vesicle** (VES-ih-kl) on the same side to form the **ejaculatory** (e-JAK-u-lah-to-re) **duct**. The right and left ejaculatory ducts travel through the body of the prostate gland and then empty into the urethra.

SEMEN

Semen (SE-men) (meaning "seed") is the mixture of sperm cells and various secretions that is expelled from the body. It is a sticky fluid with a milky appearance. The pH is in the alkaline range of 7.2 to 7.8. The secretions in semen serve several functions:

- Nourish the spermatozoa
- Transport the spermatozoa
- Neutralize the acidity of the male urethra and the female vaginal tract
- Lubricate the reproductive tract during sexual intercourse
- Prevent infection by means of antibacterial enzymes and antibodies

The glands discussed next contribute secretions to the semen **(see Fig. 20-1)**.

The Seminal Vesicles The seminal vesicles are twisted muscular tubes with many small outpouchings. They are approximately 7.5 cm (3 in.) long and are attached to the connective tissue at the posterior of the urinary bladder. The glandular lining produces a thick, yellow, alkaline secretion containing large quantities of simple sugar and other substances that provide nourishment for the spermatozoa. The seminal fluid makes up a large part of the semen's volume.

The Prostate Gland The **prostate gland** lies immediately inferior to the urinary bladder, where it surrounds the first part of the urethra. Ducts from the prostate carry its secretions into the urethra. The thin, alkaline prostatic secretion helps neutralize vaginal acidity and enhance the spermatozoa's motility. The prostate gland is also supplied with muscular tissue, which, upon signals from the nervous system, contracts to aid in the expulsion of the semen from the body.

Bulbourethral Glands The **bulbourethral** (bul-bo-u-RE-thral) **glands**, also called *Cowper glands*, are a pair of pea-sized organs located in the pelvic floor just inferior to the prostate gland. They secrete mucus to lubricate the urethra and tip of the penis during sexual stimulation. The ducts of these glands extend approximately 2.5 cm (1 in.) from each side and empty into the urethra before it extends into the penis.

Other very small glands secrete mucus into the urethra as it passes through the penis.

THE URETHRA AND PENIS

The male urethra, as discussed in Chapter 19, serves the dual purpose of conveying urine from the bladder and semen from the ejaculatory duct to the outside. Semen ejection is made possible by **erection**, the stiffening and enlargement of the penis, through which the major portion of the urethra extends. The penis is made of spongy tissue containing many blood spaces that are relatively empty when the organ is flaccid but that fill with blood and distend when the penis is erect. This tissue is subdivided into three segments, each called a **corpus** (body) **(Fig. 20-5)**. A single, ventrally located **corpus spongiosum** contains the urethra. On either side is a larger **corpus cavernosum** (pl., corpora cavernosa). At the distal end of the penis, the corpus spongiosum enlarges to form the **glans penis**, which is covered with a loose fold of skin, the **prepuce** (PRE-puse), commonly called the *foreskin*. It is the end of the foreskin that is removed in a **circumcision** (sir-kum-SIZH-un), a surgery frequently performed on male infants for religious or cultural reasons. Experts disagree on the medical value of circumcision with regard to improved cleanliness and disease prevention.

The penis and scrotum together make up the male **external genitalia** (jen-ih-TA-le-ah).

Ejaculation (e-jak-u-LA-shun) is the forceful expulsion of semen through the urethra to the outside. The process is initiated by reflex centers in the spinal cord that stimulate smooth muscle contraction in the prostate. This is followed by contraction of skeletal muscle in the pelvic floor, which provides the force needed for expulsion. During ejaculation, the involuntary sphincter at the base of the bladder closes to prevent the release of urine.

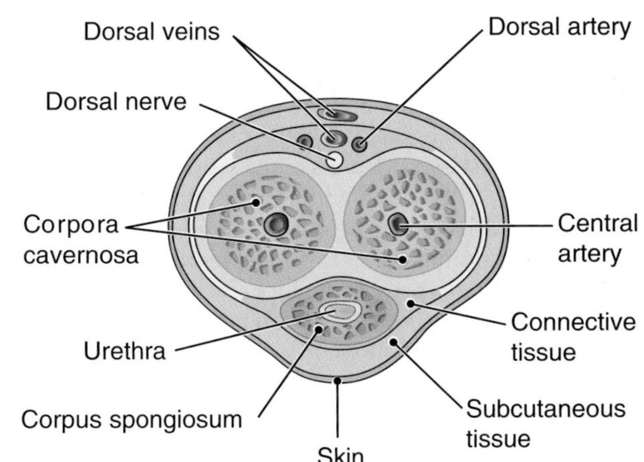

Figure 20-5 Cross-section of the penis. The subdivisions of the penis are shown along with associated vessels and nerve. **ZOOMING IN** What subdivision of the penis contains the urethra?

20

A male typically ejaculates 2 to 5 mL of semen containing 50 to 150 million sperm cells per mL. Out of the millions of spermatozoa in an ejaculation, only one, if any, can fertilize an ovum. The remainder of the cells live from only a few hours up to a maximum of 5 to 7 days.

CHECKPOINTS 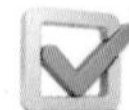

20-6 What is the order in which sperm cells travel through the ducts of the male reproductive system?

20-7 What glands, aside from the testis, contribute secretions to semen?

Hormonal Control of Male Reproduction

The activities of the testes are under the control of two hormones produced by the anterior pituitary. These hormones are named for their activity in female reproduction (described later), although they are chemically the same in both males and females.

- **Follicle-stimulating hormone** (**FSH**) stimulates the sustentacular cells and promotes the formation of spermatozoa.
- **Luteinizing hormone** (**LH**) stimulates the interstitial cells between the seminiferous tubules to produce testosterone, which is also needed for sperm cell development.

Starting at puberty, the hypothalamus begins to secrete a hormone that triggers the release of FSH and LH. These hormones are secreted continuously in the male.

The activity of the hypothalamus is in turn regulated by a negative feedback mechanism involving testosterone. As the blood level of testosterone increases, the hypothalamus secretes less releasing hormone; as the level of testosterone decreases, the hypothalamus secretes more releasing hormone (see Figure 11-3 in Chapter 11).

CHECKPOINT 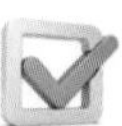

20-8 What two pituitary hormones regulate both male and female reproduction?

The Effects of Aging on Male Reproduction

A gradual decrease in the production of testosterone and spermatozoa begins as early as 20 years of age and continues throughout life. Secretions from the prostate and seminal vesicles decrease in amount and become less viscous. In a few men (less than 10%), sperm cells remain late in life, even to 80 years of age.

Erectile dysfunction may affect men at any age, but commonly increases with age. It is defined as an inability to attain or maintain an erection adequate to engage in sexual intercourse. Box 20-1 has more information on the causes and treatments of this disorder.

Box 20-1 Clinical Perspectives

Treating Erectile Dysfunction

Approximately 25 million American men and their partners are affected by **erectile dysfunction** (ED), the inability to achieve or sustain an erection long enough to have satisfying sexual intercourse. Although ED is more common in men over the age of 65, it can occur at any age and can have many causes. Until recently, ED was believed to be caused by psychological factors, such as stress or depression. It is now known that many cases of ED are caused by physical factors, including cardiovascular disease, diabetes, spinal cord injury, and damage to penile nerves during prostate surgery. Antidepressant and antihypertensive medications also can produce erectile dysfunction.

Erection results from interaction between the autonomic nervous system and penile blood vessels. Sexual arousal stimulates parasympathetic nerves in the penis to release a compound called nitric oxide (NO), which activates the vascular smooth muscle enzyme guanylyl cyclase. This enzyme catalyzes production of cyclic GMP (cGMP), a potent vasodilator that increases blood flow into the penis to cause erection. Physical factors that cause ED prevent these physiologic occurrences.

Until recently, treatment options for ED, such as penile injections, vacuum pumps, and insertion of medications into the penile urethra, were inadequate, inconvenient, and painful. Today, drugs that target the physiologic mechanisms that underlie erection are giving men who suffer from ED new hope. The best known of these is sildenafil (Viagra), which works by inhibiting the enzyme that breaks down cGMP, thus prolonging the effects of NO. Because of its short duration of action, Viagra must be taken shortly before sexual intercourse. Other drugs, such as tadalafil (Cialis) can be taken once daily, removing the need to plan the timing of sexual activity.

Although effective in about 80% of all ED cases, Viagra can cause some relatively minor side effects, including headache, nasal congestion, stomach upset, and blue-tinged vision. Viagra should never be used by men who are taking nitrate drugs to treat angina. Because nitrate drugs elevate NO levels, taking them with Viagra, a drug that prolongs the effects of NO, can cause life-threatening hypotension.

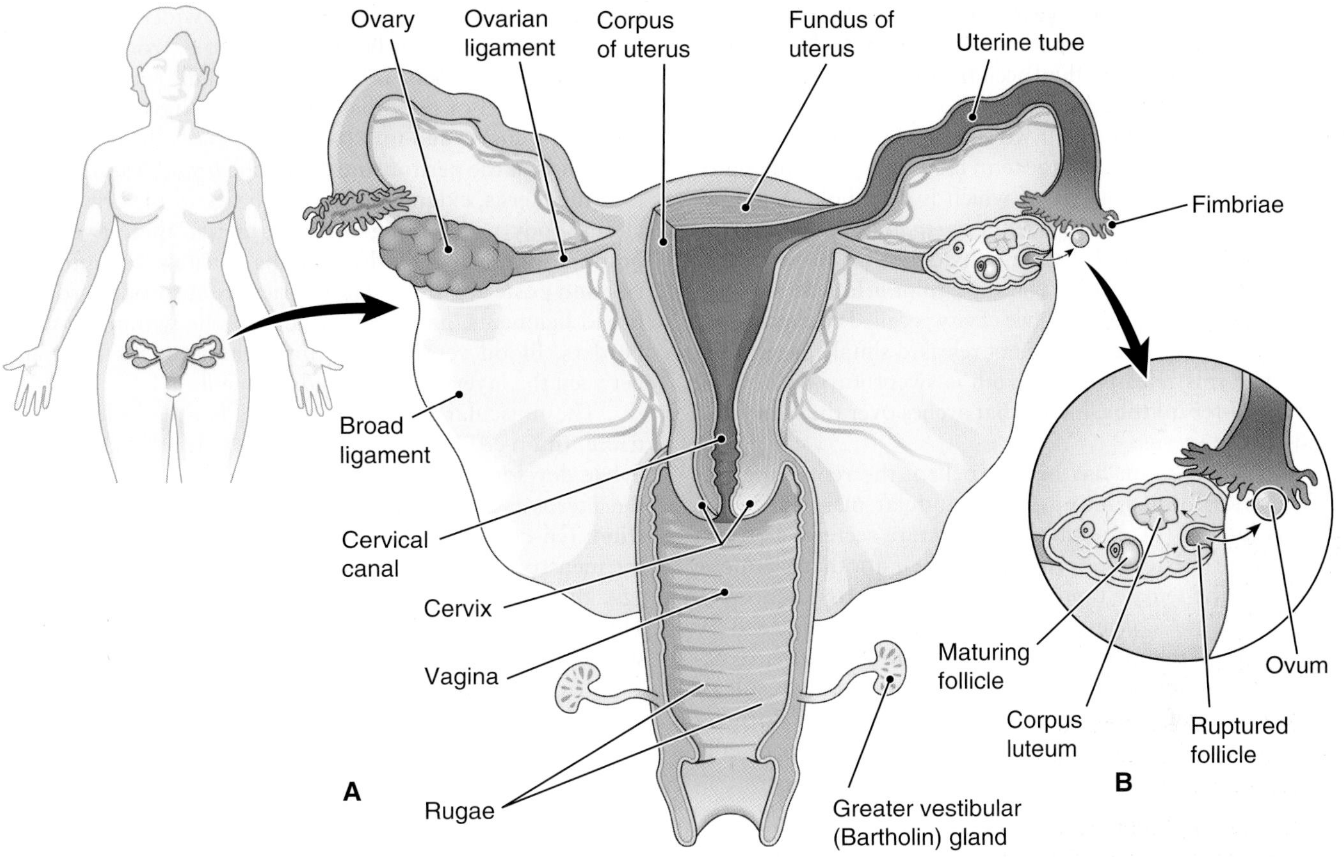

Figure 20-6 **Female reproductive system. A.** The internal portions of the female reproductive system and two of the ligaments that hold the organs in place. **B.** Stages in development of an ovarian follicle (*arrows*) and ovulation with release of the ovum from a mature follicle followed by the empty follicle's formation into the corpus luteum. ZOOMING IN What is the deepest part of the uterus called? The most inferior portion?

Benign enlargement of the prostate commonly occurs with age. This condition, known as benign prostatic hyperplasia (BPH), results from the continuous slow growth of prostate cells throughout life. As noted in Chapter 19, an enlarged prostate can put pressure on the urethra and interfere with urination. If untreated, the back pressure from retained urine can destroy kidney tissue and lead to urinary stasis in the bladder, increasing susceptibility to infection.

The Female Reproductive System

The female gonads are the paired **ovaries** (O-vah-reze), where the female gametes, or ova, are formed **(Fig. 20-6)**. The remainder of the female reproductive tract consists of an organ (uterus) to hold and nourish a developing infant, various passageways, and the external genital organs. (See **Figure A3-10** in the Dissection Atlas for a photograph of the female reproductive system.)

THE OVARIES, OVA, AND OVULATION

The ovary is a small, somewhat flattened oval body measuring approximately 4 cm (1.6 in.) in length, 2 cm (0.8 in.) in width, and 1 cm (0.4 in.) in depth. Like the testes, the ovaries descend, but only as far as the pelvic cavity. Here, they are held in place by ligaments, including the broad ligament, the ovarian ligament, and others, that attach them to the uterus and the body wall.

The outer layer of each ovary is made of a single layer of epithelium. The ova are produced beneath this layer. The ovaries of a newborn female contain more than a million potential ova. At puberty, a few hundred thousand remain.

Each ovum is contained within a small cluster of cells called an **ovarian follicle** (o-VA-re-an FOL-ih-kl) **(Fig. 20-7)**.

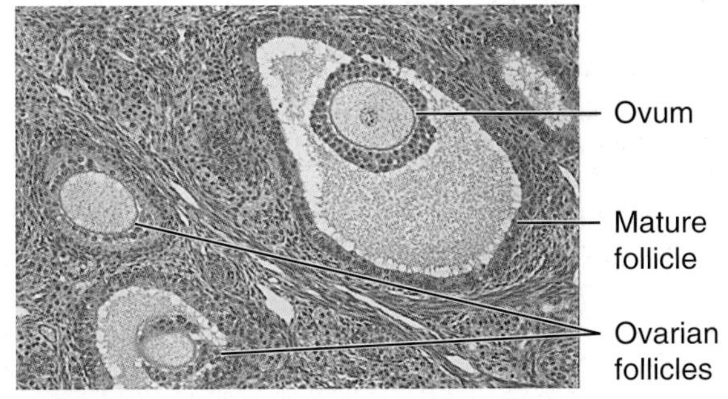

Figure 20-7 **Microscopic view of the ovary.** KEY POINT The photomicrograph shows ovarian follicles in different stages of maturation. (Courtesy of Dana Morse Bittus and BJ Cohen.)

During the reproductive years, several follicles ripen each month, but usually only one releases its ovum. As a follicle matures, it enlarges and fluid accumulates in its central cavity. During this process, cells in its wall secrete the ovarian hormone **estrogen** (ES-tro-jen), which stimulates growth of the uterine lining. (*Estrogen* is the term used for a group of related hormones, the most active of which is estradiol.) A mature ovarian follicle, formerly called a *graafian* (GRAF-e-an) *follicle,* may rupture and discharge its ovum from the ovary's surface (see Fig. 20-6B). The rupture of a follicle allowing an ovum's escape into the pelvic cavity is called **ovulation** (ov-u-LA-shun). Any ova that are not released simply degenerate.

After it is released, the ovum is swept into the nearest **uterine** (U-ter-in) **tube**, a tube that arches over the ovary and leads to the uterus.

After the ovum has been expelled, the remaining follicle is transformed into a solid glandular mass called the **corpus luteum** (LU-te-um). This structure secretes estrogen and also **progesterone** (pro-JES-ter-one), another hormone needed in the female reproductive cycle (discussed shortly). Commonly, the corpus luteum shrinks and is replaced by scar tissue. When a pregnancy occurs, however, this structure remains active for a while. Sometimes, as a result of normal ovulation, the corpus luteum persists and forms a small ovarian cyst (fluid-filled sac). This condition usually resolves without treatment.

ACCESSORY ORGANS

The accessory organs in the female are the uterine tubes, the uterus, the vagina, the greater vestibular glands, and the vulva and perineum.

The Uterine Tubes As we have noted, the tubes that transport the ova from the ovaries to the uterus are called uterine tubes. They are also known as *oviducts* (O-vih-duks) or *fallopian* (fah-LO-pe-an) *tubes.* Each is a small, muscular structure, nearly 12.5 cm (5 in.) long, extending from a point near the ovary to the uterus (womb). There is no direct connection between the ovary and uterine tube. Instead, following ovulation, the ovum is swept into the uterine tube by a current in the peritoneal fluid produced by the small, fringelike extensions called **fimbriae** (FIM-bre-e) that are located at the edge of the tube's opening into the pelvic cavity (see Fig. 20-6).

Unlike the sperm cell, the ovum cannot move by itself. Its progress through the uterine tube toward the uterus depends on the sweeping action of cilia in the tube's lining and on peristalsis of the tube. It takes about 5 days for an ovum to reach the uterus from the ovary.

The Uterus The uterine tubes lead to the **uterus** (U-ter-us), the organ in which a fetus develops to maturity. The uterus is a pear-shaped, muscular organ approximately 7.5 cm (3 in.) long, 5 cm (2 in.) wide, and 2.5 cm (1 in.) deep. (The organ is typically larger in women who have borne children and smaller in postmenopausal women.) The uterus' superior portion rests on the upper surface of the urinary bladder; the inferior portion is embedded in the pelvic floor between the bladder and the rectum. Its wider upper region is called the **corpus**, or body; the lower, narrower region is the **cervix** (SER-viks), or neck. The small, rounded region above the level of the tubal entrances is known as the **fundus** (FUN-dus) (see Fig. 20-6).

Folds of the peritoneum called the *broad ligaments* support the uterus, extending from each side of the organ to the lateral body wall. Along with the uterus, these two membranes form a partition dividing the female pelvis into anterior and posterior areas. The ovaries are suspended from the broad ligaments, and the uterine tubes lie within the upper borders. Blood vessels that supply these organs are found between the layers of the broad ligament.

The muscular wall of the uterus is called the **myometrium** (mi-o-ME-tre-um) (Fig. 20-8). In the case study, Sylvie develops a benign tumor in this layer. The lining of the uterus is a specialized epithelium known as **endometrium** (en-do-ME-tre-um). This inner layer changes during the menstrual cycle, first building up to nourish a fertilized egg, then breaking down if no fertilization has occurred. This degenerated endometrial tissue is released as the menstrual flow. The cavity inside the uterus is shaped somewhat like a capital T, but it is capable of changing shape and dilating as a fetus develops.

The Vagina The cervix leads to the **vagina** (vah-JI-nah), the distal part of the birth canal, which opens to the outside. The vagina is a muscular tube approximately 7.5 cm (3 in.) long. The cervix dips into the vagina's superior portion forming a circular recess known as the **fornix** (FOR-niks). The deepest area of the fornix, located behind the cervix, is the **posterior fornix** (Fig. 20-9). This recess in the posterior vagina lies adjacent to the most inferior portion of the peritoneal cavity, a narrow passage between the uterus and the rectum named the **cul-de-sac** (from the French meaning "bottom of the sack"). This area is also known as the *rectouterine pouch* or the *pouch of Douglas.* A rather thin layer of tissue separates the posterior fornix from this region, so that abscesses or tumors in the peritoneal cavity can sometimes be detected by vaginal examination.

The lining of the vagina is a wrinkled mucous membrane similar to that found in the stomach. The folds (rugae) permit enlargement so that childbirth usually does not tear the lining (see Fig. 20-6). In addition to being a part of the birth canal, the vagina is the organ that receives the penis during sexual intercourse. A fold of membrane called the **hymen** (HI-men) may sometimes be found at or near the vaginal (VAJ-ih-nal) canal opening (Fig. 20-10).

The Greater Vestibular Glands Just superior and lateral to the vaginal opening are the two mucus-producing **greater vestibular** (ves-TIB-u-lar) *(Bartholin)* **glands** (see Fig. 20-6). These glands secrete into an area near the vaginal opening known as the *vestibule.* Like the Cowper glands in males, these glands provide lubrication during intercourse. If a gland becomes infected, a surgical incision may be needed to reduce swelling and promote drainage.

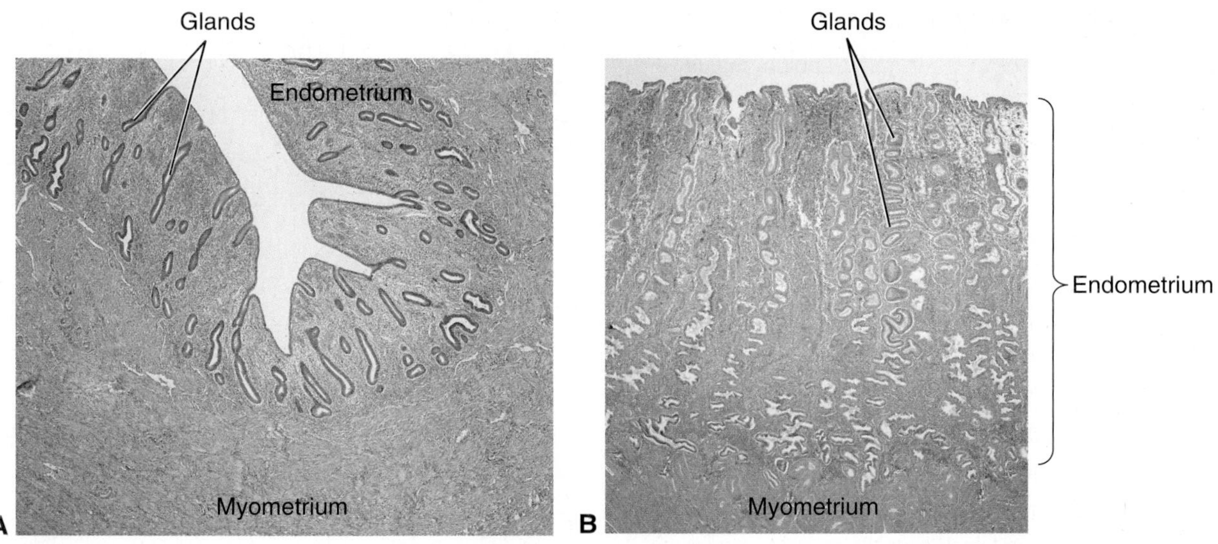

Figure 20-8 The uterus in microscopic view. KEY POINT The uterus has an outer muscular wall, the myometrium, and an inner epithelial layer, the endometrium. The photomicrographs show these layers and illustrate the changes that occur in the endometrium during the menstrual cycle. **A.** Proliferative phase (first part of cycle). The endometrium begins to repair itself following menstruation, but is relatively thin. **B.** Secretory phase (second part of cycle). The endometrium thickens and accumulates fluid under the effects of progesterone. Endometrial glands enlarge and become more active. (Reprinted with permission from Cormack DH. *Essential Histology*, 2nd ed. Philadelphia, PA: Lippincott Williams & Wilkins, 2001.) ZOOMING IN In which part of the menstrual cycle is the endometrium most highly developed?

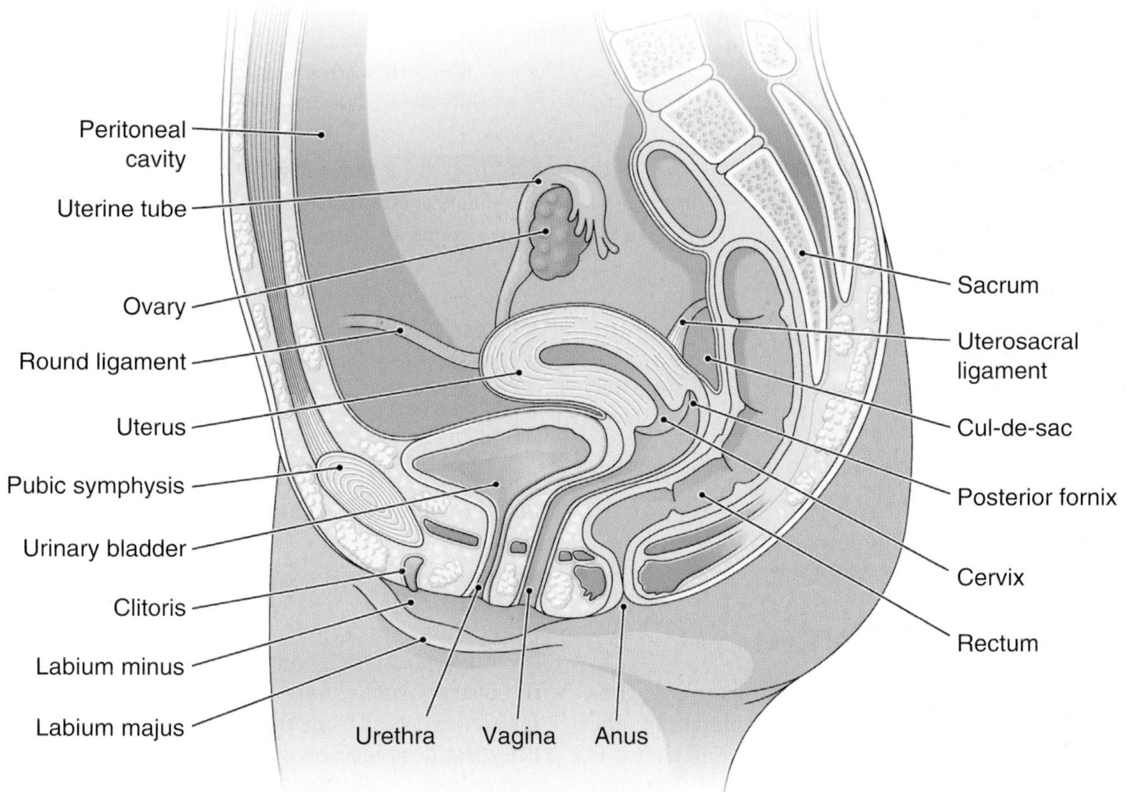

Figure 20-9 Female reproductive system (sagittal section). KEY POINT This view shows the relationship of the reproductive organs to each other and to other structures in the pelvic cavity. ZOOMING IN Which has the more anterior opening, the vagina or the urethra?

20

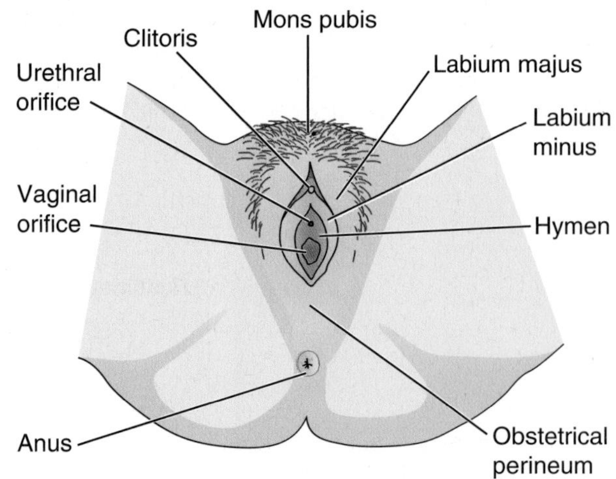

Figure 20-10 External parts of the female reproductive system. KEY POINT The external female genitalia, or vulva, includes the labia, clitoris, and mons pubis. Nearby structures are also shown.

The Vulva and the Perineum The external female genitalia make up the **vulva** (VUL-vah). This includes two pairs of lips, or **labia** (LA-be-ah), the larger *labia majora* (sing. labium majus) and smaller *labia minora* (sing. labium minus). It also includes the **clitoris** (KLIT-o-ris), a small organ of great sensitivity, as well as the openings of the urethra and vagina, and the *mons pubis*, a pad of fatty tissue over the pubic symphysis (joint) (see Fig. 20-10). Although the entire pelvic floor in both the male and female (see Fig. 8.14 in Chapter 8) is properly called the **perineum** (per-ih-NE-um), those who care for pregnant women usually refer to the limited area between the vaginal opening and the anus as the *perineum* or *obstetric perineum*.

CHECKPOINTS 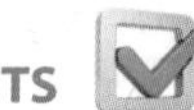

- 20-9 What is the female gamete called?
- 20-10 What is the female gonad called?
- 20-11 What structure contains each ovum?
- 20-12 What is the process of releasing an ovum from the ovary called?
- 20-13 What does the follicle become after its ovum is released?
- 20-14 In what organ does a fetus develop?

The Menstrual Cycle

In the female, as in the male, reproductive function is controlled by pituitary hormones that are regulated by the hypothalamus. Female activity differs, however, in that it is cyclic; it shows regular patterns of increases and decreases in hormone levels. These changes are regulated by hormonal feedback. The typical length of this female reproductive cycle—commonly called the **menstrual cycle**—varies between 22 and 45 days, but 28 days is taken as an average, with the first day of menstrual flow being considered the first day of the cycle (Fig. 20-11).

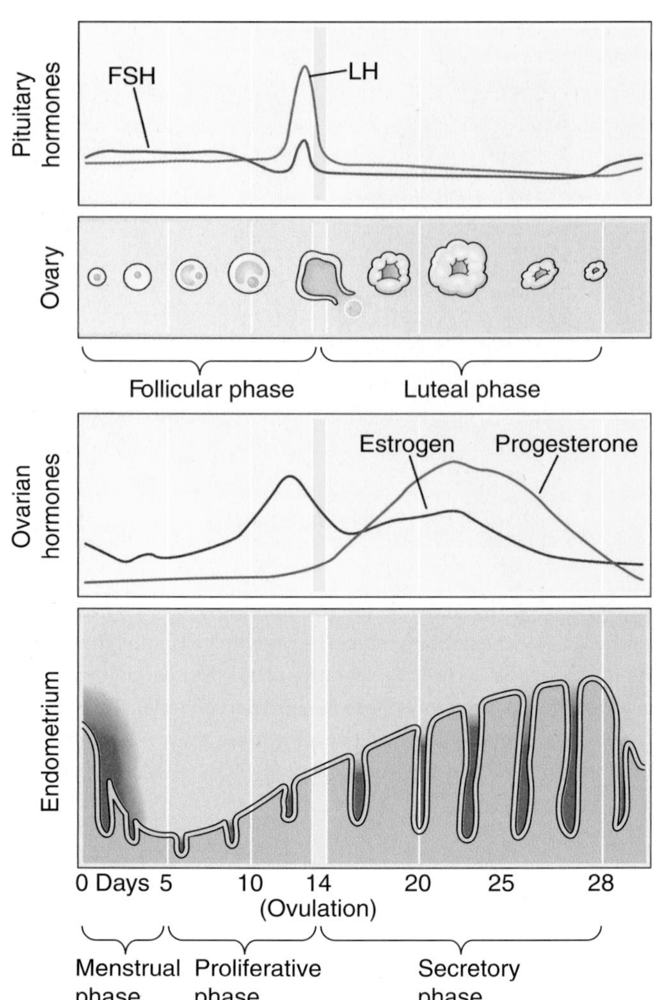

Figure 20-11 The menstrual cycle. KEY POINT Changes in pituitary and ovarian hormones, the ovary, and the uterus are shown during an average 28-day menstrual cycle with ovulation on day 14. Phases in the ovary are named for changes in follicles; phases in the uterus are named for changes in the endometrium. ZOOMING IN What ovarian hormone peaks closest to ovulation? What ovarian hormone peaks after ovulation?

BEGINNING OF THE CYCLE

At the start of each cycle, under the influence of pituitary FSH, several follicles, each containing an ovum, begin to develop in the ovary. Usually, only one of these follicles will ultimately release an ovum from the ovary in a single month. The follicle produces increasing amounts of estrogen as it matures and enlarges (see Fig. 20-11). The estrogen is carried in the bloodstream to the uterus, where it starts preparing the endometrium for a possible pregnancy. This preparation includes thickening of the endometrium and elongation of the glands that produce uterine secretions (see Fig. 20-8). Estrogen in the blood also acts as a feedback messenger to inhibit the release of FSH. When estrogen reaches high levels, it stimulates the release of LH from the pituitary (see Fig. 11-3 in Chapter 11).

OVULATION

In an average 28-day cycle, ovulation occurs on day 14 and is followed 2 weeks later by the start of the menstrual flow. However, an ovum can be released any time from day 7 to 21, thus accounting for the variation in the length of normal cycles. About 1 day before ovulation, high estrogen levels cause an **LH surge**, a sharp rise of LH in the blood. Note that there is also a small rise in FSH at this time—shown in Figure 20-11—caused by the increase in hypothalamic-releasing hormone that promotes the rise in LH. It is LH that causes ovulation. In addition, LH transforms the ruptured follicle into the corpus luteum, which produces some estrogen and large amounts of progesterone. Under the influence of these hormones, the endometrium continues to thicken, and the glands and blood vessels increase in size. The rising levels of estrogen and progesterone feed back to inhibit the release of FSH and LH from the pituitary. During this time, the ovum makes its journey to the uterus by way of the uterine tube. If the ovum is not fertilized while passing through the uterine tube, it dies within 2 to 3 days and then disintegrates.

During each menstrual cycle, changes occur in both the ovary and the uterus (see Fig. 20-11). The time before ovulation is described as the follicular phase in the ovary, because it encompasses development of the ovarian follicle. The uterus during this same time is in a proliferative phase, marked by endometrial growth. After ovulation, the ovary is in a luteal phase, with conversion of the follicle to the corpus luteum. The uterus is described as being in a secretory phase, because the endometrial glands are actively preparing the endometrium for potential implantation of a fertilized egg.

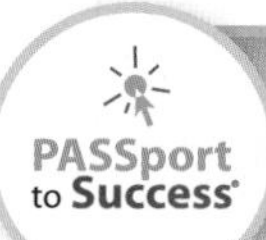

See the Student Resources on *thePoint* for a summary chart on reproductive hormones and the animation *Ovulation and Fertilization*.

THE MENSTRUAL PHASE

If fertilization does not occur, the corpus luteum degenerates, and the levels of estrogen and progesterone decrease. Without the hormones to support growth, the endometrium degenerates. Small hemorrhages appear in this tissue, producing the bloody discharge known as the **menstrual flow**, or *menses* (MEN-seze). Bits of endometrium break away and accompany the blood flow during this period of **menstruation** (men-stru-A-shun). The average duration of menstruation is 2 to 6 days.

Even before the menstrual flow ceases, the endometrium begins to repair itself through the growth of new cells. The low levels of estrogen and progesterone allow the release of FSH from the anterior pituitary. FSH causes new follicles to begin to ripen within the ovaries, and the cycle begins anew.

The activity of ovarian hormones as negative feedback messengers is the basis of hormonal methods of contraception (birth control). The estrogen and progesterone in birth control pills inhibit the release of FSH and LH from the pituitary, preventing ovulation. The menstrual period that follows withdrawal of this pharmaceutical estrogen and progesterone is anovulatory (an-OV-u-lah-tor-e); that is, it is not preceded by ovulation.

CHECKPOINT 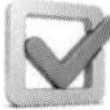

- [ ] 20-15 What are the two hormones produced in the ovaries?
- [ ] 20-16 On what day does ovulation occur in a 28-day menstrual cycle?

Menopause

Menopause (MEN-o-pawz) is the period during which menstruation ceases altogether. It ordinarily occurs gradually between the ages of 45 and 55 years and is caused by a normal decline in ovarian function. The ovary becomes chiefly scar tissue and no longer produces mature follicles or appreciable amounts of estrogen and progesterone. Eventually, the uterus, uterine tubes, vagina, and vulva all become somewhat atrophied and the vaginal mucosa becomes thinner, dryer, and more sensitive.

Menopause is an entirely normal condition, but its onset sometimes brings about effects that are temporarily disturbing. The decrease in estrogen levels can cause nervous symptoms, such as anxiety and insomnia. Because estrogen also helps maintain the vascular dilation that promotes heat loss, low levels may result in "hot flashes."

Physicians may prescribe hormone replacement therapy (HRT) to relieve the discomforts associated with menopause. This medication is usually a combination of estrogen with a synthetic progesterone (progestin), which is included to prevent overgrowth of the endometrium and the risk of endometrial cancer. Studies with the most commonly prescribed form of HRT have shown it lowers the incidence of colorectal cancer. It also lowers the incidence of hip fractures, a sign of osteoporosis. However, in addition to an increased risk of breast cancer, HRT also carries a risk of thrombosis and embolism, which is highest among women who smoke. All HRT risks increase with the duration of therapy. Therefore, treatment should be given for a short time and at the lowest effective dose. Women with a history or family history of breast cancer or circulatory problems should not take HRT.

Because of its beneficial effects, studies are continuing with estrogen alone, generally prescribed for women who have undergone a hysterectomy and do not have a uterus.

CHECKPOINT 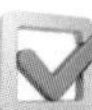

- [ ] 20-17 What is the definition of menopause?

Birth Control

Birth control is most commonly achieved by **contraception**, which is the use of artificial methods to prevent fertilization of the ovum. Birth control measures that prevent

Table 20-1 Main Methods of Birth Control Currently in Use

Method	Description	Advantages	Disadvantages
Surgical			
Vasectomy/tubal ligation	Cutting and tying of tubes carrying gametes	Nearly 100% effective; involves no chemical or mechanical devices	Not usually reversible; rare surgical complications
Hormonal			
Birth control pills	Estrogen and progestin, or progestin alone, taken orally to prevent ovulation	Highly effective; requires no last-minute preparation	Alters physiology; return to fertility may be delayed; risk of cardiovascular disease in older women who smoke or have hypertension
Birth control shot	Injection of synthetic progesterone every 3 mo to prevent ovulation	Highly effective; lasts for 3 to 4 mo	Alters physiology; same side effects as birth control pill; possible menstrual irregularity, amenorrhea
Birth control patch	Adhesive patch placed on body that administers estrogen and progestin through the skin; left on for 3 wk and removed for a fourth week	Protects long-term; less chance of incorrect use; no last-minute preparation	Alters physiology; same possible side effects as birth control pill
Birth control ring	Flexible ring inserted into vagina that releases hormones internally; left in place for 3 wk and removed for a fourth week	Long-lasting; highly effective; no last-minute preparation	Possible infections, irritation; same possible side effects as birth control pill
Barrier			
Condom	Sheath that prevents semen from contacting the female reproductive tract	Readily available; does not affect physiology; does not require medical consultation; protects against STIs	
Male	Sheath that fits over erect penis and prevents release of semen	Inexpensive	Must be applied just before intercourse; may slip or tear
Female	Sheath that fits into vagina and covers cervix	Gives women control over last-minute contraception	Relatively expensive; may be difficult or inconvenient to insert
Diaphragm (with spermicide)	Rubber cap that fits over cervix and prevents entrance of sperm	Does not affect physiology; no side effects	Must be inserted before intercourse and left in place for 6 h; requires fitting by physician
Contraceptive sponge (with spermicide)	Soft, disposable foam disk containing spermicide, which is moistened with water and inserted into the vagina	Protects against pregnancy for 24 h; nonhormonal; available without prescription; inexpensive	85%–90% effective depending on proper use; possible skin irritation
Intrauterine device (IUD)	Metal or plastic device inserted into uterus through vagina; prevents fertilization and implantation by release of copper or birth control hormones	Highly effective for 5–10 y depending on type; reversible; no last-minute preparation	Must be introduced by health professional; heavy menstrual bleeding
Other			
Spermicide	Chemicals used to kill sperm; best when used in combination with a barrier method	Available without prescription; inexpensive; does not affect physiology	May cause local irritation; must be used just before intercourse
Fertility awareness	Abstinence during fertile part of cycle as determined by menstrual history, basal body temperature, or quality of cervical mucus	Does not affect physiology; accepted by certain religions	High failure rate; requires careful record keeping

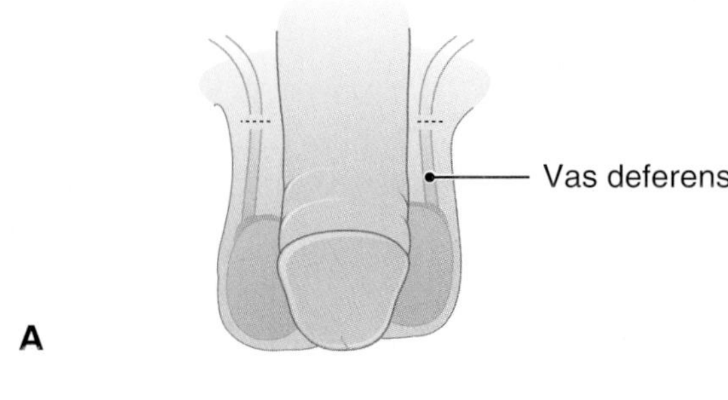

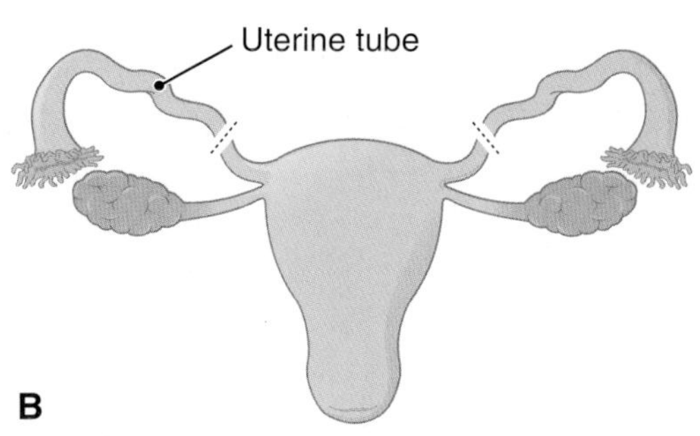

Figure 20-12 Surgical sterilization. KEY POINT The tubes that transport the gametes are cut. **A.** Vasectomy severs the ductus deferens bilaterally. **B.** Tubal ligation severs the uterine tubes bilaterally.

implantation of the fertilized ovum are also considered contraceptives, although technically they do not prevent conception and are more accurately called **abortifacients** (ah-bor-tih-FA-shents) (agents that cause abortion). Some birth control methods act by both mechanisms. Table 20-1 presents a brief description of the main contraceptive methods currently in use along with some advantages and disadvantages of each. The list is given in a rough order of decreasing effectiveness.

The surest contraceptive method is surgical sterilization. Tubal ligation and vasectomy work by severing and tying off (or cauterizing) the ducts that carry the gametes: the uterine tubes in women and the ductus deferens in men (Fig. 20-12). A man who has had a vasectomy retains the ability to produce hormones and semen as well as the ability to engage in sexual intercourse, but no fertilization can occur.

The various hormonal methods of birth control basically differ in how the hormones are administered. In addition to delivery by pills, an injection, a skin patch, or a vaginal ring, birth control hormones can be implanted as a thin rod under the skin of the upper arm. This method is highly effective and lasts for about 3 years, but it must be implanted and removed by a health professional. The emergency contraceptive pill is a synthetic progesterone (progestin) taken within 72 hours after intercourse, usually in two doses 12 hours apart. It reduces the risk of pregnancy following unprotected intercourse. This so-called "morning after pill" is intended for emergency use and not as a regular birth control method. Researchers have done trials with a male contraceptive pill, but none is on the market as yet. The male version of "the pill" also works by suppressing GnRH to inhibit release of FSH and LH, which are important in spermatogenesis. Use of testosterone as a negative feedback messenger requires regular injections and has some undesirable side effects at the doses needed. Administration of the female hormone progesterone prevents spermatogenesis, but also inhibits normal testosterone production. Studies are ongoing to find the best way to deliver the right male contraceptive hormones at safe and effective doses.

Mifepristone (RU 486) is a drug taken after conception to terminate an early pregnancy. It blocks the action of progesterone, causing the uterus to shed its lining and release the fertilized egg. It must be combined with administration of prostaglandins to expel the uterine tissue.

Note in Table 20-1 that only male and female condoms protect against the spread of STIs (see Box 20-2 for more

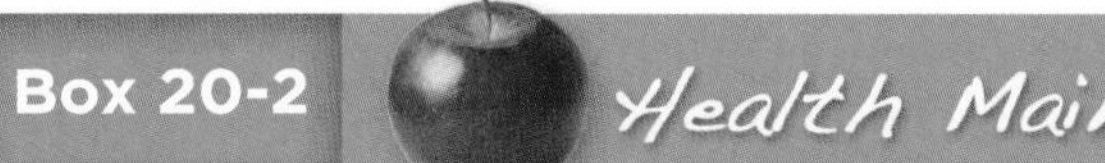

Box 20-2 *Health Maintenance*

Sexually Transmitted Infections: Lowering Your Risks

Sexually transmitted infections (STIs) such as chlamydia, gonorrhea, genital herpes, HIV, and syphilis are some of the most common infectious diseases in the United States, affecting more than 13 million men and women each year. These diseases are associated with complications such as pelvic inflammatory disease, epididymitis, infertility, liver failure, neurological disorders, cancer, and AIDS. Women are more likely to contract STIs than are men. The same mechanisms that transport sperm cells through the female reproductive tract also move infectious organisms. The surest way to prevent STIs is to avoid sexual contact with others. If you are sexually active, the following techniques can lower your risks:

- Maintain a monogamous sexual relationship with an uninfected partner.
- Correctly and consistently use a male or female condom. Although not 100% effective, condoms greatly reduce the risk of contracting an STI.
- Avoid contact with body fluids such as blood, semen, and vaginal fluids, all of which may harbor infectious organisms.
- Urinate and wash the genitals after sex. This may help remove infectious organisms before they cause disease.
- Have regular checkups for STIs. Most of the time STIs cause no symptoms, particularly in women.

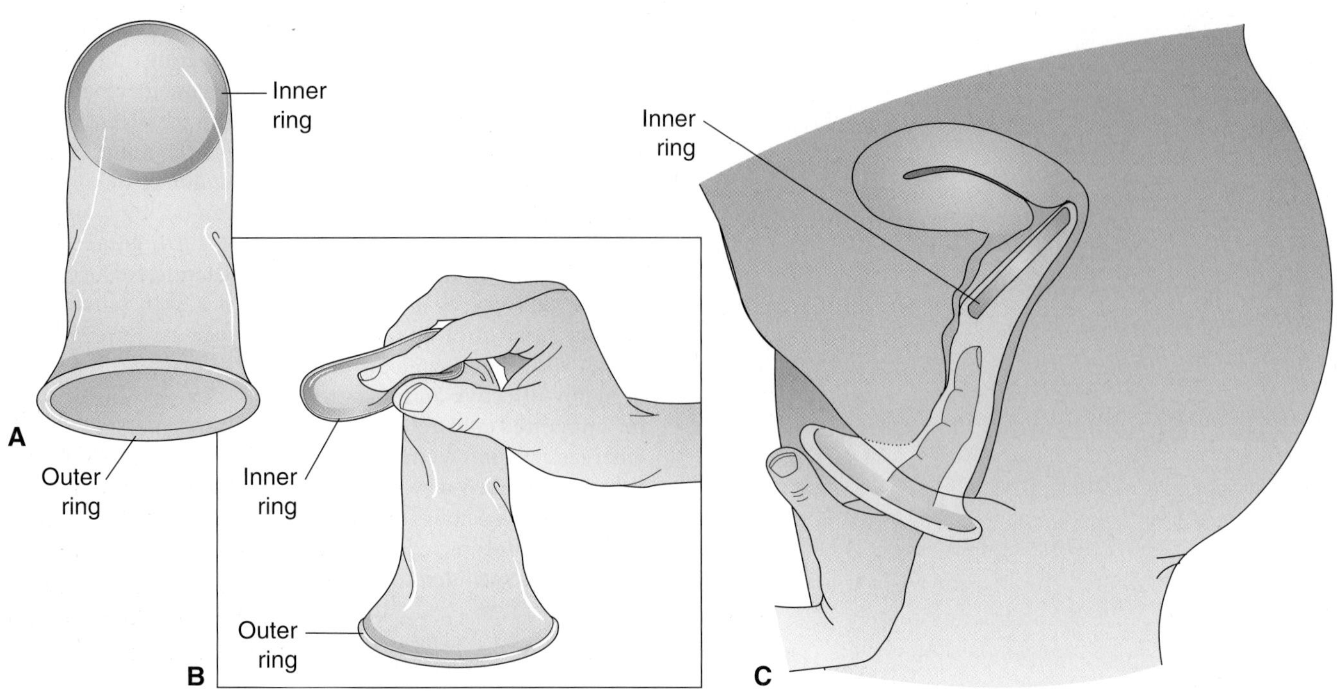

Figure 20-13 Insertion of a female condom. A. The condom has a flexible inner ring and an outer ring supporting a sheath. **B.** The flexible inner ring is compressed between the thumb and middle finger and inserted with the index finger deep into the vagina. **C.** The inner ring holds the condom in place. The outer ring remains outside the vaginal opening. (Reprinted with permission from Smeltzer SC, Bare B. *Textbook of Medical-Surgical Nursing*, 12th ed. Philadelphia, PA: Lippincott Williams & Wilkins, 2009.)

information on lowering one's risk of contracting an STI). The female condom is a sheath that fits into the vagina **(Fig. 20-13)**. A flexible inner ring inserted into the top of the vagina holds the condom in place; an outer ring remains outside the vaginal opening. While more expensive than the male condom, it gives a woman control over last-minute contraception and does not require any drugs or medical visits.

CHECKPOINT 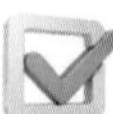

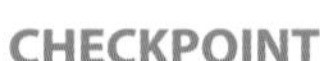

20-18 What is the definition of contraception?

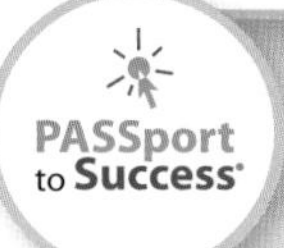

Clinics and medical offices may employ physician assistants. See the Student Resources on *thePoint* for a description of this career.

A&P in Action Revisited

Sylvie's Myomectomy

Dr. Bernard visited Sylvie in the outpatient recovery room to discuss the results of her myomectomy. "The procedure was successful," he reported. "We were able to remove the fibroid completely and repair the uterus with a hysteroscope, a type of endoscope. There are several methods available now to avoid hysterectomy in cases of myomas, and many people believe you should preserve the uterus if possible, even after childbearing years. If fibroids are larger, or more numerous, or in certain other locations in the uterus, we sometimes need to use a laparoscope or do an abdominal incision. But you're fine for now. Take it easy for the rest of the week, and don't drive for a couple of days. Call my office if you have any pain or bleeding. You should schedule a checkup in 6 months to see how you are doing."

"Thanks Doctor," Sylvie said. "I feel pretty good right now, so I assume I'll be fine. I'll be sure to let you know if I'm not."

Sylvie's case contains medical terms that can be divided into standardized parts. Each chapter in this book contains a section on "word anatomy" that gives the meanings of the prefixes, roots, and suffixes used in the chapter. Knowledge of these word elements helps you to remember scientific terms and to make guesses about the meaning of new terms. You can find the definitions of many scientific word parts in a good dictionary.

Chapter Wrap-Up

Summary Overview

A detailed chapter outline with space for note-taking is on *thePoint*. The figure below illustrates the main topics covered in this chapter.

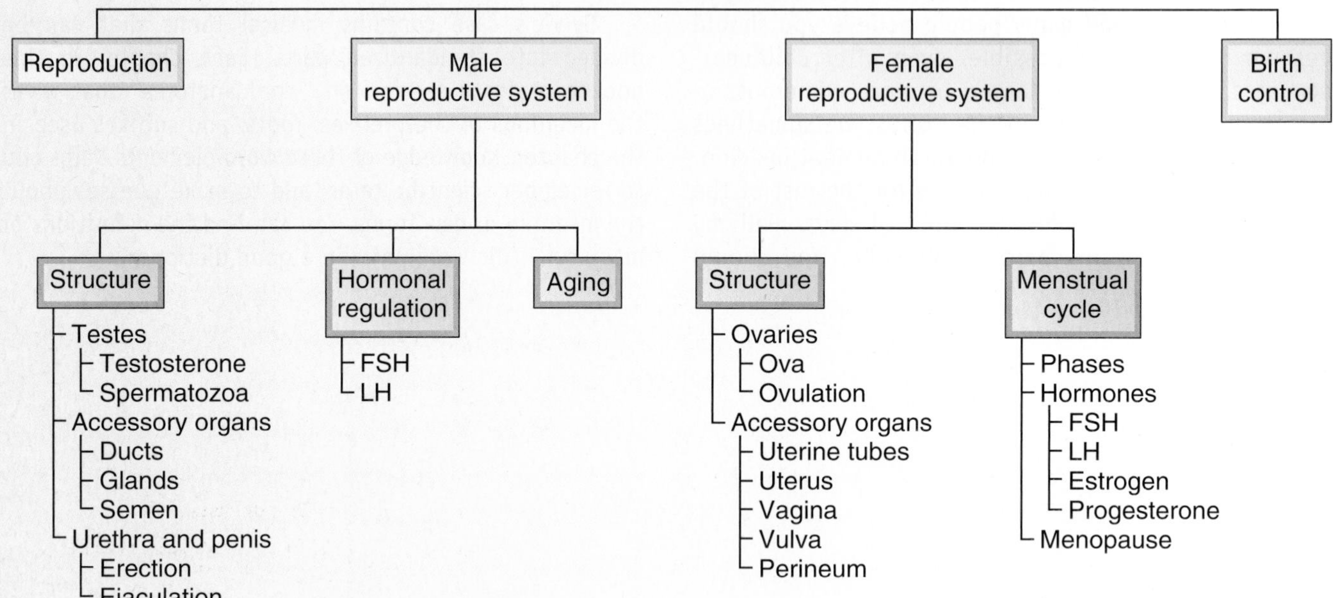

Key Terms

The terms listed below are emphasized in this chapter. Knowing them will help you organize and prioritize your learning. These and other boldface terms are defined in the Glossary with phonetic pronunciations.

corpus luteum
endometrium
estrogen
follicle
follicle-stimulating hormone (FSH)
gamete
luteinizing hormone (LH)
menopause
menses
menstruation
ovary
ovulation
ovum (pl., ova)
progesterone
semen
spermatozoon (pl., spermatozoa)
testis (pl., testes)
testosterone
uterus

Word Anatomy

Scientific terms are built from standardized word parts (prefixes, roots, and suffixes). Learning the meanings of these parts can help you remember words and interpret unfamiliar terms.

WORD PART	MEANING	EXAMPLE
The Male Reproductive System		
semin/o	semen, seed	Sperm cells are produced in the *seminiferous* tubules.
test/o	testis	The hormone *testosterone* is produced in the testis.
acr/o	extremity, end	The *acrosome* covers the head of a sperm cell.
fer	to carry	The ductus *deferens* carries spermatozoa away from (de-) the testis.
circum-	around	A cut is made around the glans to remove part of the foreskin in a *circumcision*.
The Female Reproductive System		
ov/o, ov/i	egg	An *ovum* is an egg cell.
ovar, ovari/o	ovary	An *ovarian* follicle encloses an ovum.
metr/o	uterus	The *myometrium* is the muscular (my/o) layer of the uterus.
rect/o	rectum	The *rectouterine* pouch is between the uterus and rectum.

Questions for Study and Review

BUILDING UNDERSTANDING

Fill in the Blanks

1. Gametes go through a special process of cell division called _____.
2. Spermatozoa begin their development in tiny coiled _____.
3. An ovum matures in a small fluid-filled cluster of cells called the _____.
4. The main male sex hormone is _____.
5. The process of releasing an ovum from the ovary is called _____.

Matching > Match each numbered item with the most closely related lettered item.

___ **6.** A hormone released by the pituitary that promotes follicular development in the ovary

___ **7.** A hormone released by developing follicles that promotes thickening of the endometrium

___ **8.** A hormone released by the pituitary that stimulates ovulation

___ **9.** A hormone released by the corpus luteum that promotes thickening of the endometrium

a. follicle-stimulating hormone
b. estrogen
c. luteinizing hormone
d. progesterone

Multiple Choice

___ **10.** What structure does the fetal testis travel through to descend into the scrotum?

a. spermatic cord
b. inguinal canal
c. seminiferous tubule
d. vas deferens

___ **11.** Where are the enzymes that help the sperm cell to penetrate the ovum located?

a. acrosome
b. head
c. midpiece
d. flagellum

___ **12.** Which structure contains the male urethra?

a. corpus cavernosum
b. corpus spongiosum
c. vas deferens
d. seminiferous tubules

___ **13.** What structure(s) suspend the uterus and ovaries in the pelvic cavity?

a. uterine tubes
b. broad ligaments
c. fimbriae
d. fornix

___ **14.** What is the term for the area between the vaginal opening and the anus?

a. vestibule
b. vulva
c. hymen
d. perineum

___ **15.** Which phase is promoted by decreased estrogen and progesterone levels?

a. luteal phase
b. menstrual phase
c. proliferative phase
d. secretory phase

UNDERSTANDING CONCEPTS

16. Compare and contrast the following terms:

a. asexual reproduction and sexual reproduction
b. spermatozoa and ova
c. sustentacular cell and interstitial cell
d. ovarian follicle and corpus luteum
e. myometrium and endometrium

17. Trace the pathway of sperm from the site of production to the urethra.

18. Describe the components of semen, their sites of production, and their functions.

19. List the hormones that control male reproduction and state their functions.

20. Trace the pathway of an ovum from the site of production to the site of implantation.

21. Beginning with the first day of the menstrual flow, describe the events of one complete cycle, including the role of the hormones involved.

22. Define *contraception*. Describe methods of contraception that involve (1) barriers; (2) chemicals; (3) hormones; (4) prevention of implantation.

CONCEPTUAL THINKING

23. Theoretically, it is possible for a brain-dead man to ejaculate. What anatomical and physiological feature makes this possible?

24. Jen, a middle-aged mother of three, is considering a tubal ligation, a contraceptive procedure that involves cutting the uterine tubes. Jen is worried that this might cause her to enter early menopause. Should she be worried?

25. Sylvie's case involves a myoma. Given your knowledge of word anatomy, in which layer of Sylvie's uterus is the myoma located? What type of tissue is this layer composed of?

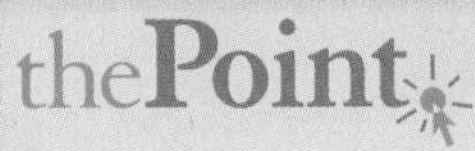

For more questions, see the learning activities on *thePoint*.

CHAPTER 21 Development and Heredity

A&P in Action

Ben's Second Case: The Genetics of Cystic Fibrosis

When 2-year-old Ben was diagnosed with cystic fibrosis (CF), his parents, Alison and David, were shocked to discover that he had inherited the genetic disease from them. At first, their attention was focused only on Ben and the treatment he would need. Later, they also began to wonder how they had passed on the disease and whether or not other children they might have would be at risk. So they made an appointment with a genetic counselor.

Ms. Clarkson explained, "All of a person's traits are inherited from his or her parents in the form of genes, bits of DNA carried on chromosomes in the gametes. CF is caused by a change, or mutation, in a gene on chromosome number 7. This gene codes for a chloride ion channel that is important in manufacturing sweat, digestive fluids, and mucus."

"But how come Ben has CF, that he inherited from us, but we don't have any signs of the disease?" Alison asked.

Ms. Clarkson replied, "A genetic disease can arise from a spontaneous mutation, but more likely, you and David are carriers of the CF gene."

"Meaning ...?" said David.

"Meaning, that you each have one CF gene, but you also have one non-CF gene—so you don't have CF." "All genetic traits—from hair color to a genetic disease—are determined by pairs of genes, one from our mother and one from our father. If even one of these genes is a so-called dominant gene, it will always be expressed. A person with a dominant disease gene will show the disease and you know it's there. However, most genetic diseases, including CF, are caused by recessive genes. These can be masked by a dominant gene so you need two copies to show the disease. You and Alison are disease free, but you each carry one CF gene that was passed on to Ben."

"Will all of our children have CF?" Alison wondered. "Should we stop here with our family?"

"Not necessarily. We could do a family study to look for CF in your relatives, and there is a lab test done on blood or saliva to identify carriers, but we can assume at this point that both of you are carriers. There's a one in four chance that any of your children will have CF. The risk is constant with each birth, whether you've had a child with CF or not. There is a prenatal test that can identify CF in a fetus, and you can choose to make family decisions based on those results. But that's for future discussions. Right now, you have to concentrate on Ben and his care."

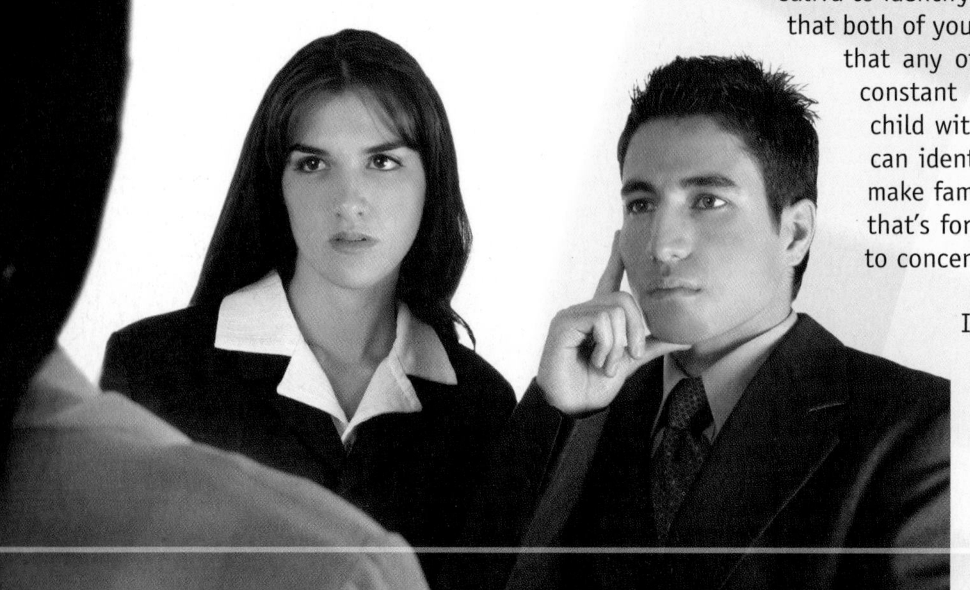

In this chapter, we learn more about heredity. Later, we see what treatment options are available for Ben.

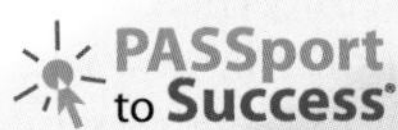

Ancillaries *At-A-Glance*

Visit *thePoint* to access the PASSport to Success and the following resources. For guidance in using these resources most effectively, see pp. ix–xviii.

Learning TOOLS

- Learning Style Self-Assessment
- Live Advise Online Student Tutoring
- Tips for Effective Studying

Learning RESOURCES

- E-book: Chapter 21
- Web Figure: Apgar scoring system
- Web Chart: Placental Hormones
- Animation: Fetal Circulation
- Health Professions: Midwife and Other Birth Assistants
- Detailed Chapter Outline
- Answers to Questions for Study and Review
- Audio Pronunciation Glossary

Learning ACTIVITIES

- Pre-Quiz
- Visual Activities
- Kinesthetic Activities
- Auditory Activities

Learning Outcomes

After careful study of this chapter, you should be able to:

1. Describe fertilization and the early development of the fertilized egg, ***p. 414***
2. Describe the structure and function of the placenta, ***p. 415***
3. Describe how fetal circulation differs from adult circulation, ***p. 415***
4. Briefly describe changes that occur in the embryo, fetus, and mother during pregnancy, ***p. 417***
5. Name the hormones active in lactation and describe the action of each, ***p. 417***
6. Cite the advantages of breast-feeding, ***p. 424***
7. Briefly describe the mechanism of gene function, ***p. 424***
8. Explain the difference between dominant and recessive genes, ***p. 425***
9. Compare *phenotype* and *genotype* and give examples of each, ***p. 425***
10. Describe what is meant by a *carrier* of a genetic trait, ***p. 425***
11. Define *meiosis* and explain its function in reproduction, ***p. 426***
12. Explain how sex is determined in humans, ***p. 427***
13. Describe what is meant by the term *sex-linked* and list several sex-linked traits, ***p. 427***
14. List several factors that may influence the expression of a gene, ***p. 428***
15. Referring to the case study, describe the inheritance of the cystic fibrosis trait, ***pp. 412, 429***
16. Show how word parts are used to build words related to development and heredity (see Word Anatomy at the end of the chapter), ***p. 431***

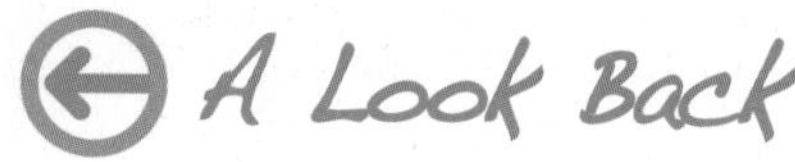

Description of the male and female reproductive tracts continues with discussion of the events that occur in a mother and fetus if fertilization takes place. We elaborate on the action of some hormones introduced in Chapter 11 as they apply to pregnancy, childbirth, and lactation. Negative feedback mechanisms control many aspects of reproduction. However, childbirth and lactation represent a different type of feedback process—positive feedback—a system that maintains rather than reverses an action.

Pregnancy

Pregnancy begins with fertilization of an ovum and ends with childbirth. During this approximately 38-week period of development, known as **gestation** (jes-TA-shun), a single fertilized egg divides repeatedly, and the new cells differentiate into all the tissues of the developing offspring. Along the way, many changes occur in the mother as well as her baby. **Obstetrics** (ob-STET-riks) (OB) is the branch of medicine that is concerned with the care of women during pregnancy, childbirth, and the 6 weeks after childbirth. A physician who specializes in obstetrics is an *obstetrician*. Some obstetricians specialize in high-risk pregnancies, as does Sue's physician in the case study.

FERTILIZATION AND THE START OF PREGNANCY

When semen is deposited in the vagina, the millions of spermatozoa immediately wriggle about in all directions, some traveling into the uterus and uterine tubes (**Fig. 21-1**). If an egg cell is present in the uterine tube, many spermatozoa cluster around it. Using enzymes, they dissolve the coating around the ovum, so that eventually one sperm cell can penetrate its plasma membrane. The nuclei of the sperm and egg then combine (**see Box 21-1**).

The result of this union is a single cell, called a **zygote** (ZI-gote), with the full human chromosome number of 46. The zygote divides rapidly into two cells and then four cells and soon forms a ball of cells called a *morula*

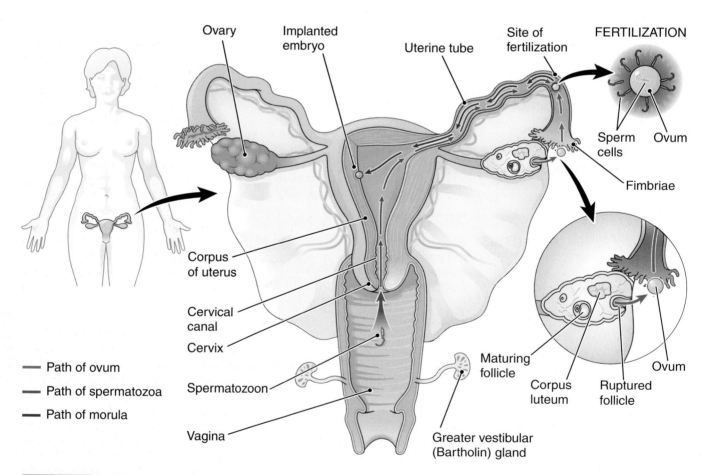

Figure 21-1 The female reproductive system. KEY POINT Arrows show the pathways of the spermatozoa, ovum, and morula, the ball of cells formed from the dividing zygote. The figure also shows fertilization and implantation of the embryo. ZOOMING IN Where is the ovum fertilized?

Box 21-1 *Clinical Perspectives*

Assisted Reproductive Technology: The "Art" of Conception

At least one in ten American couples is affected by infertility. Assisted reproductive technologies such as *in vitro* fertilization (IVF), gamete intrafallopian transfer (GIFT), and zygote intrafallopian transfer (ZIFT) can help these couples become pregnant.

In vitro fertilization refers to fertilization of an ovum outside the mother's body in a laboratory dish (*in vitro* means in glass). It is often used when a woman's uterine tubes are blocked or when a man has a low sperm count. The woman participating in IVF is given hormones to cause ovulation of several ova. These are then withdrawn with a needle and fertilized with the father's sperm. After a few divisions, some of the fertilized ova are placed in the uterus, thus bypassing the uterine tubes. Additional fertilized ova can be frozen to repeat the procedure in case of failure or for later pregnancies.

GIFT can be used when the woman has at least one normal oviduct and the man has an adequate sperm count. As in IVF, the woman is given hormones to cause ovulation of several ova, which are collected. Then, the ova and the father's sperm are placed into the uterine tube using a catheter. Thus, in GIFT, fertilization occurs inside the woman, not in a laboratory dish.

ZIFT is a combination of both IVF and GIFT. Fertilization takes place in a laboratory dish, and then the zygote is placed into the uterine tube.

Because of a lack of guidelines or restrictions in the United States in the field of assisted reproductive technology, some problems have arisen. These issues concern the use of stored embryos and gametes, use of embryos without consent, and improper screening for disease among donors. In addition, the implantation of more than one fertilized ovum has resulted in a high incidence of multiple births, even up to seven or eight offspring in a single pregnancy, a situation that imperils the survival and health of the babies.

(MOR-u-lah). During this time, the cell cluster is traveling toward the uterine cavity, pushed along by cilia lining the oviduct and by peristalsis (contractions) of the tube. After reaching the uterus, the little ball of cells burrows into the greatly thickened uterine lining and is soon implanted and completely covered. After **implantation** in the uterus, a group of cells within the dividing cluster becomes an **embryo** (EM-bre-o), the term used for the growing offspring in the early stage of gestation. The other cells within the cluster will differentiate into tissue that will support the developing **fetus** (FE-tus), the growing offspring from the beginning of the third month of gestation until birth.

THE PLACENTA

For a few days after implantation, the embryo gets nourishment from its surrounding fluids. As it grows, the embryo's increasing needs are met by the **placenta** (plah-SEN-tah), a flat, circular organ that consists of a spongy network of blood-filled sinuses and capillary-containing villi (Fig. 21-2). (*Placenta* is from a Latin word meaning "pancake.") The placenta consists of both maternal and embryonic tissue. The maternal portion is simply a well-vascularized internal portion of the endometrium. The embryonic portion is called the **chorion** (KO-re-on), which forms projections called *chorionic villi*. The chorionic villi break down the endometrial tissue, creating a network of venous sinuses filled with maternal blood. The placenta is the organ of nutrition, respiration, and excretion for the developing offspring throughout gestation. Although the blood of the mother and her offspring do not mix—each has its own blood and cardiovascular system—exchanges take place between maternal blood in the sinuses and embryonic blood in the capillaries of the chorionic villi. In this manner, gases (CO_2 and O_2) are exchanged, nutrients are provided to the developing offspring, and waste products are released into the maternal blood to be eliminated.

The Umbilical Cord The embryo is connected to the developing placenta by a stalk of tissue that eventually becomes the **umbilical** (um-BIL-ih-kal) **cord.** This structure carries blood to and from the embryo, later called the fetus. The cord encloses two arteries that carry blood low in oxygen from the fetus to the placenta, and one vein that carries blood high in oxygen from the placenta to the fetus (see Fig. 21-2). (Note that, like the pulmonary vessels, these arteries carry blood low in oxygen and this vein carries blood high in oxygen.)

Fetal Circulation The fetus has special circulatory adaptations to carry blood to and from the umbilical cord and to bypass its nonfunctional lungs. A small amount of the oxygen-rich blood traveling toward the fetus in the **umbilical vein** is delivered directly to the liver. However, most of the blood bypasses the liver and is added to the oxygen-poor blood in the inferior vena cava through a small vessel, the **ductus venosus**. Although mixed, this blood still contains enough oxygen to nourish fetal tissues. Once in the right atrium, most of the blood flows directly into the left atrium through a small hole in the atrial septum, the **foramen ovale** (o-VA-le). This blood has bypassed the right ventricle and the pulmonary circuit. Blood that does enter

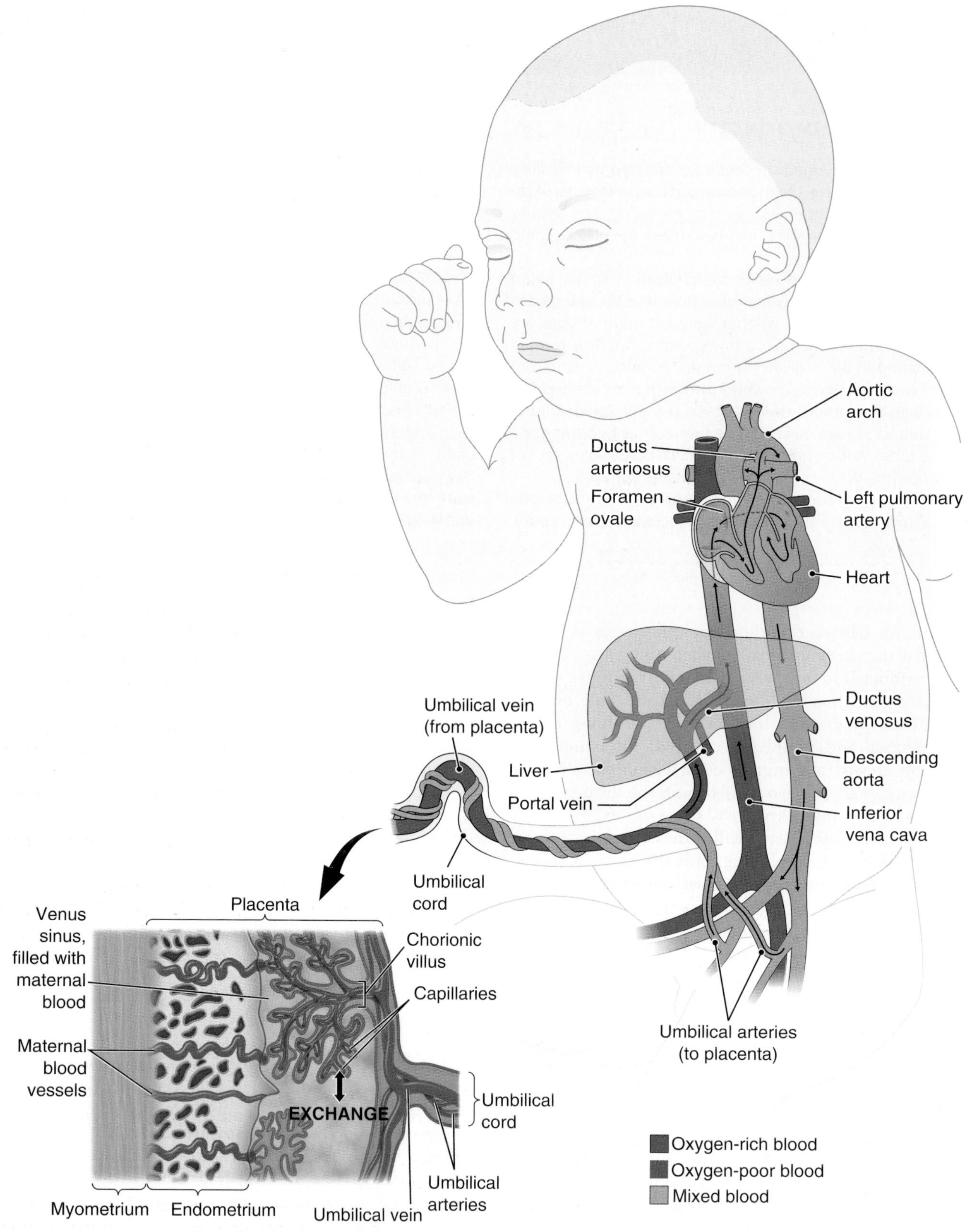

Figure 21-2 Fetal circulation and section of placenta. KEY POINT *Colors* show relative oxygen content of blood. The placenta is formed by the uterine endometrium and fetal chorion. Exchanges between fetal and maternal blood occur through the capillaries of the chorionic villi. ZOOMING IN What is signified by the purple color in this illustration?

the right ventricle is pumped into the pulmonary artery. Although a small amount of this blood goes to the lungs, most of it shunts directly into the systemic circuit through a small vessel, the **ductus arteriosus**, which connects the pulmonary artery to the descending aorta **(see Fig. 21-2)**. After traveling throughout fetal tissue, blood returns to the placenta to pick up oxygen through the two **umbilical arteries**.

After birth, when the baby's lungs are functioning, these adaptations begin to close. The foramen ovale gradually seals and the various vessels constrict into fibrous cords, usually within minutes after birth (only the proximal parts of the umbilical arteries persist as arteries to the urinary bladder).

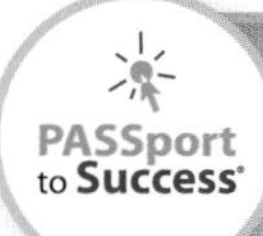

See the Student Resources on *thePoint* to view the animation *Fetal Circulation*.

HORMONES AND PREGNANCY

Beginning soon after implantation, some embryonic cells produce the hormone **human chorionic gonadotropin** (ko-re-ON-ik gon-ah-do-TRO-pin) (**hCG**). This hormone stimulates the ovarian corpus luteum, prolonging its life-span to 11 or 12 weeks and causing it to secrete increasing amounts of progesterone and estrogen. It is hCG that is used in tests as an indicator of pregnancy.

Progesterone is essential for the maintenance of pregnancy. It promotes endometrial secretions to nourish the embryo, maintains the endometrium, and decreases the uterine muscle's ability to contract, thus preventing the embryo from being expelled from the body. During pregnancy, progesterone also helps prepare the breasts for milk secretion. Estrogen promotes enlargement of the uterus and breasts.

The placenta also secretes hormones. By the 11th or 12th week of pregnancy, the corpus luteum is no longer needed; by this time, the placenta has developed the capacity to secrete adequate amounts of progesterone and estrogen, and the corpus luteum disintegrates. Miscarriages (loss of an embryo or fetus) are most likely to occur during this critical time when hormone secretion is shifting from the corpus luteum to the placenta.

Human placental lactogen (**hPL**) is another hormone secreted by the placenta during pregnancy, reaching a peak at term, the normal conclusion of pregnancy. hPL stimulates growth of the breasts to prepare the mother for milk production, or **lactation** (lak-TA-shun). More importantly, it regulates the levels of nutrients in the mother's blood to keep them available for the fetus. This second function leads to an alternate name for this hormone: human chorionic somatomammotropin, based on its ability to stimulate growth (somat/o) and the mammary glands (mamm/o).

Relaxin is a placental hormone that softens the cervix and relaxes the sacral joints and the pubic symphysis. These changes help to widen the birth canal and aid in birth.

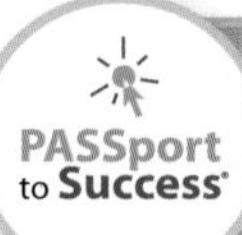

See the Student Resources on *thePoint* for a summary chart on placental hormones.

CHECKPOINTS 

- [ ] **21-1** What structure is formed by the union of an ovum and a spermatozoon?
- [ ] **21-2** What organ nourishes the developing fetus?
- [ ] **21-3** What is the function of the umbilical cord?
- [ ] **21-4** Fetal circulation is adapted to bypass what organs?

DEVELOPMENT OF THE EMBRYO

The developing offspring is referred to as an embryo for the first 8 weeks of life **(Fig. 21-3)**, and the study of growth during this period is called **embryology** (em-bre-OL-o-je). The beginnings of all body systems are established during this time. The heart and the brain are among the first organs to develop. A primitive nervous system begins to form in the third week. The heart and blood vessels originate during the second week, and the first heartbeat appears during week 4, at the same time that other muscles begin to develop.

By the end of the first month, the embryo is approximately 0.62 cm (0.25 in) long, with four small swellings at the sides called **limb buds**, which will develop into the four extremities. At this time, the heart produces a prominent bulge at the anterior of the embryo.

By the end of the second month, the embryo takes on an appearance that is recognizably human. In male embryos, the primitive testes have formed and have begun to secrete testosterone, which will direct formation of the male reproductive organs as gestation continues. **Figure 21-4** shows photographs of embryonic and early fetal development. A developing infant is especially sensitive to harmful substances and poor maternal nutrition during this early stage of pregnancy when so many important developmental events are occurring. Sue's physician, in the case study, must be sure that her medications don't harm her fetus and that she has a good diet with adequate vitamins.

DEVELOPMENT OF THE FETUS

During the period of fetal development, from the beginning of the third month until birth, the organ systems continue to grow and mature. The ovaries form in the female early in this fetal period, and at this stage they contain all the primitive cells (oocytes) that can later develop into mature ova (eggs).

For study, the entire gestation period may be divided into three equal segments or **trimesters**. The fetus's most rapid growth occurs during the second trimester (months 4 to 6). By the end of the fourth month, the fetus is almost 15 cm (6 in.) long, and its external genitalia are sufficiently developed to reveal its sex. By the seventh month, the fetus is usually approximately 35 cm (14 in.) long and weighs

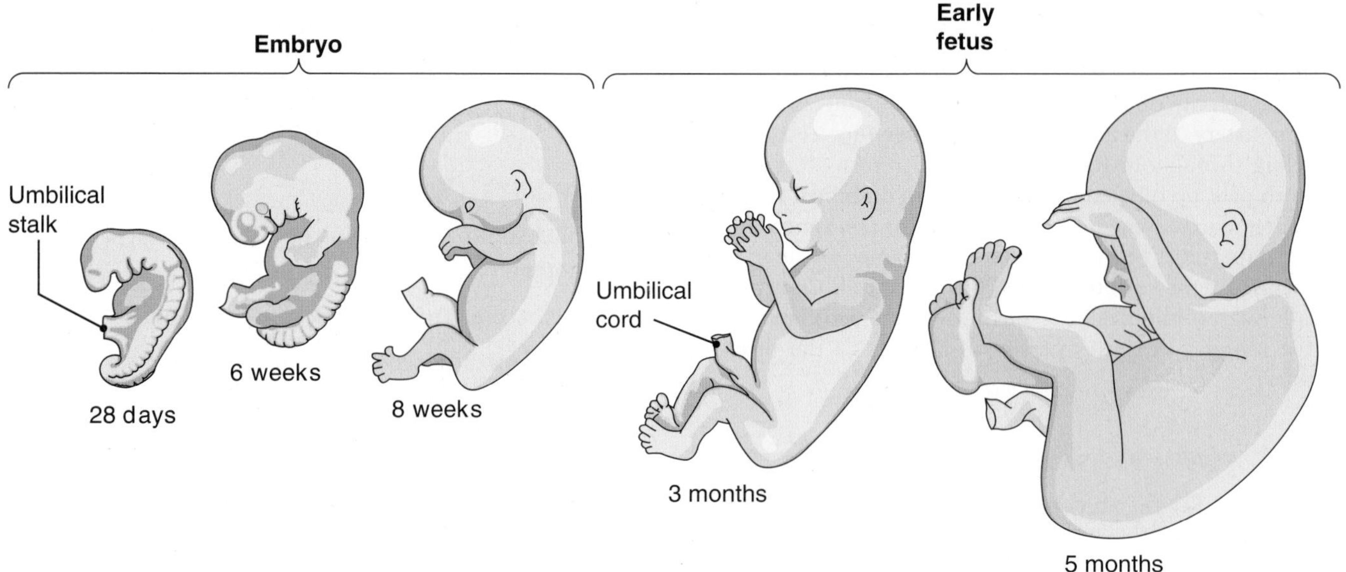

Figure 21-3 **Development of an embryo and early fetus.**

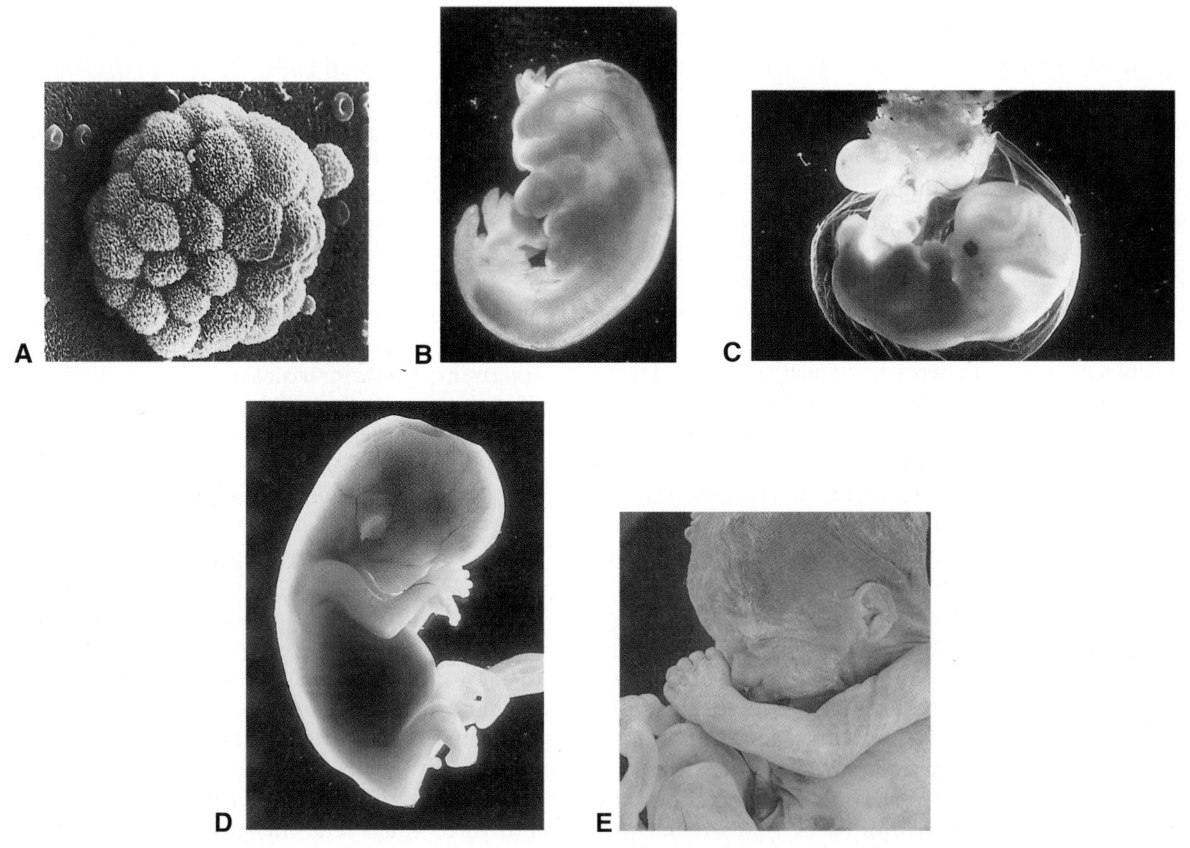

Figure 21-4 **Human embryos at different stages and early fetus.** KEY POINT The embryonic stage lasts for the first 2 months of pregnancy. Thereafter, the developing offspring is called a fetus. **A.** Implantation in uterus 7 to 8 days after conception. **B.** Embryo at 32 days. **C.** At 37 days. **D.** At 41 days. **E.** Fetus between 12 and 15 weeks. (Reprinted with permission from Pillitteri A. *Maternal and Child Health Nursing*, 6th ed. Philadelphia, PA: Lippincott Williams & Wilkins, 2009.)

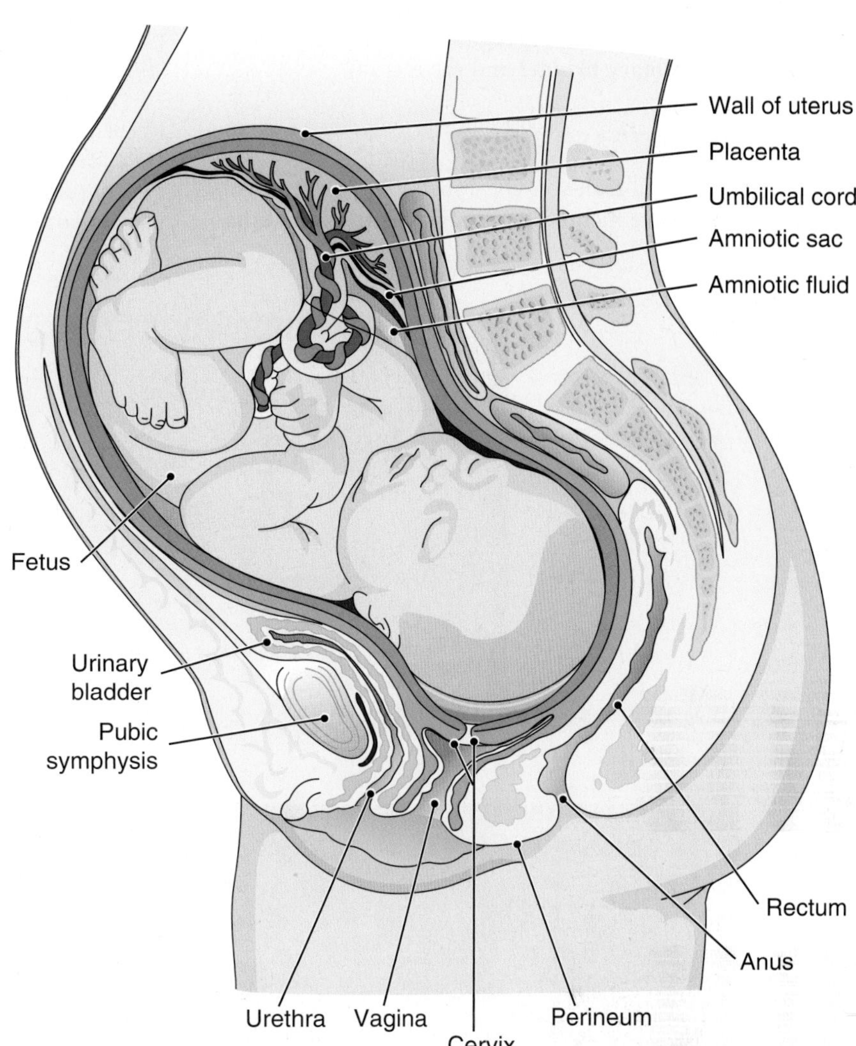

Figure 21-5 Midsagittal section of a pregnant uterus with intact fetus.
KEY POINT The fetus is contained in an amniotic sac filled with amniotic fluid.
ZOOMING IN What structure connects the fetus to the placenta?

approximately 1.1 kg (2.4 lb). At the end of pregnancy, the normal length of the fetus is 45 to 56 cm (18 to 22.5 in.), and the weight varies from 2.7 to 4.5 kg (6 to 10 lb).

The **amniotic** (am-ne-OT-ik) **sac**, which is filled with a clear liquid known as **amniotic fluid**, surrounds the fetus and serves as a protective cushion for it (Fig. 21-5). The amniotic sac ruptures at birth, an event marked by the common expression that the mother's "water broke."

During development, the fetal skin is protected by a layer of cheeselike material called the **vernix caseosa** (VER-niks ka-se-O-sah) (literally, "cheesy varnish").

THE MOTHER

The total period of pregnancy, from fertilization of the ovum to birth, is approximately 266 days, also given as 280 days or 40 weeks from the last menstrual period (LMP). During this time, the mother must supply all the food and oxygen for the fetus and eliminate its waste materials. To support the additional demands of the growing fetus, the mother's metabolism changes markedly, and several organ systems increase their output:

- The heart pumps more blood to supply the needs of the uterus and the fetus.
- The lungs provide more oxygen by increasing the rate and depth of respiration.
- The kidneys excrete nitrogenous wastes from both the fetus and the mother.
- The digestive system supplies additional nutrients for the growth of maternal organs (uterus and breasts) and fetal growth, as well as for subsequent labor and milk secretion.

Nausea and vomiting are common discomforts in early pregnancy. These most often occur upon arising or during periods of fatigue, and are more common in women who smoke. The specific cause of these symptoms is not known, but they may be due to the great changes in hormone levels that occur at this time. The nausea and vomiting usually last for only a few weeks to several months.

Urinary frequency and constipation are often present during the early stages of pregnancy and then usually disappear. They may reappear late in pregnancy as the fetus' head drops from the abdominal region down into the pelvis, pressing on the urinary bladder and the rectum.

THE USE OF ULTRASOUND IN OBSTETRICS

Ultrasonography (ul-trah-son-OG-rah-fe) is a safe, painless, and noninvasive method for studying soft tissue. It has proved extremely valuable for monitoring pregnancies and childbirth.

An ultrasound image, called a *sonogram*, is made by sending high-frequency sound waves into the body (Fig. 21-6). Each time a wave meets an interface between two tissues of different densities, an echo is produced. An instrument called a *transducer* converts the reflected sound

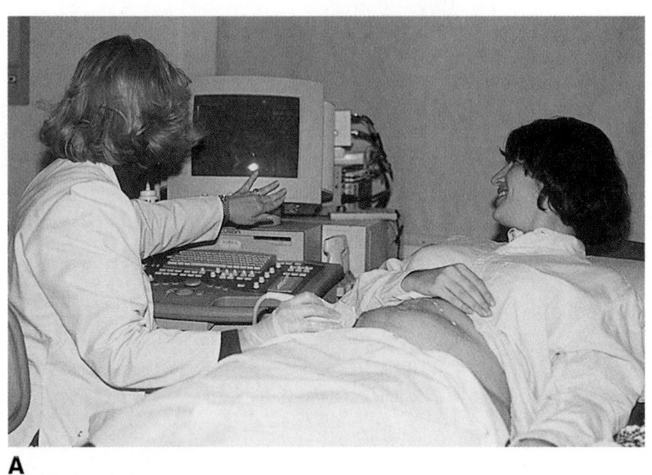

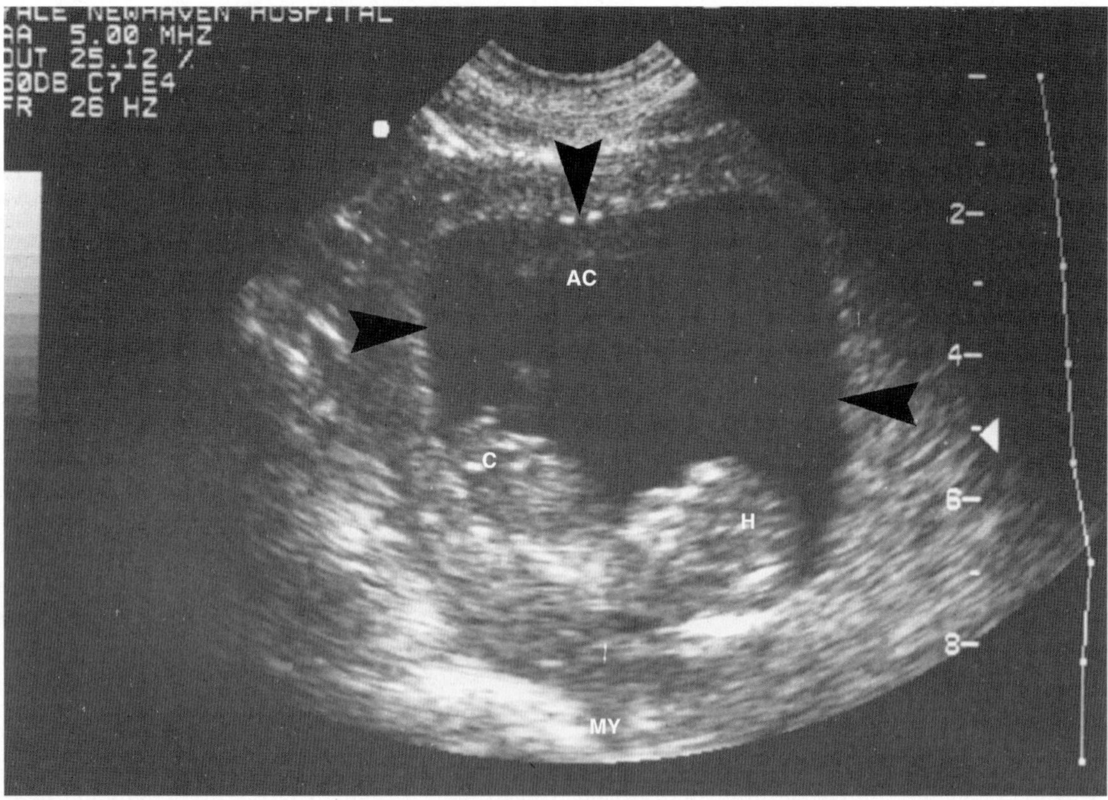

Figure 21-6 Sonography. KEY POINT Ultrasound is used to monitor pregnancy and childbirth. **A.** A sonogram is recorded as a mother views her baby on the monitor. **B.** Sonogram of a pregnant uterus at 11 weeks showing the amniotic cavity (AC) filled with amniotic fluid. The fetus is seen in longitudinal section showing the head (H) and coccyx (C). The myometrium (MY) of the uterus is also seen.
(A, Reprinted with permission from Pillitteri A. *Maternal & Child Health Nursing,* 6th ed. Philadelphia, PA: Lippincott Williams & Wilkins, 2009. B, Reprinted with permission from Scoutt L. *Clinical Anatomy by Regions*, 8th ed. Philadelphia, PA: Lippincott Williams & Wilkins, 2009.)

waves into electrical energy, and a computer is used to generate an image on a viewing screen.

Ultrasound scans can be used in obstetrics to diagnose pregnancy, judge fetal age, and determine the location of the placenta. The technique can also show the presence of excess amniotic fluid and fetal abnormalities (see Fig. 21-6B).

CHECKPOINTS 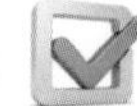

21-5 At about what time in gestation does the heartbeat first appear?

21-6 What is the name of the fluid-filled sac that holds the fetus?

21-7 What is the approximate duration of pregnancy in days from the time of fertilization?

Childbirth

The exact mechanisms that trigger the beginning of uterine contractions for childbirth are still not completely known. Some fetal and maternal factors that probably work in combination to start labor are:

- Stretching of the uterine muscle stimulates production of prostaglandin, which promotes uterine contractions.
- Pressure on the cervix from the baby stimulates release of **oxytocin** (ok-se-TO-sin) from the posterior pituitary. Oxytocin stimulates uterine contractions, and the uterine muscle becomes increasingly sensitive to this hormone late in pregnancy.
- Changes in the placenta that occur with time may contribute to the start of labor.
- Cortisol from the fetal adrenal cortex inhibits the mother's progesterone production. Increase in the relative amount of estrogen as compared to progesterone stimulates uterine contractions.

After labor begins, stimuli from the cervix and vagina induce reflex secretion of oxytocin, which in turn increases the uterine contractions.

POSITIVE FEEDBACK

The events that occur in childbirth involve **positive feedback**, a type of feedback mechanism we have not yet discussed. Positive feedback is much less common than the negative feedback illustrated many times in previous chapters. Whereas negative feedback reverses a condition to bring it back to a norm, positive feedback intensifies a response. (Think of a fist fight escalating among a group of people.) Activity continues until resources are exhausted, the stimulus is removed, or some outside force interrupts the activity. (In our fight analogy, people tire, the original fighters are separated,

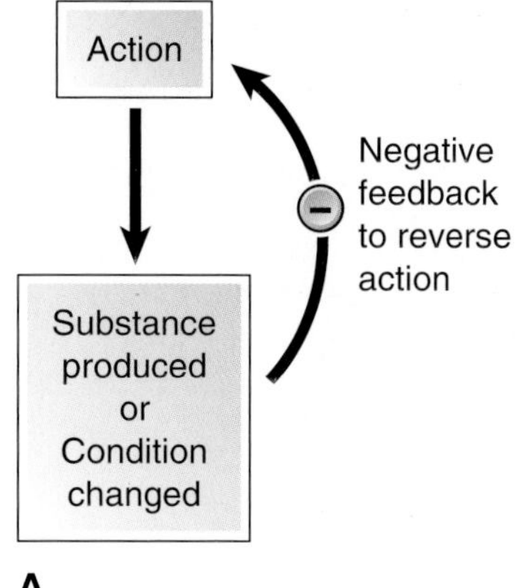

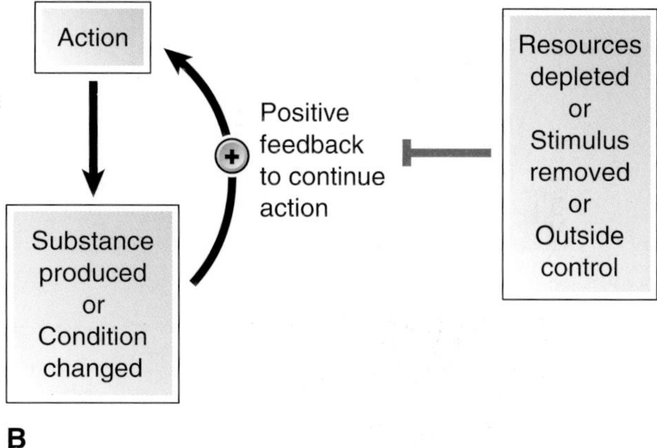

Figure 21-7 Comparison of positive and negative feedback. KEY POINT **A.** Negative feedback maintains homeostasis, bringing changes back to a norm. **B.** Positive feedback intensifies responses until the feedback loop is interrupted. ZOOMING IN What possible forces can stop a positive feedback system?

or the police arrive to break things up!). The diagrams in Figure 21-7 compare negative and positive feedback.

During childbirth, for example, cervical stretching stimulates the pituitary to release oxytocin. This hormone stimulates further uterine contractions. As contractions increase in force, the cervix is stretched even more, causing further release of oxytocin. The escalating contractions and hormone release continue until the baby is born and the stimulus is removed.

THE FOUR STAGES OF LABOR

The process by which the fetus is expelled from the uterus is known as **labor** or *parturition* (par-tu-RISH-un) (Fig. 21-8). It is divided into four stages:

1. The **first stage** begins with the onset of regular uterine contractions. With each contraction, the cervix becomes thinner and the cervical canal larger. Rupture of the amniotic sac may occur at any time, with a gush of fluid from the vagina.

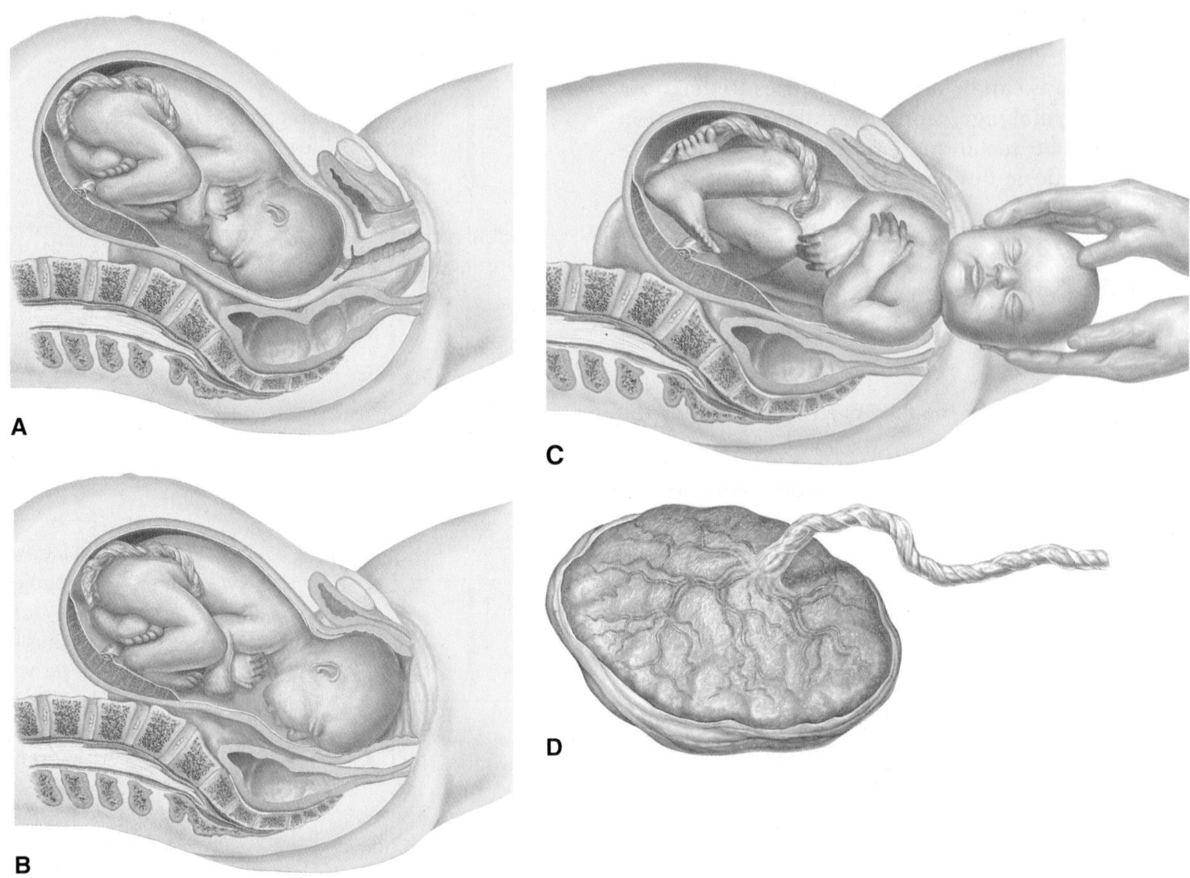

Figure 21-8 **Stages of labor.** The first stage **(A)** begins with the onset of uterine contractions; the second stage **(B,C)** begins when the cervix is completely dilated and ends with birth of the baby; the third stage **(D)** includes expulsion of the afterbirth. A fourth stage (not shown) involves control of bleeding and uterine contractions. (Reprinted with permission from Anatomical Chart Company. *OB/GYN Disorders*, Philadelphia, PA: Lippincott Williams & Wilkins, 2008.)

2. The **second stage** begins when the cervix is completely dilated and ends with the baby's birth. This stage involves the passage of the fetus, usually head first, through the cervical canal and the vagina to the outside **(see Figs. 21-8B,C)**. To prevent tissues of the pelvic floor from being torn during childbirth, as often happens, the obstetrician may cut the mother's perineum just before her infant is born; such an operation is called an **episiotomy** (eh-piz-e-OT-o-me). The area between the vagina and the anus that is cut in an episiotomy is referred to as the surgical or obstetrical perineum. (See **Fig. 20-12** in Chapter 20.)
3. The **third stage** begins after the child is born and ends with the expulsion of the *afterbirth*; that is, the placenta, the membranes of the amniotic sac, and the umbilical cord, except for a small portion remaining attached to the baby's umbilicus (um-BIL-ih-kus), or navel **(see Fig. 21-8D)**.
4. The **fourth stage** begins after expulsion of the afterbirth and constitutes a period in which bleeding is controlled. Contraction of the uterine muscle acts to close off the blood vessels leading to the placental site. If an episiotomy was performed, the obstetrician now repairs this clean cut.

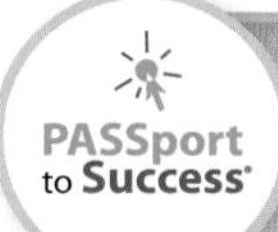

See the Student Resources on *thePoint* for information on midwives and other birth assistants.

CESAREAN SECTION

A **cesarean** (se-ZAR-re-an) **section** (C section) is an incision made in the abdominal wall and uterine wall through which the fetus is manually removed from the mother's body. A cesarean section may be required for a variety of reasons, including placental abnormalities; abnormal fetal position; disproportion between the head of the fetus and the mother's pelvis that makes vaginal birth difficult or dangerous; and other problems that may arise during pregnancy and labor.

MULTIPLE BIRTHS

Until recently, statistics indicated that twins occurred in about 1 of every 80 to 90 births, varying somewhat in different countries. Triplets occurred much less frequently, usually once in several thousand births, whereas quadruplets occurred very rarely. The birth of quintuplets represented a historic event unless the mother had taken fertility drugs. Now these fertility drugs, usually gonadotropins, are given more commonly, and the number of multiple births has increased significantly. Multiple fetuses tend to be born prematurely and therefore have a high death rate. However, better care of infants and newer treatments have resulted in more living multiple births than ever.

Twins originate in two different ways, and on this basis are divided into two types:

- **Fraternal twins** result from the fertilization of two different ova by two spermatozoa. Two completely different individuals, as distinct from each other as brothers and sisters of different ages, are produced. Each fetus has its own placenta and surrounding amniotic sac.
- **Identical twins** develop from a single zygote formed from a single ovum fertilized by a single spermatozoon. Sometime during the early stages of development, the embryonic cells separate into two units. Usually, there is a single placenta, although there must be a separate umbilical cord for each fetus. Identical twins are always the same sex and carry the same inherited traits.

Other multiple births may be fraternal, identical, or combinations of these. The tendency to multiple births seems to be hereditary.

PREGNANCY OUTCOMES

An infant born between 37 and 42 weeks of gestation is described as a **term infant.** However, a pregnancy may end before its full term has been completed. The term **live birth** is used if the baby breathes or shows any evidence of life such as heartbeat, pulsation of the umbilical cord, or movement of voluntary muscles. Infants born before the 37th week of gestation are considered **preterm**. Often these babies have low birth weight of less than 2,500 g (5.5 lb) and are immature (premature) in development. They are subject to a number of medical conditions, including anemia, jaundice, respiratory problems, and feeding difficulties.

Loss of the fetus is classified according to the duration of the pregnancy:

- The term **abortion** refers to loss of the embryo or fetus before the 20th week or weight of about 500 g (1.1 lb). This loss can be either spontaneous or induced.
    - **Spontaneous abortion** occurs naturally with no interference. The most common causes are related to an abnormality of the embryo or fetus. Other causes include abnormality of the mother's reproductive organs, infections, or chronic disorders, such as kidney disease or hypertension. **Miscarriage** is the lay term for spontaneous abortion.
    - **Induced abortion** occurs as a result of deliberate interruption of pregnancy. A **therapeutic abortion** is an abortion performed by a physician as a treatment for a variety of reasons. More liberal access to this type of abortion has dramatically reduced the incidence of death related to illegal abortion.
- The term **fetal death** refers to loss of the fetus after the eighth week of pregnancy. **Stillbirth** refers to the birth of an infant who is lifeless.

Immaturity is a leading cause of death in the newborn. After the 20th week of pregnancy, the fetus is considered **viable**, that is, able to live outside the uterus. A fetus expelled before the 24th week or before reaching a weight of 1,000 g (2.2 lb) has little more than a 50% chance of survival; one born at a point closer to the full 38 weeks of gestation stands a much better chance of living. However, increasing numbers of immature infants are being saved because of advances in neonatal intensive care.

Hospitals use the Apgar score to assess a newborn's health and predict survival. Five features, such as respiration, pulse, etc., are rated as 0, 1, or 2 at 1 minute and 5 minutes after birth. The maximum possible score on each test is 10. Infants with low scores require medical attention and have lower survival rates.

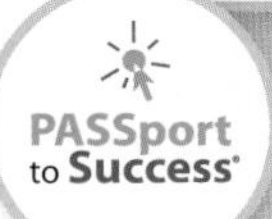

See the Student Resources on *thePoint* for the Apgar scoring system.

CHECKPOINTS 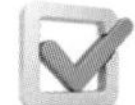

- 21-8 What is parturition?
- 21-9 What is a cesarean section?
- 21-10 What does the term *viable* mean with reference to a fetus?

The Mammary Glands and Lactation

The **mammary glands**, contained in the female breasts, are associated organs of the reproductive system. They provide nourishment for the baby after its birth. The mammary glands are similar in construction to the sweat glands. Each gland is divided into a number of lobes composed of glandular tissue and fat, and each lobe is further subdivided. Secretions from the lobes are conveyed through **lactiferous** (lak-TIF-er-us) **ducts**, all of which converge at the papilla (nipple) **(Fig. 21-9)**.

21

The mammary glands begin developing during puberty, but they do not become functional until the end of a pregnancy. As already noted, estrogen and progesterone during pregnancy help prepare the breasts for lactation, as do prolactin (PRL) from the anterior pituitary and placental lactogen (hPL). The first mammary gland secretion is a thin liquid called **colostrum** (ko-LOS-trum). It is nutritious but has a somewhat different composition from milk. Milk

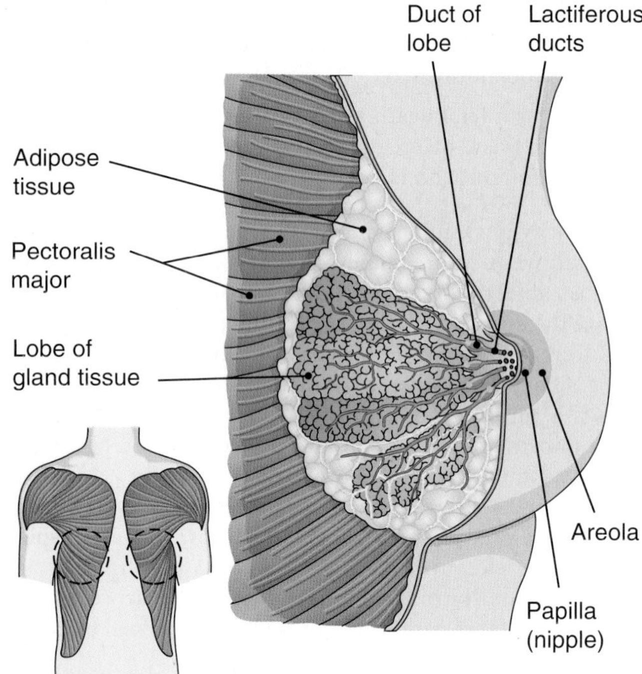

Figure 21-9 Section of the breast (mammary gland). KEY POINT The glands are divided into lobes containing milk ducts that converge at the nipple. ZOOMING IN What muscle underlies the breast?

secretion begins within a few days following birth and can continue for several years as long as milk is frequently removed by the suckling baby or by pumping. In another example of positive feedback, the nursing infant's suckling at the breast promotes release of PRL, which activates the mammary glands' secretory cells. Nursing also stimulates oxytocin release from the posterior pituitary. This hormone causes the milk ducts to contract, resulting in the ejection, or *letdown*, of milk.

The newborn baby's digestive tract is not ready for the usual adult mixed diet. Mother's milk is more desirable for the young infant than milk from other animals for several reasons, some of which are listed below:

- Infections that may be transmitted by foods exposed to the outside air are avoided by nursing.
- Both breast milk and colostrum contain maternal antibodies that help protect the baby against pathogens.
- The proportions of various nutrients and other substances in human milk are perfectly suited to the human infant, changing within a single feeding from a watery fluid that quenches the infant's thirst to a fluid rich in fat that satisfies the infant's hunger. The composition of breast milk also changes over time as the infant grows. Substitutes are not exact imitations of human milk. Nutrients are present in more desirable amounts if the mother's diet is well balanced.
- The psychological and emotional benefits of nursing are of infinite value to both the mother and the infant.

CHECKPOINT

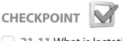

- [ ] 21-11 What is lactation?

Heredity

We are often struck by the resemblance of a baby to one or both of its parents, yet rarely do we stop to consider *how* various traits are transmitted from parents to offspring. This subject—heredity—has fascinated humans for thousands of years. The *Old Testament* contains numerous references to heredity (although the word itself was unknown in biblical times). It was not until the 19th Century, however, that methodical investigation into heredity was begun. At that time, an Austrian monk, Gregor Mendel, discovered through his experiments with garden peas that there was a precise pattern in the appearance of differences among parents and their **progeny** (PROJ-eh-ne), their offspring or descendants. Mendel's most important contribution to the understanding of heredity was the demonstration that there are independent units of heredity in the cells. Later, these independent units were given the name **genes**.

GENES AND CHROMOSOMES

Genes are actually segments of DNA contained in the threadlike chromosomes within the nucleus of each cell. (Only the mature red blood cell, which has lost its nucleus, lacks DNA.) Genes govern cells by controlling the manufacture of proteins, especially enzymes, which are necessary for all the chemical reactions that occur within the cell. They also contain the information to make the proteins that constitute structural materials, hormones, and growth factors. This is a good time to look back at Chapter 3, which has details on chromosomes, genes, and DNA **(see Figs. 3-14 and 3-15)**.

When body cells divide by the process of mitosis, the DNA that makes up the chromosomes is replicated and distributed to the daughter cells, so that each daughter cell gets exactly the same kind and number of chromosomes as were in the original cell **(see Fig. 3-18)**. Each chromosome (aside from the Y chromosome, which determines male sex) may carry thousands of genes, and each gene carries the code for a specific **trait** (characteristic). These traits constitute the physical, biochemical, and physiologic makeup of every cell in the body. (See **Box 21-2** on modern studies of the human genetic make-up.)

In humans, every nucleated cell except the gametes (reproductive cells) contains 46 chromosomes. The chromosomes exist in pairs. One member of each pair was received at the time of fertilization from the offspring's father, and one was received from the mother. The paired chromosomes, except for the pair that determines sex, are

Box 21-2 *Hot Topics*

The Human Genome Project: Reading the Book of Life

Packed tightly in nearly every one of your body cells (except the red blood cells) is a complete copy of your genome—the genetic instructions that direct all of your cellular activities. Written in the language of deoxyribonucleic acid (DNA), these instructions consist of genes parceled into 46 chromosomes that code for proteins. In 1990, a consortium of scientists from around the world set out to crack the genetic code and read the human genome, our "book of life." This monumental task, called the Human Genome Project, was completed in 2003 and succeeded in mapping the entire human genome—3 billion DNA base pairs arranged into about 20,000 to 25,000 genes. Now, scientists can pinpoint the exact location and chemical code of every gene in the body.

The human genome was decoded using a technique called sequencing. Samples of human DNA were fragmented into smaller pieces and then inserted into bacteria. As the bacteria multiplied, they produced more and more copies of the human DNA fragments, which the scientists extracted. The DNA copies were loaded into a sequencing machine capable of "reading" the string of DNA nucleotides that composed each fragment. Then, using computers, the scientists put all of the sequences from the fragments back together to get the entire human genome.

Now, scientists hope to use all these pages of the book of life to revolutionize the treatment of human disease. The information obtained from the Human Genome Project may lead to improved disease diagnosis, new drug treatments, and even gene therapy.

alike in size and appearance. Thus, each body cell has one pair of sex chromosomes and 22 pairs (44 chromosomes) that are not involved in sex determination and are known as **autosomes** (AW-to-somes).

The paired autosomes carry genes for the same traits at exactly the same sites on each. Any gene that appears at a specific site on a chromosome is called an **allele** (al-LEEL). Because our chromosomes are paired, the alleles for each trait are also paired on the matching chromosomes. For example, Ben in the case study inherits an allele from each parent that will determine whether he has cystic fibrosis or not.

DOMINANT AND RECESSIVE GENES

Another of Mendel's discoveries was that genes can be either dominant or recessive. A **dominant** gene is one that expresses its effect in the cell regardless of whether its allele on the matching chromosome is the same as or different from the dominant gene. The gene needs to be received from only one parent to be expressed in the offspring. When the matching genes for a trait are different, the alleles are described as **heterozygous** (het-er-o-ZI-gus) or hybrid.

The effect of a **recessive** gene is not evident unless its paired allele on the matching chromosome is also recessive. Thus, a recessive trait appears only if the recessive genes for that trait are received from both parents. A simple test, often done in biology labs to study genetic inheritance, is a test for the ability to taste phenylthiocarbamide (PTC), a harmless organic chemical not found in food. The ability to detect PTC's bitter taste is inherited as a dominant gene. Inability to taste it is carried by a recessive gene. Thus, nontasting appears in an offspring only if genes for nontasting are received from both parents. When both the genes for a trait are the same, that is, both dominant or both recessive, the alleles are said to be **homozygous** (ho-mo-ZI-gus) or purebred. A recessive trait only appears if a person's genes are homozygous for that trait. In contrast, a dominant trait will appear whether the genes are homozygous (both dominant) or heterozygous (one of each) because a dominant gene is always expressed if it is present.

Any characteristic that can be observed or can be tested for is part of a person's **phenotype** (FE-no-tipe). Eye color, for example, can be seen when looking at a person. Blood type is not visible but can be determined by testing and is also a part of a person's phenotype. When someone has the recessive phenotype, his or her genetic makeup, or **genotype** (JEN-o-tipe), is obviously homozygous recessive. When a dominant phenotype appears, the person's genotype can be either homozygous dominant or heterozygous, as noted above. Only genetic studies or family studies can reveal which it is.

A recessive gene is not expressed if it is present in a cell together with a dominant allele. However, the recessive gene can be passed onto offspring and may thus appear in future generations. An individual who shows no evidence of a trait but has a recessive gene for that trait is described as a **carrier** of the gene. Using genetic terminology, that person shows the dominant phenotype but has a heterozygous genotype for that trait. Using our PTC tasting example, a taster might be a carrier for the nontasting gene and could pass it on to his or her children.

DISTRIBUTION OF CHROMOSOMES TO OFFSPRING

The reproductive cells (ova and spermatozoa) are produced by a special process of cell division called **meiosis** (mi-O-sis) (Fig. 21-10). This process divides the chromosome number in half, so that each reproductive cell has 23 chromosomes instead of the 46 in other body cells. The process of meiosis begins, as does mitosis, with replication of the chromosomes. (See Fig. 3-18 in Chapter 3.) Then, these duplicated chromosomes line up across the center of the cell. However, instead of a random distribution of the 46 chromosomes, as occurs in mitosis, there is a pairing of the matching chromosomes that came from each parent (see Fig. 21-10).

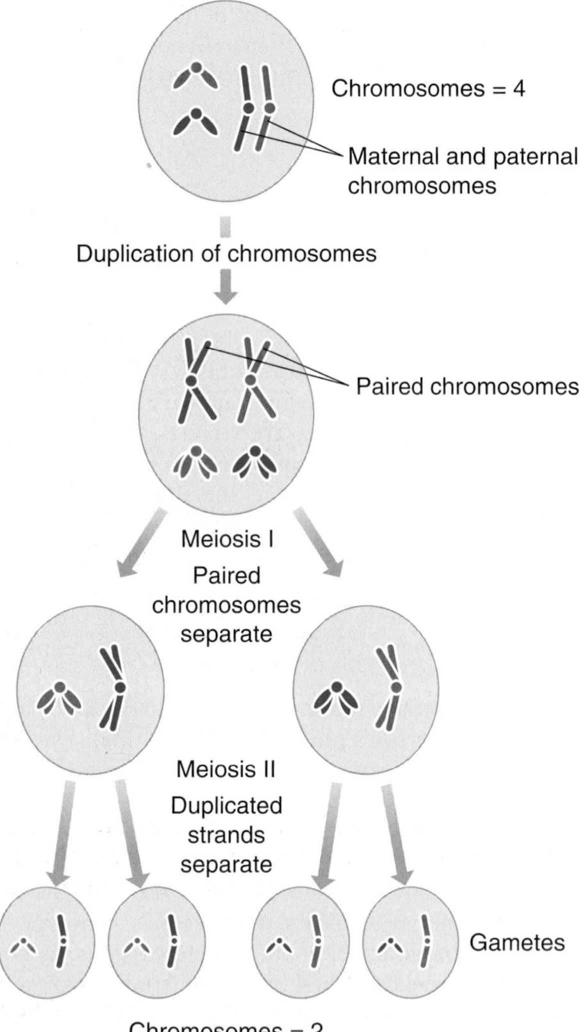

Figure 21-10 Meiosis. KEY POINT Meiosis halves the chromosome number in formation of gametes. Because the process begins with chromosome replication, two meiotic divisions are needed, first to reduce the chromosome number and then to separate the duplicated strands. The example shows a cell with a chromosome number of 4, in contrast to a human cell, which has 46 chromosomes. ZOOMING IN How many chromosomes are present in a human gamete?

The first meiotic division (meiosis I) distributes the maternal and paternal chromosomes into separate cells. Then, a second meiotic division (meiosis II) separates the strands of the duplicated chromosomes and distributes each strand to an individual gamete. In the end, each gamete receives one member of each chromosome pair that was present in the original cell.

It is very important to note that the separation of the chromosome pairs occurs at random, meaning that either member of a given pair may be included in a gamete. Looking at Figure 21-10, you will see that the color-coded maternal and paternal chromosomes are randomly distributed. This reassortment of chromosomes in the gametes leads to increased variety within the population. (In a human cell with 46 chromosomes, the chances for varying combinations are much greater than in the example shown in Figure 21-10.) Thus, children in a family resemble each other, but no two look exactly alike (unless they are identical twins), because they receive different combinations of maternal and paternal chromosomes.

Geneticists use a grid called a **Punnett square** to show all the combinations of genes that can result from a given parental cross, that is, a mating that produces offspring (Fig. 21-11). In these calculations, a capital letter is used for the dominant gene and the recessive gene is represented by the lower case of the same letter. For example, if T represents the gene for the dominant trait PTC taster, then

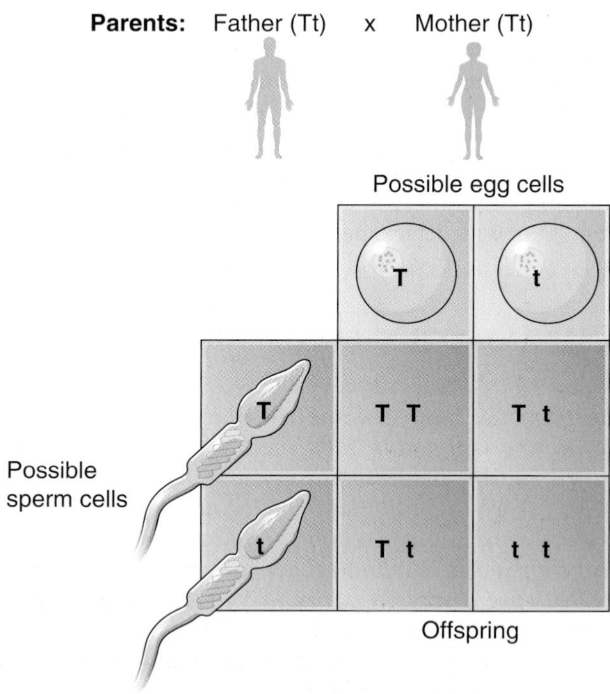

Figure 21-11 A Punnett square. KEY POINT Geneticists use this grid to show all the possible combinations of a given cross, in this case, Tt ×Tt. ZOOMING IN What percentage of children from this cross will show the recessive phenotype? What percentage will be heterozygous?

t would be the recessive gene for nontaster. In the offspring, the genotype TT is homozygous dominant and the genotype Tt is heterozygous, both of which will show the dominant phenotype taster. The homozygous recessive genotype tt will show the recessive phenotype nontaster.

A Punnett square shows all the possible gene combinations of a given cross and the theoretical ratios of all the genotypes produced. For example, in the cross shown in **Figure 21-11,** the theoretical chances of producing a baby with the genotype TT are 25% (1 in 4). The chances of producing a baby with the genotype of tt and the recessive phenotype nontaster are also 25%. The chances of producing heterozygous Tt offspring for this trait are 50% (2 in 4). In all, 75% of the offspring will have the dominant phenotype taster, because they have at least one dominant gene for the trait. In Ben's case, because CF is determined by a recessive gene, there was a 25% chance that he would have CF, because both his parents are carriers for the gene. If his parents have other children, the risk is the same with each birth.

In real life, genetic ratios may differ from the theoretical predictions, especially if the number of offspring is small. For example, the chances of having a male or female baby are 50–50 with each birth, for reasons explained shortly, but a family might have several girls before having a boy, and vice versa. The chances of seeing the predicted ratios improve as the number of offspring increases.

SEX DETERMINATION

The two chromosomes that determine the offspring's sex, unlike the autosomes (the other 22 pairs of chromosomes), are not matched in size and appearance. The female X chromosome is larger than most other chromosomes and carries genes for other characteristics in addition to that for sex. The male Y chromosome is smaller than other chromosomes and mainly determines sex. A female has two X chromosomes in each body cell; a male has one X from his mother and one Y from his father.

By the process of meiosis, each sperm cell receives either an X or a Y chromosome, whereas every ovum receives only an X chromosome **(Fig. 21-12)**. If a sperm cell with an X chromosome fertilizes an ovum, the resulting infant will be female; if a sperm with a Y chromosome fertilizes an ovum, the resulting infant will be male.

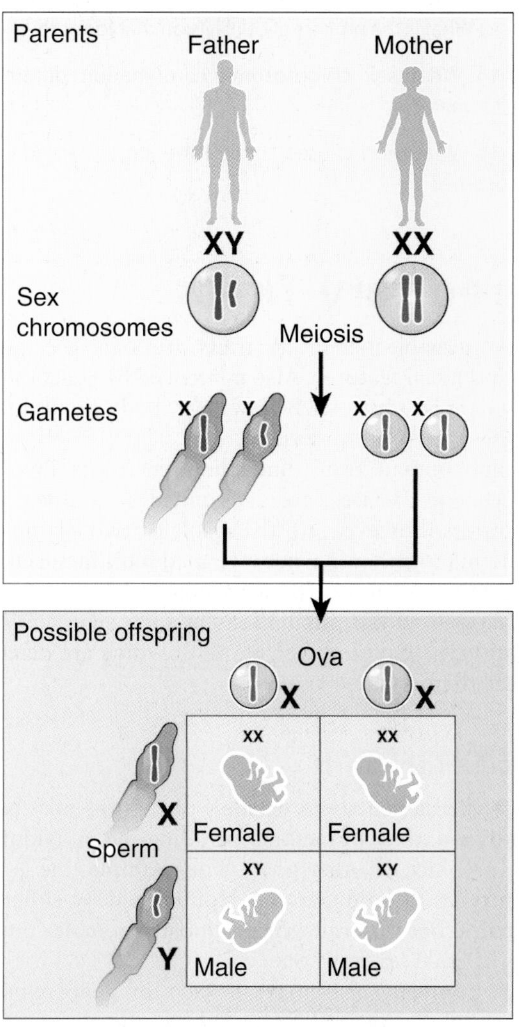

Figure 21-12 **Sex determination.** KEY POINT If an X chromosome from a male unites with an X chromosome from a female, the child is female (XX); if a Y chromosome from a male unites with an X chromosome from a female, the child is male (XY). ZOOMING IN What is the expected ration of male to female offspring in a family?

SEX-LINKED TRAITS

Any trait that is carried on a sex chromosome is said to be **sex-linked**. Because the Y chromosome carries few traits aside from sex determination, most sex-linked traits are carried on the X chromosome and are best described as *X-linked*. Examples are hemophilia, certain forms of baldness, and red-green color blindness.

Sex-linked traits appear almost exclusively in males. The reason for this is that most of these traits are recessive, and if a recessive gene is located on the X chromosome in a male it cannot be masked by a matching dominant gene. (Remember that the Y chromosome with which the X chromosome pairs is very small and carries few genes.) Thus, a male who has only one recessive gene for a trait will exhibit that characteristic, whereas a female must have two recessive genes to show the trait. The female must inherit a recessive gene for that trait from each parent and be homozygous recessive in order for the trait to appear. The daughter of a man with an X-linked disorder is always at least a carrier of the gene for that disorder, because a daughter always receives her father's single X chromosome. So, for example, if you are female and your father is color-blind, then each of your sons will have a 50/50 chance of being color-blind.

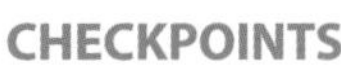
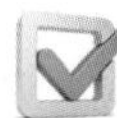

CHECKPOINTS

☐ 21-12 What is a gene? What is a gene made of?

☐ 21-13 What is the difference between a dominant and a recessive gene?

☐ **21-14** What is the process of cell division that forms the gametes?

☐ **21-15** What sex chromosome combination determines a female? A male?

☐ **21-16** What term is used to describe a trait carried on a sex chromosome?

Hereditary Traits

Some observable hereditary traits are skin, eye, and hair color and facial features. Also influenced by genetics are less clearly defined traits, such as weight, body build, life span, and susceptibility to disease.

Some human traits, including the traits involved in many genetic diseases, are determined by a single pair of genes; most, however, are the result of two or more gene pairs acting together in what is termed **multifactorial inheritance.** This type of inheritance accounts for the wide range of variations within populations in such characteristics as coloration, height, and weight, all of which are determined by more than one pair of genes.

GENE EXPRESSION

The effect of a gene on a person's phenotype may be influenced by a variety of factors, including the individual's sex or the presence of other genes. For example, the genes for certain types of baldness may be inherited by either males or females, but the traits appear mostly in males under the effects of male sex hormone.

Environment also plays a part in gene expression. For example, a person might inherit the dominant gene for freckles, but the freckles appear only when the skin is exposed to sunlight. In the case of multifactorial inheritance, gene expression might be quite complex. You inherit a potential for a given size, for example, but your actual size is additionally influenced by such factors as nutrition, development, and general state of health. The same is true of life span and susceptibility to diseases.

We should also note here that dominance is not always clear-cut. Sometimes, dominant genes are expressed together as *codominance*. Take the inheritance of blood type, for example. Genes for type A and type B are dominant over O. A person with the genotype AO is type A; a person with the genotype BO is type B. However, neither A nor B is dominant over the other. If a person inherits a gene for both A and B, his or her blood type is AB. Also, a person heterozygous for a certain trait may show some intermediate expression of the trait. The term for this type of gene interaction is *incomplete dominance.*

GENETIC MUTATION

Any change in a gene or a chromosome is termed a genetic **mutation** (mu-TA-shun). Mutations may occur spontaneously or may be induced by some agent, such as ionizing radiation or a chemical, described as a **mutagen**

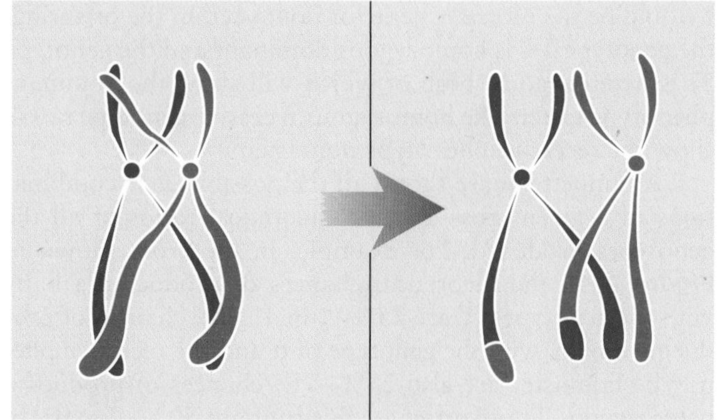

Figure 21-13 Genetic exchange. KEY POINT In cell division, chromosomes tangle and exchange sections. These exchanges may be equal, maintaining a normal genetic makeup. They may also result in losses or duplications known as mutations.

(MU-tah-jen) or mutagenic agent. Often, these changes occur during cell division (mitosis or meiosis) as chromosomes come together, reassort, and get distributed to two new cells. The long, threadlike chromosomes can intertwine and exchange segments **(Fig. 21-13)**. Sometimes these exchanges are equivalent, and the total genetic material remains normal, but sometimes genes are damaged or there is a loss, duplication, or rearrangement of the genetic material. These changes may involve a single gene, a portion of a chromosome, or whole chromosomes.

If a mutation occurs in an ovum or a spermatozoon, the altered trait may be inherited by an offspring. The vast majority of harmful mutations never are expressed because the affected fetus dies and is spontaneously aborted. Most remaining mutations are so inconsequential that they have no detectable effect. Beneficial mutations, on the other hand, tend to survive and increase as a population evolves.

MITOCHONDRIAL INHERITANCE

Although we have emphasized the nucleus as the repository of genetic material in the cell, the mitochondria also contain some hereditary material. Mitochondria, you will recall, are the cells' powerhouse organelles, converting the energy in nutrients into ATP. Because mitochondria were separate organisms early in the evolution of life and later merged with other cells, they have their own DNA and multiply independently. Mitochondrial DNA can mutate, as does nuclear DNA, and disease can be the result. Such diseases can cause serious damage to metabolically active cells in the brain, liver, muscles, kidneys, and endocrine organs. These mitochondrial genes are passed only from a mother to her offspring, because almost all the cytoplasm in the zygote is contributed by the ovum. The head of the spermatozoon, because these cells must be smaller and lighter, carries very little cytoplasm and no mitochondria.

CHECKPOINT 

☐ **21-17** What is a mutation?

A&P in Action Revisited

Managing Ben's Cystic Fibrosis

After learning Ben's diagnosis, his parents met with his pediatrician to discuss the treatment Ben would require to manage his CF. Although the doctor told them that there was no cure for CF yet, they were relieved to hear that there had been vast improvements in treatment in recent years. He explained that the goals of CF treatment were to minimize respiratory and digestive problems.

Therapies for respiratory problems in people with CF center on keeping the lungs clear of mucus that can block the respiratory passageways and provide an excellent growth medium for infectious organisms. Chest physical therapy, which involves pounding the chest and back with either one's hands or a machine, is the main method of removing mucus from the lungs and is repeated three to four times daily. Antiinflammatory and mucolytic (mucus-dissolving) drugs are also useful in loosening mucus from the lungs. Unfortunately, it is difficult to remove all of the mucus, so most people with CF have persistent lung infections, which require antibiotic treatment.

Management of digestive problems also centers on clearing the digestive tract of mucus, as well as ensuring adequate nutrition. Enemas and mucolytic medications are used to treat intestinal mucoid blockages. A high-calorie diet (low in fat and high in protein) improves growth and development and helps the immune system to resist lung infections. Oral pancreatic enzymes are taken before every meal to help the small intestine digest fats and proteins and absorb more vitamins.

In this case, Ben's parents learned about the genetic causes of and treatments for CF. It would take them some time to absorb all of this information, but they were confident that they could minimize Ben's respiratory and digestive problems. To review the respiratory system, see Chapter 16. For a review of the digestive system, see Chapter 17.

Chapter Wrap-Up

Summary Overview

A detailed chapter outline with space for note-taking is on *thePoint*. The figure below illustrates the main topics covered in this chapter.

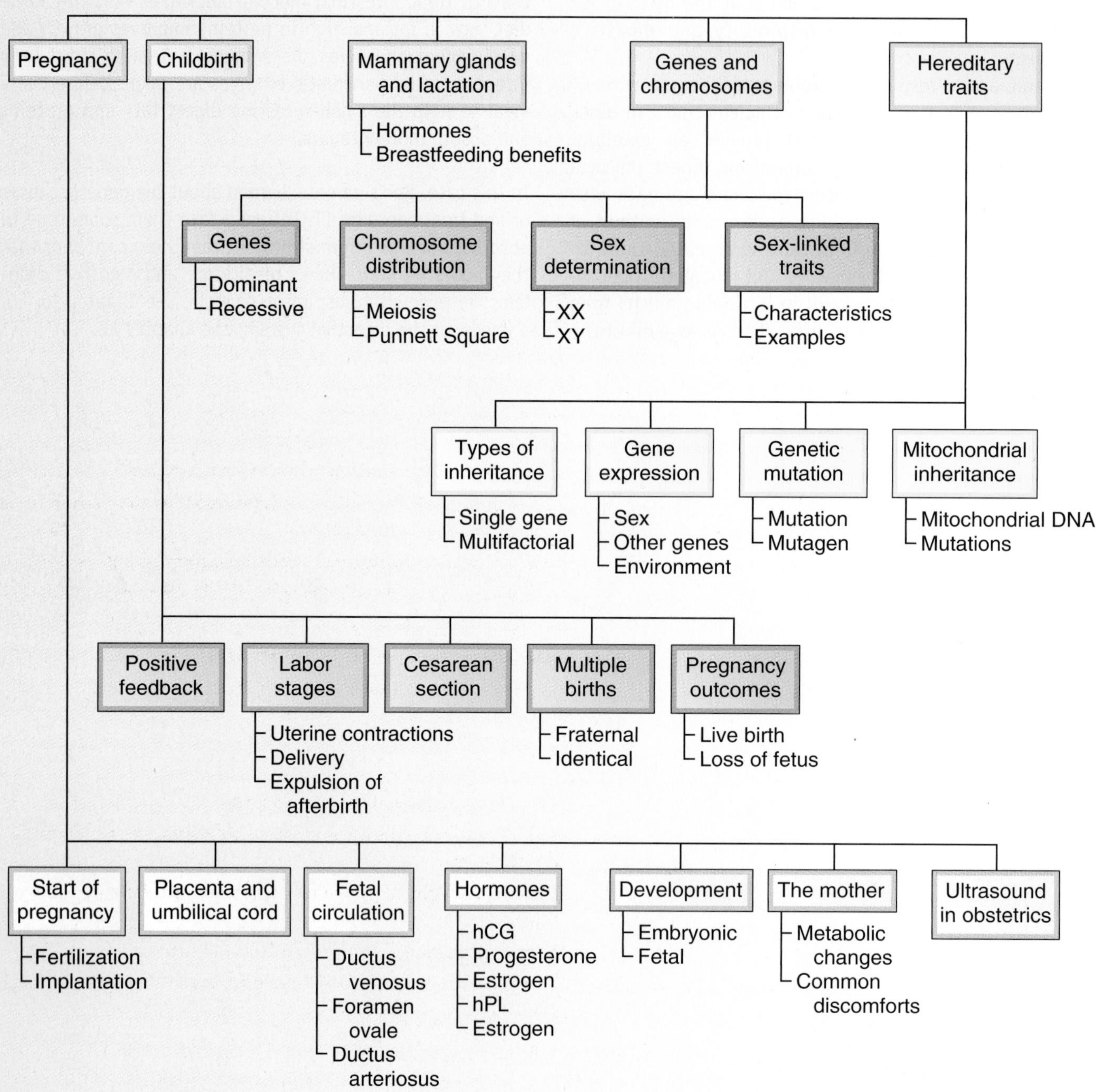

Key Terms

The terms listed below are emphasized in this chapter. Knowing they will help you organize and prioritize your learning. These and other boldface terms are defined in the Glossary with phonetic pronunciations.

abortion
allele
amniotic sac
autosome
carrier
chorion
chromosome
colostrum
dominant
embryo
fertilization
fetus
gene
genetic
genotype
gestation
heredity
heterozygous
homozygous
human chorionic gonadotropin (hCG)
implantation
lactation
meiosis
mutagen
mutation
obstetrics
oxytocin
parturition
phenotype
placenta
progeny
recessive
sex-linked
trait
umbilical cord
zygote

Word Anatomy

Scientific terms are built from standardized word parts (prefixes, roots, and suffixes). Learning the meanings of these parts can help you remember words and interpret unfamiliar terms.

WORD PART	MEANING	EXAMPLE
Pregnancy		
zyg/o	joined	An ovum and spermatozoon join to form a *zygote*.
chori/o	membrane, chorion	Human *chorionic* gonadotropin is produced by the chorion (outermost cells) of the embryo.
somat/o	body	Human chorionic *somatomammotropin* controls nutrients for the body and acts on the mammary glands (mamm/o).
Childbirth		
ox/y	sharp, acute	*Oxytocin* is a hormone that stimulates labor.
toc/o	labor	See preceding example.
Genes and Chromosomes		
chrom/o	color	*Chromosomes* color darkly with stains.
aut/o-	self	*Autosomes* are all the chromosomes aside from the two that determine sex.
heter/o	other, different	*Heterozygous* paired genes (alleles) are different from each other.
homo-	same	*Homozygous* paired genes (alleles) are the same.
phen/o	to show	Traits that can be observed or tested for make up a person's *phenotype*.
Hereditary Traits		
multi-	many	*Multifactorial* traits are determined by multiple pairs of genes.

Questions for Study and Review

BUILDING UNDERSTANDING

Fill in the Blanks

1. Fetal skin is protected by a cheeselike material called_____.
2. The first mammary secretion is called _____.
3. Sound waves can be used to safely monitor pregnancy with a technique called _____.
4. The basic unit of heredity is a(n) _____.
5. Chromosomes not involved in sex determination are known as _____.

Matching > Match each numbered item with the most closely related lettered item.

___ 6. A placental hormone that stimulates the ovaries to secrete progesterone and estrogen

___ 7. A placental hormone that regulates maternal blood nutrient levels

___ 8. A placental hormone that softens the cervix, which widens the birth canal

___ 9. A pituitary hormone that stimulates uterine contractions

___ 10. A pituitary hormone that stimulates maternal milk production

a. human placental lactogen

b. prolactin

c. oxytocin

d. relaxin

e. human chorionic gonadotropin

Multiple Choice

___ 11. What is a morula?

a. a dividing ball of cells that implants in the endometrium
b. the structure that nourishes the fetus
c. the vessel that carries blood from the embryo to the placenta
d. an abnormality of the placenta

___ 12. How long is the average total period of pregnancy, from fertilization to birth?

a. 30 weeks
b. 38 weeks
c. 40 weeks
d. 48 weeks

___ 13. With regard to identical twins, which statement is incorrect?

a. They develop from a single zygote.
b. They share one umbilical cord.
c. They are always the same sex.
d. They carry the same inherited traits.

___ 14. What do genes control the manufacture of?

a. carbohydrates
b. lipids
c. proteins
d. electrolytes

___ 15. What are paired genes for a given trait known as?

a. chromosomes
b. ribosomes
c. nucleotides
d. alleles

UNDERSTANDING CONCEPTS

16. Distinguish among the following: zygote, embryo, and fetus.
17. Explain the role of the placenta in fetal development.
18. Is blood in the umbilical arteries relatively high or low in oxygen? In the umbilical vein?
19. What is the major event of each of the four stages of parturition?
20. List several reasons why breast milk is best for baby.
21. How many chromosomes are there in a human body cell? In a human gamete?
22. Dana has one dominant allele for brown eyes (B) and one recessive allele for blue eyes (b). What is Dana's genotype? What is her phenotype?
23. Describe the process of meiosis and explain how it results in genetic variation.

CONCEPTUAL THINKING

24. If mitosis were used to produce gametes, what consequences would this have on the offspring's genotype, phenotype, and chromosome number?

25. In the case story, Ben's parents were both carriers of the cystic fibrosis trait. Using a Punnett square, calculate the possible genotypic and phenotypic combinations for their offspring.

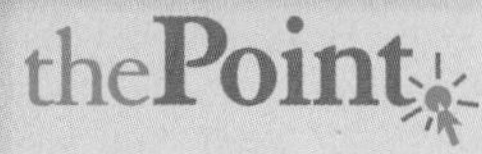

For more questions, see the learning activities on *thePoint.*

Glossary

A

abdominopelvic (ab-dom-ih-no-PEL-vik) Pertaining to the abdomen and pelvis.

abduction (ab-DUK-shun) Movement away from the midline.

abortifacient (ah-bor-tih-FA-shent) Agent that induces an abortion.

abortion (ah-BOR-shun) Loss of an embryo or fetus before the 20th week of pregnancy.

absorption (ab-SORP-shun) Transfer of digested nutrients from the digestive tract into the circulation.

accommodation (ah-kom-o-DA-shun) Coordinated changes in the lens of the eye that enable one to focus on near and far objects.

acetylcholine (as-e-til-KO-lene) **(ACh)** Neurotransmitter; released at synapses within the nervous system and at the neuromuscular junction.

acid (AH-sid) Substance that can donate a hydrogen ion to another substance.

acid-fast stain Procedure used to color cells for viewing under the microscope.

acidosis (as-ih-DO-sis) Condition that results from a decrease in the pH of body fluids.

acrosome (AK-ro-some) Caplike structure over the head of the sperm cell that helps the sperm to penetrate the ovum.

ACTH See adrenocorticotropic hormone.

actin (AK-tin) One of the two contractile proteins in muscle cells, the other being myosin.

action potential Sudden change in the electrical charge on a cell membrane, which then spreads along the membrane; nerve impulse.

active transport Movement of molecules into or out of a cell from an area where they are in lower concentration to an area where they are in higher concentration. Such movement, which is opposite to the direction of normal flow by diffusion, requires energy and transporters.

adduction (ad-DUK-shun) Movement toward the midline.

adenoids (AD-eh-noyds) Popular name for pharyngeal tonsil located in the nasopharynx.

adenosine triphosphate (ah-DEN-o-sene tri-FOS-fate) **(ATP)** Energy-storing compound found in all cells.

ADH See antidiuretic hormone.

adhesion (ad-HE-zhun) Holding together of two surfaces or parts; band of connective tissue between parts that are normally separate; molecular attraction between contacting bodies.

adipose (AD-ih-pose) Referring to fats or a type of connective tissue that stores fat.

adrenal (ah-DRE-nal) **gland** Endocrine gland located above the kidney; suprarenal gland.

adrenaline (ah-DREN-ah-lin) See epinephrine.

adrenergic (ad-ren-ER-jik) An activity or structure that responds to epinephrine (adrenaline).

adrenocorticotropic (ah-dre-no-kor-tih-ko-TRO-pik) hormone (ACTH) Hormone produced by the anterior pituitary that stimulates the adrenal cortex.

aerobic (air-O-bik) Requiring oxygen.

afferent (AF-fer-ent) Carrying toward a given point, such as a sensory neuron that carries nerve impulses toward the central nervous system.

agglutination (ah-glu-tih-NA-shun) Clumping of cells due to an antigen–antibody reaction.

agglutinin (a-GLU-tih-nin) An antibody that causes clumping or agglutination of the agent that stimulated its formation.

agonist (AG-on-ist) Muscle that contracts to perform a given movement.

agranulocyte (a-GRAN-u-lo-site) Leukocyte without visible granules in the cytoplasm when stained; lymphocyte or monocyte.

albumin (al-BU-min) Protein in blood plasma and other body fluids; helps maintain the osmotic pressure of the blood.

aldosterone (al-DOS-ter-one) Hormone released by the adrenal cortex that promotes sodium and water reabsorption in the kidneys.

alkali (AL-kah-li) Substance that can accept a hydrogen ion (H^+); substance that donates a hydroxide ion (OH^-); a base.

alkalosis (al-kah-LO-sis) Condition that results from an increase in the pH of body fluids.

allele (al-LEEL) One member of the gene pair that controls a given trait.

alveolus (al-VE-o-lus) Small sac or pouch; usually a tiny air sac in the lungs through which gases are exchanged between the outside air and the blood; tooth socket; pl., alveoli.

amino (ah-ME-no) **acid** Building block of protein.

amniotic (am-ne-OT-ik) Pertaining to the sac that surrounds and cushions the developing fetus or to the fluid that fills that sac.

amniotic (am-ne-OT-ik) **sac** Fluid-filled sac that surrounds and cushions the developing fetus.

anabolism (ah-NAB-o-lizm) Metabolic building of simple compounds into more complex substances needed by the body.

anaerobic (an-air-O-bik) Not requiring oxygen.

anaphase (AN-ah-faze) The third stage of mitosis in which chromosomes separate to opposite sides of the cell.

anastomosis (ah-nas-to-MO-sis) Communication between two structures, such as blood vessels.

anatomy (ah-NAT-o-me) Study of body structure.

anemia (ah-NE-me-ah) Abnormally low level of hemoglobin or red cells in the blood, resulting in inadequate delivery of oxygen to the tissues.

androgen (AN-dro-jen) Any male sex hormone.

angiotensin (an-je-o-TEN-sin) Substance formed in the blood by the action of the renal enzyme renin; it increases blood pressure by causing vascular constriction, stimulating the release of aldosterone from the adrenal cortex and ADH from the posterior pituitary, and increasing thirst.

anion (AN-i-on) Negatively charged particle (ion).

anoxia (ah-NOK-se-ah) See hypoxia.

ANP See atrial natriuretic peptide.

ANS See autonomic nervous system.

antagonist (an-TAG-o-nist) Muscle that has an action opposite that of a given movement or muscle; substance that opposes the action of another substance.

anterior (an-TE-re-or) Toward the front or belly surface; ventral.

antibody (AN-te-bod-e) **(Ab)** Substance produced in response to a specific antigen; immunoglobulin.

antidiuretic (an-ti-di-u-RET-ik) **hormone (ADH)** Hormone released from the posterior pituitary gland that increases water reabsorption in the kidneys, thus decreasing the urinary output.

antigen (AN-te-jen) **(Ag)** Foreign substance that induces an immune response.

antioxidant (an-te-OX-ih-dant) Substances in the diet that protect against harmful free radicals.

antipyretic (an-ti-pi-RET-ik) Drug that reduces fever.

antiserum (an-te-SE-rum) Serum containing antibodies that may be given to provide passive immunity; immune serum.

anus (A-nus) Inferior opening of the digestive tract.

aorta (a-OR-tah) The largest artery; carries blood out of the heart's left ventricle.

apex (A-peks) Pointed region of a cone-shaped structure.

apnea (AP-ne-ah) Temporary cessation of breathing.

apocrine (AP-o-krin) Referring to a gland that releases some cellular material along with its secretions.

aponeurosis (ap-o-nu-RO-sis) Broad sheet of fibrous connective tissue that attaches muscle to bone or to other muscle.

appendicular (ap-en-DIK-u-lar) **skeleton** Part of the skeleton that includes the bones of the upper extremities, lower extremities, shoulder girdle, and hips.

appendix (ah-PEN-diks) Fingerlike tube of lymphatic tissue attached to the first portion of the large intestine; vermiform (wormlike) appendix.
aquaporin (ak-kwah-POR-in) A transmembrane channel protein that regulates water movement across the plasma membrane.
aqueous (A-kwe-us) Pertaining to water; an aqueous solution is one in which water is the solvent.
aqueous (A-kwe-us) **humor** Watery fluid that fills much of the eyeball anterior to the lens.
arachnoid (ah-RAK-noyd) Middle layer of the meninges.
areolar (ah-RE-o-lar) Referring to loose connective tissue, any small space, or to an areola, a circular area of marked color.
arrector pili (ah-REK-tor PI-li) Muscle attached to a hair follicle that raises the hair.
arteriole (ar-TE-re-ole) Vessel between a small artery and a capillary.
arteriosclerosis (ar-te-re-o-skle-RO-sis) Hardening of the arteries.
artery (AR-ter-e) Vessel that carries blood away from the heart.
arthroscope (AR-thro-skope) Instrument for examining the interior of the knee and surgically repairing the knee.
articular (ar-TIK-u-lar) Pertaining to a joint.
atherosclerosis (ath-er-o-skleh-RO-sis) Hardening of the arteries due to the deposit of yellowish, fatlike material in the lining of these vessels.
atom (AT-om) Smallest subunit of a chemical element.
atomic number The number of protons in the nucleus of an element's atoms; a number characteristic of each element.
atrial natriuretic (na-tre-u-RET-ik) **peptide (ANP)** Hormone produced by the atria of the heart that lowers blood pressure by promoting excretion of sodium and water.
atrioventricular (a-tre-o-ven-TRIK-u-lar) **(AV) node** Part of the heart's conduction system.
atrium (A-tre-um) One of the heart's two upper chambers; adj., atrial.
auditory (AW-dih-tor-e) **tube** Tube that connects the middle ear cavity to the throat; eustachian tube.
autonomic (aw-to-NOM-ik) **nervous system (ANS)** The part of the nervous system that controls smooth muscle, cardiac muscle, and glands; the visceral or involuntary nervous system.
autosome (AW-to-some) Any chromosome not involved in sex determination. There are 44 autosomes (22 pairs) in humans.
AV node See atrioventricular node.
axial (AK-se-al) **skeleton** The part of the skeleton that includes the skull, spinal column, ribs, and sternum.
axilla (ak-SIL-ah) Hollow beneath the arm where it joins the body; armpit.
axon (AK-son) Fiber of a neuron that conducts impulses away from the cell body.

B

band cell Immature neutrophil.
baroreceptor (bar-o-re-SEP-ter) Receptor that responds to pressure, such as those in vessel walls that respond to stretching and help regulate blood pressure; a type of mechanoreceptor.
basal ganglia (BA-sal GANG-le-ah) Gray masses in the lower part of the forebrain that aid in motor planning; basal nuclei
base Substance that can accept a hydrogen ion (H+); substance that donates a hydroxide ion (OH^-); an alkali.
basophil (BA-so-fil) Granular white blood cell that shows large, dark blue cytoplasmic granules when stained with basic stain.
B cell Agranular white blood cell that gives rise to antibody-producing plasma cells in response to an antigen; B lymphocyte.
bicarbonate ion (bi-KAR-bon-ate I-on) Ion formed from carbonic acid along with hydrogen ion.
bile Substance produced in the liver that emulsifies fats.
bilirubin (BIL-ih-ru-bin) Pigment derived from the breakdown of hemoglobin and found in bile.
biofeedback (bi-o-FEED-bak) A method for controlling involuntary responses by means of electronic devices that monitor changes and feed information back to a person.
blood urea nitrogen (BUN) Amount of nitrogen from urea in the blood; test to evaluate kidney function.
bolus (BO-lus) A concentrated mass; the portion of food that is moved to the back of the mouth and swallowed.
Bowman capsule See glomerular capsule.
bone Hard connective tissue that makes up most of the skeleton, or any structure composed of this type of tissue.
bradycardia (brad-e-KAR-de-ah) Heart rate of less than 60 beats per minute.
brain The central controlling area of the central nervous system (**CNS**).
brain stem Portion of the brain that connects the cerebrum with the spinal cord; contains the midbrain, pons, and medulla oblongata.
Broca (bro-KAH) **area** Area of the cerebral cortex concerned with motor control of speech; motor speech area.
bronchiole (BRONG-ke-ole) Microscopic branch of a bronchus.
bronchus (BRONG-kus) Large air passageway in the lung; pl., bronchi (BRONG-ki).
buffer (BUF-er) Substance that prevents sharp changes in a solution's pH.
bulbourethral (bul-bo-u-RE-thral) **gland** Gland that secretes mucus to lubricate the urethra and tip of penis during sexual stimulation; Cowper gland.
bulk transport Movement of large amounts of material through a cell's plasma membrane.
BUN See blood urea nitrogen.
bursa (BER-sah) Small, fluid-filled sac found in an area subject to stress around bones and joints; pl., bursae (BER-se).

C

calcitonin (kal-sih-TO-nin) Thyroid hormone that acts to lower blood calcium levels and promote calcium deposition in bones, but has little or no effect at physiologic levels in humans; thyrocalcitonin.
calcitriol (kal-sih-TRI-ol) The active form of vitamin D; dihydroxycholecalciferol (di-hi-drok-se-ko-le-kal-SIF-eh-rol).
calyx (KA-liks) Cuplike extension of the renal pelvis that collects urine; pl., calyces (KA-lih-seze).
cancellous (KAN-sel-us) Referring to spongy bone tissue.
cancer (KAN-ser) Tumor that spreads to other tissues.
capillary (CAP-ih-lar-e) Microscopic vessel through which exchanges take place between the blood and the tissues.
carbohydrate (kar-bo-HI-drate) Simple sugar or compound made from simple sugars linked together, such as starch or glycogen.
carbon Element that is the basis of organic chemistry.
carbon dioxide (di-OX-ide) (CO_2) Gaseous waste product of cellular metabolism.
carbonic acid (kar-BON-ik) Acid formed when carbon dioxide dissolves in water; carbonic acid then separates into hydrogen ion and bicarbonate ion.
carbonic anhydrase (an-HI-drase) Enzyme that catalyzes the interconversion of carbon dioxide with bicarbonate ion and hydrogen ion.
cardiac (KAR-de-ak) Pertaining to the heart.
cardiovascular system (kar-dE-o-VAS-ku-lar) System consisting of the heart and blood vessels that transports blood throughout the body.
carrier Individual who has a gene that is not expressed in the phenotype but that can be passed to offspring.
cartilage (KAR-tih-lij) Type of hard connective tissue found at the ends of bones, the tip of the nose, larynx, trachea, and the embryonic skeleton.
CAT See computed tomography.
catabolism (kah-TAB-o-lizm) Metabolic breakdown of substances into simpler substances; includes the digestion of food and the oxidation of nutrient molecules for energy.
catalyst (KAT-ah-list) Substance that speeds the rate of a chemical reaction.
cataract (KAT-ah-rakt) Opacity of the eye's lens or lens capsule.
catheter (KATH-eh-ter) Tube that can be inserted into a vessel or cavity; may be used to remove fluid, such as urine or blood; v., catheterize.
cation (KAT-i-on) Positively charged particle (ion).
cauda equina (KAW-dah eh-KWI-nah) Bundle composed of the spinal nerves that arise from the terminal region of the spinal cord; the individual nerves gradually exit from their appropriate segments of the spinal column.
caudal (KAWD-al) Toward or nearer to the sacral region of the spinal column.
cavity (KAV-ih-te) Hollow space; hole.
CCK See cholecystokinin.
cecum (SE-kum) Small pouch at the beginning of the large intestine.
cell Basic unit of life.
cell membrane See plasma membrane.

cellular respiration Series of reactions by which nutrients are oxidized for energy within the cell.
central canal Channel in the center of an osteon of compact bone; channel in the center of the spinal cord that contains CSF.
central nervous system (CNS) Part of the nervous system that includes the brain and spinal cord.
centrifuge (SEN-trih-fuje) An instrument that separates materials in a mixture based on density.
centriole (SEN-tre-ole) Rod-shaped body near the nucleus of a cell; functions in cell division.
cerebellum (ser-eh-BEL-um) Small section of the brain inferior to the cerebral hemispheres; functions in coordination, balance, and muscle tone.
cerebral (SER-e-bral) **cortex** Very thin outer layer of gray matter on the surface of the cerebral hemispheres.
cerebrospinal (ser-e-bro-SPI-nal) **fluid (CSF)** Fluid that circulates in and around the brain and spinal cord.
cerebrum (SER-e-brum) Largest part of the brain; composed of two cerebral hemispheres.
cerumen (seh-RU-men) Earwax; adj., ceruminous (seh-RU-min-us).
cervix (SER-vix) Constricted portion of an organ or part, such as the lower portion of the uterus; neck; adj., cervical.
cesarean (se-ZAR-re-en) **section** Incision in the abdominal and uterine walls for delivery of a fetus; C section.
chemistry (KEM-is-tre) Study of the composition and properties of matter.
chemoreceptor (ke-mo-re-SEP-tor) Receptor that responds to chemicals in body fluids.
cholecystokinin (ko-le-sis-to-KI-nin) **(CCK)** Duodenal hormone that stimulates release of pancreatic enzymes and bile from the gallbladder.
cholesterol (ko-LES-ter-ol) Lipid synthesized by the liver that is found in all plasma membranes, in bile, myelin, steroid hormones, and elsewhere; circulates in the blood and is stored in liver and adipose tissue.
cholinergic (ko-lin-ER-jik) Activity or structure that responds to acetylcholine.
chondrocyte (KON-dro-site) Cell that produces and maintains cartilage.
chordae tendineae (KOR-de ten-DIN-e-e) Fibrous threads that stabilize the heart's AV valve flaps.
chorion (KO-re-on) Outer embryonic layer that, together with a layer of the endometrium, forms the placenta.
choroid (KO-royd) Pigmented middle layer of the eye.
choroid plexus (KO-royd PLEKS-us) Vascular network in the brain's ventricles that forms cerebrospinal fluid.
chromosome (KRO-mo-some) Dark-staining, threadlike body in a cell's nucleus; contains genes that determine hereditary traits.
chyle (kile) Milky-appearing fluid absorbed into the lymphatic system from the small intestine. It consists of lymph and droplets of digested fat.
chyme (kime) Mixture of partially digested food, water, and digestive juices that forms in the stomach.
cicatrix (SIK-ah-trix) Scar.
cilia (SIL-e-ah) Hairs or hairlike processes, such as eyelashes or microscopic extensions from a cell's surface; sing., cilium.
ciliary (SIL-e-ar-e) **muscle** Eye muscle that controls the shape of the lens.
circumduction (ser-kum-DUK-shun) Circular movement at a joint.
circumcision (sir-kum-SIJ-un) Surgery to remove the foreskin of the penis.
cisterna chyli (sis-TER-nah KI-li) Initial portion of the thoracic lymph duct, which is enlarged to form a temporary storage area.
CK See creatine kinase.
clitoris (KLIT-o-ris) Small organ of great sensitivity in the external genitalia of the female.
CNS See central nervous system.
coagulation (ko-ag-u-LA-shun) Clotting, as of blood.
cochlea (KOK-le-ah) Coiled portion of the inner ear that contains the organ of hearing.
colic (KOL-ik) Spasm of visceral muscle.
collagen (KOL-ah-jen) Flexible white protein that gives strength and resilience to connective tissue, such as bone and cartilage.
colloid (kol-OYD) Mixture in which suspended particles do not dissolve but remain distributed in the solvent because of their small size (e.g., cytoplasm); colloidal suspension.
colon (KO-lon) Main portion of the large intestine.
colostrum (ko-LOS-trum) Secretion of the mammary glands released prior to secretion of milk.
complement (KOM-ple-ment) Group of blood proteins that helps antibodies and phagocytes to destroy foreign cells.
compliance (kom-PLI-ans) Ease with which a hollow structure, such as the thorax or alveoli of the lungs, can be expanded under pressure.
compound Substance composed of two or more chemical elements.
computed tomography (to-MOG-rah-fe) **(CT)** Imaging method in which multiple radiographic views taken from different angles are analyzed by computer to show an area cross section; used to detect tumors and other abnormalities; also called computed axial tomography (CAT).
concha (KON-ka) Shell-like bone in the nasal cavity; pl., conchae (KON-ke).
condyle (KON-dile) Rounded projection, as on a bone.
cone Receptor cell in the eye's retina; used for vision in bright light.
conjunctiva (kon-junk-TI-vah) Membrane that lines the eyelid and covers the anterior part of the sclera (white of the eye).
contraception (con-trah-SEP-shun) Prevention of an ovum's fertilization or a fertilized ovum's implantation; birth control.
convergence (kon-VER-jens) Centering of both eyes on the same visual field.
cornea (KOR-ne-ah) Clear portion of the sclera that covers the anterior of the eye.
coronary (KOR-on-ar-e) Referring to the heart or to the arteries supplying blood to the heart.
corpus callosum (kal-O-sum) Thick bundle of myelinated nerve cell fibers, deep within the brain, that carries nerve impulses from one cerebral hemisphere to the other.
corpus luteum (LU-te-um) Yellow body formed from ovarian follicle after ovulation; produces progesterone.
cortex (KOR-tex) Outer layer of an organ, such as the brain, kidney, or adrenal gland.
countercurrent mechanism Mechanism for concentrating urine as it flows through the collecting ducts.
covalent (KO-va-lent) **bond** Chemical bond formed by the sharing of electrons between atoms.
cranial (KRA-ne-al) Pertaining to the cranium, the part of the skull that encloses the brain; toward the head or nearer to the head.
creatine (KRE-ah-tin) **phosphate** Compound in muscle tissue that stores energy in high-energy bonds.
creatinine (kre-AT-ih-nin) Nitrogenous waste product eliminated in urine.
creatine kinase (CK) (KRE-ah-tin KI-nase) Enzyme in muscle cells that is needed to synthesize creatine phosphate and is released in increased amounts when muscle tissue is damaged; the form specific to cardiac muscle cells is creatine kinase MB (CK-MB).
crenation (kre-NA-shun) Shrinking of a cell, as when placed in a hypertonic solution.
crista (KRIS-tah) Receptor for the sense of rotational equilibrium; pl., cristae.
cryoprecipitate (kri-o-pre-SIP-ih-tate) Precipitate formed when plasma is frozen and then thawed.
CSF See cerebrospinal fluid.
CT See computed tomography.
cutaneous (ku-TA-ne-us) Referring to the skin.
cuticle (KU-tih-kl) Extension of the stratum corneum that seals the space between the nail plate and the skin above the nail root.
cystic (SIS-tik) **duct** Duct that carries bile into and out of the gallbladder.
cystic fibrosis (SIS-tik fi-BRO-sis) Hereditary disease involving thickened secretions and electrolyte imbalances.
cytology (si-TOL-o-je) Study of cells.
cytoplasm (SI-to-plazm) Substance that fills the cell, consisting of a liquid cytosol and organelles.
cytosol (SI-to-sol) Liquid portion of the cytoplasm, consisting of nutrients, minerals, enzymes, and other materials in water.

D

deamination (de-am-ih-NA-shun) Removal of amino groups from proteins in metabolism.
decubitus (de-KU-bih-tus) Lying down.
defecation (def-eh-KA-shun) Act of eliminating undigested waste from the digestive tract.

degeneration (de-jen-er-A-shun) Breakdown, as from age, injury, or disease.
deglutition (deg-lu-TISH-un) Act of swallowing.
dehydration (de-hi-DRA-shun) Excessive loss of body fluid.
denaturation (de-nah-tu-RA-shun) Change in structure of a protein, such as an enzyme, so that it can no longer function.
dendrite (DEN-drite) Neuron fiber that conducts impulses toward the cell body.
deoxyribonucleic (de-OK-se-ri-bo-nu-kle-ik) **acid (DNA)** Genetic material of the cell; makes up the chromosomes in the cell's nucleus.
depolarization (de-po-lar-ih-ZA-shun) Sudden reduction of the electrical potential (charge) on a plasma membrane.
dermal papillae (pah-PIL-le) Extensions of the dermis that project up into the epidermis; they contain blood vessels that supply the epidermis.
dermatome (DER-mah-tome) Region of the skin supplied by a single spinal nerve.
dermis (DER-mis) True skin; deeper part of the skin.
dextrose (DEK-strose) Glucose, as found in nature.
diabetes mellitus (di-ah-BE-teze mel-LI-tus) Disease of insufficient insulin or insufficient response to insulin in which excess glucose is found in the blood and the urine; characterized by abnormal metabolism of glucose, protein, and fat.
diaphragm (DI-ah-fram) Dome-shaped muscle under the lungs that flattens during inhalation; a separating membrane or structure.
diaphysis (di-AF-ih-sis) Shaft of a long bone.
diarthrosis (di-ar-THRO-sis) Freely movable joint; synovial joint.
diastole (di-AS-to-le) Relaxation phase of the cardiac cycle; adj., diastolic (di-as-TOL-ik).
diencephalon (di-en-SEF-ah-lon) Region of the brain between the cerebral hemispheres and the midbrain; contains the thalamus, hypothalamus, and pituitary gland.
diffusion (dih-FU-zhun) Movement of molecules from a region where they are in higher concentration to a region where they are in lower concentration.
digestion (di-JEST-yun) Process of breaking down food into absorbable particles.
digestive system (di-JES-tiv) The system involved in taking in nutrients, converting them to a form the body can use, and absorbing them into the circulation.
dihydroxycholecalciferol (di-hi-drok-se-ko-le-kal-SIF-eh-rol) The active form of vitamin D.
dilation (di-LA-shun) Widening of a part, such as the pupil of the eye, a blood vessel, or the uterine cervix; dilatation.
disaccharide (di-SAK-ah-ride) Compound formed of two simple sugars linked together, such as sucrose and lactose.
dissect (dis-sekt) To cut apart or separate tissues for study.
distal (DIS-tal) Farther from a structure's origin or from a given reference point.
DNA See deoxyribonucleic acid.
dominant (DOM-ih-nant) Referring to a gene that is always expressed in the phenotype if present.
dopamine (DO-pah-mene) Neurotransmitter.
dorsal (DOR-sal) At or toward the back; posterior.
dorsiflexion (dor-sih-FLEK-shun) Bending the foot upward at the ankle.
duct Tube or vessel.
ductus arteriosus (DUK-tus ar-te-re-O-sus) Small vessel in the fetus that carries blood from the pulmonary artery to the descending aorta.
ductus deferens (DEF-er-enz) Tube that carries sperm cells from the testis to the urethra; vas deferens.
ductus venosus (ve-NO-sus) Small vessel in the fetus that carries blood from the umbilical vein to the inferior vena cava.
duodenum (du-o-DE-num) First portion of the small intestine.
dura mater (DU-rah MA-ter) Outermost layer of the meninges.
dyspnea (disp-NE-ah) Difficult or labored breathing.

E

eccrine (EK-rin) Referring to sweat glands that regulate body temperature and vent directly to the surface of the skin through a pore.
ECG See electrocardiograph.
echocardiograph (ek-o-KAR-de-o-graf) Instrument to study the heart by means of ultrasound; the record produced is an echocardiogram.
EEG See electroencephalograph.
effector (ef-FEK-tor) Muscle or gland that responds to a stimulus; effector organ.
efferent (EF-fer-ent) Carrying away from a given point, such as a motor neuron that carries nerve impulses away from the central nervous system.
ejaculation (e-jak-u-LA-shun) Expulsion of semen through the urethra.
EKG See electrocardiograph.
elasticity (e-las-TIS-ih-te) Capacity of a structure to return to its original shape after being stretched.
electrocardiograph (e-lek-tro-KAR-de-o-graf) **(ECG, EKG)** Instrument to study the heart's electric activity; record made is an electrocardiogram.
electroencephalograph (e-lek-tro-en-SEF-ah-lo-graf) **(EEG)** Instrument used to study the brain's electric activity; record made is an electroencephalogram.
electrolyte (e-LEK-tro-lite) Compound that separates into ions in solution; substance that conducts an electric current in solution.
electron (e-LEK-tron) Negatively charged particle located in an energy level outside an atom's nucleus.
electrophoresis (e-lek-tro-fo-RE-sis) Separation of components in a mixture by passing an electric current through it; components separate on the basis of their charge.
element (EL-eh-ment) One of the substances from which all matter is made; substance that cannot be decomposed into a simpler substance.
embolism (EM-bo-lizm) The condition of having an embolus (obstruction in the circulation).
embolus (EM-bo-lus) Blood clot or other obstruction in the circulation.
embryo (EM-bre-o) Developing offspring during the first 8 weeks of gestation.
emulsify (e-MUL-sih-fi) To break up fats into small particles; n., emulsification.
endocardium (en-do-KAR-de-um) Membrane that lines the heart's chambers and covers the valves.
endocrine (EN-do-krin) Referring to a gland that secretes into the bloodstream.
endocrine system System composed of glands that secrete hormones.
endocytosis (en-do-si-TO-sis) Movement of large amounts of material into a cell using vesicles (e.g., phagocytosis and pinocytosis).
endolymph (EN-do-limf) Fluid that fills the membranous labyrinth of the inner ear.
endomysium (en-do-MIS-e-um) Connective tissue around an individual muscle fiber.
endometrium (en-do-ME-tre-um) Inner layer of the uterus.
endoplasmic reticulum (en-do-PLAS-mik re-TIK-u-lum) **(ER)** Network of membranes in the cellular cytoplasm; may be smooth or rough based on absence or presence of ribosomes.
endorphin (en-DOR-fin) Pain-relieving substance released naturally from the brain.
endosteum (en-DOS-te-um) Thin membrane that lines a bone marrow cavity.
endothelium (en-do-THE-le-um) Epithelium that lines the heart, blood vessels, and lymphatic vessels.
enzyme (EN-zime) Organic catalyst; speeds the rate of a reaction but is not changed in the reaction.
eosinophil (e-o-SIN-o-fil) Granular white blood cell that shows beadlike, bright pink cytoplasmic granules when stained with acid stain.
epicardium (ep-ih-KAR-de-um) Membrane that forms the heart wall's outermost layer and is continuous with the lining of the fibrous pericardium; visceral pericardium.
epicondyle (ep-ih-KON-dile) Small projection on a bone above a condyle.
epidermis (ep-ih-DER-mis) Outermost layer of the skin.
epididymis (ep-ih-DID-ih-mis) Coiled tube on the surface of the testis in which sperm cells are stored and in which they mature.
epigastric (ep-ih-GAS-trik) Pertaining to the region just inferior to the sternum (breastbone).
epiglottis (ep-e-GLOT-is) Leaf-shaped cartilage that covers the larynx during swallowing.
epimysium (ep-ih-MIS-e-um) Sheath of fibrous connective tissue that encloses a muscle.
epinephrine (ep-ih-NEF-rin) Hormone released from the adrenal medulla; adrenaline.

epiphysis (eh-PIF-ih-sis) End of a long bone; adj., epiphyseal (ep-ih-FIZ-e-al).
episiotomy (eh-piz-e-OT-o-me) Cutting of the perineum between the vaginal opening and the anus to reduce tissue tearing in childbirth.
epithelium (ep-ih-THE-le-um) One of the four main types of tissues; forms glands, covers surfaces, and lines cavities; adj., epithelial.
EPO See erythropoietin.
equilibrium (e-kwih-LIB-re-um) Sense of balance.
ER See endoplasmic reticulum.
erythrocyte (eh-RITH-ro-site) Red blood cell.
erythropoietin (EPO) (eh-rith-ro-POY-eh-tin) Hormone released from the kidney that stimulates red blood cell production in the red bone marrow.
esophagus (eh-SOF-ah-gus) Muscular tube that carries food from the throat to the stomach.
estrogen (ES-tro-jen) Group of female sex hormones that promotes development of the uterine lining and maintains secondary sex characteristics; the main estrogen is estradiol.
eustachian (u-STA-shun) **tube** See auditory tube
eversion (e-VER-zhun) Turning outward, with reference to movement of the foot.
excitability In cells, the ability to transmit an electric current along the plasma membrane.
excretion (eks-KRE-shun) Removal and elimination of metabolic waste products from the blood.
exfoliation (eks-fo-le-A-shun) Loss of cells from the surface of tissue, such as the skin.
exhalation (eks-hah-LA-shun) Expulsion of air from the lungs; expiration.
exocrine (EK-so-krin) Referring to a gland that secretes through a duct.
exocytosis (eks-o-si-TO-sis) Movement of large amounts of material out of the cell using vesicles.
extension (eks-TEN-shun) Motion that increases the angle at a joint, returning a body part to the anatomic position.
extracellular (EK-strah-sel-u-lar) Outside the cell.
extremity (ek-STREM-ih-te) Limb; an arm or leg.

F

facilitated diffusion Movement of material across the plasma membrane as it would normally flow by diffusion but using transporters to speed movement.
fallopian (fah-LO-pe-an) **tube** See uterine tube.
fascia (FASH-e-ah) Band or sheet of fibrous connective tissue.
fascicle (FAS-ih-kl) Small bundle, as of muscle cells or nerve cell fibers.
fat Type of lipid composed of glycerol and fatty acids; triglyceride.
febrile (FEB-ril) Pertaining to fever.
feces (FE-seze) Waste material discharged from the large intestine; excrement; stool.
feedback Return of information into a system, so that it can be used to regulate that system.
fertilization (fer-til-ih-ZA-shun) Union of an ovum and a spermatozoon.
fetus (FE-tus) Developing offspring from the start of the ninth week of gestation until birth.
fever (FE-ver) Abnormally high body temperature.
fibrin (FI-brin) Blood protein that forms a blood clot.
fibrinogen (fi-BRIN-o-jen) Plasma protein that is converted to fibrin in blood clotting.
filtration (fil-TRA-shun) Movement of material through a semipermeable membrane under mechanical force, such as the force of blood pressure.
fimbriae (FIM-bre-e) Fringelike extensions of the uterine tube that sweep a released ovum into the tube.
fissure (FISH-ure) Deep groove.
flagellum (flah-JEL-lum) Long whiplike extension from a cell used for locomotion; pl., flagella.
flexion (FLEK-shun) Bending motion that decreases the angle between bones at a joint, moving a body part away from the anatomic position.
follicle (FOL-lih-kl) Sac or cavity, such as the ovarian follicle or hair follicle.
follicle-stimulating hormone (FSH) Hormone produced by the anterior pituitary that stimulates development of ova in the ovary and spermatozoa in the testes.
fontanel (fon-tah-NEL) Membranous area in the infant skull where bone has not yet formed; also spelled fontanelle; "soft spot."
foramen (fo-RA-men) Opening or passageway, as into or through a bone; pl., foramina (fo-RAM-in-ah).
foramen magnum Large opening in the skull's occipital bone through which the spinal cord passes to join the brain.
foramen ovale (o-VA-le) Small hole in the fetal atrial septum that allows blood to pass directly from the right atrium to the left atrium.
formed elements Cells and cell fragments in the blood.
fornix (FOR-niks) Recess or archlike structure.
fossa (FOS-sah) Hollow or depression, as in a bone; pl., fossae (FOS-se).
fovea (FO-ve-ah) Small pit or cup-shaped depression in a surface; the fovea centralis near the center of the retina is the point of sharpest vision.
frontal (FRONT-al) Describing a plane that divides a structure into anterior and posterior parts.
FSH See follicle-stimulating hormone.
fulcrum (FUL-krum) Pivot point in a lever system; joint in the skeletal system.
fundus (FUN-dus) The deepest portion of an organ, such as the eye or the uterus.

G

gallbladder (GAWL-blad-er) Muscular sac on the inferior surface of the liver that stores bile.
gamete (GAM-ete) Reproductive cell; ovum or spermatozoon.
gamma globulin (GLOB-u-lin) Protein fraction in the blood plasma that contains antibodies.
ganglion (GANG-le-on) Collection of nerve cell bodies located outside the central nervous system.
gastric-inhibitory peptide (GIP) Duodenal hormone that inhibits release of gastric juice and stimulates insulin release from the pancreas.
gastrin (GAS-trin) Hormone released from the stomach that stimulates stomach activity.
gastrointestinal (gas-tro-in-TES-tih-nal) **(GI)** Pertaining to the stomach and intestine or the digestive tract as a whole.
gene Hereditary factor; portion of the DNA on a chromosome.
genetic (jeh-NET-ik) Pertaining to the genes or heredity.
genitalia (jen-ih-TA-le-ah) Reproductive organs, both external and internal.
genotype (JEN-o-tipe) Genetic make-up of an organism.
gestation (jes-TA-shun) Period of development from conception to birth.
GH See growth hormone.
GI See gastrointestinal.
gingiva (JIN-jih-vah) Tissue around the teeth; gum.
glans Enlarged distal portion of the penis.
glial cells (GLI-al) Cells that support and protect the nervous system; neuroglia.
glomerular (glo-MER-u-lar) **capsule** Enlarged portion of the nephron that surrounds the glomerulus; Bowman capsule.
glomerular (glo-MER-u-lar) **filtrate** Fluid and dissolved materials that leave the blood and enter the kidney nephron through the glomerular capsule.
glomerulus (glo-MER-u-lus) Cluster of capillaries surrounded by the nephron's glomerular capsule.
glottis (GLOT-is) Space between the vocal cords.
glucagon (GLU-kah-gon) Hormone from the pancreatic islets that raises blood glucose level.
glucocorticoid (glu-ko-KOR-tih-koyd) Steroid hormone from the adrenal cortex that increases the concentration of nutrients in the blood during times of stress, e.g., cortisol.
glucose (GLU-kose) Simple sugar; main energy source for the cells; dextrose.
glycemic (gli-SE-mik) **effect** Measure of how rapidly a food raises the blood glucose level and stimulates release of insulin.
glycogen (GLI-ko-jen) Compound built from glucose molecules that is stored for energy in the liver and muscles.
glycolysis (gli-KOL-ih-sis) First, anaerobic phase of glucose's metabolic breakdown for energy.
goblet cell Single-celled gland that secretes mucus.
Golgi (GOL-je) **apparatus** System of cellular membranes that formulates special substances; also called Golgi complex.
gonad (GO-nad) Sex gland; ovary or testis.

gonadotropin (gon-ah-do-TRO-pin) Hormone that acts on a reproductive gland (ovary or testis), e.g., FSH, LH.
Graafian (GRAF-e-an) **follicle** A mature ovarian follicle.
gram (g) Basic unit of weight in the metric system.
Gram stain Procedure used to color microorganisms for viewing under the microscope.
granulocyte (GRAN-u-lo-site) Leukocyte with visible granules in the cytoplasm when stained.
gray matter Nervous tissue composed of unmyelinated fibers and cell bodies.
greater vestibular (ves-TIB-u-lar) **gland** Gland that secretes mucus into the vagina; Bartholin gland.
growth hormone (GH) Hormone produced by anterior pituitary that promotes tissue growth; somatotropin.
gustation (gus-TA-shun) Sense of taste; adj., gustatory.
gyrus (JI-rus) Raised area of the cerebral cortex; pl., gyri (JI-ri).

H

Haversian (ha-VER-shan) **canal** See central canal.
Haversian system See osteon.
heart (hart) Organ that pumps blood through the cardiovascular system.
hemapheresis (hem-ah-fer-E-sis) Return of blood components to a donor following separation and removal of desired components.
hematocrit (he-MAT-o-krit) **(Hct)** Volume percentage of red blood cells in whole blood; packed cell volume.
hemocytometer (he-mo-si-TOM-eh-ter) Device used to count blood cells under the microscope.
hemodialysis (he-mo-di-AL-ih-sis) Removal of impurities from the blood by their passage through a semipermeable membrane in a fluid bath.
hemoglobin (he-mo-GLO-bin) **(Hb)** Iron-containing protein in red blood cells that binds oxygen.
hemolysis (he-MOL-ih-sis) Rupture of red blood cells; v., hemolyze (HE-mo-lize).
hemolytic (he-mo-LIT-ik) **disease of the newborn** (**HDN**) Condition that results from Rh incompatibility between a mother and her fetus; erythroblastosis fetalis.
hemopoiesis (he-mo-poy-E-sis) Production of blood cells; hematopoiesis.
hemorrhage (HEM-eh-rij) Loss of blood.
hemostasis (he-mo-STA-sis) Stoppage of bleeding.
heparin (HEP-ah-rin) Substance that prevents blood clotting; anticoagulant.
heredity (he-RED-ih-te) Transmission of characteristics from parent to offspring by means of the genes.
hereditary (he-RED-ih-tar-e) Transmitted or transmissible through the genes; familial.
heterozygous (het-er-o-ZI-gus) Having unmatched alleles for a given trait; hybrid.
hilum (HI-lum) Indented region of an organ where vessels and nerves enter or leave.
hippocampus (hip-o-KAM-pus) Sea horse–shaped region of the limbic system that functions in learning and formation of long-term memory.
histamine (HIS-tah-mene) Substance released from tissues during an inflammatory reaction.
histology (his-TOL-o-je) Study of tissues.
homeostasis (ho-me-o-STA-sis) State of balance within the body; maintenance of body conditions within set limits.
homozygous (ho-mo-ZI-gus) Having identical alleles for a given trait; purebred.
hormone Chemical messenger secreted by a tissue that has specific regulatory effects on certain other cells.
host An organism in or on which a parasite lives.
human chorionic gonadotropin (ko-re-ON-ik gon-ah-do-TRO-pin) **(hCG)** Hormone produced by embryonic cells soon after implantation that maintains the corpus luteum.
human placental lactogen (hPL) Hormone produced by the placenta that prepares the breasts for lactation and maintains nutrient levels in maternal blood.
humoral (HU-mor-al) Pertaining to body fluids, such as immunity based on antibodies circulating in the blood.
hyaline (HI-ah-lin) Clear, glasslike; referring to a type of cartilage.
hydrolysis (hi-DROL-ih-sis) Splitting of large molecules by the addition of water, as in digestion.
hydrophilic (hi-dro-FIL-ik) Mixing with or dissolving in water, such as salts; literally "water-loving."
hydrophobic (hi-dro-FO-bik) Repelling and not dissolving in water, such as fats; literally "water-fearing."
hymen Fold of membrane near the opening of the vaginal canal.
hypercapnia (hi-per-KAP-ne-ah) Increased level of carbon dioxide in the blood.
hyperglycemia (hi-per-gli-SE-me-ah) Abnormal increase in the amount of glucose in the blood.
hyperpnea (hi-PERP-ne-ah) Increase in the depth and rate of breathing.
hypertension (hi-per-TEN-shun) High blood pressure.
hypertonic (hi-per-TON-ik) Describing a solution that is more concentrated than the fluids within a cell.
hypertrophy (hy-PER-tro-fe) Enlargement or overgrowth of an organ or part.
hyperventilation (hi-per-ven-tih-LA-shun) Increased amount of air entering the alveoli of the lungs due to deep and rapid respiration.
hypocapnia (hi-po-KAP-ne-ah) Decreased level of carbon dioxide in the blood.
hypochondriac (hi-po-KON-dre-ak) Pertaining to a region on either side of the abdomen just inferior to the ribs.
hypogastric (hi-po-GAS-trik) Pertaining to an area inferior to the stomach; most inferior midline region of the abdomen.
hypoglycemia (hi-po-gli-SE-me-ah) Abnormal decrease in the amount of glucose in the blood.
hypophysis (hi-POF-ih-sis) Pituitary gland.
hypopnea (hi-POP-ne-ah) Decrease in the rate and depth of breathing.
hypothalamus (hi-po-THAL-ah-mus) Region of the brain that controls the pituitary and controls numerous reflexes that maintain homeostasis.
hypotonic (hi-po-TON-ik) Describing a solution that is less concentrated than the fluids within a cell.
hypoventilation (hi-po-ven-tih-LA-shun) Insufficient amount of air entering the alveoli.
hypoxemia (hi-pok-SE-me-ah) Lower than normal concentration of oxygen in arterial blood.
hypoxia (hi-POK-se-ah) Lower than normal level of oxygen in the tissues.

I

ileum (IL-e-um) Most distal portion of the small intestine.
ileus (IL-e-us) Intestinal obstruction caused by lack of peristalsis or by muscle contraction.
iliac (IL-e-ak) Pertaining to the ilium, the upper portion of the hipbone; pertaining to the most inferior, lateral regions of the abdomen.
immune (ih-MUNE) **system** Complex of cellular and molecular components that provides defense against foreign cells and substances as well as abnormal body cells.
immunity (ih-MU-nih-te) Power of an individual to resist or overcome the effects of a disease or other harmful agent.
immunization (ih-mu-nih-ZA-shun) Use of a vaccine to produce immunity; vaccination.
immunoglobulin (im-mu-no-GLOB-u-lin) **(Ig)** See antibody.
implantation (im-plan-TA-shun) Embedding of a fertilized ovum into the uterine lining.
inferior (in-FE-re-or) Below or lower.
inferior vena cava (VE-nah KA-vah) Large vein that drains the lower body and empties into the heart's right atrium.
infundibulum (in-fun-DIB-u-lum) Stalk that connects the pituitary gland to the brain's hypothalamus.
ingestion (in-JES-chun) Intake of food.
inguinal (IN-gwih-nal) Pertaining to the groin region or the region of the inguinal canal.
inhalation (in-hah-LA-shun) Drawing of air into the lungs; inspiration.
insertion (in-SER-shun) Muscle attachment connected to a movable part.
insulin (IN-su-lin) Hormone from the pancreatic islets that lowers blood glucose level.
integument (in-TEG-u-ment) Skin; adj., integumentary.
integumentary system The skin and all its associated structures.
intercalated (in-TER-cah-la-ted) **disk** A modified plasma membrane in cardiac tissue that allows rapid transfer of electric impulses between cells.
intercellular (in-ter-SEL-u-lar) Between cells.

intercostal (in-ter-KOS-tal) Between the ribs.
interferon (in-ter-FERE-on) **(IFN)** Group of substances released from virus-infected cells that prevent spread of infection to other cells; also nonspecifically boosts the immune system.
interleukin (in-ter-LU-kin) Substance released by a T cell, macrophage, or endothelial cell that stimulates other immune system cells.
interneuron (in-ter-NU-ron) Nerve cell that transmits impulses within the central nervous system.
interphase (IN-ter-faze) Stage in a cell's life between one mitosis and the next when the cell is not dividing.
interstitial (in-ter-STISH-al) Between; pertaining to an organ's spaces or structures between active tissues.
intestine (in-TES-tin) Organ of the digestive tract between the stomach and the anus, consisting of the small and large intestine.
intracellular (in-trah-SEL-u-lar) Within a cell.
inversion (in-VER-zhun) Turning inward, with reference to movement of the foot.
ion (I-on) Charged particle formed when an electrolyte goes into solution.
ionic bond Chemical bond formed by the exchange of electrons between atoms.
iris (I-ris) Circular colored region of the eye around the pupil.
islets (I-lets) Groups of cells in the pancreas that produce hormones; islets of Langerhans (LAHNG-er-hanz).
isometric (i-so-MET-rik) **contraction** Muscle contraction in which there is no change in muscle length but an increase in muscle tension, as in pushing against an immovable force.
isotonic (i-so-TON-ik) Describing a solution that has the same concentration as the fluid within a cell.
isotonic contraction Muscle contraction in which the tone within the muscle remains the same but the muscle shortens to produce movement.
isotope (I-so-tope) Form of an element that has the same atomic number as another form of that element but a different atomic weight; isotopes differ in their numbers of neutrons.
isthmus (IS-mus) Narrow band, such as the band that connects the two lobes of the thyroid gland.

J

jejunum (je-JU-num) Second portion of the small intestine.
joint Area of junction between two or more bones; articulation.
juxtaglomerular (juks-tah-glo-MER-u-lar) **(JG) apparatus** Structure in the kidney composed of cells of the afferent arteriole and distal tubule that secretes the enzyme renin when blood pressure decreases below a certain level.

K

keratin (KER-ah-tin) Protein that thickens and protects the skin; makes up hair and nails.
kidney (KID-ne) Organ of excretion.
kilocalorie (kil-o-KAL-o-re) **(kcal)** Measure of the energy content of food; technically, the amount of heat needed to raise l kg of water 1°C; Calorie (C).
kinesthesia (kin-es-THE-ze-ah) Sense of body movement.
Kupffer (KOOP-fer) **cells** Macrophages in the liver that help to fight infection.

L

labium (LA-be-um) Lip; pl., labia (LA-be-ah).
labyrinth (LAB-ih-rinth) Inner ear, named for its complex shape; maze.
lacrimal (LAK-rih-mal) Referring to tears or the tear glands.
lacrimal (LAK-rih-mal) **apparatus** Lacrimal (tear) gland and its associated ducts.
lacrimal gland Gland above the eye that secretes tears.
lactation (lak-TA-shun) Secretion of milk.
lacteal (LAK-te-al) Lymphatic capillary that drains digested fats from the villi of the small intestine.
lactic (LAK-tik) **acid** Organic acid that accumulates in muscle cells metabolizing nutrients anaerobically.
laryngopharynx (lah-rin-go-FAR-inks) Lowest portion of the pharynx, opening into the larynx and esophagus.
larynx (LAR-inks) Structure between the pharynx and trachea that contains the vocal cords; voice box.
lateral (LAT-er-al) Farther from the midline; toward the side.
lens Biconvex structure of the eye that changes in thickness to accommodate near and far vision; crystalline lens.
leptin (LEP-tin) Hormone produced by adipocytes that aids in weight control by decreasing food intake and increasing energy expenditure.
leukocyte (LU-ko-site) White blood cell.
LH See luteinizing hormone.
ligament (LIG-ah-ment) Band of connective tissue that connects a bone to another bone; thickened portion or fold of the peritoneum that supports an organ or attaches it to another organ.
ligand (LIG-and) Substance that binds to a receptor in the plasma membrane; participates in receptor-mediated endocytosis.
limbic (LIM-bik) **system** Area between the brain's cerebrum and diencephalon that is involved in emotional states and behavior.
lipid (LIP-id) Type of organic compound, one example of which is a fat.
liter (LE-ter) **(L)** Basic unit of volume in the metric system; 1,000 mL; 1.06 qt.
liver (LIV-er) Large gland inferior to the diaphragm in the superior right abdomen; has many functions, including bile secretion, detoxification, storage, and interconversion of nutrients.
loop of Henle (HEN-le) See nephron loop.
lumbar (LUM-bar) Pertaining to the region of the spine between the thoracic vertebrae and the sacrum.
lumen (LU-men) Central opening of an organ or vessel.
lung Organ of respiration.
lunula (LU-nu-la) Pale half-moon–shaped area at the proximal end of the nail.
luteinizing (LU-te-in-i-zing) **hormone (LH)** Hormone produced by the anterior pituitary that induces ovulation and formation of the corpus luteum in females; in males, it stimulates cells in the testes to produce testosterone.
lymph (limf) Fluid in the lymphatic system.
lymph node Mass of lymphoid tissue along the path of a lymphatic vessel that filters lymph and harbors white blood cells active in immunity.
lymphatic duct (lim-FAH-tic) One of two large vessels draining lymph from the lymphatic system into the venous system.
lymphatic system System consisting of the lymphatic vessels and lymphoid tissue; involved in immunity, digestion, and fluid balance.
lymphocyte (LIM-fo-site) Agranular white blood cell that functions in immunity.
lysosome (LI-so-some) Cell organelle that contains digestive enzymes.

M

macrophage (MAK-ro-faj) Large phagocytic cell that develops from a monocyte; presents antigen to lymphocytes in immune response.
macula (MAK-u-lah) Spot; flat, discolored spot on the skin, such as a freckle or measles lesion; also called macule; small yellow spot in the eye's retina that contains the fovea, the point of sharpest vision; equilibrium receptor in the vestibule of the inner ear.
magnetic resonance imaging (MRI) Method for studying tissue based on nuclear movement after exposure to radio waves in a powerful magnetic field.
major histocompatibility complex (MHC) Group of genes that codes for specific proteins (antigens) on cellular surfaces; these antigens are important in cross-matching for tissue transplantation; they are also important in immune reactions.
MALT Mucosal-associated lymphoid tissue; tissue in the mucous membranes that helps fight infection.
mammary (MAM-er-e) **gland** Milk-secreting portion of the breast.
mast cell White blood cell related to a basophil that is present in tissues; active in inflammatory and allergic reactions.
mastication (mas-tih-KA-shun) Act of chewing.
matrix (MA-triks) The nonliving background material in a tissue; the intercellular material.
meatus (me-A-tus) Short channel or passageway, such the external opening of a canal or a channel in bone.
medial (ME-de-al) Nearer the midline of the body.
mediastinum (me-de-as-TI-num) Region between the lungs and the organs and vessels it contains.
medulla (meh-DUL-lah) Inner region of an organ; marrow.
medullary (MED-u-lar-e) **cavity** Channel at the center of a long bone that contains yellow bone marrow.
medulla oblongata (ob-long-GAH-tah) Part of the brain stem that connects the brain to the spinal cord.

megakaryocyte (meg-ah-KAR-e-o-site) Very large cell that gives rise to blood platelets.
meibomian (mi-BO-me-an) **gland** Gland that produces a secretion that lubricates the eyelashes.
meiosis (mi-O-sis) Process of cell division that halves the chromosome number in the formation of the reproductive cells.
melanin (MEL-ah-nin) Dark pigment found in the skin, hair, parts of the eye, and certain parts of the brain.
melanocyte (MEL-ah-no-site) Cell that produces melanin.
melatonin (mel-ah-TO-nin) Hormone produced by the pineal gland.
membrane (MEM-brane) Thin sheet of tissue.
membrane potential (po-TEN-shal) Difference in electric charge on either side of a plasma membrane; transmembrane potential.
Mendelian (men-DE-le-en) **laws** Principles of heredity discovered by an Austrian monk named Gregor Mendel.
meninges (men-IN-jeze) Three layers of fibrous membranes that cover the brain and spinal cord.
menopause (MEN-o-pawz) Time during which menstruation ceases.
menses (MEN-seze) Monthly flow of blood from the female reproductive tract.
menstruation (men-stru-A-shun) Period of menstrual flow.
mesentery (MES-en-ter-e) Membranous peritoneal ligament that attaches the small intestine to the dorsal abdominal wall.
mesocolon (mes-o-KO-lon) Peritoneal ligament that attaches the colon to the dorsal abdominal wall.
mesothelium (mes-o-THE-le-um) Epithelial tissue found in serous membranes.
metabolic rate Rate at which energy is released from nutrients in the cells.
metabolic syndrome Condition related to type 2 diabetes mellitus with insulin resistance, obesity, hyperglycemia, high blood pressure, and metabolic disturbances; also called syndrome X.
metabolism (meh-TAB-o-lizm) All the physical and chemical processes by which an organism is maintained.
metaphase (MET-ah-faze) Second stage of mitosis, during which the chromosomes line up across the equator of the cell.
meter (ME-ter) **(m)** Basic unit of length in the metric system; 1.1 yards.
MHC See Major histocompatibility complex.
microbiology (mi-kro-bi-OL-o-je) Study of microscopic organisms.
micrometer (MI-kro-me-ter) **(mcm)** 1/1,000th of a millimeter; an instrument for measuring through a **microscope** (pronounced mi-KROM-eh-ter).
microorganism (mi-kro-OR-gan-izm) Microscopic organism.
microscope (MI-kro-skope) Magnifying instrument used to examine cells and other structures not visible with the naked eye; examples are the compound light microscope, transmission electron microscope (TEM), and scanning electron microscope (SEM).
microvilli (mi-kro-VIL-li) Small projections of the plasma membrane that increase surface area; sing., microvillus.
micturition (mik-tu-RISH-un) Act of urination; voiding of the urinary bladder.
midbrain Upper portion of the brainstem.
mineral (MIN-er-al) Inorganic substance; in the diet, an element needed in small amounts for health.
mineralocorticoid (min-er-al-o-KOR-tih-koyd) Steroid hormone from the adrenal cortex that regulates electrolyte balance, e.g., aldosterone.
mitochondria (mi-to-KON-dre-ah) Cellular organelles that manufacture ATP with the energy released from the oxidation of nutrients; sing., mitochondrion.
mitosis (mi-TO-sis) Type of cell division that produces two daughter cells exactly like the parent cell.
mitral (MI-tral) **valve** Valve between the heart's left atrium and left ventricle; left AV valve; bicuspid valve.
mixture Blend of two or more substances.
molecule (MOL-eh-kule) Particle formed by chemical bonding of two or more atoms; smallest subunit of a compound.
monocyte (MON-o-site) Phagocytic agranular white blood cell that differentiates into a macrophage.
monomer (MON-o-mer) Building block or single unit of a larger molecule.
monosaccharide (mon-o-SAK-ah-ride) Simple sugar; basic unit of carbohydrates.
motor (MO-tor) Describing structures or activities involved in transmitting impulses away from the central nervous system; efferent.
motor end plate Region of a muscle cell membrane that receives nervous stimulation.
motor unit Group consisting of a single neuron and all the muscle fibers it stimulates.
mouth Proximal opening of the digestive tract where food is ingested, chewed, mixed with saliva, and swallowed.
MRI See magnetic resonance imaging.
mucosa (mu-KO-sah) Lining membrane that produces mucus; mucous membrane.
mucus (MU-kus) Thick protective fluid secreted by mucous membranes and glands; adj., mucous.
multiple (SKLE-ro-SIS) **sclerosis** Disease that affects the myelin sheath around axons leading to neuron degeneration.
murmur Abnormal heart sound.
muscle (MUS-l) Tissue that contracts to produce movement or tension; includes skeletal, smooth, and cardiac types; adj., muscular.
muscular (MUS-ku-lar) **system** The system of skeletal muscles that moves the skeleton, supports and protects the organs, and maintains posture.
mutagen (MU-tah-jen) Agent that causes mutation; adj., mutagenic (mu-tah-JEN-ik).
mutation (mu-TA-shun) Change in a gene or a chromosome.
myelin (MI-el-in) Fatty material that covers and insulates the axons of some neurons.
myocardium (mi-o-KAR-de-um) Middle layer of the heart wall; heart muscle.
myoglobin (MI-o-glo-bin) Compound that stores oxygen in muscle cells.
myoma (mi-O-mah) Usually benign tumor of the uterus; fibroma; fibroid.
myometrium (mi-o-ME-tre-um) Muscular layer of the uterus.
myosin (MI-o-sin) One of the two contractile proteins in muscle cells, the other being actin.

N

nasopharynx (na-zo-FAR-inks) Upper portion of the pharynx located posterior to the nasal cavity.
natural killer (NK) cell Type of lymphocyte that can nonspecifically destroy abnormal cells.
negative feedback Self-regulating system in which the result of an action reverses that action; a method for keeping body conditions within a normal range and maintaining homeostasis.
nephron (NEF-ron) Microscopic functional unit of the kidney.
nephron loop Hairpin-shaped segment of the renal tubule between the proximal and distal tubules; loop of Henle.
nerve Bundle of neuron fibers outside the central nervous system.
nerve impulse Electric charge that spreads along the membrane of a neuron; action potential.
nervous system (NER-vus) The system that transports information in the body by means of electric impulses.
neurilemma (nu-rih-LEM-mah) Thin sheath that covers certain peripheral axons; aids in axon regeneration.
neuroglia (nu-ROG-le-ah) Supporting and protective cells of the nervous system; glial cells.
neuromuscular junction Point at which a neuron's axon contacts a muscle cell.
neuron (NU-ron) Conducting cell of the nervous system.
neurotransmitter (nu-ro-TRANS-mit-er) Chemical released from the ending of an axon that enables a nerve impulse to cross a synapse.
neutron (NU-tron) Noncharged particle in an atom's nucleus.
neutrophil (NU-tro-fil) Phagocytic granular white blood cell; polymorph; poly; PMN; seg.
nevus (NE-vus) Mole or birthmark.
nitrogen (NI-tro-jen) Chemical element found in all proteins.
node Small mass of tissue, such as a lymph node; space between cells in the myelin sheath.
norepinephrine (nor-epi-ih-NEF-rin) Neurotransmitter similar in composition and action to the hormone epinephrine; noradrenaline.
normal saline Isotonic or physiologic salt solution.
nucleic acid (nu-KLE-ik) Complex organic substance composed of nucleotides that makes up DNA and RNA.
nucleolus (nu-KLE-o-lus) Small unit within the nucleus that assembles ribosomes.

nucleotide (NU-kle-o-tide) Building block of DNA and RNA; one is also a component of ATP.

nucleus (NU-kle-us) Largest cellular organelle, containing the DNA, which directs all cell activities; group of neurons in the central nervous system; in chemistry, the central part of an atom.

O

olfaction (ol-FAK-shun) Sense of smell; adj., olfactory.

omentum (o-MEN-tum) Portion of the peritoneum; greater omentum extends over the anterior abdomen; lesser omentum extends between the stomach and liver.

ophthalmic (of-THAL-mik) Pertaining to the eye.

ophthalmoscope (of-THAL-mo-skope) Instrument for examining the posterior (fundus) of the eye.

organ (OR-gan) Body part containing two or more tissues functioning together for specific purposes.

organ of Corti (KOR-te) See spiral organ.

organelle (or-gan-EL) Specialized subdivision within a cell.

organic (or-GAN-ik) Referring to the typically large and complex carbon compounds found in living things; contain hydrogen and usually oxygen as well as other elements.

organism (OR-gan-izm) Any organized living thing, such as a plant, animal, or microorganism.

origin (OR-ih-jin) Source; beginning; muscle attachment connected to a nonmoving part.

oropharynx (o-ro-FAR-inks) Middle portion of the pharynx, located behind the mouth.

orthopnea (or-THOP-ne-ah) Difficulty in breathing that is relieved by sitting in an upright position.

osmosis (os-MO-sis) Diffusion of water through a semipermeable membrane.

osmotic (os-MOT-ik) **pressure** Tendency of a solution to draw water into it; directly related to a solution's concentration.

osseus (OS-e-us) Pertaining to bone tissue.

ossicle (OS-ih-kl) One of three small bones of the middle ear: malleus, incus, or stapes.

ossification (os-ih-fih-KA-shun) Process of bone formation.

osteoblast (OS-te-o-blast) Bone-forming cell.

osteoclast (OS-te-o-clast) Cell that breaks down bone.

osteocyte (OS-te-o-site) Mature bone cell; maintains bone but does not produce new bone tissue.

osteon (OS-te-on) Subunit of compact bone, consisting of concentric rings of bone tissue around a central channel; haversian system.

otolithic (o-to-LITH-ik) **membrane** Gelatinous material in which equilibrium receptor cells in the vestibule of the inner ear are embedded.

otoliths (O-to-liths) Crystals that add weight to the otolithic membrane of equilibrium receptors in the vestibule of the inner ear.

ovarian follicle (o-VA-re-an FOL-ih-kl) Cluster of cells containing an ovum. A follicle can mature during a menstrual cycle and release its ovum.

ovary (O-vah-re) Female reproductive gland.

oviduct (O-vih-dukt) See uterine tube.

ovulation (ov-u-LA-shun) Release of an ovum from a mature ovarian follicle (graafian follicle).

ovum (O-vum) Female reproductive cell or gamete; pl., ova.

oxidation (ok-sih-DA-shun) Chemical breakdown of nutrients for energy.

oxygen (OK-sih-jen) (O_2) Gas needed to break down nutrients completely for energy within the cell.

oxytocin (ok-se-TO-sin) Hormone from the posterior pituitary that causes uterine contraction and milk ejection ("letdown") from the breasts.

P

pacemaker Group of cells or artificial device that sets activity rate; in the heart, the sinoatrial (SA) node that normally initiates contractions.

palate (PAL-at) Roof of the oral cavity; anterior portion is hard palate, posterior portion is soft palate.

pancreas (PAN-kre-as) Large, elongated gland behind the stomach; produces digestive enzymes and hormones (e.g., insulin, glucagon).

papilla (pah-PIL-ah) Small nipplelike projection or elevation.

papillary muscles (PAP-ih-lar-e) Columnar muscles in the heart's ventricular walls that anchor and pull on the chordae tendineae to prevent the valve flaps from everting when the ventricles contract.

papule (PAP-ule) Firm, raised lesion of the skin.

parasympathetic nervous system Craniosacral division of the autonomic nervous system; generally reverses the fight-or-flight (stress) response.

parathyroid (par-ah-THI-royd) **gland** Any of four to six small glands embedded in the capsule enclosing the thyroid gland; produces parathyroid hormone, which raises blood calcium level by causing calcium release from bones and calcium retention in the kidney.

parietal (pah-RI-eh-tal) Pertaining to the wall of a space or cavity.

parturition (par-tu-RISH-un) Childbirth; labor.

pelvis (PEL-vis) Basinlike structure, such as the lower portion of the abdomen or the upper flared portion of the ureter (renal pelvis).

penis (PE-nis) Male organ of urination and sexual intercourse.

perforating canal Channel across a long bone that contains blood vessels and nerves; Volkmann canal.

pericardium (per-ih-KAR-de-um) Fibrous sac lined with serous membrane that encloses the heart.

perichondrium (per-ih-KON-dre-um) Layer of connective tissue that covers cartilage.

perilymph (PER-e-limf) Fluid that fills the inner ear's bony labyrinth.

perimysium (per-ih-MIS-e-um) Connective tissue around a fascicle of muscle tissue.

perineum (per-ih-NE-um) Pelvic floor; external region between the anus and genital organs.

periosteum (per-e-OS-te-um) Connective tissue membrane covering a bone.

peripheral (peh-RIF-er-al) Located away from a center or central structure.

peripheral nervous system (PNS) All the nerves and nervous tissue outside the central nervous system.

peristalsis (per-ih-STAL-sis) Wavelike movements in the wall of an organ or duct that propel its contents forward.

peritoneum (per-ih-to-NE-um) Serous membrane that lines the abdominal cavity and forms outer layer of abdominal organs; forms supporting ligaments for some organs.

peroxisome (per-OK-sih-some) Cell organelle that enzymatically destroys harmful substances produced in metabolism.

Peyer (PI-er) **patches** Clusters of lymphatic nodules in the mucous membranes lining the distal small intestine.

pH Symbol indicating hydrogen ion (H^+) concentration; scale that measures the relative acidity and alkalinity (basicity) of a solution.

phagocyte (FAG-o-site) Cell capable of engulfing large particles, such as foreign matter or cellular debris, through the plasma membrane.

phagocytosis (fag-o-si-TO-sis) Engulfing of large particles through the plasma membrane.

pharynx (FAR-inks) Throat; passageway between the mouth and esophagus.

phenotype (FE-no-tipe) All the characteristics of an organism that can be seen or tested for.

phospholipid (fos-fo-LIP-id) Complex lipid containing phosphorus; major component of the plasma membrane.

phrenic (FREN-ik) Pertaining to the diaphragm.

phrenic nerve Nerve that activates the diaphragm.

physiology (fiz-e-OL-o-je) Study of the function of living organisms.

pia mater (PI-ah MA-ter) Innermost layer of the meninges.

pineal (PIN-e-al) **gland** Gland in the brain that is regulated by light; involved in sleep–wake cycles.

pinna (PIN-nah) Outer projecting portion of the ear; auricle.

pinocytosis (pi-no-si-TO-sis) Intake of small particles and droplets by a cell's plasma membrane.

pituitary (pih-TU-ih-tar-e) **gland** Endocrine gland located under and controlled by the hypothalamus; releases hormones that control other glands; hypophysis.

placenta (plah-SEN-tah) Structure that nourishes and maintains the developing fetus during pregnancy.

plasma (PLAZ-mah) Liquid portion of the blood.

plasma cell Cell derived from a B cell that produces antibodies.

plasma membrane Outer covering of a cell; regulates what enters and leaves cell; cell membrane.

plasmapheresis (plas-mah-fer-E-sis) Separation and removal of plasma from donated blood and return of the formed elements to the donor.

platelet (PLATE-let) Cell fragment that forms a plug to stop bleeding and acts in blood clotting; thrombocyte.
pleura (PLU-rah) Serous membrane that lines the chest cavity and covers the lungs.
plexus (PLEK-sus) Network of vessels or nerves.
PNS See peripheral nervous system.
polysaccharide (pol-e-SAK-ah-ride) Compound formed from many simple sugars linked together (e.g., starch, glycogen).
pons (ponz) Area of the brain between the midbrain and medulla; connects the cerebellum with the rest of the central nervous system.
portal system Venous system that carries blood to a second capillary bed through which it circulates before returning to the heart.
positive feedback Control system in which an action or the product of an action maintains or intensifies that action. The action stops when materials are depleted, the stimulus is removed, or an outside force interrupts the action.
positron emission tomography (to-MOG-rah-fe) (PET) Imaging method that uses a radioactive substance to show activity in an organ.
posterior (pos-TE-re-or) Toward the back; dorsal.
potential (po-TEN-shal) Electric charge, as on the plasma membrane of a neuron or other cell; potential difference, membrane potential, or transmembrane potential.
precipitation (pre-sip-ih-TA-shun) Settling out of a solid previously held in solution or suspension in a liquid; in immunity, clumping of small particles as a result of an antigen–antibody reaction; seen as a cloudiness.
prefix A word part that comes before a root and modifies its meaning.
pregnancy (PREG-nan-se) Period during which an embryo or fetus is developing in the body.
prepuce (PRE-puse) Loose fold of skin that covers the glans penis; foreskin.
presbycusis (pres-be-KU-sis) Slowly progressive hearing loss that often accompanies aging.
presbyopia (pres-be-O-pe-ah) Loss of visual accommodation that occurs with age, leading to farsightedness.
preterm (PRE-term) Referring to an infant born before the 37th week of gestation.
PRL see prolactin.
progeny (PROJ-eh-ne) Offspring, descendent.
progesterone (pro-JES-ter-one) Hormone produced by the corpus luteum and placenta; maintains the uterine lining for pregnancy.
prolactin (pro-LAK-tin) Hormone from the anterior pituitary that stimulates milk production in the mammary glands; PRL.
prone Face down or palm down.
prophase (PRO-faze) First stage of mitosis, during which the chromosomes become visible and the organelles disappear.
prophylaxis (pro-fih-LAK-sis) Prevention of disease.
proprioceptor (pro-pre-o-SEP-tor) Sensory receptor that aids in judging body position and changes in position; located in muscles, tendons, and joints.
prostaglandin (pros-tah-GLAN-din) Any of a group of hormones produced by many cells; these hormones have a variety of effects.
prostate (PROS-tate) **gland** Gland that surrounds the urethra below the bladder and contributes secretions to the semen.
protein (PRO-tene) Organic compound made of amino acids, which contain nitrogen in addition to carbon, hydrogen, and oxygen (some contain sulfur or phosphorus as well); found as structural materials and metabolically active compounds, such as enzymes, some hormones, pigments, antibodies, and others.
prothrombin (pro-THROM-bin) Clotting factor; converted to thrombin during blood clotting.
prothrombinase (pro-THROM-bih-nase) Blood clotting factor that converts prothrombin to thrombin.
proton (PRO-ton) Positively charged particle in an atom's nucleus.
proximal (PROK-sih-mal) Nearer to point of origin or to a reference point.
puerperal (pu-ER-per-al) Related to childbirth.
pulmonary circuit Pathway that carries blood from the heart to the lungs to pick up oxygen and release carbon dioxide and then returns the blood to the heart.
pulse Wave of increased pressure in the vessels produced by heart contraction.
pulse pressure Difference between systolic and diastolic pressures.
pupil (PU-pil) Opening in the center of the eye through which light enters.
Purkinje (pur-KIN-je) **fibers** Part of the heart's conduction system; conduction myofibers.
pus Mixture of bacteria and leukocytes formed in response to infection.
pylorus (pi-LOR-us) Distal region of the stomach that leads to the pyloric sphincter.
pyruvic (pi-RU-vik) **acid** Intermediate product in the breakdown of glucose for energy.

R

radioactivity (ra-de-o-ak-TIV-ih-te) Emission of atomic particles from an element.
radiography (ra-de-og-rah-fe) Production of an image by passage of x-rays through the body onto sensitized film; record produced is a radiograph.
receptor (re-SEP-tor) Specialized cell or ending of a sensory neuron that can be excited by a stimulus. Protein in the plasma membrane or other part of a cell that binds a chemical signal (e.g., hormone, neurotransmitter) resulting in a change in cellular activity.
recessive (re-SES-iv) Referring to a gene that is not expressed in the phenotype if a dominant gene for the same trait is present.
reflex (RE-fleks) Simple, rapid, automatic response involving few neurons.
reflex arc (ark) Pathway through the nervous system from stimulus to response; commonly involves a sensory receptor, sensory neuron, central neuron(s), motor neuron, and effector.
refraction (re-FRAK-shun) Bending of light rays as they pass from one medium to another of a different density.
relaxin (re-LAKS-in) Placental hormone that softens the cervix and relaxes the pelvic joints.
renal tubule Coiled and looped portion of a nephron between the glomerular capsule and the collecting duct.
renin (RE-nin) Enzyme released from the kidney's juxtaglomerular apparatus that indirectly increases blood pressure by activating angiotensin.
repolarization (re-po-lar-ih-ZA-shun) Sudden return to the original charge on a plasma membrane following depolarization.
resorption (re-SORP-shun) Loss of substance from a solid tissue, such as bone or a tooth and return of the components to the blood.
respiration (res-pih-RA-shun) Process by which oxygen is obtained from the environment and delivered to the cells as carbon dioxide is removed from the tissues and released to the environment.
respiratory system System consisting of the lungs and breathing passages involved in exchange of oxygen and carbon dioxide between the outside air and the blood.
reticular (reh-TIK-u-lar) **formation** Network in the limbic system that governs wakefulness and sleep.
retina (RET-ih-nah) Innermost layer of the eye; contains light-sensitive cells (rods and cones).
retroperitoneal (ret-ro-per-ih-to-NE-al) Behind the peritoneum, as are the kidneys, pancreas, and abdominal aorta.
Rh factor Red cell antigen; D antigen.
rhodopsin (ro-DOP-sin) Light-sensitive pigment in the rods of the eye.
rib One of the slender curved bones that make up most of the thorax; costa; adj., costal.
ribonucleic (RI-bo-nu-kle-ik) **acid (RNA)** Substance needed for protein manufacture in the cell.
ribosome (RI-bo-some) Small body in the cell's cytoplasm that is a site of protein manufacture.
RNA See ribonucleic acid.
rod Receptor cell in the retina of the eye; used for vision in dim light.
roentgenogram (rent-GEN-o-gram) Image produced by means of x-rays; radiograph.
root (rute) a basic part; an attached or embedded part. See also word root.
rotation (ro-TA-shun) Twisting or turning of a bone on its own axis.
rugae (RU-je) Folds in the lining of an organ, such as the stomach or urinary bladder; sing., ruga (RU-gah).

S

SA node See sinoatrial node.
saliva (sah-LI-vah) Secretion of the salivary glands; moistens food and contains an enzyme that digests starch.

salt Compound formed by reaction between an acid and a base (e.g., NaCl, table salt).

saltatory (SAL-tah-to-re) **conduction** Transmission of an electric impulse from node to node along a myelinated fiber; faster than continuous conduction along the entire membrane.

sagittal (SAJ-ih-tal) Describing a plane that divides a structure into right and left portions.

sarcoplasmic reticulum (sar-ko-PLAS-mik re-TIK-u-lum) **(SR)** Intracellular membrane in muscle cells that is equivalent to the endoplasmic reticulum (ER) in other cells; stores calcium needed for muscle contraction.

saturated fat Fat that has more hydrogen atoms and fewer double bonds between carbons than do unsaturated fats.

scar Fibrous connective tissue that replaces normal tissues destroyed by injury or disease; cicatrix (SIK-ah-triks).

Schwann (shvahn) **cell** Cell in the nervous system that produces the myelin sheath around peripheral axons.

sclera (SKLE-rah) Outermost layer of the eye; made of tough connective tissue; "white" of the eye.

scrotum (SKRO-tum) Sac in which testes are suspended.

sebaceous (seh-BA-chus) Pertaining to sebum, an oily substance secreted by skin glands.

sebum (SE-bum) Oily secretion that lubricates the skin; adj., sebaceous (se-BA-shus).

secretin (se-KRE-tin) Hormone from the duodenum that stimulates pancreatic release of water and bicarbonate.

segmentation (seg-men-TA-shun) Alternating contraction and relaxation of the circular muscle in the small intestine's wall, which mix its contents with digestive juices and move them through the organ.

selectively permeable Describing a membrane that regulates what can pass through (e.g., a cell's plasma membrane).

sella turcica (SEL-ah TUR-sih-ka) Saddlelike depression in the floor of the skull that holds the pituitary gland.

semen (SE-men) Mixture of sperm cells and secretions from several glands of the male reproductive tract.

semicircular canal Bony canal in the internal ear that contains some receptors for the sense of equilibrium; there are three semicircular canals in each ear.

semilunar (sem-e-LU-nar) Shaped like a half-moon, such as the flaps of the pulmonary and aortic valves.

seminal vesicle (VES-ih-kl) Gland that contributes secretions to the semen.

seminiferous (seh-mih-NIF-er-us) **tubules** Tubules in which sperm cells develop in the testis.

semipermeable (sem-e-PER-me-ah-bl) Capable of being penetrated by some substances and not others.

sensory (SEN-so-re) Describing cells or activities involved in transmitting impulses toward the central nervous system; afferent.

sensory adaptation Gradual loss of sensation when sensory receptors are exposed to continuous stimulation.

sensory receptor Part of the nervous system that detects a stimulus.

septum (SEP-tum) Dividing wall, as between the chambers of the heart or the nasal cavities.

serosa (se-RO-sah) Serous membrane; epithelial membrane that secretes a thin, watery fluid.

serotonin (ser-o-TO-nin) Neurotransmitter and vasoconstrictor.

Sertoli cells See sustentacular cells.

serum (SE-rum) Liquid portion of blood without clotting factors; thin, watery fluid; adj., serous (SE-rus).

sex-linked Referring to a gene carried on a sex chromosome, usually the X chromosome.

sinoatrial (si-no-A-tre-al) **(SA) node** Tissue in the right atrium's upper wall that sets the rate of heart contractions; the heart's pacemaker.

sinus (SI-nus) Cavity or channel, such as the paranasal sinuses in the skull bones.

sinus rhythm Normal heart rhythm originating at the SA node.

sinusoid (SI-nus-oyd) Enlarged capillary that serves as a blood channel.

skeletal (SKEL-eh-tal) **system** The body system that includes the bones and joints.

skeleton (SKEL-eh-ton) Bony framework of the body; adj., skeletal.

skull Bony framework of the head.

solute (SOL-ute) Substance that is dissolved in another substance (the solvent).

solution (so-LU-shun) Homogeneous mixture of one substance dissolved in another; the components in a mixture are evenly distributed and cannot be distinguished from each other.

solvent (SOL-vent) Substance in which another substance (the solute) is dissolved.

somatic (so-MAT-ik) **nervous system** Division of the nervous system that controls voluntary activities and stimulates skeletal muscle.

somatotropin (so-mah-to-TRO-pin) Growth hormone.

specific gravity Weight of a substance as compared to the weight of an equal volume of pure water.

spermatic (sper-MAT-ik) **cord** Cord that extends through the inguinal canal and suspends the testis; contains blood vessels, nerves, and ductus deferens.

spermatozoon (sper-mah-to-ZO-on) Male reproductive cell or gamete; pl., spermatozoa; sperm cell.

sphincter (SFINK-ter) Muscular ring that regulates the size of an opening.

sphygmomanometer (sfig-mo-mah-NOM-eh-ter) Device used to measure blood pressure; blood pressure apparatus or cuff.

spinal cord Nervous tissue contained in the spinal column; major relay area between the brain and the peripheral nervous system.

spiral (SPI-ral) **organ** Receptor for hearing located in the cochlea of the internal ear; organ of Corti.

spirometer (spi-ROM-eh-ter) Instrument for recording lung volumes; tracing obtained is a spirogram.

spleen Lymphoid organ in the upper left region of the abdomen.

squamous (SKWA-mus) Flat and irregular, as in squamous epithelium.

SR See sarcoplasmic reticulum.

stain (stane) Dye that aids in viewing structures under the microscope.

stem cell Cell that has the potential to develop into different types of cells.

sterilization (ster-ih-li-ZA-shun) Procedure that makes an individual incapable of reproduction.

steroid (STE-royd) Category of lipids that includes the hormones of the sex glands and the adrenal cortex.

stethoscope (STETH-o-skope) Instrument for conveying sounds from the patient's body to the examiner's ears.

stimulus (STIM-u-lus) Change in the external or internal environment that produces a response.

stomach (STUM-ak) Organ of the digestive tract that stores food, mixes it with digestive juices, and moves it into the small intestine.

stratified In multiple layers (strata).

stratum (STRA-tum) A layer; pl., strata.

stratum basale (bas-A-le) Deepest layer of the epidermis; layer that produces new epidermal cells; stratum germinativum.

stratum corneum (KOR-ne-um) The thick uppermost layer of the epidermis.

striations (stri-A-shuns) Stripes or bands, as seen in skeletal muscle and cardiac muscle.

stroke Damage to the brain due to lack of oxygen; usually caused by a blood clot in a vessel (thrombus) or rupture of a vessel; cerebrovascular accident (CVA).

subcutaneous (sub-ku-TA-ne-us) Under the skin.

submucosa (sub-mu-KO-sah) Layer of connective tissue beneath the mucosa.

substrate Substance on which an enzyme works.

sudoriferous (su-do-RIF-er-us) Producing sweat; referring to the sweat glands.

suffix A word part that follows a root and modifies its meaning.

sulcus (SUL-kus) Shallow groove, as between convolutions of the cerebral cortex; pl., sulci (SUL-si).

superior (su-PE-re-or) Above; in a higher position.

superior vena cava (VE-nah KA-vah) Large vein that drains the upper part of the body and empties into the heart's right atrium.

supine (SU-pine) Face up or palm up.

surfactant (sur-FAK-tant) Substance in the alveoli that prevents their collapse by reducing surface tension of the fluid lining them.

suspension (sus-PEN-shun) Heterogeneous mixture that will separate unless shaken.

suspensory ligaments Filaments attached to the ciliary muscle of the eye that hold the lens in place and can be used to change its shape.

sustentacular (sus-ten-TAK-u-lar) **cells** Cells in the seminiferous tubules that aid in development of spermatozoa; Sertoli cells.

suture (SU-chur) Type of joint in which bone surfaces are closely united, as in the skull; stitch used in surgery to bring parts together; to stitch parts together in surgery.

sympathetic nervous system Thoracolumbar division of the autonomic nervous system; stimulates a fight-or-flight (stress) response.
synapse (SIN-aps) Junction between two neurons or between a neuron and an effector.
synarthrosis (sin-ar-THRO-sis) Immovable joint.
synergist (SIN-er-jist) Substance or structure that enhances the work of another. A muscle that works with a prime mover to produce a given movement.
synovial (sin-O-ve-al) Pertaining to a thick, lubricating fluid found in joints, bursae, and tendon sheaths; pertaining to a freely movable (diarthrotic) joint.
system (SIS-tem) Group of organs functioning together for the same general purposes.
systemic (sis-TEM-ik) Referring to a generalized infection or condition.
systemic circuit Pathway that carries blood to all tissues of the body to deliver oxygen and pick up.
systole (SIS-to-le) Contraction phase of the cardiac cycle; adj., systolic (sis-TOL-ik).

T

tachycardia (tak-e-KAR-de-ah) Heart rate more than 100 beats per minute in an adult.
tachypnea (tak-IP-ne-ah) Increased rate of respiration.
tactile (TAK-til) Pertaining to the sense of touch.
target tissue Tissue that is capable of responding to a specific hormone.
T cell Lymphocyte active in immunity that matures in the thymus gland; may destroy foreign cells directly, help in or regulate the immune response; T lymphocyte.
tectorial (tek-TO-re-al) **membrane** Membrane overlying the sensory (hair) cells in the spiral organ of hearing.
telophase (TEL-o-faze) Final stage of mitosis, during which new nuclei form and the cell contents usually divide.
tendon (TEN-don) Cord of fibrous connective tissue that attaches a muscle to a bone.
teniae (TEN-e-e) **coli** Bands of smooth muscle in the wall of the large intestine.
testis (TES-tis) Male reproductive gland; pl., testes (TES-teze).
testosterone (tes-TOS-ter-one) Male sex hormone produced in the testes; promotes sperm cell development and maintains secondary sex characteristics.
thalamus (THAL-ah-mus) Region of the brain located in the diencephalon; chief relay center for sensory impulses traveling to the cerebral cortex.
thorax (THO-raks) Chest; adj., thoracic (tho-RAS-ik).
thrombocyte (THROM-bo-site) Blood platelet; cell fragment that participates in clotting.
thrombolytic (throm-bo-LIT-ik) Dissolving blood clots.
thrombosis (throm-BO-sis) Condition of having a thrombus (blood clot in a vessel).
thrombus (THROM-bus) Blood clot within a vessel.
thymosin (THI-mo-sin) Hormone produced by the thymus gland.
thymus (THI-mus) Lymphoid organ in the upper portion of the chest; site of T cell development.
thyroid (THI-royd) Endocrine gland in the neck.
thyroid-stimulating hormone (TSH) Hormone produced by the anterior pituitary that stimulates the thyroid gland; thyrotropin.
thyroxine (thi-ROK-sin) Hormone produced by the thyroid gland; increases metabolic rate and needed for normal growth; T_4.
tissue Group of similar cells that performs a specialized function.
tonicity (to-NIS-ih-te) Osmotic pressure of a solution in relation to that of a cell.
tonsil (TON-sil) Mass of lymphoid tissue in the region of the pharynx.
tonus (TO-nus) Partially contracted state of muscle; also, tone.
toxin (TOK-sin) Poison.
toxoid (TOK-soyd) Altered toxin used to produce active immunity.
trachea (TRA-ke-ah) Tube that extends from the larynx to the bronchi; windpipe.
tract Bundle of neuron fibers within the central nervous system.
trait Characteristic.
transfusion (trans-FU-zhun) Introduction of blood or blood components directly into the bloodstream of a recipient.
transverse Describing a plane that divides a structure into superior and inferior parts.
tricuspid (tri-KUS-pid) **valve** Valve between the heart's right atrium and right ventricle.
triglyceride (tri-GLIS-er-ide) Simple fat composed of glycerol and three fatty acids.
trigone (TRI-gone) Triangular-shaped region in the floor of the bladder that remains stable as the bladder fills.
triiodothyronine (tri-i-o-do-THI-ro-nin) Thyroid hormone that functions with thyroxine to raise cellular metabolism; T_3.
tropomyosin (tro-po-MI-o-sin) Protein that works with troponin to regulate contraction in skeletal muscle.
troponin (tro-PO-nin) Protein that works with tropomyosin to regulate contraction in skeletal muscle.
TSH See thyroid-stimulating hormone.
tympanic (tim-PAN-ik) **membrane** Membrane between the external and middle ear that transmits sound waves to the bones of the middle ear; eardrum.

U

ultrasound (UL-trah-sound) Very high-frequency sound waves; used in medical imaging to visualize soft structures.
umbilical (um-BIL-ih-kal) **cord** Structure that connects the fetus with the placenta; contains vessels that carry blood between the fetus and placenta.
umbilicus (um-BIL-ih-kus) Small scar on the abdomen that marks the former attachment of the umbilical cord to the fetus; navel.
universal solvent Term used for water because it dissolves more substances than any other solvent.
unsaturated fat Fat that has fewer hydrogen atoms and more double bonds between carbons than do saturated fats.
urea (u-RE-ah) Nitrogenous waste product excreted in the urine; end product of protein metabolism.
ureter (U-re-ter) Tube that carries urine from the kidney to the urinary bladder.
urethra (u-RE-thrah) Tube that carries urine from the urinary bladder to the outside of the body.
urinalysis (u-rin-AL-ih-sis) Laboratory examination of urine's physical and chemical properties.
urinary bladder Hollow organ that stores urine until it is eliminated.
urinary (U-rin-ar-e) **system** The system involved in elimination of soluble waste, water balance, and regulation of body fluids.
urination (u-rin-A-shun) Voiding of urine; micturition.
urine (U-rin) Liquid waste excreted by the kidneys.
uterine (U-ter-in) **tube** Tube that carries ova from the ovary to the uterus; oviduct; fallopian tube.
uterus (U-ter-us) Muscular, pear-shaped organ in the female pelvis within which the fetus develops during pregnancy; adj., uterine.
uvea (U-ve-ah) Middle coat of the eye, including the choroid, iris, and ciliary body; vascular and pigmented structures of the eye.
uvula (U-vu-lah) Soft, fleshy, V-shaped mass that hangs from the soft palate.

V

vaccination (vak-sin-A-shun) Administration of a vaccine to protect against a specific disease; immunization.
vaccine (vak-SENE) Substance used to produce active immunity; usually, a suspension of attenuated or killed pathogens or some component of a pathogen given by inoculation to prevent a specific disease.
vagina (vah-JI-nah) Distal part of the birth canal that opens to the outside of the body; female organ of sexual intercourse.
valence (VA-lens) Combining power of an atom; number of electrons lost, gained, or shared by atoms of an element in chemical reactions.
valve Structure that prevents fluid from flowing backward, as in the heart, veins, and lymphatic vessels.
vas deferens (DEF-er-enz) Tube that carries sperm cells from the testis to the urethra; ductus deferens.
vascular (VAS-ku-lar) Pertaining to blood vessels.
vasectomy (vah-SEK-to-me) Surgical removal of part or all of the ductus (vas) deferens; usually done on both sides to produce sterility.
vasoconstriction (vas-o-kon-STRIK-shun) Decrease in a blood vessel's lumen diameter.

vasodilation (vas-o-di-LA-shun) Increase in a blood vessel's lumen diameter.
vein (vane) Vessel that carries blood toward the heart.
vena cava (VE-nah KA-vah) Large vein that carries blood into the heart's right atrium; superior vena cava or inferior vena cava.
venous sinus (VE-nus SI-nus) Large channel that drains blood low in oxygen.
ventilation (ven-tih-LA-shun) Movement of air into and out of the lungs.
ventral (VEN-tral) At or toward the front or belly surface; anterior.
ventricle (VEN-trih-kl) Cavity or chamber; one of the heart's two lower chambers; one of the brain's four chambers in which cerebrospinal fluid is produced; adj., ventricular (ven-TRIK-u-lar).
venule (VEN-ule) Vessel between a capillary and a vein.
vernix caseosa (VEr-niks ka-se-O-sah) Cheeselike sebaceous secretion that covers a newborn.
vertebra (VER-teh-brah) Bone of the spinal column; pl., vertebrae (VER-teh-bre).
vesicle (VES-ih-kl) Small sac filled with fluid.
vesicular transport Use of vesicles to move large amounts of material through a cell's plasma membrane.
vestibular apparatus (ves-TIB-u-lar) Part of the inner ear concerned with equilibrium; consists of the semicircular canals and vestibule.
vestibular (ves-TIB-u-lar) **folds** Folds of mucous membrane superior to the vocal cords in the larynx. They close off the glottis during swallowing and straining down; false vocal cords.
vestibule (VES-tih-bule) Any space at the entrance to a canal or organ; in the inner ear, area that contains some receptors for the sense of equilibrium.
villi (VIL-li) Small fingerlike projections from the surface of a membrane; projections in the lining of the small intestine through which digested food is absorbed; sing., villus.
viscera (VIS-er-ah) Organs in the ventral body cavities, especially the abdominal organs; adj., visceral.
viscosity (vis-KOS-ih-te) Thickness, as of the blood or other fluid.
vitamin (VI-tah-min) Organic compound needed in small amounts for health.
vitreous (VIT-re-us) **body** Soft, jellylike substance that fills the eyeball and holds the shape of the eye; vitreous humor.
vocal cords Folds of mucous membrane in the larynx used in producing speech; vocal folds.
Volkmann canal See perforating canal.

W

Wernicke (VER-nih-ke) **area** Portion of the cerebral cortex concerned with speech recognition and the meaning of words.
white matter Nervous tissue composed of myelinated fibers.
word root The main part of a word to which prefixes and suffixes may be attached.

X

x-ray Ray or radiation of extremely short wavelength that can penetrate opaque substances and affect photographic plates and fluorescent screens.

Z

zygote (ZI-gote) Fertilized ovum; cell formed by the union of a sperm and an egg.

ssary of Word Parts

Use of Word Parts in Scientific Terminology

Scientific terminology, the special language of scientific and health occupations, is based on an understanding of a few relatively basic elements. These elements—roots, prefixes, and suffixes—form the foundation of almost all scientific terms. A useful way to familiarize yourself with each term is to learn to pronounce it correctly and say it aloud several times. Soon, it will become an integral part of your vocabulary.

The foundation of a word is the word root. Examples of word roots are *abdomin*, referring to the belly region and *aden*, pertaining to a gland. A word root is often followed by a vowel to facilitate pronunciation when an ending is added, as in *abdomino* and *adeno*. We then refer to it as a "combining form," and it usually appears in texts with a slash before the vowel, as in *abdomin/o* and *aden/o*.

A prefix is a part of a word that precedes the word root and changes its meaning. For example, the prefix *mal-* in malnutrition means "abnormal." A suffix, or word ending, is a part that follows the word root and adds to or changes its meaning. The suffix *-rhea* means "profuse flow" or "discharge," as in diarrhea, a condition characterized by excessive discharge of liquid stools.

Many scientific words are compound words; that is, they are made up of more than one root or combining form. Examples of such compound words are *cardiovascular* (pertaining to the heart and blood vessels) and *hydrophobic* (repelling and not dissolving in water; literally "water-fearing"), and many other complex words, such as *sternoclavicular* (indicating relations to both the sternum and the clavicle).

A general knowledge of language structure and spelling rules is also helpful in mastering scientific terminology. For example, adjectives include words that end in *-al*, as in sternal (the noun is sternum), and words that end in*-ous*, as in mucous (the noun is mucus).

The following list includes some of the most commonly used word roots, prefixes, and suffixes, as well as examples of their use. Prefixes are followed by a hyphen; suffixes are preceded by a hyphen; and word roots have no hyphen. Commonly used combining vowels are added to most roots following a slash.

Word Parts

a-, an- not, without: *aphasia, atrophy, anemia, anuria*
ab- away from: *abduction, aboral*
abdomin/o belly or abdominal area: *abdominocentesis, abdominoscopy*
acous, acus hearing, sound: *acoustic, presbyacusis*
acr/o- end, extremity: *acromegaly, acromion*
actin/o, actin/i relation to raylike structures or, more commonly, to light or roentgen (x-) rays, or some other type of radiation: *actiniform, actinodermatitis*
ad- (sometimes converted to *ac-, af-, ag-, ap-, as-, at-,*) toward, added to, near: *adrenal, accretion, agglomerated, afferent*
aden/o gland: *adenectomy, adenitis, adenocarcinoma*
aer/o air, gas, oxygen: *aerobic, aerate*
-agogue inducing, leading, stimulating: *cholagogue, galactagogue*
-al pertaining to, resembling: *skeletal, surgical, ileal*
alb/i- white: *albinism, albinuria*
alge, alg/o, alges/i pain: *algetic, algophobia, analgesic*
-algia pain, painful condition: *myalgia, neuralgia*
amb/i- both, on two sides: *ambidextrous, ambivalent*
ambly- dimness, dullness: *amblyopia*
amphi- on both sides, around, double: *amphiarthrosis, amphibian*
amyl/o starch: *amylase, amyloid*
an- not, without: *anaerobic, anoxia, anemic*
ana- upward, back, again, excessive: *anatomy, anastomosis, anabolism*
andr/o male: *androgen, androgenous*
angi/o vessel: *angiogram, angiotensin*
ant/i- against; to prevent, suppress, or destroy: *antarthritic, antibiotic, anticoagulant*
ante- before, ahead of: *antenatal, antepartum*
anter/o- position ahead of or in front of (i.e., anterior to) another part: *anterolateral, anteroventral*
-apheresis take away, withdraw: *hemapheresis, plasmapheresis*
ap/o- separation, derivation from: *apocrine, apoptosis, apophysis*
aqu/e water: *aqueous, aquatic, aqueduct*
-ar pertaining to, resembling: *muscular, nuclear*
arthr/o joint or articulation: *arthrolysis, arthrostomy, arthritis*
-ary pertaining to, resembling: *salivary, dietary, urinary*
-ase enzyme: *lipase, protease*
-asis *See* –sis
atel/o- imperfect: *atelectasis*
ather/o gruel: *atherosclerosis, atheroma*
audi/o sound, hearing: *audiogenic, audiometry, audiovisual*
aut/o- self: *autistic, autodigestion, autoimmune*

bar/o pressure: *baroreceptor, barometer*
bas/o- alkaline: *basic, basophilic*
bi- two, twice: *bifurcate, bisexual*
bil/i bile: *biliary, bilirubin*
bio- life, living organism: *biopsy, antibiotic*
blast/o, -blast early stage of a cell, immature cell: *blastula, blastophore, erythroblast*
bleph, blephar/o eyelid, eyelash: *blepharism, blepharitis, blepharospasm*
brachi, brachi/o arm: *brachial, brachiocephalic, brachiotomy*
brachy- short: *brachydactylia, brachyesophagus*
brady- slow: *bradycardia*
bronch/o-, bronch/i bronchus: ***bronchiectasis, bronchoscope***
bucc cheek: *buccal*

capn/o carbon dioxide: *hypocapnia, hypercapnia*
carcin/o cancer: *carcinogenic, carcinoma*
cardi/o, cardi/a heart: *carditis, cardiac, cardiologist*
cata- down: *catabolism, catalyst*
-cele swelling; enlarged space or cavity: *cystocele, meningocele, rectocele*
celi/o abdomen: *celiac, celiocentesis*
centi- relating to 100 (used in naming units of measurements): *centigrade, centimeter*
-centesis perforation, tapping: *aminocentesis, paracentesis*
cephal/o head: *cephalalgia, cephalopelvic*
cerebr/o brain: *cerobrospinal, cerebrum*
cervi neck: *cervical, cervix*
cheil/o lips; brim or edge: *cheilitis, cheilosis*
chem/o, chem/i chemistry, chemical: *chemotherapy, chemocautery, chemoreceptor*
chir/o, cheir/o hand: *cheiralgia, cheiromegaly, chiropractic*
chol/e, chol/o bile, gall: *chologogue, cholecyst, cholelith*
cholecyst/o gallbladder: *cholecystitis, cholecystokinin*
chondr/o, chondri/o cartilage: *chondric, chondrocyte, chondroma*
chori/o membrane: *chorion, choroid, choriocarcinoma*
chrom/o, chromat/o color: *chromosome, chromatin, chromophilic*
-cid, -cide to cut, kill, destroy: *bactericidal, germicide, suicide*
circum- around, surrounding: *circumorbital, circumrenal, circumduction*
-clast break: *osteoclast*
clav/o, cleid/o clavicle: *cleidomastoid, subclavian*
co- with, together: *cofactor, cohesion, coinfection*
colp/o vagina: *colpectasia, colposcope, colpotomy*
con- with: *concentric, concentrate, conduct*
contra- opposed, against: *contraindication, contralateral*
corne/o horny: *corneum, cornified, cornea*
cortic/o cortex: *cortical, corticotropic, cortisone*
cost/a, cost/o- ribs: *intercostal, costosternal*
counter- against, opposite to: *counteract, counterirritation, countertraction*
crani/o skull: *cranium, craniotomy*
cry/o- cold: *cryalgesia, cryogenic, cryotherapy*
crypt/o- hidden, concealed: *cryptic, cryptogenic, cryptorchidism*
-cusis hearing: *acusis, presbyacusis*

cut- skin: *subcutaneous*
cyan/o- blue: *cyanosis, cyanogen*
cyst/i, cyst/o sac, bladder: *cystitis, cystoscope*
cyt/o, -cyte cell: *cytology, cytoplasm, osteocyte*

dactyl/o digits (usually fingers, but sometimes toes): *dactylitis, polydactyly*
de- remove: *detoxify, dehydration*
dendr tree: *dendrite*
dent/o, dent/i tooth: *dentition, dentin, dentifrice*
derm/o, dermat/o skin: *dermatitis, dermatology, dermatosis*
di- twice, double: *dimorphism, dibasic, dihybrid*
dipl/o- double: *diplopia, diplococcus*
dia- through, between, across, apart: *diaphragm, diaphysis*
dis- apart, away from: *disarticulation, distal*
dors/i, dors/o- back (in the human, this combining form is the same as poster/o-): *dorsal, dorsiflexion, dorso-nuchal*
dys- disordered, difficult, painful: *dysentery, dysphagia, dyspnea*

e- out: *enucleation, evisceration, ejection*
-ectasis expansion, dilation, stretching: *angiectasis, bronchiectasis*
ecto- outside, external: *ectoderm, ectogenous*
-ectomy surgical removal or destruction by other means: *appendectomy, thyroidectomy*
edem swelling: *edema, edematous*
-emia condition of blood: *glycemia, hyperemia*
encephal/o brain: *encephalitis, encephalogram*
end/o- in, within, innermost: *endarterial, endocardium, endothelium*
enter/o intestine: *enteritis, enterocolitis*
epi- on, upon: *epicardium, epidermis*
equi- equal: *equidistant, equivalent, equilibrium*
erg/o work: *ergonomic, energy, synergy*
eryth-, erythr/o red: *erythema, erythrocyte*
-esthesia sensation: *anesthesia, paresthesia*
eu- well, normal, good: *euphoria, eupnea*
ex/o- outside, out of, away from: *excretion, exocrine, exophthalmic*
extra- beyond, outside of, in addition to: *extracellular, extrasystole, extravasation*

fasci fibrous connective tissue layers: *fascia, fascitis, fascicle*
fer, -ferent to bear, to carry: *afferent, efferent, transfer*
fibr/o threadlike structures, fibers: *fibrillation, fibroblast, fibrositis*

gastr/o stomach: *gastritis, gastroenterostomy*
-gen an agent that produces or originates: *allergen, pathogen, fibrinogen*
-genic produced from, producing: *neurogenic, pyogenic, psychogenic*
genit/o organs of reproduction: *genitoplasty, genitourinary*
gen/o- a relationship to reproduction or sex: *genealogy, generate, genetic, genotype*
-geny manner of origin, development or production: *ontogeny, progeny*
gest/o gestation, pregnancy: *progesterone, gestagen*
glio, -glia gluey material; specifically, the support tissue of the central nervous system: *glioma, neuroglia*
gloss/o tongue: *glossitis, glossopharyngeal*
glyc/o- relating to sugar, glucose, sweet: *glycemia, glycosuria*
gnath/o related to the jaw: *prognathic, gnathoplasty*
gnos to perceive, recognize: *agnostic, prognosis, diagnosis*
gon seed, knee: *gonad, gonarthritis*
-gram record, that which is recorded: *electrocardiogram, electroencephalogram*
graph/o, -graph instrument for recording, writing: *electrocardiograph, electroencephalograph, micrograph*
-graphy process of recording data: *photography, radiography*
gyn/o, gyne, gynec/o female, woman: *gynecology, gynecomastia, gynoplasty*
gyr/o circle: *gyroscope, gyrus, gyration*

hema, hemo, hemat/o blood: *hematoma, hematuria, hemorrhage*
hemi- one half: *hemisphere, heminephrectomy, hemiplegia*
hepat/o liver: *hepatitis, hepatogenous*
heter/o- other, different: *heterogenous, heterosexual, heterochromia*
hist/o, histi/o tissue: *histology, histiocyte*
homeo-, homo- unchanging, the same: *homeostasis, homosexual*
hydr/o water: *hydrolysis, hydrocephalus*
hyper- above, over, excessive: *hyperesthesia, hyperglycemia, hypertrophy*
hypo- deficient, below, beneath: *hypochondrium, hypodermic, hypogastrium*
hyster/o uterus: *hysterectomy*
-ia state of, condition of: *myopia, hypochondria, ischemia*
-iatrics, -trics medical specialty: *pediatrics, obstetrics*
iatr/o physician, medicine: *iatrogenic*
-ic pertaining to, resembling: *metric, psychiatric, geriatric*
idio- self, one's own, separate, distinct: *idiopathic, idiosyncrasy*
-ile pertaining to, resembling: *febrile, virile*
im-, in- in, into, lacking: *implantation, infiltration, inanimate*
infra- below, inferior: *infraspinous, infracortical*
insul/o pancreatic islet, island: *insulin, insulation, insulinoma*
inter- between: *intercostal, interstitial*
intra- within a part or structure: *intracranial, intracellular, intraocular*
isch suppression: *ischemia*
-ism state of: *alcoholism, hyperthyroidism*
iso- same, equal: *isotonic, isometric*
-ist one who specializes in a field of study: *cardiologist, gastroenterologist*
-itis inflammation: *dermatitis, keratitis, neuritis*

juxta- next to: *juxtaglomerular, juxtaposition*

kary/o nucleus: *karyotype, karyoplasm*
kerat/o cornea of the eye, certain cornified tissues: *keratin, keratitis, keratoplasty*
kine movement: *kinetic, kinesiology, kinesthesia*

lacri- tear: *lacrimal*
lact/o milk: *lactation, lactogenic*
laryng/o larynx: *laryngeal, laryngectomy, laryngitis*
later/o- side: *lateral*
-lemma sheath: *neurilemma, sarcolemma*
leuk/o- (also written as *leuc-, leuco-*) white, colorless: *leukocyte, leukoplakia*
lip/o lipid, fat: *lipase, lipoma*
lig- bind: *ligament, ligature, ligand*
lingu/o tongue: *lingual, linguadental*
lith/o stone (calculus): *lithiasis, lithotripsy*
-logy study of: *physiology, gynecology*
lute/o yellow: *macula lutea, corpus luteum*
lymph/o lymph, lymphatic system, lymphocyte: *lymphoid, lymphedema*
lyso-, -lysis, -lytic: loosening, dissolving, separating: *hemolysis, paralysis, lysosome*

macr/o- large, abnormal length: *macrophage, macroblast*. See also -mega, megal/o-
mal- bad, diseased, disordered, abnormal: *malnutrition, malocclusion, malunion*
malac/o, -malacia softening: *malacoma, osteomalacia*
mamm/o breast, mammary gland: *mammogram, mammoplasty, mammal*
man/o pressure: *manometer, sphygmomanometer*
mast/o breast: *mastectomy, mastitis*
meg/a-, megal/o, -megaly unusually or excessively large: *megacolon, megaloblast, splenomegaly, megakaryocyte*
melan/o dark, black: *melanin, melanocyte, melanoma*
men/o physiologic uterine bleeding, menses: *menstrual, menorrhagia, menopause*
mening/o membranes covering the brain and spinal cord: *meningitis, meningocele*
mes/a, mes/o- middle, midline: *mesencephalon, mesoderm*
meta- change, beyond, after, over, near: *metabolism, metacarpal, metaplasia*
-meter, metr/o measure: *hemocytometer, sphygmomanometer, spirometer, isometric*
metr/o uterus: *endometrium, metroptosis, metrorrhagia*
micro- very small: *microscope, microbiology, microsurgery, micrometer*

mon/o- single, one: *monocyte, mononucleosis*
morph/o shape, form: *morphogenesis, morphology*
multi- many: *multiple, multifactorial, multipara*
my/o muscle: *myenteron, myocardium, myometrium*
myc/o, mycet fungus: *mycid, mycete, mycology, mycosis, mycelium*
myel/o marrow (often used in reference to the spinal cord): *myeloid, myeloblast, osteomyelitis, poliomyelitis*
myring/o tympanic membrane: *myringotomy, myringitis*
myx/o mucus: *myxoma, myxovirus*

narc/o stupor: *narcosis, narcolepsy, narcotic*
nas/o nose: *nasopharynx, paranasal*
natri sodium: *hyponatremia, natriuretic*
necr/o death, corpse: *necrosis*
neo- new: *neoplasm, neonatal*
neph, nephr/o kidney: *nephrectomy, nephron*
neur/o, neur/i nerve, nervous tissue: *neuron, neuralgia, neuroma*
neutr/o neutral: *neutrophil, neutropenia*
noct/i night: *noctambulation, nocturia, noctiphobia*

ocul/o eye: *oculist, oculomotor, oculomycosis*
odont/o tooth, teeth: *odontalgia, orthodontics*
-odynia pain, tenderness: *myodynia, neurodynia*
-oid like, resembling: *lymphoid, myeloid*
olig/o- few, a deficiency: *oligospermia, oliguria*
-oma tumor, swelling: *hematoma, sarcoma*
-one ending for steroid hormone: *testosterone, progesterone*
onych/o nails: *paronychia, onychoma*
oo, ovum, egg: *oocyte, oogenesis* (do not confuse with oophor-)
oophor/o ovary: *oophorectomy, oophoritis, oophorocystectomy*. See also ovar-
ophthalm/o eye: *ophthalmia, ophthalmologist, ophthalmoscope*
-opia disorder of the eye or vision: *heterotropia, myopia, hyperopia*
or/o mouth: *oropharynx, oral*
orchi/o, orchid/o testis: *orchitis, cryptorchidism*
orth/o- straight, normal: *orthopedics, orthopnea, orthosis*
-ory pertaining to, resembling: *respiratory, circulatory*
oscill/o to swing to and fro: *oscilloscope*
osmo- osmosis: *osmoreceptor, osmotic*
oss/i, osse/o, oste/o bone, bone tissue: *osseous, ossicle, osteocyte, osteomyelitis*
ot/o ear: *otalgia, otitis, otomycosis*
-ous pertaining to, resembling: *fibrous, venous, androgynous*
ov/o egg, ovum: *oviduct, ovulation*
ovar, ovari/o ovary: *ovarian, ovariectomy*. See also oophor
ox-, -oxia pertaining to oxygen: *hypoxemia, hypoxia, anoxia*
oxy sharp, acute: *oxygen, oxytocia*

pan- all: *pandemic, panacea*
papill/o nipple: *papilloma, papillary*
para- near, beyond, apart from, beside: *paramedical, parametrium, parathyroid, parasagittal*
pariet/o wall: *parietal*
path/o, -pathy disease, abnormal condition: *pathogen, pathology, neuropathy*
ped/o, pedia child, foot: *pedophobia, pediatrician, pedialgia*
-penia lack of: *leukopenia, thrombocytopenia*
per- through, excessively: *percutaneous, perfusion*
peri- around: *pericardium, perichondrium*
-pexy fixation: *nephropexy, proctopexy*
phag/o to eat, to ingest: *phagocyte, phagosome*
-phagia, -phagy eating, swallowing: *aphagia, dysphagia*
-phasia speech, ability to talk: *aphasia, dysphasia*
phen/o to show: *phenotype*
-phil, -philic to like, have an affinity for: *eosinophilia, hemophilia, hydrophilic*
phleb/o vein: *phlebitis, phlebotomy*
-phobia fear, dread, abnormal aversion: *phobic, acrophobia, hydrophobia*
phot/o light: *photoreceptor, photophobia*
phren/o diaphragm: *phrenic, phrenicotomy*
physi/o natural, physical: *physiology, physician*
pil/e, pil/i, pil/o hair, resembling hair: *pileous, piliation, pilonidal*
pin/o to drink: *pinocytosis*
-plasty molding, surgical formation: *cystoplasty, gastroplasty, kineplasty*
-plegia stroke, paralysis: *paraplegia, hemiplegia*
pleur/o side, rib, pleura: *pleurisy, pleurotomy*
-pnea air, breathing: *dyspnea, eupnea*
pneum/o, pneumat/o air, gas, respiration: *pneumothorax, pneumograph, pneumatocele*
pneumon/o lung: *pneumonia, pneumonectomy*
pod/o foot: *podiatry, pododynia*
-poiesis making, forming: *erythropoiesis, hematopoiesis*
polio- gray, gray matter: *polioencephalitis, poliomyelitis*
poly- many: *polyarthritis, polycystic, polycythemia*
post- behind, after, following: *postnatal, postocular, postpartum*
pre- before, ahead of: *precancerous, preclinical, prenatal*
presby- old age: *presbycusis, presbyopia*
pro- before, in front of, in favor of: *prodromal, prosencephalon, prolapse, prothrombin*
proct/o rectum: *proctitis, proctocele, proctologist*
propri/o own: *proprioception*
pseud/o false: *pseudoarthrosis, pseudostratified, pseudopod*
psych/o mind: *psychosomatic, psychotherapy*
-ptosis downward displacement, falling, prolapse: *blepharoptosis, enteroptosis, nephroptosis*
pulm/o, pulmon/o lung: *pulmonic, pulmonology*
py/o pus: *pyuria, pyogenic, pyorrhea*
pyel/o renal pelvis: *pyelitis, pyelogram, pyelonephrosis*
pyr/o fire, fever: *pyrogen, antipyretic, pyromania*

quadr/i- four: *quadriceps, quadriplegic*

rachi/o spine: *rachicentesis, rachischisis*
radio- emission of rays or radiation: *radioactive, radiography, radiology*
re- again, back: *reabsorption, reaction, regenerate*
rect/o rectum: *rectal, rectouterine*
ren/o kidney: *renal, renopathy*
reticul/o network: *reticulum, reticular*
retro- backward, located behind: *retrocecal, retroperitoneal*
rhin/o nose: *rhinitis, rhinoplasty*
-rhage, -rhagia* bursting forth, excessive flow: *hemorrhage, menorrhagia*
-rhaphy* suturing or sewing up a gap or defect in a part: *herniorrhaphy, gastrorrhaphy, cystorrhaphy*
-rhea* flow, discharge: *diarrhea, gonorrhea, seborrhea*

sacchar/o sugar: *monosaccharide, polysaccharide*
salping/o tube: *salpingitis, salpingoscopy*
sarc/o flesh: *sarcolemma, sarcoplasm, sarcomere*
scler/o hard, hardness; *scleroderma, sclerosis*
scoli/o- twisted, crooked: *scoliosis, scoliosometer*
-scope instrument used to look into or examine a part: *bronchoscope, endoscope, arthroscope*
semi- partial, half: *semipermeable, semicoma*
semin/o semen, seed: *seminiferous, seminal*
sep, septic poison, rot, decay: *sepsis, septicemia*
sin/o cavity, sinus: *sinusitis, sinusoid, sinoatrial*
-sis condition or process, usually abnormal: *dermatosis, osteoporosis*
soma-, somat/o, -some body: *somatic, somatotype, somatotropin*
son/o sound: *sonogram, sonography*
sphygm/o pulse: *sphygmomanometer*
spir/o breathing: *spirometer, inspiration, expiration*
splanchn/o- internal organs: *splanchnic, splanchnoptosis*
splen/o spleen: *splenectomy, splenic*
staphyl/o grapelike cluster: *staphylococcus*
stat, -stasis stand, stoppage, remaining at rest: *hemostasis, static, homeostasis*
sten/o- contracted, narrowed: *stenosis*
sthen/o, -sthenia, -sthenic strength: *asthenic, calisthenics, neurasthenia*
steth/o chest: *stethoscope*
stoma, stomat/o mouth: *stomatitis*
-stomy surgical creation of an opening into a hollow organ or an opening between two organs: *colostomy, tracheostomy, gastroenterostomy*
strept/o chain: *streptococcus, streptobacillus*

---

*When a suffix beginning with *rh* is added to a word root, the *r* is doubled.

sub- under, below, near, almost: *subclavian, subcutaneous, subluxation*
super- over, above, excessive: *superego, supernatant, superficial*
supra- above, over, superior: *supranasal, suprarenal*
sym-, syn- with, together: *symphysis, synapse*
syring/o fistula, tube, cavity: *syringectomy, syringomyelia*

tach/o-, tachy- rapid: *tachycardia, tachypnea*
tars/o eyelid, foot: *tarsitis, tarsoplasty, tarsoptosis*
-taxia, -taxis order, arrangement: *ataxia, chemotaxis, thermotaxis*
tel/o end: *telophase, telomere*
tens- stretch, pull: *extension, tensor*
terat/o malformed fetus: *teratogen, teratogenic*
test/o testis: *testosterone, testicular*
tetr/a four: *tetralogy, tetraplegia*
therm/o-, -thermy heat: *thermalgesia, thermocautery, diathermy, thermometer*
thromb/o blood clot: *thrombosis, thrombocyte*
toc/o labor: *eutocia, dystocia, oxytocin*
tom/o, -tomy incision of, cutting: *anatomy, phlebotomy, laparotomy*
ton/o tone, tension: *tonicity, tonic*
tox, toxic/o poison: *toxin, cytotoxic, toxemia, toxicology*
trache/o trachea, windpipe: *tracheal, tracheitis, tracheotomy*
trans- across, through, beyond: *transorbital, transpiration, transplant, transport*

tri- three: *triad, triceps*
trich/o hair: *trichiasis, trichosis, trichology*
troph/o, -trophic, -trophy nutrition, nurture: *atrophic, hypertrophy*
trop/o, -tropin, -tropic turning toward, acting on, influencing, changing: *thyrotropin, adrenocorticotropic, gonadotropic*
tympan/o drum: *tympanic, tympanum*

ultra- beyond or excessive: *ultrasound, ultraviolent, ultrastructure*
uni- one: *unilateral, uniovular, unicellular*
-uria urine: *glycosuria, hematuria, pyuria*
ur/o urine, urinary tract: *urology, urogenital*

vas/o vessel, duct: *vascular, vasectomy, vasodilation*
viscer/o internal organs, viscera: *visceral, visceroptosis*
vitre/o glasslike: *vitreous*

xer/o dryness: *xeroderma, xerophthalmia, xerosis*

-y condition of: *tetany, atony, dysentery*

zyg/o joined: *zygote, heterozygous, monozygotic*

Appendix 1

Periodic Table of the Elements

The periodic table lists the chemical elements according to their atomic numbers. The boxes in the table have information about the elements, as shown by the example at the top of the chart. The upper number in each box is the atomic number, which represents the number of protons in the nucleus of the atom. Under the name of the element is its chemical symbol, an abbreviation of its modern or Latin name. The Latin names of four common elements are shown below the chart. The bottom number in each box gives the atomic weight (mass) of that element's atoms compared with the weight of carbon atoms. Atomic weight is the sum of the weights of the protons and neutrons in the nucleus.

All the elements in a column share similar chemical properties based on the number of electrons in their outermost energy levels. Those in column VIII are nonreactive (inert) and are referred to as noble gases. The 26 elements found in the body are color coded according to quantity (see totals above the chart). Carbon, hydrogen, oxygen, and nitrogen make up 96% of body weight. The first three of these are present in all carbohydrates, lipids, proteins, and nucleic acids. Nitrogen is an additional component of all proteins. Nine other elements make up almost all the rest of body weight. The remaining 13 elements are present in very small amounts and are referred to as trace elements. Although needed in very small quantities, they are essential for good health, as they are parts of enzymes and other compounds used in metabolism.

PERIODIC TABLE OF THE ELEMENTS

96% of body weight

3.9% of body weight

0.1% of body weight

Notation:

6 Carbon C 12.01	Atomic number Name Symbol Atomic weight

I	II											III	IV	V	VI	VII	VIII
1 Hydrogen **H** 1.01																	2 Helium **He** 4.00
3 Lithium **Li** 6.94	4 Beryllium **Be** 9.01											5 Boron **B** 10.81	6 Carbon **C** 12.01	7 Nitrogen **N** 14.01	8 Oxygen **O** 16.00	9 Fluorine **F** 19.00	10 Neon **Ne** 20.18
11 Sodium **Na** 22.99	12 Magnesium **Mg** 24.31											13 Aluminum **Al** 26.98	14 Silicon **Si** 28.09	15 Phosphorus **P** 30.97	16 Sulfur **S** 32.07	17 Chlorine **Cl** 35.45	18 Argon **Ar** 39.95
19 Potassium **K** 39.10	20 Calcium **Ca** 40.08	21 Scandium **Sc** 44.96	22 Titanium **Ti** 47.88	23 Vanadium **V** 50.94	24 Chromium **Cr** 52.00	25 Manganese **Mn** 54.94	26 Iron **Fe** 55.85	27 Cobalt **Co** 58.93	28 Nickel **Ni** 58.69	29 Copper **Cu** 63.55	30 Zinc **Zn** 65.39	31 Gallium **Ga** 69.72	32 Germanium **Ge** 72.59	33 Arsenic **As** 74.92	34 Selenium **Se** 78.96	35 Bromine **Br** 79.90	36 Krypton **Kr** 83.80
37 Rubidium **Rb** 85.47	38 Strontium **Sr** 87.62	39 Yttrium **Y** 88.91	40 Zirconium **Zr** 91.22	41 Niobium **Nb** 92.91	42 Molybdenum **Mo** 95.94	43 Technetium **Tc** (98)	44 Ruthenium **Ru** 101.1	45 Rhodium **Rh** 102.9	46 Palladium **Pd** 106.4	47 Silver **Ag** 107.9	48 Cadmium **Cd** 112.4	49 Indium **In** 114.8	50 Tin **Sn** 118.7	51 Antimony **Sb** 121.8	52 Tellurium **Te** 127.6	53 Iodine **I** 126.9	54 Xenon **Xe** 131.3
55 Cesium **Cs** 132.91	56 Barium **Ba** 137.34		72 Hafnium **Hf** 178.5	73 Tantalum **Ta** 180.9	74 Tungsten **W** 183.9	75 Rhenium **Re** 186.2	76 Osmium **Os** 190.2	77 Iridium **Ir** 192.2	78 Platinum **Pt** 195.1	79 Gold **Au** 196.9	80 Mercury **Hg** 200.6	81 Thallium **Tl** 204.4	82 Lead **Pb** 207.2	83 Bismuth **Bi** 209.0	84 Polonium **Po** (210)	85 Astatine **At** (210)	86 Radon **Rn** (222)
87 Francium **Fr** (223)	88 Radium **Ra** (226)		104 Rutherfordium **Rf** (257)	105 Dubnium **Db** (260)	106 Seaborgium **Sg** (263)	107 Bohrium **Bh** (262)	108 Hassium **Hs** (265)	109 Meitnerium **Mt** (267)	110 Darmstadtium **Ds** (271)	111 Unnamed (272)	112 Unnamed (277)						

57-71 Lanthanides	57 Lanthanum **La** 138.9	58 Cerium **Ce** 140.1	59 Praseodymium **Pr** 140.9	60 Neodymium **Nd** 144.2	61 Promethium **Pm** (145)	62 Samarium **Sm** (150.4)	63 Europium **Eu** 152.0	64 Gadolinium **Gd** 157.3	65 Terbium **Tb** 158.9	66 Dysprosium **Dy** 162.5	67 Holmium **Ho** 164.9	68 Erbium **Er** 167.3	69 Thulium **Tm** 168.9	70 Ytterbium **Yb** 173.0	71 Lutetium **Lu** 175.0
89-103 Actinides	89 Actinium **Ac** (227)	90 Thorium **Th** 232.0	91 Protactinium **Pa** (231)	92 Uranium **U** (238)	93 Neptunium **Np** (237)	94 Plutonium **Pu** (244)	95 Americium **Am** (243)	96 Curium **Cm** (247)	97 Berkelium **Bk** (247)	98 Californium **Cf** (251)	99 Einsteinium **Es** (254)	100 Fermium **Fm** (257)	101 Mendelevium **Md** (256)	102 Nobelium **No** (259)	103 Lawrencium **Lr** (257)

Name	Latin name	Symbol
Copper	*cuprium*	Cu
Iron	*ferrum*	Fe
Potassium	*kalium*	K
Sodium	*natrium*	Na

Appendix 2

Answers to Chapter Checkpoint and Zooming In Questions

Chapter 1

Answers to Checkpoint Questions

1-1 Study of body structure is anatomy; study of body function is physiology.

1-2 Organs working together combine to form systems.

1-3 Catabolism and anabolism are the two types of metabolic reactions. In catabolism, complex substances are broken down into simpler compounds. In anabolism, simple compounds are used to manufacture materials needed for body functions.

1-4 Extracellular fluid is located outside of cells; intracellular fluid is located within cells.

1-5 Negative feedback is the main method used to maintain homeostasis.

1-6 Proximal describes a location closer to an origin. The elbow is proximal to the wrist.

1-7 The three planes in which the body can be cut are sagittal, frontal (coronal), and transverse (horizontal).

1-8 The two main body cavities are the dorsal and ventral cavities.

1-9 The three central regions of the abdomen are the epigastric, umbilical, and hypogastric regions. The three left and right regions are the hypochondriac, lumbar, and iliac (inguinal) regions.

Answers to Zooming In Questions

1-6 The figures are standing in the anatomic position.

1-7 The transverse (horizontal) plane divides the body into superior and inferior parts. The frontal (coronal) plane divides the body into anterior and posterior parts.

1-10 The ventral cavity contains the diaphragm.

1-13 The umbilical, hypogastric, left lumbar, and left iliac (inguinal) regions are represented in the left lower quadrant.

Chapter 2

Answers to Checkpoint Questions

2-1 Atoms are subunits of elements.

2-2 Three types of particles found in atoms are protons, neutrons, and electrons.

2-3 The two types of chemical bonds are ionic bonds and covalent bonds. Ionic bonds result from the transfer of electrons from one atom to another. Covalent bonds are formed by the sharing of electrons between atoms.

2-4 When an electrolyte goes into solution, it separates into charged particles called ions (cations and anions).

2-5 Molecules are units composed of two or more covalently bonded atoms. Compounds are substances composed of two or more different elements.

2-6 In a solution, the solute dissolves and remains evenly distributed (the mixture is homogeneous); in a suspension, the material in suspension does not dissolve and settles out unless the mixture is shaken (the mixture is heterogeneous).

2-7 Water is the most abundant compound in the body.

2-8 A value of 7.0 is neutral on the pH scale. An acid measures lower than 7.0; a base measures higher than 7.0.

2-9 A buffer is a substance that maintains a steady pH of a solution.

2-10 Isotopes that give off radiation are termed radioactive or radioisotopes.

2-11 Carbon is the basis of organic chemistry.

2-12 The three main categories of organic compounds are carbohydrates, lipids, and proteins.

2-13 An enzyme is a catalyst that speeds the rate of chemical reactions in the body.

2-14 A nucleotide contains a sugar, a phosphate group, and a nitrogenous base. DNA, RNA, and ATP are examples of compounds composed of nucleotides.

Answers to Zooming In Questions

2-1 The number of protons is equal to the number of electrons. There are eight protons and eight electrons in an oxygen atom.

2-2 Oxygen needs two electrons to complete its outermost energy level. Magnesium needs to lose two electrons to achieve an outermost energy level.

2-3 Sodium has one electron in its outermost energy level. Chlorine has seven electrons in its outermost energy level.

2-4 Two electrons are needed to complete the energy level of each hydrogen atom.

2-5 Two hydrogen atoms bond with an oxygen atom to form water.

2-6 The amount of hydroxide ion (OH^-) in a solution decreases when the amount of hydrogen ion (H^+) increases.

2-8 The building blocks (monomers) of disaccharides and polysaccharides are monosaccharides.

2-9 There are three carbon atoms in glycerol.

2-10 The amino group of an amino acid contains nitrogen.

2-11 The shape of an enzyme after the reaction is the same as it was before the reaction.

2-12 The prefix *tri-* means three.

Chapter 3

Answers to Checkpoint Questions

3-1 The cell shows organization, metabolism, responsiveness, homeostasis, growth, and reproduction.

3-2 Three types of microscopes are the compound light microscope, transmission electron microscope (TEM), and scanning electron microscope (SEM).

3-3 The main substance of the plasma membrane is phospholipids. The three types of materials found within the membrane are cholesterol, carbohydrates (glycoproteins and glycolipids), and proteins.

3-4 The membrane potential is an electric charge (voltage differential) on the membrane. It is maintained by ions on either side of the membrane.

3-5 The cell organelles are specialized structures that perform different tasks.

3-6 The nucleus is called the cell's control center because it contains chromosomes, hereditary units that control all cellular activities.

3-7 The two types of organelles used for movement are cilia, which are small and hairlike, and the flagellum, which is long and whiplike.

3-8 Diffusion, facilitated diffusion, osmosis, and filtration do not require cellular energy; active transport and bulk transport require cellular energy. Bulk transport includes endocytosis (phagocytosis, pinocytosis, receptor-mediated endocytosis) and exocytosis.

3-9 An isotonic solution has the same concentration as the intracellular fluid; a hypotonic solution is less concentrated; a hypertonic solution is more concentrated.

3-10 The building blocks of nucleic acids are nucleotides.

3-11 DNA codes for proteins in the cell.

3-12 The three types of RNA active in protein synthesis are messenger RNA (mRNA), ribosomal RNA (rRNA), and transfer RNA (tRNA).

3-13 Before mitosis can occur, the DNA must replicate (double). Replication occurs during interphase.

3-14 The four stages of mitosis are prophase, metaphase, anaphase, and telophase.

Answers to Zooming In Questions

3-1 **A**: The transmission electron microscope (TEM). **B** shows the most internal structure. The scanning electron microscope (SEM). **C** shows the cilia in three dimensions.

3-2 Ribosomes attached to the ER make it look rough. Cytosol is the liquid part of the cytoplasm.

3-3 The plasma membrane is described as a bilayer because it is in two layers.

3-4 Large, negatively charged protein ions contribute to the negative charge along the intracellular membrane.

3-5 Epithelial cells (B) would best cover a large surface area because they are flat.

3-7 An increase in the number of transporters would increase the rate of facilitated diffusion. A decrease in the number of transporters would decrease the rate of facilitated diffusion.

3-8 If the solute could pass through the membrane in this system, the solute and solvent molecules would equalize on the two sides of the membrane, and the fluid level would be the same on both sides.

3-9 If the concentration of solute was increased on side B of this system, the osmotic pressure would increase.

3-10 If lost blood were replaced with pure water, red blood cells would swell because the blood would become hypotonic to the cells.

3-12 A lysosome would likely help to destroy a particle taken in by phagocytosis.

3-15 The nucleotides pair up so that there is one large nucleotide and one smaller nucleotide in each pair.

3-18 If the original cell has 46 chromosomes, each daughter cell will have 46 chromosomes after mitosis.

Chapter 4

Answers to Checkpoint Questions

4-1 The three basic shapes of epithelium are squamous (flat and irregular), cuboidal (square), and columnar (long and narrow).

4-2 Exocrine glands secrete into a nearby organ, cavity, or to the surface of the skin and generally secrete through ducts. Endocrine glands secrete directly into surrounding tissue fluids and into the blood.

4-3 The intercellular material in connective tissue is the matrix.

4-4 Collagen makes up the main fibers in connective tissue.

4-5 Circulating connective tissues are blood and lymph. Generalized connective tissues are loose (areolar, adipose) and dense, as found in membranes, capsules, ligaments, and tendons. Structural connective tissues are cartilage and bone.

4-6 The three types of muscle tissues are skeletal (voluntary), cardiac, and smooth (visceral) muscle.

4-7 The basic cell of the nervous system is the neuron, and it carries nerve impulses.

4-8 The nonconducting support cells of the nervous system are neuroglia (glial cells).

4-9 The three types of epithelial membranes are the cutaneous membrane (skin), serous membranes, and mucous membranes.

Answers to Zooming In Questions

4-1 The epithelial cells are in a single layer.

4-2 Stratified epithelium protects underlying tissue from wear and tear.

4-4 Of the tissues shown, areolar connective tissue has the most fibers; adipose tissue is modified for storage.

Chapter 5

Answers to Checkpoint Questions

5-1 The skin and its associated structures make up the integumentary system.

5-2 The superficial layer of the skin is the epidermis; the deeper layer is the dermis.

5-3 The subcutaneous layer is composed of loose connective tissue and adipose (fat) tissue.

5-4 The sebaceous glands produce an oily secretion called *sebum*.

5-5 The sweat glands are the sudoriferous glands.

5-6 A hair develops within a sheath called the *hair follicle*.

5-7 The active cells that produce a nail are located in the nail root in the proximal end of the nail.

5-8 Keratin and sebum help to prevent dehydration.

5-9 Temperature is regulated through the skin by dilation (widening) and constriction (narrowing) of blood vessels and by evaporation of perspiration from the body surface.

5-10 Melanin, hemoglobin, and carotene are the main pigments that impart color to the skin.

5-11 Epithelial and connective tissues repair themselves most easily.

Answers to Zooming In Questions

5-1 The epidermis is supplied with oxygen and nutrients from blood vessels in the dermis. The subcutaneous layer is located beneath the skin.

5-4 The sebaceous glands and apocrine sweat glands secrete to the outside through the hair follicles. The sweat glands are made of simple cuboidal epithelium.

Chapter 6

Answers to Checkpoint Questions

6-1 The shaft of a long bone is the diaphysis; the end of a long bone is the epiphysis.

6-2 Compact bone makes up the main shaft of a long bone and the outer layer of other bones; spongy (cancellous) bone makes up the ends of the long bones and the center of other bones. It also lines the medullary cavity of the long bones.

6-3 The cells found in bone are osteoblasts, which build bone tissue, osteocytes, which maintain bone, and osteoclasts, which break down (resorb) bone.

6-4 Calcium compounds are deposited in the matrix of bone to harden it.

6-5 The epiphyseal plates are the secondary growth centers of a long bone.

6-6 The markings on bones help to form joints, are points for muscle attachments, and allow passage of nerves and blood vessels.

6-7 The skeleton of the trunk consists of the vertebral column and the bones of the thorax, which are the ribs and sternum.

6-8 The five regions of the vertebral column are the cervical vertebrae, thoracic vertebrae, lumbar vertebrae, sacrum, and coccyx.

6-9 The bones of the shoulder girdle, hip, and extremities make up the appendicular skeleton.

6-10 The three types of joints, classified according to the material between the adjoining bones are fibrous, cartilaginous, and synovial.

6-11 A synovial joint or diarthrosis is the most freely movable type of joint.

Answers to Zooming In Questions

6-2 The membrane on the outside of a long bone is the periosteum; the membrane on the inside of a long bone is the endosteum.

6-3 The cells in the spaces (lacunae) of compact bone are osteocytes.

6-5 A suture is the type of joint between bones of the skull. The maxilla and palatine bones make up each side of the hard palate. A foramen is a hole.

6-6 The ethmoid makes up the superior and middle conchae.

6-7 The anterior fontanel is the largest fontanel.

6-8 The cervical and lumbar vertebrae form a convex curve; the thoracic and sacral vertebrae form a concave curve.

6-9 The lumbar vertebrae are the largest and heaviest because they bear the most weight.

6-10 The atlas and axis are missing a body.

6-11 The costal cartilages attach to the ribs.

6-12 The prefix *supra-* means above; the prefix *infra-* means below.

6-13 The medial bone of the forearm is the ulna.

6-15 The olecranon of the ulna forms the bony prominence of the elbow.

6-16 There are 14 phalanges on each hand.

6-17 The ischium is nicknamed the "sit bone."

6-19 The fibula is the lateral bone of the leg; the tibia is weight bearing.

6-20 The calcaneus is the heel bone; the talus forms a joint with the tibia.

6-21 The greater trochanter is a point for ligament attachment; articular (hyaline) cartilage covers the ends of a bone.

Chapter 7

Answers to Checkpoint Questions

7-1 The three types of muscle are smooth muscle, cardiac muscle, and skeletal muscle.

7-2 The three main functions of skeletal muscle are movement of the skeleton, maintenance of posture, and generation of heat.

7-3 The neuromuscular junction (NMJ) is the special synapse where a nerve cell makes contact with a muscle cell.

7-4 Acetylcholine (ACh) is the neurotransmitter involved in the stimulation of skeletal muscle cells.

7-5 Excitability and contractility are the two properties of muscle cells that are needed for response to a stimulus.

7-6 Actin and myosin are the filaments that interact to produce a muscle contraction.

7-7 Calcium is needed to allow actin and myosin to interact.

7-8 ATP is the compound produced by the oxidation of nutrients that supplies the energy for muscle contraction.

7-9 Lactic acid accumulates during anaerobic metabolism.

7-10 The two main types of muscle contraction are isotonic and isometric contractions.

7-11 The origin is the muscle's attachment to a less movable part of the skeleton; the insertion is the attachment to a movable part of the skeleton.

7-12 The muscle that produces a movement is the prime mover; the muscle that produces the opposite movement is the antagonist.

7-13 A third-class lever represents the action of most muscles. In this system, the fulcrum is behind the point of effort and the weight.

7-14 The diaphragm is the muscle most important in breathing.

7-15 The muscles of the abdominal wall are strengthened by having the muscle fibers run in different directions.

Answers to Zooming In Questions

7-1 The endomysium is the innermost layer of connective tissue in a skeletal muscle. Perimysium surrounds a fascicle of muscle fibers.

7-4 The actin and myosin filaments do not change in length as muscle contracts, they simply overlap more.

7-6 Contraction of the biceps brachii produces flexion at the elbow.

7-7 In a third-class lever system, the fulcrum is behind the point of effort and the weight.

7-10 The frontalis, temporalis, nasalis, and zygomaticus are named for the bones they are near.

7-11 Carpi means wrist; digitorum means fingers.

7-13 Rectus means straight; oblique means at an angle.

7-15 Four muscles make up the quadriceps femoris.

7-16 The Achilles tendon inserts on the calcaneus (heel bone).

Chapter 8

Answers to Checkpoint Questions

8-1 The two structural divisions of the nervous system are the central and peripheral nervous systems.

8-2 The somatic nervous system is voluntary and controls skeletal muscle; the autonomic (visceral) nervous system is involuntary and controls involuntary muscles (cardiac and smooth muscle) and glands.

8-3 A dendrite is a neuron fiber that carries impulses toward the cell body; an axon is a neuron fiber that carries impulses away from the cell body.

8-4 Myelinated fibers are white; unmyelinated tissue is gray.

8-5 A nerve is a bundle of neuron fibers in the peripheral nervous system; a tract is a bundle of neuron fibers in the central nervous system.

8-6 Sensory (afferent) nerves convey impulses toward the CNS; Motor (efferent) nerves convey impulses away from the CNS.

8-7 Neuroglia (glial cells) are the nonconducting cells of the nervous system that protect, nourish, and support the neurons.

8-8 The two stages of an action potential are depolarization, when the charge on the membrane reverses, and repolarization, when the charge returns to the resting state.

8-9 Sodium ion (Na^+) and potassium ion (K^+) are the two ions involved in generating an action potential.

8-10 Neurotransmitters are the chemicals that carry information across the synaptic cleft.

8-11 The gray mater forms an H-shaped section in the center of the cord and extends in two pairs of columns called the dorsal and ventral horns. The white matter is located around the gray matter.

8-12 Tracts in the white matter of the spinal cord carry impulses to and from the brain. Ascending tracts conduct toward the brain; descending tracts conduct away from the brain.

8-13 There are 31 pairs of spinal nerves.

8-14 The dorsal root of a spinal nerve contains sensory fibers; the ventral root contains motor fibers.

8-15 A pathway through the nervous system from a stimulus to an effector is a reflex arc.

8-16 There are two neurons in each motor pathway of the autonomic nervous system (ANS).

8-17 The sympathetic system stimulates a stress response; the parasympathetic system reverses a stress response.

Answers to Zooming In Questions

8-1 The brain and spinal cord make up the central nervous system; the cranial nerves and spinal nerves make up the peripheral nervous system.

8-2 The neuron shown is a motor neuron because it is carrying information away from the CNS toward an effector organ. It is part of the somatic nervous system, because the effector is skeletal muscle.

8-5 The endoneurium is the deepest layer of connective tissue in a nerve; the epineurium is the outermost layer.

8-8 The charge on the membrane reverses at the point of an action potential.

8-11 The spinal cord is not as long as the spinal column. There are seven cervical vertebrae and eight cervical spinal nerves.

8-12 The sacral spinal nerves (S1) carry impulses from the skin of the toes. The cervical spinal nerves (C6, 7, 8) carry impulses from the skin of the anterior hand and fingers.

8-13 The reflex arc shown is a somatic reflex arc, as it involves a skeletal muscle effector. An interneuron is located between the sensory and motor neurons in the CNS.

8-14 The parasympathetic system has ganglia closer to the effector organs.

Chapter 9

Answers to Checkpoint Questions

9-1 The main divisions of the brain are the cerebrum, diencephalon, brain stem, and cerebellum.

9-2 The three layers of the meninges are the dura mater, arachnoid, and pia mater.

9-3 CSF is produced in the ventricles of the brain. The two lateral ventricles are in the cerebral hemispheres, the third ventricle is in the diencephalon, and the fourth is between the brain stem and the cerebellum.

9-4 The frontal, parietal, temporal, and occipital are the four surface lobes of each cerebral hemisphere.

9-5 The cerebral cortex is the outer layer of gray matter of the cerebral hemispheres where higher functions occur.

9-6 The thalamus of the diencephalons directs sensory input to the cerebral cortex; the hypothalamus helps to maintain homeostasis.

9-7 The three subdivisions of the brain stem are the midbrain, pons, and medulla oblongata.

9-8 The cerebellum aids in coordination of voluntary muscles, maintenance of balance, and maintenance of muscle tone.

9-9 There are 12 pairs of cranial nerves.

9-10 Cranial nerves may be sensory, motor, or mixed. A mixed nerve has both sensory and motor fibers.

Answers to Zooming In Questions

9-1 The cerebrum is the largest part of the brain. The brain stem, specifically the medulla oblongata, connects with the spinal cord.

9-2 The dural (venous) sinuses are formed where the dura mater divides into two layers. There are three layers of meninges.

9-3 The fourth ventricle is continuous with the central canal of the spinal cord.

9-4 The largest ventricles are the lateral ventricles in the cerebral hemispheres.

9-5 The central sulcus separates the frontal from the parietal lobe; the lateral sulcus separates the temporal from the frontal and parietal lobes.

9-6 The primary sensory area is posterior to the central sulcus. The primary motor area is anterior to the central sulcus.

9-7 The pituitary gland is attached to the hypothalamus.

Chapter 10

Answers to Checkpoint Questions

10-1 A sensory receptor is a part of the nervous system that responds to a stimulus.

10-2 Based on types of stimulus, there are chemoreceptors that respond to chemicals in solution; photoreceptors that respond to light; thermoreceptors that respond to temperature; mechanoreceptors that respond to movement.

10-3 The general senses are widely distributed; the special senses are in specialized sense organs.

10-4 When a sensory receptor adapts to a stimulus it fails to respond.

10-5 Structures that protect the eye include the skull bones, eyelid, eyelash, eyebrow, conjunctiva, and lacrimal gland.

10-6 The fibrous tunic includes the cornea and sclera; the vascular tunic includes the choroid, suspensory ligaments, and iris; the nervous tunic is the retina.

10-7 The structures that refract light as it passes through the eye are the cornea, aqueous humor, lens, and vitreous body.

10-8 The rods and cones are the receptor cells of the retina.

10-9 The extrinsic eye muscles pull on the eyeball so that both eyes center on one visual field, a process known as convergence.

10-10 The iris adjusts the size of the pupil to regulate the amount of light that enters the eye.

10-11 The ciliary muscle adjusts the thickness of the lens to accommodate for near vision.

10-12 Cranial nerve II is the optic nerve. It carries impulses from the retinal rods and cones to the brain.

10-13 The ossicles of the middle ear are three small bones, the malleus, incus, and stapes, which transmit sound waves from the tympanic membrane to the inner ear.

10-14 The organ of hearing is the spiral organ (organ of Corti) located in the cochlear duct within the cochlea.

10-15 The equilibrium receptors are located in the vestibule and semicircular canals, together called the vestibular apparatus.

10-16 The senses of taste and smell are the special senses that respond to chemical stimuli.

10-17 Touch, pressure, temperature, position (proprioception), and pain are the general senses.

10-18 Proprioceptors are the receptors that respond to change in position. They are located in muscles, tendons, and joints.

Answers to Zooming In Questions

10-3 The cornea is the anterior structure continuous with the sclera.

10-6 Location and direction of fibers are characteristics used in naming the extrinsic eye muscles.

10-7 The circular muscles of the iris contract to make the pupil smaller; the radial muscles contract to make the pupil larger.

10-8 The suspensory ligaments of the ciliary muscle hold the lens in place.

10-10 The oculomotor nerve (III) controls eye movements.

10-11 The tympanic membrane separates the outer ear from the middle ear.

10-12 The vestibulocochlear nerve (VIII) is formed by merger of the cochlear and vestibular nerves.

10-13 The cochlear duct contains the spiral organ.

10-14 The cilia on the macular cells bend when the fluid around them moves.

Chapter 11

Answers to Checkpoint Questions

11-1 Hormones are chemicals that have specific regulatory effects on certain cells or organs in the body. Some of their effects are to regulate growth, metabolism, reproduction, and behavior.

11-2 Negative feedback is the main method used to regulate the secretion of hormones.

11-3 The hypothalamus controls the pituitary.

11-4 Growth hormone (GH), thyroid-stimulating hormone (TSH), adrenocorticotropic hormone (ACTH), prolactin (PRL), follicle-stimulating hormone (FSH), and luteinizing hormone (LH) are the hormones from the anterior pituitary.

11-5 Antidiuretic hormone (ADH) and oxytocin are released from the posterior pituitary.

11-6 Thyroid hormones increase the metabolic rate in cells.

11-7 Iodine is needed to produce thyroid hormones.

11-8 Calcium is regulated by parathyroid hormone and calcitriol.

11-9 Epinephrine (adrenaline) is the main hormone produced by the adrenal medulla.

11-10 Glucocorticoids, mineralocorticoids, and sex hormones are released by the adrenal cortex.

11-11 Cortisol raises blood glucose levels.

11-12 Insulin and glucagon produced by the pancreatic islets regulate glucose levels.

11-13 Secondary sex characteristics are features associated with gender other than reproductive activity.

11-14 The stomach, small intestine, kidney, brain, heart, thymus, and placenta are some organs other than the endocrine glands that produce hormones.

11-15 Epinephrine, ACTH, cortisol, growth hormone, thyroid hormones, sex hormones, and insulin are some hormones released in time of stress.

Answers to Zooming In Questions

11-1 The anterior pituitary controls the thyroid gland.

11-3 The infundibulum connects the hypothalamus and the pituitary gland.

11-4 The larynx is superior to the thyroid; the trachea is inferior to the thyroid.

11-6 The outer region of the adrenal is the cortex; the inner region is the medulla.

11-8 Insulin and glucagon mainly influence the liver and skeletal muscles.

Chapter 12

Answers to Checkpoint Questions

12-1 Some substances transported in blood are oxygen, carbon dioxide, nutrients, electrolytes, vitamins, hormones, urea, and toxins.

12-2 The pH range of the blood is 7.35 to 7.45.

12-3 The two main components of blood are the liquid portion, or plasma, and the formed elements, which include the cells and cell fragments.

12-4 Protein is the most abundant type of substance in plasma aside from water.

12-5 All blood cells form in red bone marrow.

12-6 Hematopoietic stem cells give rise to all blood cells.

12-7 The main function of hemoglobin is to carry oxygen in the blood.

12-8 The granular leukocytes are neutrophils, eosinophils, and basophils. The agranular leukocytes are lymphocytes and monocytes.

12-9 The main function of leukocytes is to destroy pathogens. They also remove other foreign material and cellular debris.

12-10 Platelets are essential to blood clotting (coagulation).

12-11 Fibrin forms a meshwork that traps cells and plasma to form a clot.

12-12 Plasma has clotting factors; serum does not.

12-13 The four ABO blood type groups are A, B, AB, and O.

12-14 The blood antigens most often involved in incompatibility reactions are the A antigen, B antigen, and Rh (D) antigen.

12-15 Blood is commonly separated into its component parts by a centrifuge.

12-16 A hematocrit is the percentage of red cell volume in whole blood.

12-17 Hemoglobin is expressed as grams per deciliter (dL) of whole blood or as a percentage of a given standard, usually the average male normal of 15.6 g hemoglobin per dL.

Answers to Zooming In Questions

12-2 Erythrocytes (red blood cells) are the most numerous cells in the blood.

12-3 Erythrocytes are described as biconcave because they have an inward depression on both sides.

12-5 Simple squamous epithelium makes up the capillary wall.

12-7 The suffix *-ase* indicates that prothrombinase is an enzyme. The prefix *pro-* indicates that prothrombin is a precursor.

12-8 No. To test for Rh antigen, you have to use anti-Rh serum. The two types of antigens are independent.

Chapter 13

Answers to Checkpoint Questions

13-1 The innermost layer of the heart wall is the endocardium; the middle layer is the myocardium; the outermost layer is the epicardium.

13-2 The pericardium is the sac that encloses the heart.

13-3 The atrium is the heart's upper receiving chamber on each side. The ventricle is the lower pumping chamber on each side.

13-4 The valves direct the flow of blood through the heart.

13-5 The coronary circulation is the system that supplies blood to the myocardium.

13-6 Systole is the contraction phase of the cardiac cycle. Diastole is the relaxation phase.

13-7 Cardiac output is the amount of blood pumped by each ventricle in 1 minute. It is determined by the stroke volume, the amount of blood ejected from the ventricle with each beat, and by the heart rate, the number of times the heart beats per minute.

13-8 The scientific name for the pacemaker is the sinoatrial (SA) node.

13-9 The autonomic nervous system is the main influence on the rate and strength of heart contractions.

13-10 A heart murmur is an abnormal heart sound.

13-11 ECG (EKG) stands for electrocardiogram or electrocardiography.

13-12 Catheterization is the use of a thin tube threaded through a vessel for diagnosis or repair.

Answers to Zooming In Questions

13-1 The left lung is smaller than the right because the heart is located more toward the left in the thorax.

13-2 The myocardium is the thickest layer of the heart wall.

13-4 The left ventricle has the thickest wall.

13-5 The right AV valve has three cusps; the left AV valve has two cusps.

13-6 The great cardiac vein is the largest cardiac vein. It leads into the coronary sinus and then into the right atrium.

13-8 The AV (tricuspid and mitral) valves close when the ventricles contract. The semilunar (pulmonary and aortic valves) open when the ventricles contract.

13-9 The internodal pathways connect the SA and AV nodes.

13-10 The vagus nerve (cranial nerve X) carries parasympathetic impulses to the heart.

13-11 The length of the cardiac cycle shown in this diagram is 0.8 seconds.

Chapter 14

Answers to Checkpoint Questions

14-1 The five types of blood vessels are arteries, arterioles, capillaries, venules, and veins.

14-2 The pulmonary circuit carries blood from the heart to the lungs to pick up oxygen and then back to the heart; the systemic circuit carries blood to and from all remaining tissues in the body.

14-3 Smooth muscle makes up the middle tunic of arteries and veins. Smooth muscle is involuntary muscle controlled by the autonomic nervous system.

14-4 A single layer of squamous epithelium makes up the wall of a capillary.

14-5 The aorta is divided into the ascending aorta, aortic arch, thoracic aorta, and abdominal aorta. The thoracic aorta and abdominal aorta make up the descending aorta.

14-6 The brachiocephalic, left common carotid, and left subclavian arteries are the three branches of the aortic arch.

14-7 The brachiocephalic artery supplies the arm and head on the right side.

14-8 An anastomosis is a communication between two vessels.

14-9 Superficial veins are near the surface; deep veins are closer to the interior and generally parallel the arteries.

14-10 The superior vena cava and inferior vena cava drain the systemic circuit and empty into the right atrium.

14-11 A venous sinus is a large channel that drains blood low in oxygen.

14-12 The hepatic portal system takes blood from the abdominal organs to the liver.

14-13 Blood pressure helps to push material out of a capillary; blood osmotic pressure helps to draw materials into a capillary.

14-14 Vasodilation (widening) and vasoconstriction (narrowing) are the two types of vasomotor changes.

14-15 Vasomotor activities are regulated in the medulla of the brain stem.

14-16 Pulse is the wave of pressure that begins at the heart and travels along the arteries.

14-17 Blood pressure is the force exerted by blood against the walls of the vessels.

14-18 Blood vessel diameter, as regulated by vasomotor activities, is the most important factor in determination of peripheral resistance. Other factors are blood viscosity and blood vessel length.

14-19 Systolic and diastolic pressures are measured when taking blood pressure.

Answers to Zooming In Questions

14-1 Arteries carry blood away from the heart. Veins carry blood toward the heart.

14-2 Veins have valves that control blood flow.

14-3 An artery has a thicker wall than a vein of comparable size.

14-4 There is one brachiocephalic artery.

14-5 The left and right common iliac arteries branch from the terminal aorta.

14-7 There are two brachiocephalic veins.

14-8 The hepatic veins drain into the inferior vena cava.

14-10 The proximal valve is closer to the heart.

14-11 Pulse pressure drops to 0 in the arterioles.

Chapter 15

Answers to Checkpoint Questions

15-1 The lymphatic system helps maintain fluid balance by bringing excess fluid and proteins from the tissues to the blood; protects against foreign material and foreign or abnormal cells; absorbs fats from the small intestine.

15-2 The lymphatic capillaries are more permeable than blood capillaries and begin blindly. They are closed at one end and do not bridge two vessels.

15-3 The two main lymphatic vessels are the right lymphatic duct and the thoracic duct.

15-4 Lymph nodes filter lymph. They also have lymphocytes to fight infection.

15-5 The spleen filters blood.

15-6 T cells of the immune system develop in the thymus.

15-7 Tonsils are located in the vicinity of the pharynx (throat).

15-8 The unbroken skin, mucous membranes, body secretions, and reflexes to expel microorganisms constitute the first line of defense against the invasion of pathogens.

15-9 Phagocytosis, natural killer cells, inflammation, fever, interferon, and complement are factors in the second line of defense against infection.

15-10 Complement is a group of blood proteins that aid in immunity both nonspecifically and specifically.

15-11 Acquired immunity is specific against particular disease agents and develops during a person's lifetime.

15-12 An antigen is any foreign substance, usually a protein that induces an immune response.

15-13 The four types of T cells are cytotoxic, helper, regulatory, and memory T cells.

15-14 Antigen-presenting cells take in and digest a foreign antigen. They then display fragments of the antigen in their plasma membrane along with self (MHC) antigens that a T cell can recognize.

15-15 An antibody is a substance produced in response to an antigen.

15-16 Plasma cells, derived from B cells, produce antibodies.

15-17 Natural immunity develops from contact with a disease organism or passage of antibodies through the placenta or mother's milk. Artificial acquired immunity develops from immunization with a vaccine or administration of an immune serum.

15-18 Active acquired immunity develops from contact with a disease organism either naturally or in a vaccine. Passive acquired immunity is obtained by antibodies from an outside source, either through the placenta and mother's milk or as an immune serum.

Answers to Zooming In Questions

15-1 A vein receives lymph collected from the body.

15-3 Mammary, axillary, subscapular, and interpectoral nodes are some nodes that receive lymph drainage from the breast.

15-4 An afferent vessel carries lymph into a node; an efferent vessel carries lymph out of a node.

15-8 Increased blood flow causes the heat, redness, swelling, and pain characteristic of inflammation.

15-10 Digestive enzymes are contained in the lysosome that joins the phagocytic vesicle.

15-11 Plasma cells and memory cells develop from activated B cells.

Chapter 16

Answers to Checkpoint Questions

16-1 The four phases of respiration are pulmonary ventilation, external gas exchange, gas transport in the blood, and internal gas exchange.

16-2 As air passes over the nasal mucosa it is filtered, warmed, and moistened.

16-3 The three regions of the pharynx are the nasopharynx, oropharynx, and laryngopharynx.

16-4 The scientific name for the throat is pharynx; for the voice box is larynx; for the windpipe is trachea.

16-5 The cells that line the respiratory passageways have cilia to move fluid with entrapped impurities upward to be eliminated from the respiratory system.

16-6 Gas exchange in the lungs occurs in the alveoli.

16-7 The membrane that encloses the lung in the pleura.

16-8 Inhalation (inspiration) and exhalation (expiration) are the two phases of quiet breathing. Inhalation is active and exhalation is passive.

16-9 A gas's partial pressure on either side of a membrane determines its direction of diffusion. Partial pressure is expressed in millimeters of mercury (mm Hg).

16-10 Hemoglobin holds almost all of the oxygen carried in the blood.

16-11 The main form in which carbon dioxide is carried in the blood is as bicarbonate ion.

16-12 The centers that set the basic pattern of respiration are in the medulla of the brain stem.

16-13 The phrenic nerve is the motor nerve that controls the diaphragm.

16-14 Carbon dioxide is the main chemical controller of respiration.

Answers to Zooming In Questions

16-1 Blood travels to the lungs from the right side of the heart; blood returns to the left side of the heart.

16-2 The heart is located in the medial depression of the left lung.

16-4 The epiglottis is named for its position above the glottis.

16-6 The external and internal intercostal muscles are located between the ribs.

16-7 Gas pressure decreases as the volume of its container increases.

16-8 Residual volume cannot be measured with a spirometer, nor can total lung capacity and functional residual capacity.

Chapter 17

Answers to Checkpoint Questions

17-1 Food must be broken down by digestion into particles small enough to pass through the plasma membrane.

17-2 The digestive tract typically has a wall composed of a mucous membrane (mucosa), a submucosa, smooth muscle (muscularis externa), and a serous membrane (serosa).

17-3 The peritoneum is the large serous membrane that lines the abdominopelvic cavity and covers the organs it contains.

17-4 There are 20 baby teeth, which are also called deciduous teeth.

17-5 Proteins are digested in the stomach.

17-6 The three divisions of the small intestine are the duodenum, jejunum, and ileum.

17-7 Most digestion takes place in the small intestine under the effects of digestive juices from the small intestine and the accessory organs. Most absorption of digested food and water also occurs in the small intestine.

17-8 The divisions of the large intestine are the cecum, ascending colon, transverse colon, descending colon, sigmoid colon, and rectum.

17-9 The large intestine reabsorbs some water and stores, forms, and eliminates the stool. It also houses bacteria that provide some vitamins.

17-10 The salivary glands are the parotid, anterior and inferior to the ear; submandibular (submaxillary), near the body of the lower jaw; and sublingual, under the tongue.

17-11 The liver secretes bile, which emulsifies fats, that is, breaks it down into small particles.

17-12 The gallbladder stores bile.

17-13 The pancreas secretes sodium bicarbonate, which neutralizes the acidic chyme from the stomach.

17-14 The pancreas produces the most complete digestive secretions.

17-15 Absorption is the movement of digested nutrients into the circulation.

17-16 The two types of control over the digestive process are nervous control and hormonal control.

17-17 Hunger is the desire for food that can be satisfied by the ingestion of a filling meal. Appetite is a desire for food that is unrelated to a need for food.

Answers to Zooming In Questions

17-1 Smooth muscle (circular and longitudinal) is between the submucosa and the serous membrane in the digestive tract wall.

17-2 The mesentery is the part of the peritoneum around the small intestine.

17-3 The salivary glands are the accessory organs that secrete into the mouth.

17-5 The gingiva is the gum.

17-6 The oblique muscle layer is an additional muscle layer in the stomach that is not found in the rest of the digestive tract.

17-7 The ileum of the small intestine joins the cecum at the ileocecal valve.

17-8 The sublingual salivary glands are directly below the tongue.

17-9 The accessory organs shown secrete into the duodenum.

Chapter 18

Answers to Checkpoint Questions

18-1 The two phases of metabolism are catabolism, the breakdown of compounds into simpler components, and anabolism, the building of simple compounds into needed substances.

18-2 Cellular respiration is the series of reactions that releases energy from nutrients in the cell.

18-3 Glucose and fatty acids are the two main energy sources for the cells.

18-4 An essential amino acid or fatty acid cannot be made metabolically and must be taken in as part of the diet.

18-5 Minerals are chemical elements, and vitamins are complex organic substances.

18-6 The normal range of blood glucose is 85 to 125 mg/dL.

18-7 Typical recommendations are 55% to 60% carbohydrate; 30% or less fat; 15% to 20% protein.

18-8 Saturated fats have no double-bonded carbons and have the maximum number of hydrogen atoms possible. Unsaturated fats have one or more double-bonded carbons and less than the maximum number of hydrogen atoms possible.

18-9 Alcohol replaces nutrients and does not yield any useful end products. In excess, it can damage the liver, tie up necessary enzymes, and acidify body fluids. It contributes to obesity and malnutrition as well as cancer, ulcers, fetal alcohol syndrome, and accidental injury.

18-10 Some factors that affect heat production are exercise, hormone production, food intake, and age.

18-11 The hypothalamus of the brain is responsible for regulating body temperature.

18-12 Normal body temperature is 36.2°C to 37.6°C (97°F to 100°F).

Answers to Zooming In Questions

18-1 Pyruvic acid produces lactic acid under anaerobic conditions; it produces CO_2 and H_2O when metabolized completely using oxygen.

18-5 The BMI is 24 (77 ÷ 3.2 = 24).

18-6 If the fan speed is increased in (B), convection, heat loss will increase. If environmental humidity increases (C), evaporation, heat loss will decrease.

Chapter 19

Answers to Checkpoint Questions

19-1 The urinary system consists of two kidneys, two ureters, the bladder, and the urethra.

19-2 Systems other than the urinary system that eliminate waste include the digestive, respiratory, and integumentary systems.

19-3 The retroperitoneal space is posterior to the peritoneum.

19-4 The renal artery supplies blood to the kidney and the renal vein drains blood from the kidney.

19-5 The outer region of the kidney is the renal cortex; the inner region is the renal medulla.

19-6 The nephron is the functional unit of the kidney.

19-7 The glomerulus is the coil of capillaries in the glomerular (Bowman) capsule.

19-8 Glomerular filtration is the movement of materials under pressure from the blood into the nephron's glomerular capsule.

19-9 The four processes involved in the formation of urine are glomerular filtration, tubular reabsorption, tubular secretion, and the countercurrent mechanism for concentrating the urine.

19-10 The JG apparatus produces renin when blood pressure drops. The signal for renin production is low sodium in the filtrate leaving the nephron.

19-11 The ureter carries urine from the kidney to the bladder.

19-12 The openings of the ureters and the urethra from the bladder trigone.

19-13 The urethra carries urine from the bladder to the outside.

19-14 Nitrogen waste, electrolyte, and pigments are normal constituents of urine.

19-15 Body fluids are grouped into intracellular fluid and extracellular fluid.

19-16 Water is lost from the body through the kidneys, the skin, the lungs, and the intestinal tract.

19-17 The control center for the sense of thirst is located in the brain's hypothalamus.

19-18 Sodium is the main cation in extracellular fluid. Potassium is the main cation in intracellular fluid.

19-19 Chloride is the main anion in extracellular fluid.

19-20 Some electrolytes are lost through the feces and sweat. The kidneys have the main job of balancing electrolytes. Several hormones, such as aldosterone, ADH, ANP, parathyroid hormone, and vitamin D, are also involved.

19-21 The acid–base balance of body fluids is maintained by buffer systems, respiration, and kidney function.

Answers to Zooming In Questions

19-1 The aorta supplies blood to the renal artery. The inferior vena cava receives blood from the renal vein.

19-2 The outer region of the kidney is the renal cortex. The inner region of the kidney is the renal medulla.

19-3 The proximal tubule is closer to the glomerular capsule. The distal tubule is farther away from the glomerular capsule.

19-7 The peritubular capillaries absorb materials that leave the nephron.

19-9 The urethra passes through the prostate gland in the male.

19-10 Water is lost through the skin, lungs, kidneys, and intestine.

19-11 The most water lost in a day is through urine.

19-12 Sodium and chloride are highest in extracellular fluid; potassium and phosphate are highest in intracellular fluids.

Chapter 20

Answers to Checkpoint Questions

20-1 Meiosis is the process of cell division that halves the chromosome number in a cell to produce a gamete.

20-2 The spermatozoon, or sperm cell, is the male gamete (sex cell).

20-3 The testis is the male gonad.

20-4 Testosterone is the main male sex hormone.

20-5 The main subdivisions of the sperm cell are the head, midpiece, and tail (flagellum).

20-6 Sperm cells leave the seminiferous tubules within the testis and then travel through the epididymis, ductus (vas) deferens, ejaculatory duct, and urethra.

20-7 Glands that contribute secretions to the semen, aside from the testes, are the seminal vesicles, prostate, and bulbourethral glands.

20-8 Follicle-stimulating hormone (FSH) and luteinizing hormone (LH) are the pituitary hormones that regulate male and female reproduction.

20-9 The ovum (egg) is the female gamete.

20-10 The ovary is the female gonad.

20-11 The ovarian follicle contains each ovum.

20-12 Ovulation is the process of releasing an ovum from the ovary.

20-13 The follicle becomes the corpus luteum after ovulation.

20-14 The fetus develops in the uterus.

20-15 The two hormones produced in the ovaries are estrogen and progesterone.

20-16 In a 28-day menstrual cycle, ovulation occurs on day 14.

20-17 Menopause is the period during which menstruation ceases.

20-18 Contraception is the use of artificial methods to prevent fertilization of the ovum or implantation of the fertilized ovum.

Answers to Zooming In Questions

20-1 The four glands that empty secretions into the urethra are the testes, seminal vesicles, prostate, and bulbourethral glands. The ductus (vas) deferens receives secretions from the epididymis.

20-3 The interstitial cells are located between the seminiferous tubules.

20-4 Mitochondria are the organelles that provide energy for sperm cell motility.

20-5 The corpus spongiosum of the penis contains the urethra.

20-6 The fundus of the uterus is the deepest part. The cervix is the most inferior portion.

20-8 The endometrium is most highly developed in the second part (the secretory phase) of the menstrual cycle.

20-9 The opening of the urethra is anterior to the opening of the vagina.

20-11 Estrogen peaks closest to ovulation. Progesterone peaks after ovulation.

Chapter 21

Answers to Checkpoint Questions

21-1 A zygote is formed by the union of an ovum and a spermatozoon.

21-2 The placenta nourishes the developing fetus.

21-3 The umbilical cord carries blood between the fetus and the placenta.

21-4 Fetal circulation is adapted to bypass the lungs.

21-5 The heartbeat first appears during the fourth week of gestation.

21-6 The amniotic sac is the fluid-filled sac that holds the fetus.

21-7 The approximate length of pregnancy in days from the time of fertilization is 266.

21-8 Parturition is the process of labor and childbirth.

21-9 A cesarean section is an incision made in the abdominal wall and the uterine wall for removal of a fetus.

21-10 The term *viable* with reference to a fetus means able to live outside the uterus.

21-11 Lactation is the secretion of milk from the mammary glands.

21-12 A gene is an independent unit of heredity. Each is a segment of DNA contained in a chromosome.

21-13 A dominant gene is always expressed, regardless of the gene on the matching chromosome. A recessive gene is only expressed if the gene on the matching chromosome is also recessive.

21-14 Meiosis is the process of cell division that forms the gametes.

21-15 The sex chromosome combination that determines a female is XX; that for a male is XY.

21-16 A trait carried on a sex chromosome is described as sex-linked.

21-17 A mutation is a change in a cell's genetic material (a gene or chromosome).

Answers to Zooming In Questions

21-1 The ovum is fertilized in the uterine tube.

21-2 The purple color signifies a mixture of blood that is low and high in oxygen.

21-5 The umbilical cord connects the fetus to the placenta.

21-7 Depletion of materials, removal of the stimulus, or an outside force can stop positive feedback.

21-9 The pectoralis major underlies the breast.

21-10 A human gamete has 23 chromosomes.

21-11 25% of children will show the recessive phenotype blond hair. 50% of children will be heterozygous.

21-12 The expected ratio of male to female offspring in a family is 50:50.

Appendix 3

Dissection Atlas

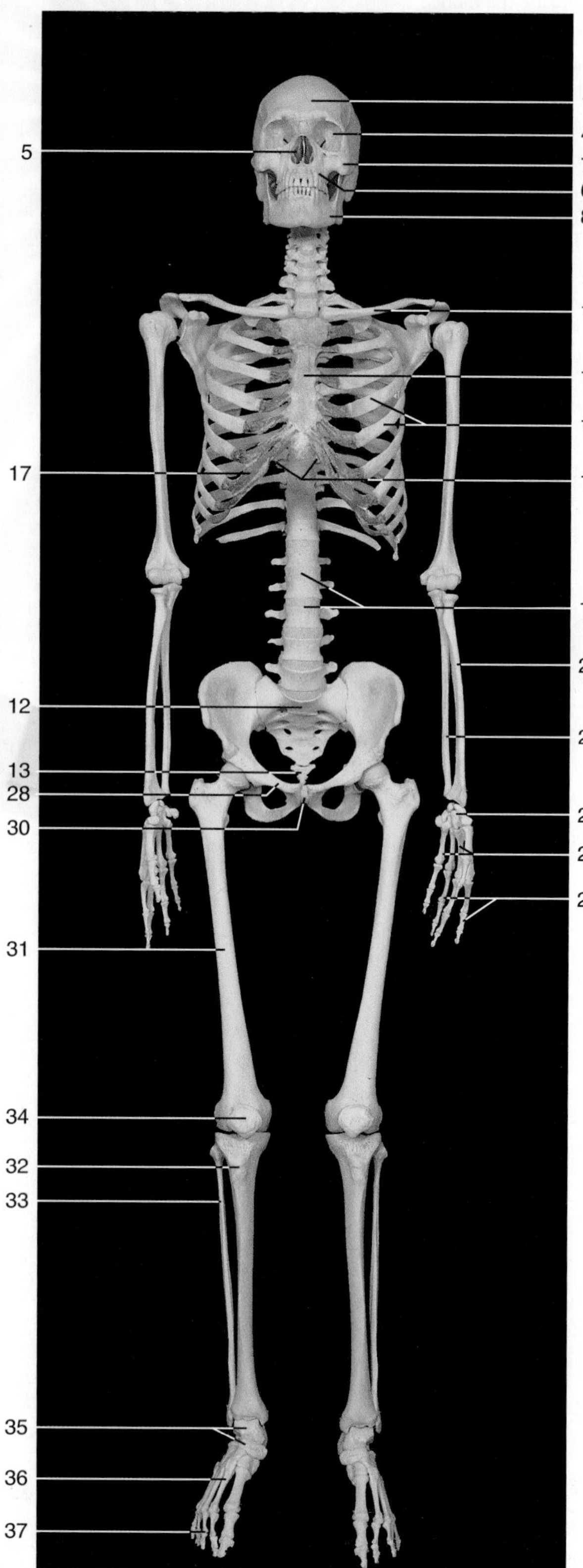

Axial skeleton

Head

1 Frontal bone
4 Orbit
5 Nasal cavity
6 Maxilla
7 Zygomatic bone
8 Mandible

Trunk and thorax

Vertebral column

12 Sacrum
13 Coccyx
14 Intervertebral discs

Thorax

15 Sternum
16 Ribs
17 Coastal cartilage
18 Infrasternal angle

Appendicular skeleton

Upper limb and shoulder girdle

19 Clavicle
22 Radius
23 Ulna
24 Carpal bones
25 Metacarpal bones
26 Phalanges of the hand

Lower limb and pelvis

28 Pubis
30 Symphysis pubis
31 Femur
32 Tibia
33 Fibula
34 Patella
35 Tarsal bones
36 Metatarsal bones
37 Phalanges of the foot

Figure A3-1 Skeleton of a female adult (anterior aspect). (Reprinted with permission from Rohen JW, Yokochi C, Lütjen-Drecoll E. *Color Atlas of Anatomy*, 6th ed. Stuttgart, New York, NY: Schattauer, 2006.)

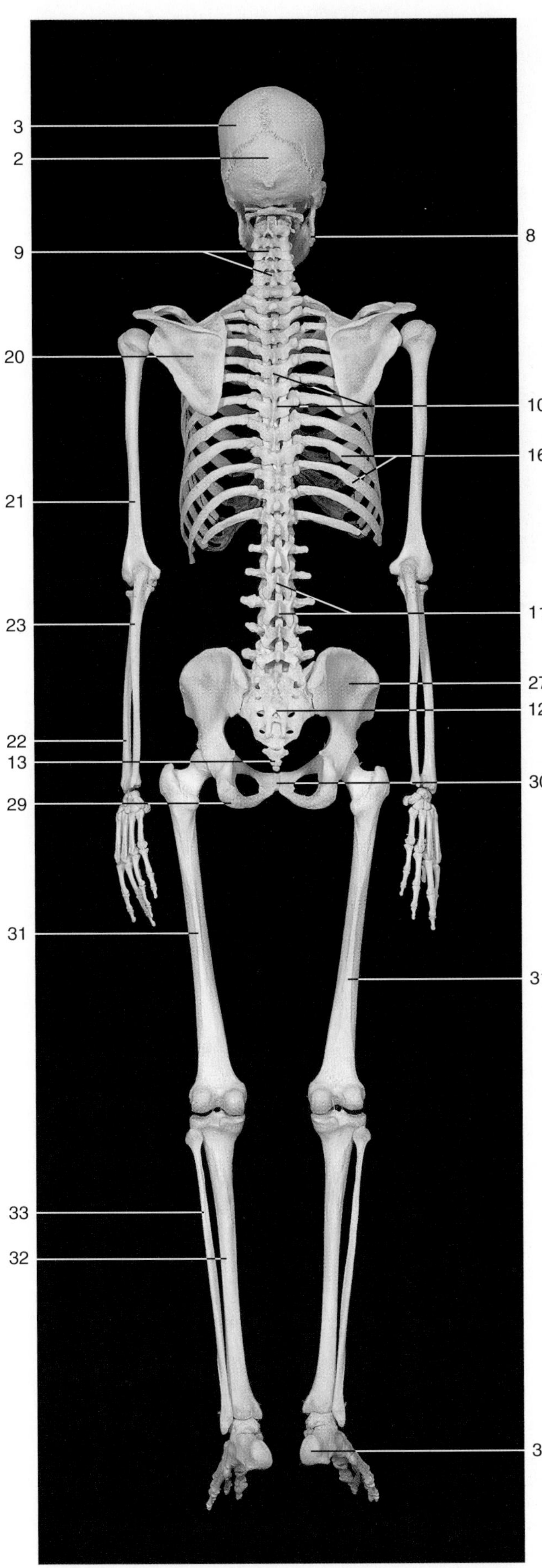

Axial skeleton

Head

2 Occipital bone
3 Parietal bone
8 Mandible

Trunk and thorax

Vertebral column

9 Cervical vertebrae
10 Thoracic vertebrae
11 Lumbar vertebrae
12 Sacrum
13 Coccyx

Thorax

16 Ribs

Appendicular skeleton

Upper limb and shoulder girdle

20 Scapula
21 Humerus
22 Radius
23 Ulna

Lower limb and pelvis

27 Ilium
29 Ischium
30 Symphysis pubis
31 Femur
32 Tibia
33 Fibula
38 Calcaneus

Figure A3-2 Skeleton of a female adult (posterior aspect). (Reprinted with permission from Rohen JW, Yokochi C, Lütjen-Drecoll E. *Color Atlas of Anatomy,* 6th ed. Stuttgart, New York, NY: Schattauer, 2006.)

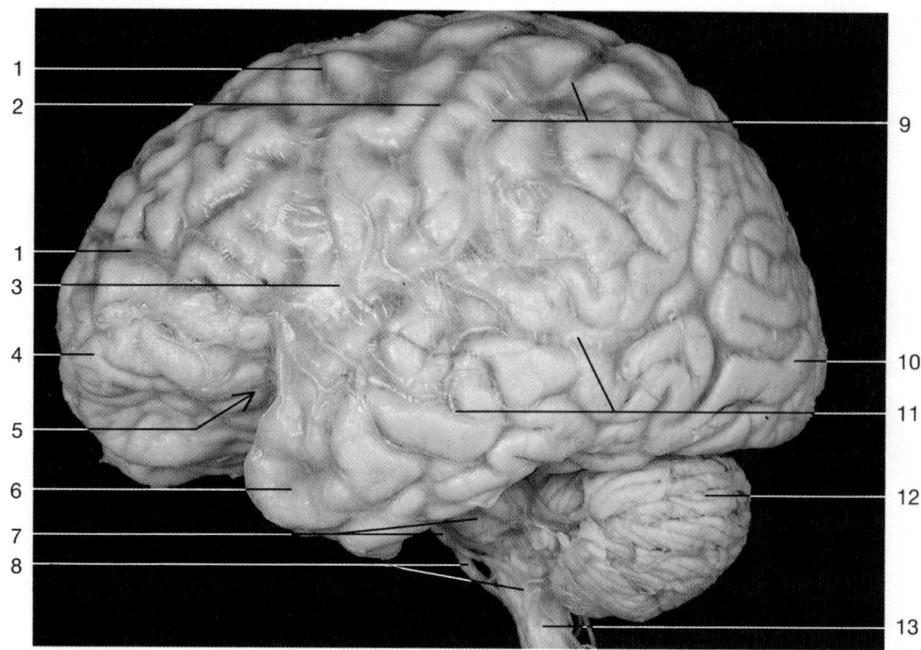

1 Superior cerebral veins
2 Position of central sulcus
3 Position of lateral sulcus
4 Frontal lobe
5 Lateral sulcus (*arrow*)
6 Temporal lobe
7 Pons and basilar artery
8 Vertebral arteries
9 Superior anastomotic vein
10 Occipital lobe
11 Inferior cerebral veins
12 Hemisphere of cerebellum
13 Medulla oblongata

Figure A3-3 Brain with pia mater and arachnoid. Frontal pole to the left (lateral aspect). (Reprinted with permission from Rohen JW, Yokochi C, Lütjen-Drecoll E. *Color Atlas of Anatomy*, 6th ed. Stuttgart, New York, NY: Schattauer, 2006.)

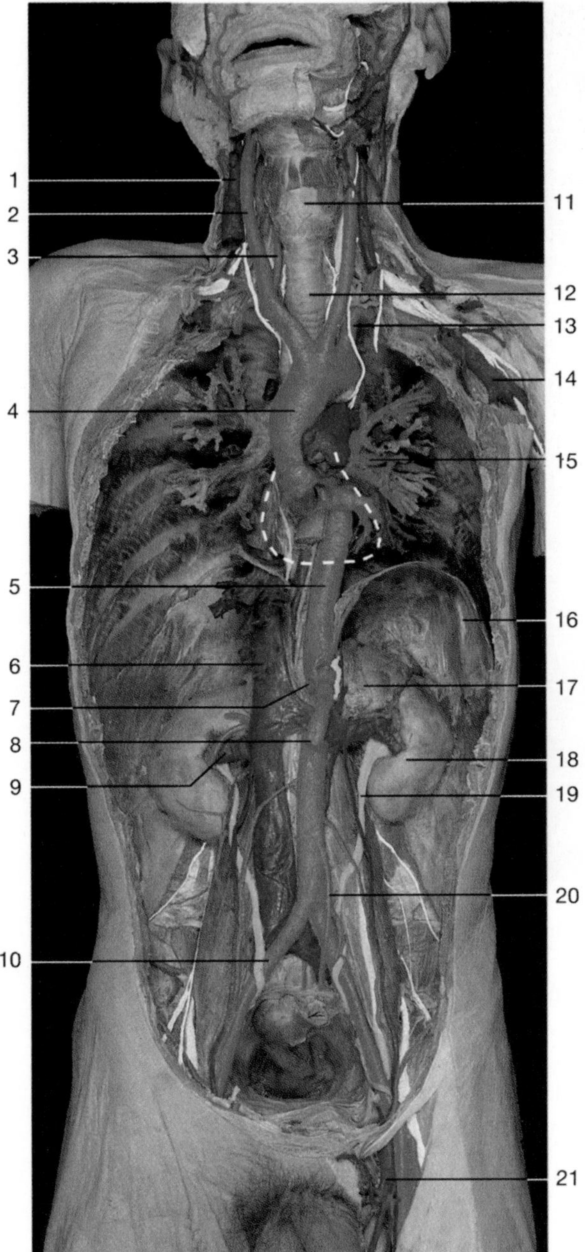

1 Internal jugular vein
2 Common carotid artery
3 Vertebral artery
4 Ascending aorta
5 Descending aorta
6 Inferior vena cava
7 Celiac trunk
8 Superior mesenteric artery
9 Renal vein
10 Common iliac artery
11 Larynx
12 Trachea
13 Left subclavian artery
14 Left axillary vein
15 Pulmonary veins
16 Diaphragm
17 Suprarenal gland
18 Kidney
19 Ureter
20 Inferior mesenteric artery
21 Femoral vein

Figure A3-4 Major vessels of the trunk. The position of the heart is indicated by the *dotted line*. (Reprinted with permission from Rohen JW, Yokochi C, Lütjen-Drecoll E. *Color Atlas of Anatomy*, 6th ed. Stuttgart, New York, NY: Schattauer, 2006.)

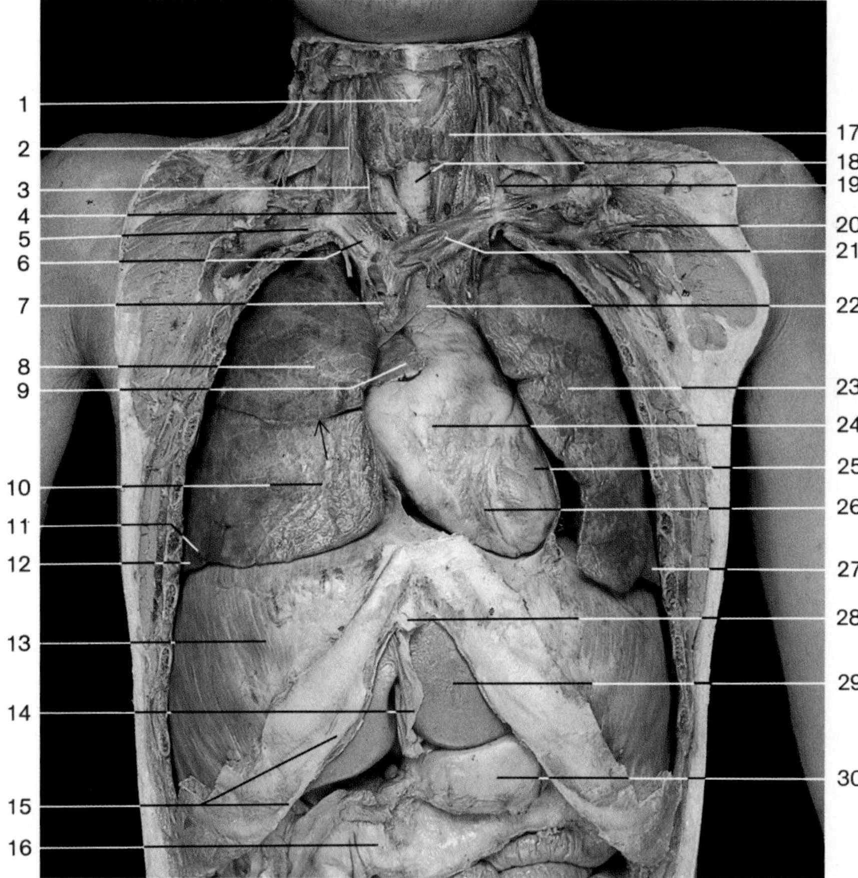

1 Cricothyroid muscle
2 Right internal jugular vein
3 Vagus nerve
4 Right common carotid artery
5 Right subclavian vein
6 Right brachiocephalic vein
7 Superior vena cava
8 Upper lobe of right lung
9 Right auricle
10 Middle lobe of right lung
11 Oblique fissure of right lung
12 Lower lobe of right lung
13 Diaphragm
14 Falciform ligament
15 Costal margin
16 Transverse colon
17 Thyroid gland
18 Trachea
19 Left internal jugular vein
20 Left cephalic vein
21 Left brachiocephalic vein
22 Pericardium (cut edge)
23 Upper lobe of left lung
24 Right ventricle
25 Left ventricle
26 Anterior interventricular sulcus
27 Lower lobe of left lung
28 Xiphoid process
29 Liver
30 Stomach

Figure A3-5 Positions of thoracic organs. The anterior thoracic wall has been removed. *Arrow*: horizontal fissure of the right lung. (Reprinted with permission from Rohen JW, Yokochi C, Lütjen-Drecoll E. *Color Atlas of Anatomy*, 6th ed. Stuttgart, New York, NY: Schattauer, 2006.)

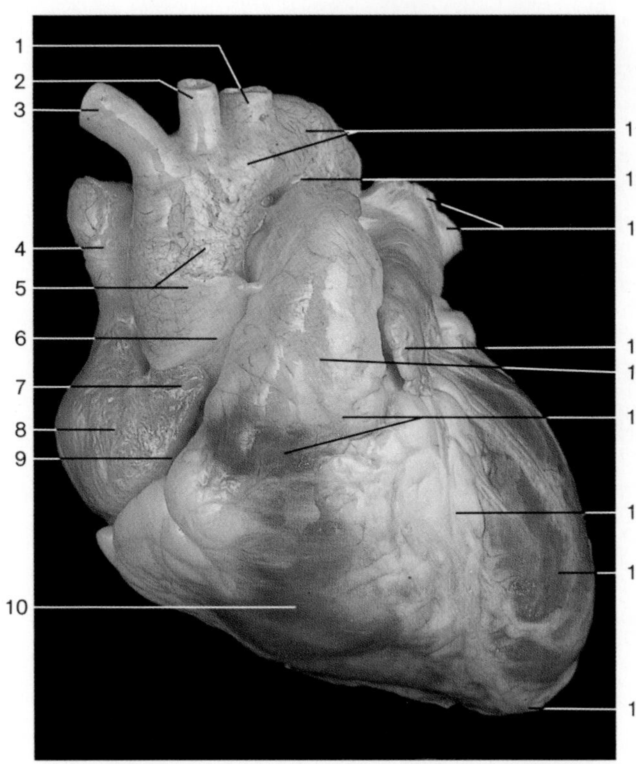

1 Left subclavian artery
2 Left common carotid artery
3 Brachiocephalic trunk
4 Superior vena cava
5 Ascending aorta
6 Bulb of the aorta
7 Right auricle
8 Right atrium
9 Coronary sulcus
10 Right ventricle
11 Aortic arch
12 Ligamentum arteriosum
13 Left pulmonary veins
14 Left auricle
15 Pulmonary trunk
16 Sinus of pulmonary trunk
17 Anterior interventricular sulcus
18 Left ventricle
19 Apex of the heart

Figure A3-6 Heart of a 30-year-old woman (anterior aspect). (Reprinted with permission from Rohen JW, Yokochi C, Lütjen-Drecoll E. *Color Atlas of Anatomy*, 6th ed. Stuttgart, New York, NY: Schattauer, 2006.)

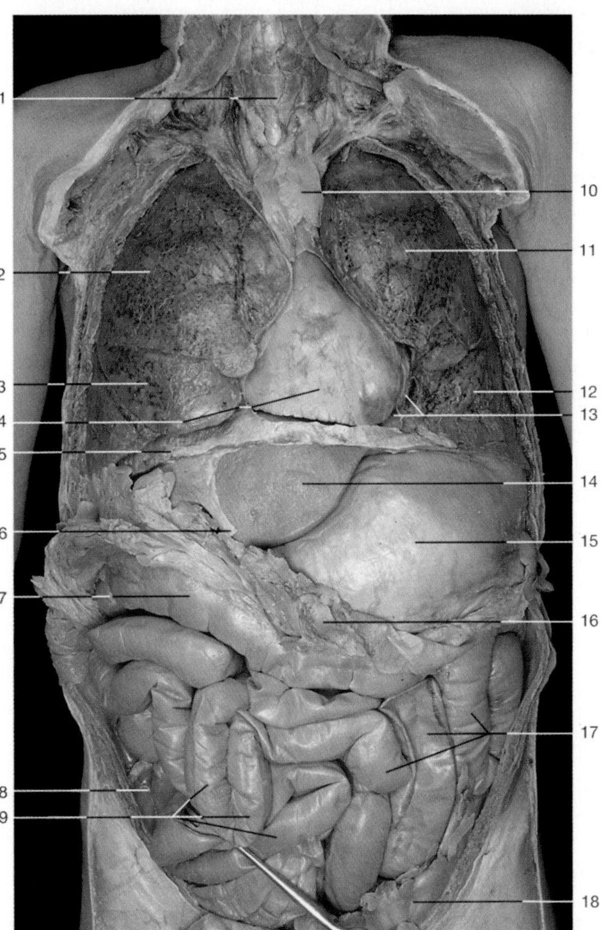

1 Thyroid gland
2 Upper lobe of right lung
3 Middle lobe of right lung
4 Heart
5 Diaphragm
6 Round ligament of liver (ligamentum teres)
7 Transverse colon
8 Cecum
9 Small intestine (ileum)
10 Thymus
11 Upper lobe of left lung
12 Lower lobe of left lung
13 Pericardium (cut edge)
14 Liver (left lobe)
15 Stomach
16 Greater omentum
17 Small intestine (jejunum)
18 Sigmoid colon

Figure A3-7 Abdominal organs in situ. The greater omentum has been partly removed or reflected. (Reprinted with permission from Rohen JW, Yokochi C, Lütjen-Drecoll E. *Color Atlas of Anatomy*, 6th ed. Stuttgart, New York, NY: Schattauer, 2006.)

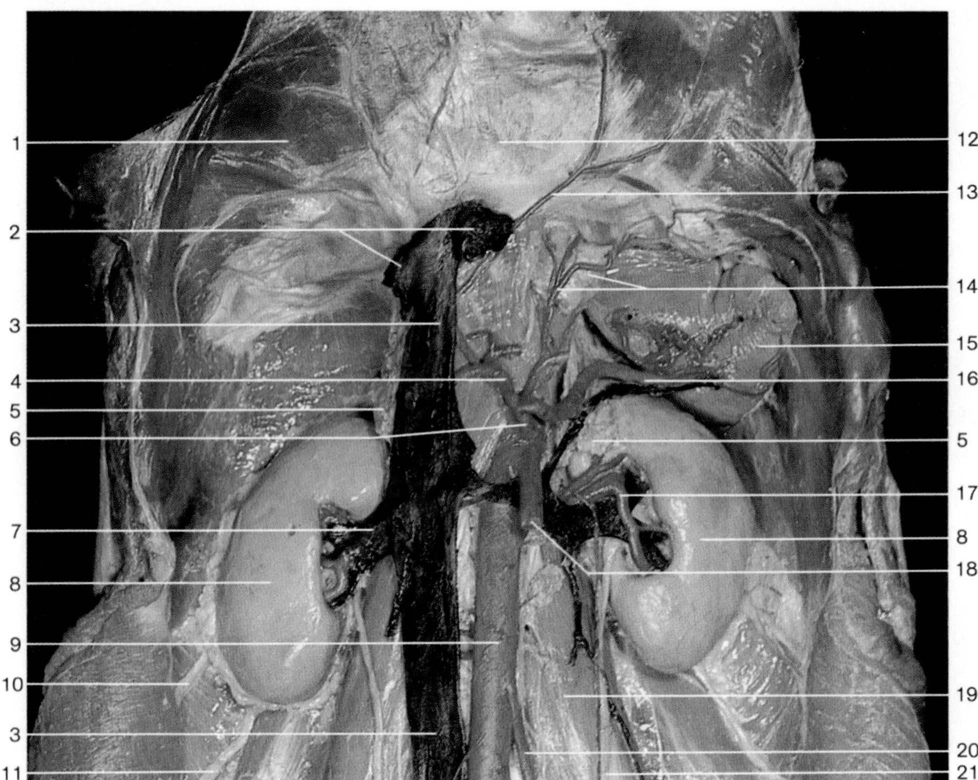

1 Diaphragm
2 Hepatic veins
3 Inferior vena cava
4 Common hepatic artery
5 Suprarenal gland
6 Celiac trunk
7 Right renal vein
8 Kidney
9 Abdominal aorta
10 Subcostal nerve
11 Iliohypogastric nerve
12 Central tendon of diaphragm
13 Inferior phrenic artery
14 Cardiac part of stomach
15 Spleen
16 Splenic artery
17 Superior renal artery
18 Superior mesenteric artery
19 Psoas major muscle
20 Inferior mesenteric artery
21 Ureter

Figure A3-8 Retroperitoneal organs, kidneys, and suprarenal glands in situ (anterior aspect). *Red*, arteries; *blue*, veins. (Reprinted with permission from Rohen JW, Yokochi C, Lütjen-Drecoll E. *Color Atlas of Anatomy*, 6th ed. Stuttgart, New York, NY: Schattauer, 2006.)

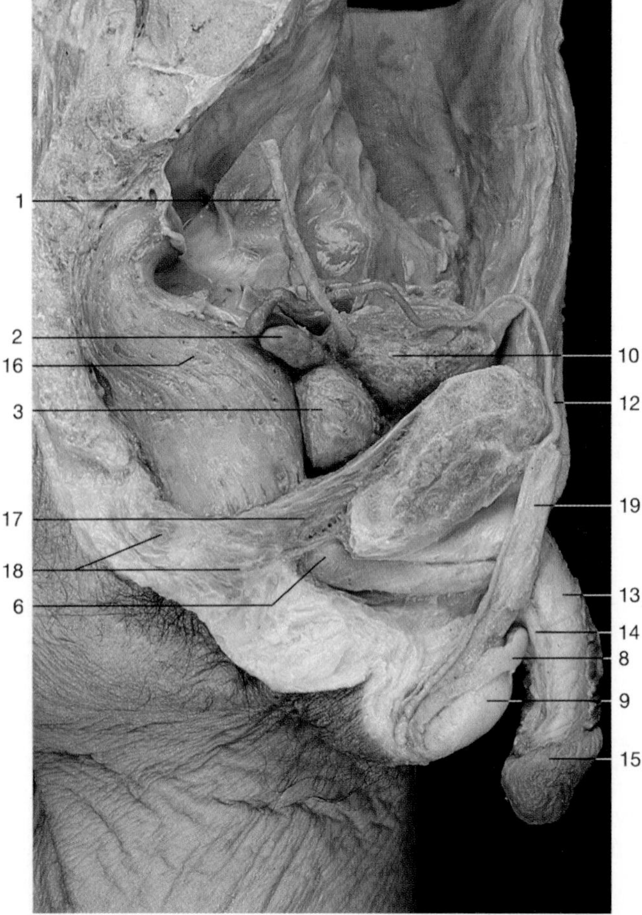

1 Ureter
2 Seminal vesicle
3 Prostate gland
6 Bulb of penis
8 Epididymis
9 Testis
10 Urinary bladder
12 Ductus deferens
13 Corpus cavernosum of penis
14 Corpus spongiosum of penis
15 Glans penis
16 Ampulla of rectum
17 Levator ani muscle
18 Anal canal and external anal sphincter muscle
19 Spermatic cord (cut)

Figure A3-9 Male genital organs in situ (right lateral aspect). (Reprinted with permission from Rohen JW, Yokochi C, Lütjen-Drecoll E. *Color Atlas of Anatomy*, 6th ed. Stuttgart, New York, NY: Schattauer, 2006.)

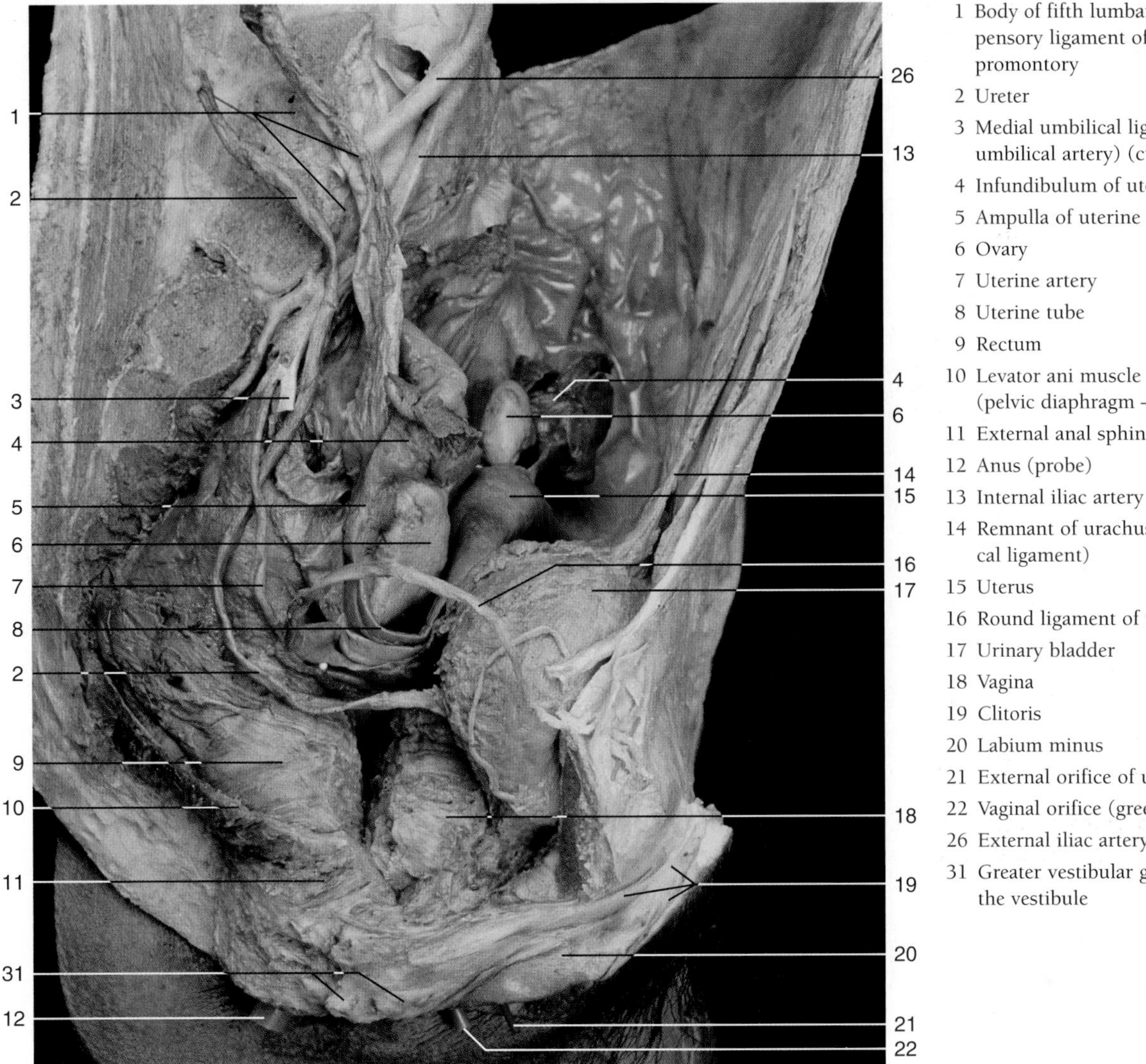

1 Body of fifth lumbar vertebra, suspensory ligament of ovary, and sacral promontory
2 Ureter
3 Medial umbilical ligament (remnant of umbilical artery) (cut)
4 Infundibulum of uterine tube
5 Ampulla of uterine tube
6 Ovary
7 Uterine artery
8 Uterine tube
9 Rectum
10 Levator ani muscle (pelvic diaphragm – cut edge)
11 External anal sphincter muscle
12 Anus (probe)
13 Internal iliac artery
14 Remnant of urachus (median umbilical ligament)
15 Uterus
16 Round ligament of uterus
17 Urinary bladder
18 Vagina
19 Clitoris
20 Labium minus
21 External orifice of urethra (red probe)
22 Vaginal orifice (green probe)
26 External iliac artery
31 Greater vestibular gland and bulb of the vestibule

Figure A3-10 Female internal genital organs in situ. Right half of the pelvis and sacrum have been removed. (Reprinted with permission from Rohen JW, Yokochi C, Lütjen-Drecoll E. *Color Atlas of Anatomy*, 6th ed. Stuttgart, New York, NY: Schattauer, 2006.)

Index

Page numbers in *italics* denote figures; page numbers followed by *t* denote tables; and page numbers followed by *B* denote boxes.

B

C

D

E

M

N

O

P

Q

R

S